STUDY GUIDE FOR

Lippincott Williams & Wilkins'

COMPREHENSIVE
Medical Assisting

STUDY GUIDE FOR

Lippincott Williams & Wilkins'

COMPREHENSIVE
Medical Assisting

FOURTH EDITION

Judy Kronenberger, RN, CMA, PhD

Professor and Program Director, Medical Assistant Technology
Sinclair Community College
Dayton, Ohio

Laura Southard Durham, BS, CMA

Medical Assisting Technologies Program Coordinator (Retired)
Forsyth Technical Community College
Winston-Salem, North Carolina

Denise Woodson, MA, MT(ASCP)SC

Academic Coordinator
Health Sciences and Nursing
Smarthinking, Inc.
Richmond, Virginia

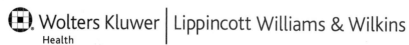

Wolters Kluwer | Lippincott Williams & Wilkins
Health

Philadelphia • Baltimore • New York • London
Buenos Aires • Hong Kong • Sydney • Tokyo

Acquisitions Editor: Kelley Squazzo
Senior Product Manager: Amy Millholen
Design Coordinator: Stephen Druding
Marketing Manager: Shauna Kelley
Compositor: SPi Global
Printer: Data Reproductions Corporation

ISBN: 9781451115727

13

1 2 3 4 5 6 7 8 9 10

DRC0312

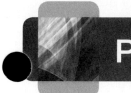

Preface

Welcome to the *Study Guide for Lippincott Williams & Wilkins' Comprehensive Medical Assisting, Fourth Edition*. In this edition, we have aligned the exercises and activities with the most current (2008) Medical Assisting Education Review Board (MAERB) of the American Association of Medical Assistants (AAMA) curriculum standards. Program directors, instructors, and students will know which activities in this *Study Guide* support comprehension of knowledge from the textbook (cognitive domain), which support the practice and skills needed to become a competent entry-level medical assistant (psychomotor domain), and which exercises encourage critical thinking and professional behaviors in the medical office (affective domain). This *Study Guide* is unique in a number of ways and offers features that are not found in most Medical Assisting study guides.

The *Study Guide* is divided into sections that coincide with the textbook: Administrative, Clinical, Laboratory, and Career Strategies. Parts I-IV include exercises that reinforce the knowledge and skills required of all Medical Assistants. Part V includes activities to "put it all together" as a potential medical office employee. All chapters have been updated and revised and we believe the extensive revision of the Clinical Laboratory chapters will be especially helpful.

Each chapter includes the following:

- **Learning Outcomes**—Learning outcomes are listed at the beginning of the chapter and are divided into AAMA/CAAHEP categories (Cognitive, Psychomotor, Affective) and ABHES competencies.
- **A Variety of Question Formats**—To meet the needs of a variety of learning styles and to reinforce content and knowledge, each chapter of the *Study Guide* includes multiple choice, matching, short answer, completion, and where applicable,

calculation-type questions. These formats will help you retain new information, reinforce previously learned content, and build confidence.

- **Case Studies for Critical Thinking**—These scenarios and questions are designed with real-world situations in mind and are intended to promote conversation about possible responses, not just one correct answer! These questions will be valuable to students who confront these types of situations during externship and graduates who encounter similar situations after employment.
- **Procedure Skill Sheets**—Every procedure in the textbook has a procedure skill sheet in the *Study Guide*. These procedures have been updated and revised in this edition and include steps on interacting with diverse patients, such as those who are visually or hearing impaired, those who do not speak English or who speak English as a second language (ESL), and patients who may have developmental challenges.
- **Putting it all Together**—Chapter 47 in the textbook allows students in the final stages of their educational program to take a comprehensive examination, and Chapter 47 in the *Study Guide* gives students the opportunity to reinforce information learned throughout their program. This final *Study Guide* chapter includes documentation skills practice for a multitude of situations and active learning activities to engage students with previously learned knowledge.

This *Study Guide* has been developed in response to numerous requests from students and instructors for a concise, understandable, and interactive resource that covers the skills necessary to become a successful Medical Assistant. We hope you find the exercises and tools in this book productive and useful towards your goal of becoming the best Medical Assistant possible!

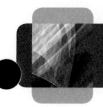

Contents

PART IV
The Clinical Laboratory

PART V
Career Strategies

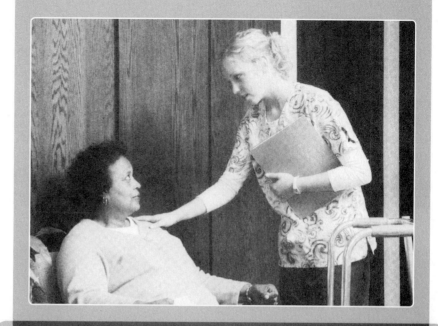

Introduction to Medical Assisting

ONE

Understanding the Profession

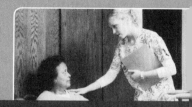

Medicine and Medical Assisting

Learning Outcomes

Cognitive Domain

1. Spell and define the key terms
2. Summarize a brief history of modern medicine
3. Explain the system of health care in the United States
4. Discuss the typical medical office
5. List medical specialties a medical assistant may encounter
6. List settings in which medical assistants may be employed
7. List the duties of a medical assistant
8. Describe the desired characteristics of a medical assistant
9. Discuss legal scope of practice for medical assistants
10. Compare and contrast physician and medical assistant roles in terms of standard of care
11. Recognize the role of patient advocacy in the practice of medical assisting
12. Identify the role of self boundaries in the health care environment
13. Differentiate between adaptive and non-adaptive coping mechanisms
14. Identify members of the health care team
15. Explain the pathways of education for medical assistants
16. Discuss the importance of program accreditation
17. Name and describe the two nationally recognized accrediting agencies for medical assisting education programs
18. Explain the benefits and avenues of certification for the medical assistant
19. Discuss licensure and certification as it applies to health care providers
20. List the benefits of membership in a professional organization
21. Identify the effect peronal ethics may have on professional performance
22. Compare personal, professional, and organizational ethics
23. Discuss all levels of governmental legislation and regulation as they apply to medical assisting practice, including FDA and DEA regulations

Psychomotor Domain

1. Perform within scope of practice
2. Practice within the standard of care for a medical assistant
3. Develop a plan for separation of personal and professional ethics
4. Respond to issues of confidentiality
5. Document accurately in the patient record

Affective Domain

1. Demonstrate awareness of the consequences of not working within the legal scope of practice
2. Apply ethical behaviors, including honesty and integrity in performance of medical assisting practice

3. Examine the impact personal ethics and morals may have on the individual's practice

ABHES Competencies

1. Comprehend the current employment outlook for the medical assistant
2. Compare and contrast the allied health professions and understand their relation to medical assisting
3. Understand medical assistant credentialing requirements and the process to obtain the credential. Comprehend the importance of credentialing
4. Have knowledge of the general responsibilities of the medical assistant
5. Define scope of practice for the medical assistant, and comprehend the conditions for practice within the state that the medical assistant is employed

6. Demonstrate professionalism by:
   a. Exhibiting dependability, punctuality, and a positive work ethic
   b. Exhibiting a positive attitude and a sense of responsibility
   c. Maintaining confidentiality at all times
   d. Being cognizant of ethical boundaries
   e. Exhibiting initiative
   f. Adapting to change
   g. Expressing a responsible attitude
   h. Being courteous and diplomatic
   i. Conducting work within scope of education, training, and ability
7. Comply with federal, state, and local health laws and regulations
8. Analyze the effect of hereditary, cultural, and environmental influences

Name: _____   Date: _____   Grade: _____

COG MULTIPLE CHOICE

1. Julia is a student in her last year of a medical assisting program. What must she complete before graduating?

   a. Certification

   b. An associate's degree

   c. An externship

   d. Curriculum

2. Who is eligible to take the RMA examination? Circle all that apply.

   a. Medical assistants who have been employed as medical instructors for a minimum of 5 years

   b. Medical assistants who have been employed in the profession for a minimum of 5 years

   c. Graduates from ABHES-accredited medical assisting programs

   d. Graduates from CAAHEP-accredited medical assisting programs

3. Marie and Pierre Curie revolutionized the principles of:

   a. nursing.

   b. disease.

   c. infection.

   d. physics.

   e. radioactivity.

4. The medical assistant's role will expand over time because of:

   a. a growing population.

   b. the risk of disease and infection.

   c. advances in medicine and technology.

   d. a financial boom.

   e. more effective training programs.

5. What drives the management practices of the outpatient medical facility?

   a. The desire to compete with other medical facilities

   b. The need to adhere to government rules and regulations

   c. The attempt to fit into mainstream medical opinion

   d. The effort to retain medical employees

   e. The focus on hiring specialized health care workers

6. Which of the following tasks is the administrative team responsible for in the medical office?

   a. Physical examinations

   b. Financial aspects of the practice

   c. Laboratory test processing

   d. Minor office surgery

   e. Drawing blood

7. Which of the following is a clinical duty?

   a. Scheduling appointments

   b. Obtaining medical histories

   c. Handling telephone calls

   d. Filing insurance forms

   e. Implementing ICD-9 and CPT coding for insurance claims

8. Empathy is the ability to:

   a. care deeply for the health and welfare of patients.

   b. keep your temper in check.

   c. show all patients good manners.

   d. remain calm in an emergency.

   e. feel pity for sick patients.

9. If a patient refers to you as a "nurse," you should:

   a. call the physician.

   b. ignore the mistake.

   c. politely correct him or her.

   d. send him or her home.

   e. ask the nurse to come into the room.

10. A group of specialized people who are brought together to meet the needs of the patient is called:

    a. multiskilled.

    b. multifaceted.

    c. multitasked.

    d. multidisciplinary.

    e. multitrained.

11. A medical assistant falls into the category of:

    a. nurse.

    b. physician assistant.

    c. medical office manager.

    d. allied health professional.

    e. all of the above.

12. The discovery of which vaccine opened the door to an emphasis on preventing disease rather than simply trying to cure preventable illnesses?

    a. Smallpox

    b. Cowpox

    c. Puerperal fever

    d. Typhoid

    e. Influenza

13. "Scope of practice" refers to:

    a. the tasks a person is trained to do.

    b. the tasks an employer allows an employee to perform.

    c. limitations placed on employees by law.

    d. a concept that varies from state to state.

    e. all of the above.

14. All accredited programs must include a(n):

    a. medical terminology course.

    b. computer course.

    c. externship.

    d. certification examination.

    e. multidisciplinary program.

15. What is the requirement for admission to the CMA examination?

    a. Successful completion of 60 CEUs

    b. Successful completion of an externship

    c. Graduation from high school

    d. Graduation from an accredited medical assisting program

    e. Successful completion of a GED program

16. An oncologist diagnoses and treats:

    a. disorders of the musculoskeletal system.

    b. disorders of the ear, nose, and throat.

    c. pregnant women.

    d. the aging population.

    e. benign and malignant tumors.

17. A CMA is required to recertify every:

    a. 1 year.

    b. 2 years.

    c. 5 years.

    d. 10 years.

    e. 15 years.

18. Which organization offers the RMA examination?

    a. American Medical Technologists

    b. American Association of Medical Assistants

    c. American Academy of Professional Coders

    d. American Health Information Management Association

    e. American Board of Medical Specialties

19. Which of the following is a benefit of association membership?

   a. Time off from work

   b. Networking opportunities

   c. Hotel expenses

   d. Free health insurance

   e. Externship placement

20. Which specialist diagnoses and treats disorders of the stomach and intestines?

   a. Endocrinologist

   b. Gastroenterologist

   c. Gerontologist

   d. Podiatrist

   e. Internist

21. A goal of regenerative medicine is to:

   a. replace the need for organ donation.

   b. slow the healing process.

   c. provide more health care jobs.

   d. sell organs commercially.

   e. win the Nobel Prize in the medicine category.

22. "Standard of care" refers to:

   a. the focus of medicine.

   b. generally accepted guidelines and principles that health care practitioners follow in the practice of medicine.

   c. a physician's specialty.

   d. a concept that only applies to physicians.

   e. a policy that was written by Hippocrates.

COG MATCHING   Grade: _____

Match the following key terms to their definitions.

Key Terms

23. _____ caduceus

24. _____ medical assistant

25. _____ outpatient

26. _____ specialty

27. _____ clinical

28. _____ administrative

29. _____ laboratory

30. _____ multidisciplinary

31. _____ inpatient

32. _____ externship

Definitions

a. completed by a CMA every 5 years by either taking the examination again or by acquiring 60 CEU

b. describing a medical facility where patients receive care but are not admitted overnight

c. a subcategory of medicine that a physician chooses to practice upon graduation from medical school

d. referring to a team of specialized professionals who are brought together to meet the needs of the patient

e. regarding a medical facility that treats patients and keeps them overnight, often accompanied by surgery or other procedure

f. a medical symbol showing a wand or staff with two serpents coiled around it

33. _____ accreditation

34. _____ certification

35. _____ recertification

g. voluntary process that involves a testing procedure to prove an individual's baseline competency in a particular area

h. regarding tasks that involve direct patient care

i. an educational course during which the student works in the field gaining hands-on experience

j. a multiskilled health care professional who performs a variety of tasks in a medical setting

k. a nongovernmental professional peer review process that provides technical assistance and evaluates educational programs for quality based on pre-established academic and administrative standards

l. regarding tasks that involve scientific testing

m. regarding tasks that focus on office procedures

COG **SHORT ANSWER**   Grade: _____

36. What is the purpose of the Centers for Medicare and Medicaid Services?

_____

_____

_____

37. The following are three specialists who may employ medical assistants. Describe what each does.

a. allergist: _____

b. internist: _____

c. gynecologist: _____

COG IDENTIFICATION

Grade: _____

As a medical assistant, you must be "multiskilled," or skilled at completing many different tasks. Almost all the tasks you will complete fall into one of two categories: administrative and clinical. But what's the difference between administrative and clinical tasks? Read each selection below and determine whether the task requires your clinical or administrative skills, then place a C or an A beside the task.

38. _____ preparing patients for examinations

39. _____ maintaining medical records

40. _____ ensuring good public relations

41. _____ obtaining medical histories

42. _____ preparing and sterilizing instruments

43. _____ screening sales representatives

AFF SHORT ANSWER

Grade: _____

44. What qualities do you possess that would make you a valuable member of your professional organization?

_____

_____

_____

45. List the characteristics that you possess that will make you a successful medical assistant.

_____

_____

_____

46. List any personal characteristics you believe you could improve.

_____

_____

_____

47. Describe the personal appearance of a professional medical assistant.

_____

_____

_____

48. What are the two accrediting bodies for the medical assisting education arena?

_____

_____

_____

49. What is the importance of having adaptive coping mechanisms in place? Give an example of a situation in which such tools would be helpful.

_____

_____

_____

50. How would you answer the question, "Legally, who is responsible for the actions of CMAs or RMAs as they perform their skills?"

_____

_____

_____

51. You are a CMA in a busy Ob/Gyn practice. You have been asked to orient a high school student who was hired to help up front and in medical records in the afternoons. She wants a career in health care but is unsure if she would be happier in a doctor's office or a hospital. She is debating between becoming a CMA or a CNA but is confused about the difference. She asks for your help in deciding what profession to choose. How would you explain the difference in the two careers?

_____

_____

_____

52. Why is the ability to respect patient confidentiality essential to the role of the medical assistant?

_____

_____

_____

53. The medical office in which you work treats a variety of patients, from all ages and backgrounds. Why should you work with a multidisciplinary health care team? What are the benefits to the patients?

_____

_____

_____

WHAT WOULD YOU DO?   Grade: _____

54. You are preparing a patient for her examination, but the physician is running behind schedule. The patient is becoming anxious and asks you to perform the examination, instead of the physician. You tell her that you will go check how much longer the physician will be. But she responds, "Can't you just perform the exam? Aren't you like a nurse?" How should you respond?

_____

_____

_____

55. The patient who asked you to perform the examination now refuses to wait for the physician. Even though she has a serious heart condition requiring monthly checkups, she leaves without being treated by the physician. You need to write a note that will be included in her chart and in an incident report. What would you say?

_____

_____

_____

COG AFF PSY **ACTIVE LEARNING**   Grade: _____

56. Review the list of specialists who employ medical assistants in textbook Table 1-2. Choose one specialty that interests you. Perform research on what kinds of procedures the specialist performs. Then consider what kinds of tasks a medical assistant employed by this specialist might perform. Write a letter to this specialist explaining why you would want to work in this kind of office. Be sure to include specific references to the tasks and procedures that interest you based on your research.

_____

_____

_____

57. Scope of practice for medical assistants can vary from state to state. In some states, CMAs are not allowed to perform invasive procedures, such as injections or phlebotomy. Go to the Web site for your state and research the laws in your state regarding the medical assistant's scope of practice. Why is it important to understand your scope of practice before beginning work in a new medical office?

_____

_____

_____

AFF **CASE STUDY FOR CRITICAL THINKING A**   Grade: _____

You are a CMA in a family practice where many of your friends and neighbors are patients. One of them is being treated for breast cancer. It seems as though everywhere you go, someone asks about her condition. They are just concerned, and so are you. You really want to give them an update on her treatment, but you know that is prohibited.

58. What is your best action? Choose all appropriate actions from the list below.

   a. Ask the patient if she minds letting you give updates to their mutual friends.

   b. Tell them that you would be violating a federal law if you discuss her care, but they should call her to find out.

   c. Tell them what they want to know. After all, they are asking because they care.

   d. Offer to help your friend/patient join a Web site that will allow her to update her friends.

AFF **CASE STUDY FOR CRITICAL THINKING B**   Grade: _____

You start your new position as a CMA for a busy pediatric practice. You are unsure of your job responsibilities, but the office manager expects you to "hit the ground running." Your first day is busy, and you are asked to handle the phones. Your first caller is a mother who is worried about her child's fever.

59. Your best response is:

   a. Don't worry. I'm sure she will be fine.

   b. Let me check the office protocol for children with fever. I will call you back.

   c. Today is my first day; I don't know, but I think she will be fine.

   d. You will need to make an appointment.

   e. I'll put you through to the doctor immediately.

60. What action could have prevented this uncomfortable situation?

   a. Having the opportunity to observe the office for a few weeks before starting

   b. Having read the policy and procedure manual before starting work

   c. Having more experience in the medical assisting field

   d. Paying better attention in class

   e. Refusing to answer the phone

61. You ask another CMA what you should do, and her response is, "I thought you were a CMA; you should know what to do." What is your next best action?

   a. Go immediately to your supervisor for guidance.

   b. Tell another co-worker what she said and ask what she thinks you should do.

   c. Start looking for another job.

   d. Tell her that if the facility had trained you properly, you would have known what to do.

   e. Tell her that you are doing your best, and you are sure you will get up to speed soon.

AFF **CASE STUDY FOR CRITICAL THINKING C**   Grade: _____

Mrs. Esposito approaches Jan, a medical assistant, at the front desk. Jan has recently treated Mrs. Esposito's son, Manuel, for a foot injury. Mrs. Esposito has just arrived in the United States and, with broken English, asks Jan if she may have her son's medical records to show Manuel's soccer coach that he will be unable to play for the rest of the season. Jan tries to explain to Mrs. Esposito that because her son is 18 years old and legally an adult, she must have his permission to release his medical records. Mrs. Esposito is frustrated and angry. Using Spanish translating software, Jan calmly attempts to explain that the physician would be happy to write a note for Manuel to give to his soccer coach explaining his injuries. After a great deal of time and effort, Mrs. Esposito thanks her for this information and apologizes for becoming angry.

62. From the list below, choose the characteristic of a professional medical assistant that Jan exhibited in the above scenario.

    a. Accuracy

    b. Proper hygiene

    c. The ability to respect patient confidentiality

    d. Honesty

63. What was the best action for Jan when she learned that Mrs. Esposito did not speak much English?

    a. Look in the Yellow Pages for a translator

    b. Try to find a Spanish translating software online

    c. Enlist the assistance of a fellow employee who speaks fluent Spanish

    d. Tell Mrs. Esposito to come back when she can bring a translator

64. When dealing with an angry person such as Mrs. Esposito, the most important action is to:

    a. Raise your voice so she will hear you

    b. Treat her as she is treating you

    c. Remain calm

    d. Notify the office manager of a problem

65. When responding to a request for the release of medical information, your first action should be to:

    a. explain the policy to the patient

    b. check for the patient's signed authorization

    c. ask the physician

    d. copy the records

Law and Ethics

Learning Outcomes

Cognitive Domain

1. Spell and define the key terms
2. Discuss all levels of governmental legislation and regulation as they apply to medical assisting practice, including the Food and Drug Administration and the Drug Enforcement Agency
3. Compare criminal and civil law as it applies to the practicing medical assistant
4. Provide an example of tort law as it would apply to a medical assistant
5. List the elements and types of contractual agreements and describe the difference in implied and express contracts
6. List four items that must be included in a contract termination or withdrawal letter
7. List six items that must be included in an informed consent form and explain who may sign consent forms
8. List five legally required disclosures that must be reported to specified authorities
9. Describe the four elements that must be proven in a medical legal suit
10. Describe four possible defenses against litigation for the medical professional
11. Explain the theory of respondeat superior, or law of agency, and how it applies to the medical assistant
12. Outline the laws regarding employment and safety issues in the medical office
13. Identify how the Americans with Disabilties Act applies to the medical assisting profession
14. Differentiate between legal, ethical and moral issues affecting health care
15. Explain how the following impact the medical assistant's practice and give examples
    a. Negligence
    b. Malpractice
    c. Statute of limitations
    d. Good Samaritan Act
    e. Uniform Anatomical Gift Act
    f. Living will/advanced directives
    g. Medical durable power of attorney
16. List the seven American Medical Association principles of ethics
17. List the five ethical principles of ethical and moral conduct outlined by the American Association of Medical Assistants
18. Recognize the role of patient advocacy in the practice of medical assisting
19. Describe the purpose of the Self-Determination Act
20. Explore issue of confidentiality as it applies to the medical assistant
21. Describe the implications of the Health Insurance Portability and Accountability Act for the medical assistant in various medical settings
22. Summarize the Patients' Bill of Rights
23. Discuss licensure and certification as it applies to health care providers
24. Describe liability, professional, personal, injury, and third party insurance

Psychomotor Domain

1. Monitor federal and state health care legislation (Procedure 2-1)
2. Incorporate the Patients' Bill of Rights into personal practice and medical office policies and procedures
3. Apply local, state, and federal health care legislation and regulation appropriate to the medical assisting practice setting

Affective Domain

1. Demonstrate sensitivity to patient rights
2. Recognize the importance of local, state, and federal legislation and regulations in the practice setting

ABHES Competencies

1. Comply with federal, state, and local health laws and regulations
2. Institute federal and state guidelines when releasing medical records or information
3. Follow established policies when initiating or terminating medical treatment
4. Understand the importance of maintaining liability coverage once employed in the industry

Name: _____   Date: _____   Grade: _____

COG MULTIPLE CHOICE

1. The branch of law concerned with issues of citizen welfare and safety is:

   a. private law.

   b. criminal law.

   c. constitutional law.

   d. administrative law.

   e. civil law.

2. Which branch of law covers injuries suffered because of another person's wrongdoings resulting from a breach of legal duty?

   a. Tort law

   b. Contract law

   c. Property law

   d. Commercial law

   e. Administrative law

3. Choose all of the true statements below regarding the Drug Enforcement Agency (DEA).

   a. The DEA regulates the sale and use of drugs.

   b. The DEA regulates the quality of drugs made in the United States.

   c. Providers who prescribe and/or dispense drugs are required to register with the DEA.

   d. Physicians must report inventory of narcotic medications on hand every month to the DEA.

   e. The DEA is a branch of the Department of Justice.

   f. Drug laws are federal and do not vary from state to state.

4. The Health Insurance Portability and Accountability Act of 1996 deals with the patient's right to:

   a. privacy.

   b. choose a physician.

   c. get information prior to a treatment.

   d. interrupt a treatment considered disadvantageous.

   e. refuse treatment.

5. Which of the following can lead a patient to file a suit for abandonment against a physician?

   a. The physician verbally asks to end the relationship with the patient.

   b. A suitable substitute is not available for care after termination of the contract.

   c. The patient disagrees with the reasons given by the physician for the termination.

   d. Termination happens 35 days after the physician's withdrawal letter is received.

   e. The physician transfers the patient's medical records to another physician of the patient's choice.

Scenario for questions 6 and 7: A man is found lying unconscious outside the physician's office. You alert several colleagues, who go outside to assess the man's condition. It is clear that he will be unable to sign a consent form for treatment.

6. How should the physician handle the unconscious man?

   a. Implied consent should be used until the man can give informed consent.

   b. A health care surrogate should be solicited to provide informed consent.

   c. The hospital administration should evaluate the situation and give consent.

   d. The physician should proceed with no-risk procedures until informed consent is given.

   e. The physician should wait for a friend or family member to give consent on the patient's behalf.

7. Once the man wakes up and gives his express consent to a treatment, this implies that he:

   a. no longer needs assistance.

   b. verbally agrees in front of witnesses on an emergency treatment.

   c. authorizes the physician to exchange the patient's information with other physicians.

   d. trusts the physician with emergency procedures that can be deemed necessary at a later time.

   e. is now familiar with the possible risks of the procedure.

8. A diagnosis of cancer must be reported to the Department of Health and Human Services to:

   a. alert the closest family members.

   b. protect the patient's right to treatment.

   c. investigate possible carcinogens in the environment.

   d. check coverage options with the insurance company.

   e. provide research for a national study.

9. What is the difference between licensure and certification?

   a. Licensure is accessible to medical assistants.

   b. Certification standards are recognized nationally.

   c. Licensure indicates education requirements are met.

   d. Certification limits the scope of activity of a physician.

   e. Licensure allows a professional to practice in any state.

10. The Good Samaritan Act covers:

    a. emergency care provided by a medical assistant.

    b. compensated emergency care outside the formal practice.

    c. sensible emergency practice administered outside the office.

    d. emergency practice administered in the hospital to uninsured patients.

    e. emergency care administered in the physician's office before the patient is registered.

11. The term *malfeasance* refers to:

    a. failure to administer treatment in time.

    b. administration of inappropriate treatment.

    c. administration of treatment performed incorrectly.

    d. failure to administer treatment in the best possible conditions.

    e. the physical touching of a patient without consent.

12. Which tort pertains to care administered without the patient's consent?

    a. Duress

    b. Assault

    c. Tort of outrage

    d. Undue influence

    e. Invasion of privacy

13. The statute of limitation indicates:

    a. the privacy rights of a minor receiving care.

    b. the risks that are presented to a patient before treatment.

    c. the responsibilities of a physician toward his or her patients.

    d. the right of a physician to have another physician care for his or her patients while out of the office.

    e. the time span during which a patient can file a suit against a caregiver.

14. The court may assess contributory negligence when a:

    a. team of physicians incorrectly diagnoses the patient.

    b. physician's malpractice is aggravated by the patient.

    c. patient does not follow the physician's prescribed treatment properly.

    d. patient gives inaccurate information that leads to wrong treatment.

    e. physician is entirely responsible for the patient's injury.

15. Which of these best describes the principle of patient advocacy?

    a. A medical assistant must adhere to his or her own code of conduct.

    b. A medical assistant must act first and foremost in the interest of the patient.

    c. A medical assistant must make sure the patient's information remains confidential.

    d. A medical assistant must make sure to act as a mediator between the physician and the patient.

    e. A medical assistant should only perform procedures that agree with his personal ethics.

16. Which of these is the basic principle of bioethics?

   a. All patients are entitled to the best possible treatment.

   b. Moral issues must be evaluated according to the patient's specific circumstances.

   c. Members of the medical community should never compromise their religious beliefs.

   d. The medical community must agree on a code of moral standards to apply to controversial cases.

   e. Moral issues are guidelines that the medical community is legally bound to follow.

17. What is the American Medical Association's regulation on artificial insemination?

   a. Both husband and wife must agree to the procedure.

   b. The donor has the right to contact the couple after the child is born.

   c. The procedure can only be performed legally in certain states.

   d. A donor can be selected only after the husband has tried the procedure unsuccessfully.

   e. The couple requesting the procedure has the right to gain information about possible donors.

18. What does the Self-Determination Act of 1991 establish?

   a. The physician has the last word on interruption of treatment.

   b. A person has the right to make end-of-life decisions in advance.

   c. The physician must follow advance directives from a patient verbatim.

   d. Family members cannot make decisions about terminating a patient's treatment.

   e. If a patient cannot make his or her own decision, a close family member can do so on his or her behalf.

19. Which of these patients would be unable to sign a consent form?

   a. A 17-year-old patient requesting information about a sexually transmitted disease

   b. A pregnant 15-year-old patient

   c. A 16-year-old boy who works full time

   d. A 17-year-old girl who requires knee surgery

   e. A married 21-year-old patient

20. In a comparative negligence case, how are damages awarded?

   a. The plaintiff receives damages based on a percentage of their contribution to the negligence.

   b. The defendant does not have to pay the plaintiff anything.

   c. The plaintiff and defendant share 50% of the court costs and receive no damages.

   d. The plaintiff has to pay damages to the defendant for defamation of character.

   e. The plaintiff receives 100% of the damages awarded.

21. Which of these laws protects you from exposure to bloodborne pathogens and other body fluids in the workplace?

   a. Civil Rights Act of 1964

   b. Self-Determination Act of 1991

   c. Occupational Safety and Health Act

   d. Americans with Disabilities Act

   e. Clinical Laboratory Improvement Act

22. The Food and Drug Administration is:

   a. not affiliated with the federal government.

   b. regulated by the Department of Health, Education and Welfare.

   c. regulates the manufacture, sale and distribution of drugs in the United States.

   d. not charged with assessing quality in the manufacture of drugs.

   e. divided among states.

COG MATCHING

Grade: _____

Match the following key terms to their definitions.

Key Terms	Definitions
23. ____ abandonment	**a.** a deceitful act with the intention to conceal the truth
24. ____ slander	**b.** process of filing or contesting a lawsuit
25. ____ assault	**c.** traditional laws outlined in the Constitution
26. ____ battery	**d.** a theory meaning that the previous decision stands
27. ____ ethics	**e.** a person under the age of majority but married or self-supporting
28. ____ tort law	**f.** previous court decisions
29. ____ civil law	**g.** a branch of law that focuses on issues between private citizens
30. ____ common law	**h.** governs the righting of wrongs suffered as a result of another person's wrong-doing
31. ____ defamation of character	
32. ____ defendant	**i.** a substitute physician
33. ____ deposition	**j.** an arrangement that gives the patient's representative the ability to make health care decisions for the patient
34. ____ durable power of attorney	**k.** sharing fees for the referral of patients to certain colleagues
35. ____ emancipated minor	**l.** the accuser in a lawsuit
36. ____ fee splitting	**m.** failure to take reasonable precautions to prevent harm to a patient
37. ____ fraud	**n.** the accused party in a lawsuit
38. ____ libel	**o.** a doctrine meaning "the thing speaks for itself"
39. ____ litigation	**p.** the unauthorized attempt to threaten or touch another person without consent
40. ____ locum tenens	**q.** the physical touching of a patient without consent
41. ____ malpractice	**r.** malicious or false statements about a person's character or reputation
42. ____ negligence	**s.** written statements that damage a person's character or reputation
43. ____ plaintiff	**t.** a process in which one party questions another party under oath
44. ____ precedents	**u.** an action by a professional health care worker that harms a patient
45. ____ res ipsa loquitur	**v.** a doctrine meaning "the thing has been decided"
46. ____ res judicata	**w.** a doctrine meaning "let the master answer," also known as the *law of agency*
47. ____ respondeat superior	**x.** guidelines specifying right or wrong that are enforced by peer review and professional organizations
48. ____ stare decisis	**y.** withdrawal by a physician from a contractual relationship with a patient without proper notification
	z. oral statements that damage a person's character or reputation

SHORT ANSWER   Grade: _____

49. List six items that must be included in an informed consent form and explain who may sign consent forms.

_____

_____

_____

50. List five legally required disclosures that must be reported to specified authorities.

_____

_____

_____

51. List nine principles cited in the American Medical Association's principles of ethics.

_____

_____

_____

52. List the five ethical principles of ethical and moral conduct outlined by the American Association of Medical Assistants.

_____

_____

_____

COG IDENTIFICATION   Grade: _____

The Americans with Disabilities Act (ADA) prohibits discrimination against people with disabilities in employment practice. Take a look at the scenarios in this chart and assess whether or not the ADA is being followed correctly. Place a check mark in the appropriate box.

Scenario	ADA-Compliance	ADA-Noncompliance
53. A physician's office extends an offer of employment to a man in a wheelchair but says that due to a shortage of parking, the office cannot offer him a parking space in the garage.		
54. A 46-year-old woman is refused a position on the basis that she is HIV positive.		
55. A mentally ill man with a history of violence is refused a job in a busy office.		
56. A small office with 10 employees chooses a healthy woman over a disabled woman because the office cannot afford to adapt the facilities in the workplace.		
57. A patient's wheelchair-bound husband cannot accompany her to her physician's visits because there is no handicap entrance for visitors.		
58. A job applicant with a severe speech impediment is rejected for a position as an emergency room receptionist.		

Some situations require a report to be filed with the Department of Health with or without the patient's consent. Read the scenarios in the chart below and decide which ones are legally required disclosures.

Scenario	Legally Required Disclosure	No Action Needed
59. A 35-year-old woman gives birth to a healthy baby girl.		
60. A physician diagnoses a patient with meningococcal meningitis.		
61. A 43-year-old man falls off a ladder and breaks his leg. He spends 3 weeks in the hospital.		
62. A teenager is involved in a hit-and-run accident. He is rushed to the hospital, but dies the next day.		
63. A 2-year-old girl is diagnosed with measles.		
64. A man is diagnosed with a sexually transmitted disease and asks the physician to keep the information confidential.		
65. A woman visits the physician's office and tells him she has mumps, but when he examines her, he discovers it is influenza.		

COG IDENTIFICATION   Grade: _____

66. Which of the following must be included in a patient consent form? Circle all that apply.

    a. Name of the physician performing the procedure

    b. Alternatives to the procedure and their risks

    c. Date the procedure will take place

    d. Probable effect on the patient's condition if the procedure is not performed

    e. Potential risks from the procedure

    f. Patient's next of kin

    g. Any exclusions that the patient requests

    h. Success rate of the procedure

67. Dr. Janeway has decided to terminate his patient, Mrs. King. The office manager drafted the following letter to Mrs. King. However, when you review the letter, you find that there are errors. Read the letter below and then explain the three problems with this letter in the space below.

Dear Mrs. King,

Because you have consistently refused to follow the dietary restrictions and to take the medication necessary to control your high blood pressure, I feel I am no longer able to provide your medical care. This termination is effective immediately.

Because you do not seem to take your medical condition seriously, I'm not sure that any other physician would want to treat you either. I will hold on to your medical records for 30 days and then they will be destroyed.

                                    Sincerely,
                                    Anthony Janeway, MD

a. _____

b. _____

c. _____

ACTIVE LEARNING

68. Research two recent medical malpractice cases on the Internet. Write a brief outline of each case and make a record of whether the tort was intentional or unintentional, and what the outcome of the case was. Compare the cases to see if there is a common theme.

69. Visit a physician's office and make a list of steps that have been taken to comply with the law. For example, if the physician charges for canceling appointments without notice, there is probably a sign by the reception desk to warn patients of the fee. How many other legal requirements can you find? Are there any that are missing?

70. As technology develops, new laws have to be written to protect the rights of patients who use it. Stem cell research is a particularly gray area and has raised many interesting ethical dilemmas. Research some recent legal cases regarding stem cell research, and write a report on some of the ethical issues the cases have raised.

71. You are a medical assistant in a busy office, and the physician has been called away on an emergency. Some of the patients have been waiting for over 2 hours, and one of them urgently needs a physical checkup for a job application. Although you are not officially qualified, you feel confident that you are able to carry out the examination by yourself. Six months later, the patient files a malpractice suit because you failed to notice a lump in her throat that turned out to be cancerous. Describe the law of agency and explain whether it would help you in the lawsuit.

AFF WHAT WOULD YOU DO?   Grade: _____

72. A family member calls to inquire about a patient's condition. You know that the patient has not given written consent for information to be passed on, but you recognize the person's voice and remember that she came in with the patient the previous day. Explain what you would say and why.

_____

_____

_____

_____

COG IDENTIFICATION

Grade: _____

73. Mrs. Stevens visits Dr. Johnson's office with neck pain. Dr. Johnson examines her and recommends that she see a specialist. Several months later, Mrs. Stevens sues Dr. Johnson for malpractice, claiming that when he examined her, he made her neck pain worse. In court, she provides pictures of her neck that show severe bruising. A specialist confirms that muscle damage has restricted Mrs. Stevens from going about her daily life. Which of the four elements needed in a medical lawsuit has Mrs. Stevens failed to prove? Circle all that apply.

   a. Duty

   b. Dereliction of duty

   c. Direct cause

   d. Damage

AFF PATIENT EDUCATION

Grade: _____

74. You have a patient who has just been diagnosed with a sexually transmitted disease. After the physician leaves the office, the patient turns to you and begs you to keep the information confidential. It is obvious that the patient is worried and embarrassed. Explain how you would inform the patient about legally required disclosures and what you would say.

   _____

   _____

   _____

   _____

AFF **CASE STUDY FOR CRITICAL THINKING A** Grade: _____

Pamela Dorsett is a patient at Highland Oaks Family Practice. She is a 40-year-old woman who has five children and a house full of cats. She brings her children in for immunizations, but otherwise you rarely see them. She walks into the office on a busy Monday morning with all five children. They are surrounded by a pungent smell of cat feces. The children are dirty and it appears are being neglected. All five of them have runny noses. She wants the doctor to see them now because she has transportation problems. You are the receptionist that day. Remember, pick the BEST answer.

75. The doctor is legally obligated to see the children at some point because:

    a. the children look neglected.

    b. there is a legal contract in place.

    c. medical ethics dictate it.

    d. all of the above.

76. If child neglect is suspected, the physician is required by federal law to:

    a. talk to the mother about her care.

    b. try to contact a family member.

    c. do nothing, as mandated by HIPAA.

    d. report the suspicions to authorities.

77. What would your first action be?

    a. Try to work the five children into the busy schedule.

    b. Consult with the providers.

    c. Make future appointments as soon as possible.

    d. Have them wait until the end of the day after all scheduled patients have been seen.

COG **AFF** **CASE STUDY FOR CRITICAL THINKING B**   Grade: _____

As a medical assistant, you will be involved in some administrative issues. Read the following scenarios and assess whether the American Medical Association standards for office management are being met. Place a check mark in the appropriate box.

Scenario	Standards Met	Standards Not Met
78. Dr. Benson tells his medical assistant to cancel Mrs. Burke's tests because she recently lost her job and will be unable to pay for them.		
79. Mr. Grant canceled his appointment with less than 24 hours' notice. He was charged a fee as noted in a sign by the receptionist's desk.		
80. Mrs. O'Malley asks Dr. Jones to help her fill out an insurance form. The form is a four-page document that takes Dr. Jones an hour to fill out. Dr. Jones charges Mrs. O'Malley $15 for filling out the form.		
81. Dr. Harris dies suddenly, and his staff tell patients that the office will close and that copies of their medical records will be transferred to another physician.		
82. Mr. Davies owes the physician's office several thousand dollars. He is moving and asks the office to transfer his medical records to his new physician. The office refuses on the grounds that Mr. Davies has not paid his bill.		
83. Mrs. Jones comes into the office for a vaccination. The physician tells the medical assistant to charge her $10 less than other patients because she is elderly and cannot afford the standard charges.		

PSY **PROCEDURE 2-1**	**Monitoring Federal and State Regulations, Changes, and Updates**

Name: _____ Date: _____ Time: _____ Grade: _____

EQUIPMENT: Computer, Internet connection, search engine or Web site list

KEY: 4 = Satisfactory   0 = Unsatisfactory   NA = This step is not counted

PROCEDURE STEPS	SELF	PARTNER	INSTRUCTOR
1. Using a search engine, go to the homepage for your state government (Example: http://www.nc.gov) and/or other related sites such as: Centers for Disease Control and Prevention (CDC), Occupational Safety and Health Act (OSHA), your state medical society, and the American Medical Association (AMA).	☐	☐	☐
2. Input keywords such as: Health care finances, allied health professionals, outpatient medical care, Medicare, etc.	☐	☐	☐
3. Create and enforce a policy for timely dissemination of information received by fax or e-mail from outside agencies.	☐	☐	☐
4. Circulate information gathered to all appropriate employees with an avenue for sharing information. Any information obtained should be shared.	☐	☐	☐
5. Post changes in policies and procedures in a designated area of the office.	☐	☐	☐
6. **AFF** Explain what you would say to a fellow employee who responds to a change in a current law with, "I will just keep doing it the old way. Who is going to care?"	☐	☐	☐

CALCULATION

Total Possible Points: _____

Total Points Earned: _____ Multiplied by 100 = _____ Divided by Total Possible Points = _____ %

PASS   **FAIL**   **COMMENTS:**

☐   ☐

Student's signature _____ Date _____

Partner's signature _____ Date _____

Instructor's signature _____ Date _____

Communication Skills

Learning Outcomes

Cognitive Domain

1. Spell and define the key terms
2. List two major forms of communication
3. Identify styles and types of verbal communication
4. Identify nonverbal communication
5. Recognize communication barriers
6. Identify techniques for overcoming communication barriers
7. Recognize the elements of oral communication using a sender-receiver process
8. Identify resources and adaptations that are required based on individual needs, i.e., culture and environment, developmental life stage, language, and physical threats to communication
9. Discuss the role of cultural, social, and ethnic diversity in ethical performance of medical assisting practice
10. Discuss the role of assertiveness in effective professional communication
11. Explain how various components of communication can affect the meaning of verbal messages
12. Define active listening
13. List and describe the six interviewing techniques
14. Give an example of how cultural differences may affect communication
15. Discuss how to handle communication problems caused by language barriers
16. List two methods that you can use to promote communication among hearing-, sight-, and speech-impaired patients
17. Discuss how to handle an angry or distressed patient
18. List five actions that you can take to improve communication with a child
19. Discuss your role in communicating with a grieving patient or family member
20. List the five stages of grief as outlined by Elisabeth Kübler-Ross
21. Discuss the key elements of interdisciplinary communication
22. Explore issue of confidentiality as it applies to the medical assistant

Psychomotor Domain

1. Respond to nonverbal communication
2. Use reflection, restatement and clarification techniques to obtain a patient history

Affective Domain

1. Apply active listening skills
2. Use appropriate body language and other nonverbal skills in communicating with patients, family, and staff
3. Demonstrate awareness of the territorial boundaries of the person with whom you are communicating
4. Demonstrate sensitivity appropriate to the message being delivered
5. Demonstrate awareness of how an individual's personal appearance affects anticipated responses
6. Demonstrate recognition of the patient's level of understanding in communications
7. Analyze communication in providing appropriate responses/feedback
8. Recognize and protect personal boundaries in communicating with others
9. Demonstrate respect for individual diversity, incorporating awareness of one's own biases in areas including gender, race, religion, and economic standing
10. Demonstrate empathy in communicating with patients, family, and staff

11. Demonstrate sensitivity in communicating with both providers and patients
12. Respond to issues of confidentiality

ABHES Competencies

1. Identify and respond appropriately when working with/caring for patients with special needs
2. Use empathy when treating terminally ill patients
3. Identify common stages that terminally ill patients go through and list organizations/support groups that can assist patients and family members of patients struggling with terminal illness
4. Advocate on behalf of family/patients, having the ability to deal and communicate with family
5. Analyze the effect of hereditary, cultural, and environmental influences
6. Locate resources and information for patients and employers
7. Be attentive, listen, and learn
8. Be impartial and show empathy when dealing with patients
9. Communicate on the recipient's level of comprehension
10. Serve as liaison between physician and others
11. Recognize and respond to verbal and nonverbal communication

Name: _____   Date: _____   Grade: _____

COG MULTIPLE CHOICE

Circle the letter preceding the correct answer.

1. Laughing, sobbing, and sighing are examples of:

   a. kinesics.

   b. proxemics.

   c. nonlanguage.

   d. paralanguage.

   e. clarification.

2. Hearing impairment that involves problems with either nerves or the cochlea is called:

   a. anacusis.

   b. conductive.

   c. presbyacusis.

   d. sensorineural.

   e. dysphasia.

3. Sally needs to obtain information from her patient about the medications he is taking. Which of the following open-ended questions is phrased in a way that will elicit the information that Sally needs?

   a. Are you taking your medications?

   b. What medications are you taking?

   c. Have you taken any medications?

   d. Did you take your medications today?

   e. Have you taken medications in the past?

4. Which of the following shows the proper sequence of the sender-receiver process?

   a. Person to send message, message to be sent, person to receive message

   b. Message to be received, person to send message, message to be sent

   c. Message to be sent, person to receive message, person to send message

   d. Person to receive message, person to send message, message to be sent

   e. Person to send message, person to receive message, message to be sent

5. "Those people always get head lice." This statement is an example of:

   a. culture.

   b. demeanor.

   c. discrimination.

   d. stereotyping.

   e. prejudice.

6. What can you do as a medical assistant to communicate effectively with a patient when there is a language barrier?

   a. Find an interpreter who can translate for the patient.

   b. Raise your voice so the patient can focus more on what you are saying.

   c. Give the patient the name and address of a physician who speaks the same language.

   d. Assess the patient and give the physician your best opinion about what is bothering the patient.

   e. Suggest that the patient find another physician who is better equipped to communicate with the patient.

7. When dealing with patients who present communication challenges, such as hearing-impaired or sight-impaired patients, it is best to:

   a. talk about the patient directly with a family member to find out what the problem is.

   b. conduct the interview alone with the patient because he needs to be able to take care of himself.

   c. address the patient's questions in the waiting room, where other people can try to help the patient communicate.

   d. refer the patient to a practice that specializes in working with hearing- and sight-impaired patients.

   e. make sure the patient feels like he is part of the process, even if his condition requires a family member's help.

8. A hearing-impaired patient's test results are in. It is important that the patient gets the results quickly. How should you get the results to the patient?

    a. Mail the test results via priority mail.

    b. Call the patient on a TDD/TTY phone and type in the results.

    c. Drive to the patient's house at lunchtime to deliver the results.

    d. Call an emergency contact of the patient and ask him or her to have the patient make an appointment.

    e. Send the patient a fax containing the test results.

9. Which of the following statements about grieving is true?

    a. The grieving period is approximately 30 days.

    b. Different cultures and individuals demonstrate grief in different ways.

    c. The best way to grieve is through wailing because it lets the emotion out.

    d. The five stages of grief must be followed in that specific order for healing to begin.

    e. Everyone grieves in his or her own way, but all of us go through the stages at the same time.

10. *Proxemics* refers to the:

    a. pitch of a person's voice.

    b. facial expressions a person makes.

    c. physical proximity that people tolerate.

    d. the combination of verbal and nonverbal communication.

    e. the ability of a patient to comprehend difficult messages.

11. Which of the following situations would result in a breach of patient confidentiality?

    a. Shredding unwanted notes that contain patient information

    b. Discussing a patient's lab results with a coworker in the hospital cafeteria

    c. Keeping the glass window between the waiting room and reception desk closed

    d. Shutting down your computer when you leave every night

    e. Paging the physician on an intercom to let him or her know a patient is waiting on the phone for results

12. "Those results can't be true. The doctor must have mixed me up with another patient." This statement reflects which of the following stages of grieving?

    a. Anger

    b. Denial

    c. Depression

    d. Bargaining

    e. Acceptance

13. Which of the following statements about communication is correct?

    a. Communication can be either verbal or nonverbal.

    b. Written messages can be interpreted through paralanguage.

    c. Verbal communication involves both oral communication and body language.

    d. Body language is the most important form of communication.

    e. Touch should be avoided in all forms of communication because it makes the recipient of the message uncomfortable.

14. During a patient interview, repeating what you have heard the patient say using an open-ended statement is called:

    a. clarifying.

    b. reflecting.

    c. summarizing.

    d. paraphrasing.

    e. allowing silences.

15. What should you do during a patient interview if there is silence?

    a. Silence should not be allowed during a patient interview.

    b. Immediately start talking so the patient does not feel awkward.

    c. Fill in charts that need to be completed until the patient is ready.

    d. Wait for the physician to arrive to speak with the patient.

    e. Gather your thoughts and think of any additional questions you have.

16. The physician is behind schedule, and a patient is angry that her appointment is late. The best way to deal with the patient is to:

    a. tell her anything that will calm her down.

    b. ignore her until the problem is solved.

    c. threaten that the physician will no longer treat her if she continues to complain.

    d. keep her informed of when the physician will be able to see her.

    e. ask her why it is such a big deal.

17. Why is it helpful to ask open-ended questions during a patient interview?

    a. They let the patient give yes or no answers.

    b. They let the patient develop an answer and explain it.

    c. They let the patient respond quickly using few words.

    d. They provide simple answers that are easy to note in the chart.

    e. They let the patient give his or her own feelings and opinions on the subject.

18. Difficulty with speech is called:

    a. dysphasia.

    b. dysphonia.

    c. nyctalopia.

    d. strabismus.

    e. myopia.

19. One particular physician runs behind schedule most of the time. His CMA has to work until he finishes seeing his patients, but her child must be picked up from day-care by 6:00 p.m. Which statement below represents one of an assertive person?

    a. I won't work late another day! My hours are 8:00 a.m. to 5:00 p.m.

    b. Sorry, doctor, I'm out of here to pick up my child. Someone else will have to stay.

    c. My daughter must be picked up by 6:00 every day. Could we look at the possibility of taking turns staying late? I could make arrangements for one day out of the week.

    d. Since you are the reason we run late, you should take care of the patients yourself.

    e. I can't believe you're asking me to stay late again. I am going to find another job.

20. The limit of personal space is generally considered to be a:

    a. 1-foot radius.

    b. 3-foot radius.

    c. 5-foot radius.

    d. 10-foot radius.

    e. 15-foot radius.

COG MATCHING

Grade: _____

Match the following key terms to their definitions.

Key Terms

21. __m__ anacusis
22. __k__ bias
23. __j__ clarification
24. __c__ cultures
25. __q__ demeanor
26. __s__ discrimination
27. __f__ dysphasia
28. __r__ dysphonia
29. __h__ feedback
30. __o__ grief
31. __a__ messages
32. __l__ mourning
33. __g__ nonlanguage
34. __p__ paralanguage
35. __i__ paraphrasing
36. __e__ presbyacusis
37. __t__ reflecting
38. __d__ stereotyping
39. __n__ summarizing
40. __b__ therapeutic

Definitions

a. information

b. something that is beneficial to a patient

c. a group of people who share a way of life and beliefs

d. holding an opinion of all members of a particular culture, race, religion, or age group based on oversimplified or negative characterizations

e. loss of hearing associated with aging

f. difficulty speaking

g. sounds that include laughing, sobbing, sighing, or grunting to convey information

h. the response to a message

i. restating what a person said using your own words or phrases

j. removal of confusion or uncertainty

k. formation of an opinion without foundation or reason

l. a demonstration of the signs of grief

m. complete hearing loss

n. briefly reviewing information discussed to determine the patient's comprehension

o. great sadness caused by a loss

p. voice tone, quality, volume, pitch, and range

q. the way a person looks, behaves, and conducts himself

r. a voice impairment that is caused by a physical condition, such as oral surgery

s. the act of not treating a patient fairly or respectfully because of his cultural, social, or personal values

t. repeating what one heard using open-ended questions

COG IDENTIFICATION   Grade: _____

41. The two main forms of communication are verbal communication and nonverbal communication. Read each form of communication below and place an "A" for verbal or a "B" for nonverbal in the space provided.

    a. _____ A patient sighs while explaining her symptoms.

    b. _____ A patient shrugs his shoulders after being told he needs to lose weight.

    c. _____ A patient's eyes dart around the room during an explanation of a procedure.

    d. _____ A physician writes "take two aspirin every 8 hours."

    e. _____ A mother is given a sheet of paper describing what to expect of her baby during months 6–9.

    f. _____ A physician puts her hand on a patient's shoulder before delivering test results.

COG PSY SHORT ANSWER   Grade: _____

42. List five local resources that can assist a grieving patient or family member. Include the name of the agency, type of help that it offers, and its phone number.

_____

_____

_____

43. Why is it important to respect cultural diversity?

_____

_____

_____

44. List the five stages of grief as outlined by Elisabeth Kübler-Ross.

_____

_____

_____

45. List five actions that you can take to improve communication with a child.

_____

_____

_____

46. List two methods that you can use to promote communication among hearing-, sight-, and speech-impaired patients.

_____

_____

_____

47. List and describe the six interviewing techniques.

_____

_____

_____

48. List two major forms of communication.

_____

_____

_____

49. What is the difference between aggressiveness and assertiveness?

_____

_____

_____

AFF **WHAT WOULD YOU DO?**   Grade: _____

50. You are working in the reception area of a busy medical practice. Patients come and go all day long, and it is your responsibility to move the flow along. One particularly busy day, you are registering an 89-year-old man. You ask him to read and sign an authorization to release records to Medicare. He says that he cannot see the form and asks if his wife can sign. His nonverbal cues make you wonder if he can read and write. From the list below, choose all appropriate actions.

  a. Ask him if he would like the number for an adult literacy program.

  b. Tell him that his wife can sign for him, but she should also read the authorization for him.

  c. Have his wife initial the "signature" and then you sign as a witness.

  d. Tell him to make an "X" if he cannot write.

  e. Tell him to sign the form without reading it.

51. A patient calls the office with symptoms and a condition that you are not familiar with. She has used some terms that you do not understand. When you relay the message to the physician, how should you communicate the patient's problem?

  _____

  _____

  _____

COG **AFF** **IDENTIFICATION**   Grade: _____

52. Read the list of nonverbal communication cues below. Beside each one, list the problem or issue this action might indicate:

  a. Crossed arms_____

  b. Slumping in chair _____

  c. A child hiding behind mother _____

  d. Hand clenching _____

53. Physicians use the information obtained during a patient interview to help them assess the patient's health. Patients will be more willing to provide information during a professionally conducted interview. Read each of the following statements describing patient interviews. Answer "yes" if the statement describes a correct interview practice; answer "no" if it describes an incorrect interview practice. Provide an explanation on how to correct the problem for all no answers.

   a. Patient interviews can be conducted in an exam room or in the waiting room. _____

   b. Answering a phone call in the middle of a new patient interview is acceptable if it is a call you have been waiting for. _____

   c. It is important to maintain eye contact with the patient, so you do not write any patient responses down until the interview is over. _____

   d. You confirm which blood pressure medication and what dosage the patient is taking. _____

   e. There is nothing wrong with skipping questions in a patient interview that may make the patient feel uncomfortable. _____

   f. Introducing yourself to the patient is a nice way to start an interview. _____

COG TRUE OR FALSE?   Grade: _____

Determine whether the following statements are true or false. If false, explain why.

54. When the office is busy, it is okay to refer to patients by their medical conditions, for example, "stomach pain in room 1."

_____

55. If an older adult patient does not have a ride home, a staff member in the office should offer him or her one.

_____

56. When talking with patients, do not reveal too many personal details about your life.

_____

57. It is inappropriate to carry on personal conversations with other staff members in front of a patient.

_____

PSY **ACTIVE LEARNING**   Grade: _____

58. Practice active listening with a partner. Have your partner tell you a detailed story that you have never heard before or explain a topic that you are unfamiliar with. After he or she has finished, wait silently for 2 minutes. Then, try to repeat the story or steps back to your partner. Next, reverse roles and let your partner listen while you tell a story or explain a concept.

_____

_____

_____

59. If you work in a pediatric office, you will certainly spend a good deal of time communicating with children. To help strengthen your communication skills with children, find a local preschool or elementary school teacher who has experience working with children. Interview this teacher about his or her communication techniques and write a list of 10 tips for communicating with children.

_____

_____

_____

AFF **CASE STUDY FOR CRITICAL THINKING A**   Grade: _____

You are working in a geriatric office taking patients back, and one of your patients is a Spanish-speaking woman who comes into the office with her son and daughter. Her body language indicates fear and worry. She appears very shy and depends on her son and daughter for assistance. They speak a little bit of English, but it is difficult to communicate with them.

60. Your first duty is to interview the patient about her medical history. Of the following steps, circle the ones you should take to get information.

   a. Speak in a normal tone and volume.

   b. Speak directly to the son and daughter.

   c. When asking a question about eyesight, point to your eyes.

   d. Use abbreviations and slang terms for medical tests.

   e. Ask the woman's son to be the interpreter and her daughter to wait outside.

   f. Use complex medical language to explain procedures.

   g. Use a Spanish-to-English dictionary.

61. The physician will be doing a complete exam on the patient. She must change into a gown. You have everyone but her daughter leave the exam room. You hand a gown to her daughter who starts toward her mother to help the patient change. The patient backs up into the corner of the room. Of the following actions, which ONE is the most appropriate?

   a. Take the gown from the daughter and give it to the patient.

   b. Leave the room and let the daughter handle it.

   c. Tell her that she will be covered and you have a blanket for her if she is cold.

   d. Tell the physician that the patient would not undress and let him or her handle it.

   e. Give the patient a big hug—that should make her feel better.

62. Following a difficult exam, the physician notes a suspicious mole on the patient's back. He instructs you to get her an appointment with a dermatologist. You explain to the three of them that you will make an appointment. You ask them if they have a preference, and they appear confused. Circle all appropriate actions in the list below.

   a. Give them a patient brochure on moles.

   b. Make an appointment in 2 weeks for them to return with a translator.

   c. Make the appointment, and write down the name and address of the facility.

   d. Give the patient a big hug and tell her what a brave girl she was.

   e. Use a Spanish-to-English dictionary to try to explain.

AFF **CASE STUDY FOR CRITICAL THINKING B**   Grade: _____

63. Your physician is treating a 7-year-old girl who needs to have her tonsils removed. Her mother has 60% hearing loss and depends on lip-reading to communicate. You need to have her sign paperwork and explain the child's need for a pre-anesthesia appointment at the hospital. Circle the suggestions below that will help you to communicate with her.

   a. Gently touch the patient to get her attention.

   b. Exaggerate your facial movements.

   c. Eliminate all distractions.

   d. Enunciate clearly.

   e. Use short sentences with short words.

   f. Speak loudly.

   g. Give the patient written instructions.

   h. Turn toward the light so your face is illuminated.

   i. Talk face-to-face with the patient, not at an angle.

64. Protocol dictates that the child has a history and physical exam before her surgery. She is obviously afraid and confused about what is happening. Circle the actions listed below that would be appropriate when communicating with the child.

a. Tell the child when you need to touch him or her and what you are going to do.

b. Talk loudly and sternly so the child will stay focused on you and not other distractions in the office.

c. Work quickly and let him or her be surprised by what you do.

d. Rephrase questions until the child understands.

e. Be playful to help gain the child's cooperation.

f. Try to speak to children at their eye level.

Patient Education

Cognitive Domain

1. Spell and define the key terms
2. Explain the medical assistant's role in patient education
3. Define the five steps in the patient education process
4. Identify five conditions that are needed for patient education to occur
5. Explain Maslow's hierarchy of human needs
6. List five factors that may hinder patient education and at least two methods to compensate for each of these factors
7. Discuss five preventive medicine guidelines that you should teach your patients
8. Explain the kinds of information that should be included in patient teaching about medication therapy
9. Explain your role in teaching patients about alternative medicine therapies
10. List and explain relaxation techniques that you and patients can learn to help with stress management
11. Describe how to prepare a teaching plan
12. List potential sources of patient education materials
13. Locate community resources and list ways of organizing and disseminating information
14. Recognize communication barriers
15. Identify techniques for overcoming communication barriers
16. Identify resources and adaptations that are required based on individual needs i.e.

culture and environment, developmental life stage, language, and physical threats to communication

Psychomotor Domain

1. Document patient education (Procedure 4-1)
2. Develop and maintain a current list of community resources related to the patient's health care needs (Procedure 4-2)

Affective Domain

1. Use language/verbal skills that enable patients' understanding
2. Demonstrate respect for diversity in approaching patients and families
3. Demonstrate empathy in communicating with patients, family and staff
4. Demonstrate sensitivity appropriate to the message being delivered
5. Demonstrate recognition of the patient's level of understanding in communications
6. Demonstrate sensitivity to patient rights

ABHES Competencies

1. Identify and respond appropriately when working/caring for patients with special needs
2. Adapt to individualized needs
3. Communicate on the recipient's level of comprehension
4. Be impartial and show empathy when dealing with patients

Name: _____   Date: _____   Grade: _____

COG MULTIPLE CHOICE

Circle the BEST answer.

1. During assessment, the most comprehensive source from which to obtain patient information is the:

   a. physician's notes.

   b. immunization record.

   c. medical record.

   d. family member.

   e. nurse.

2. When teaching a patient with many chronic health problems, it is important to

   a. focus on each problem separately.

   b. tell them that your grandmother has many of the same problems.

   c. bond with him or her.

   d. have the patient come back another time with a family member.

   e. have the physician talk to him or her.

3. Which of the following is an example of a psychomotor skill that a patient may perform?

   a. Telling the physician about his or her symptoms

   b. Explaining how a part of the body is feeling

   c. Walking around with a crutch

   d. Watching television in the waiting room

   e. Listening to a physician's instructions

4. Which part of Maslow's pyramid is the point at which a patient has satisfied all basic needs and feels he or she has control over his or her life?

   a. Safety and security

   b. Esteem

   c. Self-actualization

   d. Affection

   e. Physiologic

5. Noncompliance occurs when the patient:

   a. experiences a decrease in symptoms healed.

   b. forgets to pay his or her bill.

   c. refuses to follow the physician's orders.

   d. requests a new medical assistant to assist the physician.

   e. agrees with the physician.

6. The power of believing that something will make you better when there is no chemical reaction that warrants such improvement is:

   a. self-relaxation.

   b. positive stress.

   c. acupuncture.

   d. placebo.

   e. visualization.

7. Patient education should consist of multiple techniques or approaches so:

   a. the patient can apply his or her new knowledge to real-life events.

   b. the patient will learn and retain more.

   c. the patient will understand that there are many ways to look at an issue.

   d. the patient will know where you stand on his or her health care options.

   e. the patient will have a wider choice of treatments.

8. One mental health illness that can hinder patient education is:

   a. diabetes.

   b. Lyme disease.

   c. obstructive pulmonary disease.

   d. Alzheimer disease.

   e. anemia.

9. Health assessment forms that assess a patient's education level may also help you determine a patient's ability to:

   a. read.

   b. listen.

   c. communicate.

   d. respond.

   e. evaluate.

10. Before developing a medication schedule, you should evaluate the patient's:

    a. prescribed medication.

    b. side effects.

    c. changes in bodily functions.

    d. daily routine.

    e. bowel movements.

11. Which is an example of a recommended preventive procedure?

    a. Regular teeth whitening

    b. Childhood immunizations

    c. Daily exercise

    d. Yearly lung cancer evaluations

    e. Occasional antibiotics

12. Which of the following is true of herbal supplements?

    a. A medical assistant can recommend that a patient start taking herbal supplements without the physician's approval.

    b. A health store clerk is a good source of information on supplements.

    c. Products that claim to detoxify the whole body are generally effective.

    d. Supplements will not interfere with blood sugar levels because they are not medication.

    e. Patients should be advised that because a product is natural does not mean it is safe.

13. One example of a physiologic response to negative stress is:

    a. elevated mood.

    b. hunger pangs.

    c. headache.

    d. profuse bleeding.

    e. energy boost.

14. In Maslow's hierarchy of needs, air, water, food, and rest are considered:

    a. affection needs.

    b. safety and security needs.

    c. esteem needs.

    d. self-actualization needs.

    e. physiologic needs.

15. When explaining the benefits and risks of a proposed treatment to a patient who uses American Sign Language to communicate, the physician must:

    a. be sure the patient is given the information in writing.

    b. provide a sign language interpreter if the patient does not bring one.

    c. make the patient feel comfortable.

    d. use a notepad to communicate.

    e. let the medical assistant handle it.

16. Humans use defense mechanisms to:

    a. cope with painful problems.

    b. increase their sense of accomplishment.

    c. decrease effects of chronic physical pain.

    d. learn to get along well with others.

    e. explain complicated emotions to medical staff.

17. Support groups give patients the opportunity to:

    a. exchange and compare medical records.

    b. meet and share ideas with others who are experiencing the same issues.

    c. spread the good word about the medical office.

    d. obtain their basic physiologic needs.

    e. learn more about malpractice suits.

18. When selecting teaching material, you should first:

   a. choose preprinted material.

   b. create your own material.

   c. assess your patient's general level of understanding.

   d. let the patient find a book from the clinic library.

   e. ask the patient to create a list of specific questions.

19. Acupressure is different from acupuncture because:

   a. it does not use needles.

   b. it is not an alternative medicine.

   c. it cannot be used with cancer patients.

   d. it does not require any licensure.

   e. it is less effective.

20. If your community does not have a central agency for information and resources, then you should create a(n):

   a. hierarchy of needs.

   b. teaching plan.

   c. telephone directory.

   d. information sheet.

   e. flowchart.

21. Suppose you want to teach a patient about the need to adopt a low-sugar diet because of diabetes, but the patient doesn't believe that diabetes is a serious health problem. If education is to be effective, then which of the following must the patient accept? Circle all that apply.

   a. Diabetes has to be managed.

   b. There is a correlation between high sugar intake and diabetes.

   c. Diabetes isn't as serious as other diseases.

   d. Diabetes management requires dietary changes.

   e. It is possible to consume large quantities of high-sugar foods, but only occasionally.

COG MATCHING   Grade: _____

Match the following key terms to their definitions.

Key Terms

22. _____ alternative treatment

23. _____ assessment

24. _____ coping mechanisms

25. _____ dissemination

26. _____ documentation

27. _____ evaluation

28. _____ implementation

29. _____ learning objectives

30. _____ noncompliance

31. _____ placebo effect

32. _____ planning

Definitions

a. involves using the information you have gathered to determine how you will approach the patient's learning needs

b. skill that requires the patient to physically perform a task

c. the process that indicates how well patients are adapting or applying new information to their lives

d. produced by illness or injury and may result in physiological and psychological effects

e. includes procedures or tasks that will be discussed or performed at various points in the program to help achieve the goal

f. the process of distributing information on community resources

g. includes recording of all teachings that occurred

h. the patient's inability or refusal to follow a prescribed order

i. involves gathering information about the patient's present health care needs and abilities

33. _____ psychomotor

34. _____ stress

j. psychological defenses employed to help deal with the painful and difficult problems life can bring

k. the power of believing that something will make you better when there is no chemical reaction that warrants such improvement

l. the expected outcomes for the teaching process

m. an option or substitute to the standard medical treatment such as acupuncture

SHORT ANSWER   Grade: _____

35. List three potential sources of patient education materials.

_____

_____

_____

36. List and explain three relaxation techniques that you and patients can learn to help with stress management.

_____

_____

_____

AFF WHAT WOULD YOU DO?   Grade: _____

37. You work in a pediatric practice. A mother brings her 6-month-old son in for a routine checkup. The child has a visible lump on the right side of his head, just above his ear. The mother states that the child fell off a twin bed when she was changing his diaper. After examining the child, the physician asks you to instruct the mother in safety and also have her watch the baby closely for the next few days for signs of concussion.

   A. What resources might be available to you?

_____

_____

   B. How might you evaluate the mother's barriers to communication and understanding?

_____

_____

C. What method of instruction would you use for this situation?

_____

_____

D. What would your teaching plan need to include?

_____

_____

E. What measures should be taken if the child's injuries were consistent with possible abuse?

_____

_____

F. Why is patient education important?

_____

_____

38. Write a sentence explaining why, as a medical assistant, you must set aside your own personal feelings and life experiences when educating patients.

_____

_____

_____

COG **IDENTIFICATION**   Grade: _____

List the five factors that can hinder patient education.

39. _____

40. _____

41. _____

42. _____

43. _____

COG **PSY** **ACTIVE LEARNING** Grade: _____

44. Juggling school with other commitments may occasionally cause negative stress in your life. Make a list of how you experience stress in your daily life. Then, choose one of the three relaxation techniques discussed in this chapter. Practice that technique and then write a paragraph describing the "pros" and "cons" of the chosen technique.

_____

_____

_____

45. Develop a teaching plan for a family member or friend. For example, if your mother has asthma, then do research on the Internet to find information and resources about asthma. Remember to include all of the elements of a teaching plan. Practice your teaching techniques by educating a family member or friend about a particular illness or disease.

_____

_____

_____

46. Choose a health concern that may require external support. For example, a patient fighting cancer may wish to join a support group or other organization for help. Search the Internet for local, state, and national agencies that provide information, support, and services to patients with your chosen need. Then, compile this information in an informative and creative brochure, pamphlet, or other learning tool.

_____

_____

_____

COG **PSY** **PATIENT EDUCATION** Grade: _____

47. A patient wants to use alternative medicine in addition to medicine prescribed by the physician. What should you do?

_____

_____

48. A patient in your care is suffering physiologic effects from negative stress brought on by chronic back pain. What types of coping strategies would you recommend to the patient and why?

_____

_____

_____

49. Julia is an 8-year-old patient who has been diagnosed with type 1 diabetes. The medical office has a preprinted teaching plan entitled "Living with Type 2 Diabetes." Should you use this plan or develop your own? Explain.

_____

_____

_____

TRUE OR FALSE?   Grade: _____

Determine whether the following statements are true or false. If false, explain why.

50. Patients benefit from the use of teaching aids that they can take home and use as reference material.

_____

51. If a patient asks you a question and you're not sure of the answer, then you should give your best guess.

_____

52. A patient must have his basic needs met before self-actualization may occur.

_____

53. Visualization is a relaxation technique that involves deep-breathing and physical exercise.

_____

AFF CASE STUDY FOR CRITICAL THINKING A

Grade: _____

A 5-year-old girl in your pediatric practice has just been diagnosed with juvenile diabetes. Your physician asks you to assist the patient's parents with resources available to them.

54. From the following list, circle the BEST resource.

   a. Materials from a pharmaceutical company

   b. Other patients who have this problem

   c. The official website of the American Diabetes Association

   d. Another pediatrician's office

   e. American Medical Technologists, Inc.

55. When developing a teaching plan, circle the most appropriate entry under Learning Objectives?

   a. Patient not involved in training due to age

   b. Patient's mother describes the body's use of insulin

   c. See documentation of patient education in chart

   d. Gave patient instructional video: "Your Child and Diabetes"

   e. Patient understands disease

AFF CASE STUDY FOR CRITICAL THINKING B

Grade: _____

Your physician instructs you to come up with a plan for Mr. Johns who has been diagnosed with hypercholesterolemia. He needs to change his eating habits and lifestyle drastically. You plan to help him form a plan for making these changes.

56. Patients should be encouraged to take an active approach to their health and health care education. To assist Mr. Johns effectively, which of the following must you do? Circle all that apply.

   a. Help Mr. Johns accept his illness.

   b. Expect Mr. Johns to follow your instructions without further explanation.

   c. Involve Mr. Johns in the process of gaining knowledge.

   d. Provide Mr. Johns with positive reinforcement.

   e. Give Mr. Johns the most in-depth professional textbooks you can find.

57. Your plan for Mr. Johns should include all of the following EXCEPT:

    a. A timeline for a gradually progressing walking program

    b. recipes for low-fat dishes

    c. pamphlets with information about his condition

    d. documentation of your instruction

    e. a list of his medications

58. Ms. Jasinski is an older adult patient who has recently lost several relatives and friends. She lives alone, feels disconnected from others and, as a result, her health has begun to deteriorate. Brian, a medical assistant, gives Ms. Jasinski a friendly hug when he sees her during patient visits. He talks to her and listens to her stories. He has also encouraged her to join a senior citizens' group. Circle which of Maslow's hierarchy of needs has Brian helped fulfill for Ms. Jasinski?

    a. physiological

    b. safety and security

    c. affection and belonging

    d. self-actualization

PSY **PROCEDURE 4-1**   **Document Patient Education**

Name: _____   Date: _____   Time: _____   Grade: _____

EQUIPMENT/SUPPLIES: Patient's chart, pen

STANDARDS: Given the needed equipment and a place to work, the student will perform this skill with _____% accuracy in a total of _____ minutes. *(Your instructor will tell you what the percentage and time limits will be before you begin.)*

KEY: 4 = Satisfactory   0 = Unsatisfactory   NA = This step is not counted

PROCEDURE STEPS	SELF	PARTNER	INSTRUCTOR
1. Record the date and time of teaching.	☐	☐	☐
2. Record the information taught.	☐	☐	☐
3. Record the manner in which the information was taught.	☐	☐	☐
4. Record your evaluation of your teaching.	☐	☐	☐
5. Record any additional teaching planned.	☐	☐	☐
6. **AFF** Explain what you would do if you forgot to document an action you took during the patient education process.	☐	☐	☐

_____
_____
_____
_____
_____

Note: The medical assistant may sign his or her name in the patient record using only the "CMA" credential if the office has a signature log denoting the entire credential as "CMA(AAMA)."

CALCULATION

Total Possible Points: _____

Total Points Earned: _____ Multiplied by 100 = _____ Divided by Total Possible Points = _____ %

PASS   **FAIL**   **COMMENTS:**

☐   ☐

Student's signature _____ Date _____

Partner's signature _____ Date _____

Instructor's signature _____ Date _____

PSY PROCEDURE 4-2 | **Develop and Maintain a Current List of Community Resources Related to Patients' Healthcare Needs**

Name: _____ Date: _____ Time: _____ Grade: _____

EQUIPMENT/SUPPLIES: Phone book, Internet, newspaper

STANDARDS: Given the needed equipment and a place to work, the student will perform this skill with _____% accuracy in a total of _____ minutes. *(Your instructor will tell you what the percentage and time limits will be before you begin.)*

KEY: 4 = Satisfactory   0 = Unsatisfactory   NA = This step is not counted

PROCEDURE STEPS	SELF	PARTNER	INSTRUCTOR
1. Assess the patient's needs for the following: **a.** Education **b.** Someone to talk to **c.** Financial information **d.** Support groups **e.** Home health needs	☐	☐	☐
2. Check the local telephone book for local and state resources.	☐	☐	☐
3. Check for Web sites for the city and/or county in which the patient lives.	☐	☐	☐
4. Be prepared with materials already on hand.	☐	☐	☐
5. Give the patient the contact information in writing.	☐	☐	☐
6. Document actions and the information given to the patient.	☐	☐	☐
7. Instruct the patient to contact the office if he has any difficulty.	☐	☐	☐
8. **AFF** Explain what suggestions or assistance you would offer to a patient who would benefit from online patient education resources but does not own a computer.	☐	☐	☐

CALCULATION

Total Possible Points: _____

Total Points Earned: _____ Multiplied by 100 = _____ Divided by Total Possible Points = _____ %

PASS   **FAIL**   **COMMENTS:**

☐   ☐

Student's signature _____ Date _____

Partner's signature _____ Date _____

Instructor's signature _____ Date _____

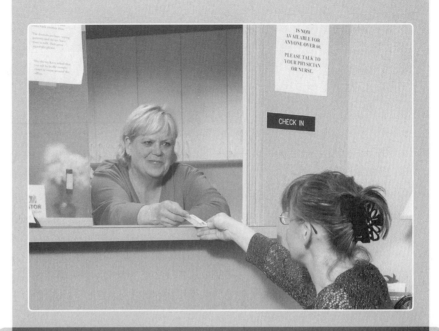

PART

II

The
Administrative
Medical
Assistant

TWO

Fundamentals of Administrative Medical Assisting

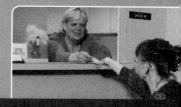

CHAPTER

5

The First Contact: Telephone and Reception

Learning Outcomes

Cognitive Domain

1. Spell and define the key terms
2. Explain the importance of displaying a professional image to all patients
3. List six duties of the medical office receptionist
4. List four sources from which messages can be retrieved
5. Discuss various steps that can be taken to promote good ergonomics
6. Describe the basic guidelines for waiting room environments
7. Describe the proper method for maintaining infection control standards in the waiting room
8. Discuss the five basic guidelines for telephone use
9. Describe the types of incoming telephone calls received by the medical office
10. Discuss how to identify and handle callers with medical emergencies
11. Describe how to triage incoming calls
12. List the information that should be given to an emergency medical service dispatcher
13. Describe the types of telephone services and special features
14. Discuss applications of electronic technology in effective communication

Psychomotor Domain

1. Handle incoming calls (Procedure 5-1)
   - Demonstrate telephone techniques

2. Call Emergency Medical Services (Procedure 5-2)
   - Demonstrate self awareness in responding to emergency situations
   - Recognize the effects of stress on all persons involved in emergency situations
3. Explain general office policies (Procedure 5-3)
   - Report relevant information to others succinctly and accurately
4. Verify eligibility for managed care services

Affective Domain

1. Demonstrate empathy in communicating with patients, family, and staff
2. Implement time management principles to maintain effective office function
3. Communicate in language the patient can understand regarding managed care and insurance plans
4. Demonstrate awareness of the consequences of not working within the legal scope of practice
5. Demonstrate sensitivity in communicating with both providers and patients
6. Demonstrate sensitivity to patient rights

ABHES Competencies

1. Use proper telephone technique
2. Receive, organize, prioritize, and transmit information expediently
3. Apply electronic technology

Name: _____   Date: _____   Grade: _____

COG MULTIPLE CHOICE

1. Which of the following creates a professional image?

   a. Arguing with a patient

   b. Clean, pressed clothing

   c. Brightly colored fingernails

   d. Referring to the physicians by his or her first name

   e. Expensive flowery perfume

2. How can you exercise diplomacy?

   a. Treat patients as they treat you.

   b. Treat patients as you would like to be treated.

   c. Ignore patients who complain about their illnesses.

   d. Answer patients' questions about other patients they see in the waiting room.

   e. Disclose confidential information if a patient or relative asks for it tactfully.

3. When preparing the charts for the day, the charts should be put in order by:

   a. age.

   b. last name.

   c. chart number.

   d. reason for visit.

   e. appointment time.

4. The receptionist should check phone messages:

   a. at night before leaving.

   b. in the morning when coming in.

   c. when on the phone and knowing a call has gone to voice mail.

   d. only after breaks, because each call coming in should be answered.

   e. when the office opens, after breaks, and periodically throughout the day.

5. Triaging calls is important because:

   a. it reduces the amount of time that callers wait.

   b. it places the calls in order of most urgent to least urgent.

   c. it lets the receptionist take care of the calls as quickly as possible.

   d. it puts the calls in time order so the receptionist knows who called first.

   e. it makes it easier for the receptionist to see which calls will be the easiest to handle.

6. There is a sign in the pediatrician's office that says "Do not throw dirty diapers in the garbage." Which of the following choices best explains the reason for the sign?

   a. Dirty diapers cannot be recycled.

   b. Dirty diapers are biohazardous waste.

   c. Dirty diapers could leave an offensive odor.

   d. Dirty diapers could make the garbage too heavy.

   e. Dirty diapers take up too much room in the garbage.

7. Chewing gum or eating while on the phone could interfere with a person's:

   a. diction.

   b. attitude.

   c. ergonomics.

   d. expression.

   e. pronunciation.

8. Which of the following activities should a receptionist do in the morning to prepare the office for patients?

   a. Vacuum the office.

   b. Stock office supplies.

   c. Disinfect examination rooms.

   d. Turn on printers and copiers.

   e. Clean the patient restrooms.

9. Which of the following statements about telephone courtesy is correct?

a. If two lines are ringing at once, answer one call and let the other go to voice mail.

b. If you are on the other line, it is acceptable to let the phone ring until you can answer it.

c. If a caller is upset, leaving him or her on hold will help improve the caller's attitude.

d. If you need to answer another line, ask if the caller would mind holding and wait for a response.

e. If someone is on hold for more than 90 seconds, he or she must leave a message and someone will call them back.

10. An ergonomic workstation is beneficial because it:

a. prevents injuries to employees.

b. educates patients about disease.

c. maintains patients' confidentiality.

d. creates a soothing, relaxed atmosphere.

e. prevents the spread of contagious diseases.

11. Which feature fosters a positive waiting room environment?

a. Abstract artwork on the walls

b. Only sofas for patients to sit in

c. Soap operas on the waiting room television

d. Prominent display of the office fax machine

e. Patient education materials in the reception area

12. When a patient calls the office and wants to be seen for chest pain, your first action should be

a. Ask if he or she also has shortness of breath, nausea, and/or profuse sweating.

b. Tell him or her to hang up and call 911.

c. Asks the patient's name in case he or she loses consciousness.

d. Tell the patient to make sure his front door is unlocked.

e. Give the patient an appointment for the next day.

13. A 5-year-old girl has just come into the office with her mother. She has the flu and is vomiting into a plastic bag. Which of the following should the receptionist do?

a. Get the patient into an examination room.

b. Call the hospital and request an ambulance.

c. Tell her to sit near the bathroom so she can vomit in the toilet.

d. Place a new plastic bag in your garbage can and ask the girl to use it.

e. Ask the patient to wait outside and you will get her when it is her turn.

14. An angry patient calls the office demanding to speak to the physician. The physician is not in the office. What should the receptionist do?

a. Page the physician immediately.

b. Try to calm the patient and take a message.

c. Give the caller the physician's cell phone number.

d. Tell the patient to calm down and call back in an hour.

e. Place the patient on hold until he or she has calmed down.

15. Which of the following statements about e-mail is true?

a. Patient e-mails should be deleted from the computer.

b. The receptionist does not generally have access to e-mail.

c. Actions taken in regard to e-mail do not need to be documented.

d. Patients should not e-mail the office under any circumstances.

e. E-mails should not be printed because the wrong person could view them.

16. The best technique for preventing the spread of disease is:

    a. washing your hands after any contact with patients.

    b. placing very sick patients immediately in an exam room.

    c. removing all reading materials or toys from the waiting room.

    d. keeping the window to the reception area closed at all times.

    e. preventing patients from changing channels on the TV in the waiting room.

17. One way to ensure patient privacy in the reception area is to:

    a. take all the patient's information at the front desk.

    b. ask the patient's permission before placing her name on the sign-in sheet.

    c. use computers in examination rooms only.

    d. make telephone calls regarding referrals at the front desk.

    e. close the privacy window when you are not speaking with a patient.

18. When receiving a call from a lab regarding a patient's test results, you should post the information:

    a. as an e-mail to the physician.

    b. in the receptionist's notebook.

    c. in the front of the patient's chart.

    d. as an e-mail to the patient's insurance company.

    e. in the front of the physician's appointment book.

19. In case of an emergency in the physician's office, who is usually responsible for calling emergency medical services (EMS)?

    a. Physician

    b. Dispatcher

    c. Receptionist

    d. Clinical staff

    e. Patient's relatives

20. When calling EMS for a patient who has an abnormal EKG, which of the following should be given first?

    a. The patient's name and age

    b. Your location

    c. The patient's insurance carrier

    d. The patient's problem

    e. Where they will be taking the patient

COG MATCHING

Grade: _____

Match the following key terms to their definitions.

Key Terms

21. _____ attitude

22. _____ closed captioning

23. _____ diction

24. _____ diplomacy

25. _____ emergency medical service (EMS)

26. _____ ergonomic

27. _____ receptionist

28. _____ teletypewriter (TTY)

29. _____ triage

Definitions

a. a person who performs administrative tasks and greets patients as they arrive at an office

b. the art of handling people with tact and genuine concern

c. a group of health care workers who care for sick and injured patients on the way to a hospital

d. printed words displayed on a television screen to help people with hearing disabilities or impairments

e. describing a workstation designed to prevent work-related injuries

f. the style of speaking and enunciating words

g. the sorting of patients into categories based on their level of sickness or injury

h. a state of mind or feeling regarding some matter

i. a special machine that allows communication on a telephone with a hearing-impaired person

COG SHORT ANSWER

Grade: _____

30. List the four sources of messages to be collected by the receptionist.

_____

_____

_____

_____

31. Why is it important to keep the waiting area neat and clean?

_____

_____

_____

_____

32. List the types of incoming calls received by the medical office.

_____

_____

_____

_____

33. Infection control is important to prevent the spread of disease among patients. List three things a medical assistant can do to help with infection control.

_____

_____

_____

_____

34. List four things you can do to maintain patient confidentiality within the reception area and waiting room.

_____

_____

_____

_____

35. You are training a new receptionist. She doesn't understand why triaging calls is important. How would you explain this to her?

_____

_____

_____

_____

PSY **IDENTIFICATION**   Grade: _____

36. The waiting room should be a comfortable and safe place for patients to wait. Review the list of guidelines below and determine which contribute to a comfortable and safe waiting room environment. Place a check in the "Yes" column for those guidelines that contribute to a comfortable and safe waiting room and place a check in the "No" column for those that do not.

Task	Yes	No
a. Sofas are preferable because they fit more people.		
b. Provide only chairs without arms.		
c. Bright, primary colors are more suitable and cheery.		
d. The room should be well ventilated and kept at a comfortable temperature.		
e. Soothing background music is acceptable.		
f. Reading material, like current magazines, should be provided.		
g. Patients should be allowed to control the television.		
h. In an office for adults, anything can be watched on the television.		
i. Closed captioning should be offered to patients with hearing impairments who want to watch television.		

37. A patient comes into the office with a severe bloody nose. He leaves bloody tissues in the waiting room and got blood on a magazine and a chair. Your supervisor says to you, "Come on! Get some gloves. We've got to clean this right away." Why do you need gloves? Why is it important that the waiting room be cleaned immediately?

_____

_____

_____

_____

COG **TRUE OR FALSE?**   Grade: _____

As a receptionist, you'll be answering incoming calls. Review the statements below and place a check in the "True" column for those that are true and place a check in the "False" column for those that are false.

Incoming Calls	True	False
38. Always ask new patients for their phone number in case you need to call them back.		
39. Always give patients an exact quote for services if asked.		
40. Patient information cannot be given to anyone without the patient's consent.		
41. All laboratory results phoned into the office must be immediately brought to the physician's attention.		
42. When a nursing home calls with a satisfactory report about a patient, you should take the information down, record it in the patient's chart, and place it on the physician's desk for review.		
43. Never discuss unsatisfactory test results with a patient unless the doctor directs you to do so.		
44. Medical assistants are not allowed to take care of prescription refill requests.		

PSY **TRIAGE**   Grade: _____

45. Triage the following calls by writing the letters in the proper order. _____

  a. Line 1: A school nurse calls with a question about a medical form.

  b. Line 2: A mother calls about her child who is having an asthma attack.

  c. Line 3: A father calls with a question about his daughter's medication.

  d. Line 4: A patient calls complaining about a sore throat.

COG **SHORT ANSWER**   Grade: _____

46. A woman calls the office frantic because she thinks she is having a heart attack. What information should you try to get first from the caller?

_____

_____

_____

_____

47. A patient in your office is having trouble breathing. You have been asked to call EMS. What five pieces of information will you need before you make the call?

_____

_____

_____

_____

48. Dr. Porter is in a meeting, but he has instructed you to communicate with him via cell phone when you get the test results back for a certain patient. However, he does not like to have his cell phone ring while he is in meetings. How will you communicate with him?

_____

_____

_____

_____

49. It is an exceptionally hot day in the spring. Because the air conditioner is not on yet, you take a chair from the waiting room and prop the door open with it. You also move the boxes that were delivered earlier away from the window so the air comes in. How is this a violation of the Americans with Disabilities Act?

_____

_____

_____

_____

50. You receive a call from a patient who complains of being short of breath. What questions will you ask to determine whether this is an emergency?

_____

_____

_____

_____

AFF PSY **ACTIVE LEARNING**   Grade: _____

51. Working with two classmates, role-play a medical emergency in the physician's office waiting room. Have one person play the role of the patient, the second person play the role of the receptionist, and the third person play the role of the EMS call operator. The patient should describe his or her condition, and the receptionist is responsible for conveying these details to EMS. Switch roles so that everyone gets a chance to play each role.

AFF **WHAT WOULD YOU DO?**   Grade: _____

52. Your office shows videos about healthy living, exercise, and nutrition throughout the day. It seems that most of the adults watch and enjoy the programming. One crowded afternoon, a patient comes up to the desk to complain that the programming is distracting and he would prefer having the television turned off. However, there are people in the room watching the television. What would you say to the upset patient?

_____

_____

_____

_____

53. Mrs. Gonzalez calls to schedule her annual checkup. She is put on hold, and when the receptionist comes back to her call, she is upset that she was placed on hold. When she comes in for her appointment, she says that the receptionist should deal with every call individually and that no one should be placed on hold. How would you explain the phone call triage system to her?

_____

_____

_____

_____

AFF **CASE STUDY FOR CRITICAL THINKING**   Grade: _____

You are working for a pediatrician. A mother arrives carrying an 18-month-old child with symptoms of a respiratory illness. You ask for her insurance card and she yells, "take care of my child first." You are willing to rearrange the usual order of things, but when you direct her to sit in the sick-child area, as per office protocol, the mother refuses, stating, "I don't want my child to get sicker." Circle the appropriate response from the lists below each question.

54. What might you say to make the mother give you the insurance information?

    a. I am required to update your chart, including your insurance information, at each visit *before* you see the physician.

    b. The physician will not see your child until I see your card.

    c. You are being very difficult. Can we start over?

    d. I'll hold the child while you get your card out.

55. What is your best action regarding the waiting area?

    a. Tell the physician.

    b. Calmly explain the policy and why you have it.

    c. Even though you will be putting her ahead of others, put the child in an open exam room.

    d. Ask the mother to leave.

    e. Tell her to take the child to the emergency room.

56. What is the most important thing you can do to make difficult situations like this better?

    a. Place signs in the waiting area about behavior.

    b. Make sure your work area is clean and neat.

    c. Make sure you always have someone else with you in the reception area.

    d. Remain calm and act professionally.

    e. Stand your ground with the angry person.

PSY PROCEDURE 5-1 | Handling Incoming Calls

Name: _____ Date: _____ Time: _____ Grade: _____

EQUIPMENT/SUPPLIES: Telephone, telephone message pad, writing utensil (pen or pencil), headset (if applicable)

STANDARDS: Given the needed equipment and a place to work, the student will perform this skill with _____ % accuracy in a total of _____ minutes. *(Your instructor will tell you what the percentage and time limits will be before you begin.)*

KEY: 4 = Satisfactory   0 = Unsatisfactory   NA = this step is not counted

PROCEDURE STEPS	SELF	PARTNER	INSTRUCTOR
1. Gather the needed equipment.	☐	☐	☐
2. Answer the phone within two rings.	☐	☐	☐
3. Greet caller with proper identification (your name and the name of the office).	☐	☐	☐
4. Identify the nature or reason for the call in a timely manner.	☐	☐	☐
5. Triage the call appropriately.	☐	☐	☐
6. Communicate in a professional manner and with unhurried speech.	☐	☐	☐
7. Clarify information as needed.	☐	☐	☐
8. Record the message on a message pad. Include the name of caller, date, time, telephone number where the caller can be reached, description of the caller's concerns, and person to whom the message is routed.	☐	☐	☐
9. Give the caller an approximate time for a return call.	☐	☐	☐
10. Ask the caller whether he or she has any additional questions or needs any other help.	☐	☐	☐
11. Allow the caller to disconnect first.	☐	☐	☐
12. Put the message in an assigned place.	☐	☐	☐
13. Complete the task within 10 minutes.	☐	☐	☐
14. **AFF** Explain how you would respond to a patient who is obviously angry.	☐	☐	☐

_____

_____

_____

_____

CALCULATION

Total Possible Points: _____

Total Points Earned: _____ Multiplied by 100 = _____ Divided by Total Possible Points = _____ %

PASS   **FAIL**   **COMMENTS:**

☐   ☐

Student's signature _____ Date _____

Partner's signature _____ Date _____

Instructor's signature _____ Date _____

PSY PROCEDURE 5-2 | Calling Emergency Medical Services

Name: _____ Date: _____ Time: _____ Grade: _____

EQUIPMENT/SUPPLIES: Telephone, patient information, writing utensil (pen, pencil)

STANDARDS: Given the needed equipment and a place to work, the student will perform this skill with _____ % accuracy in a total of _____ minutes. *(Your instructor will tell you what the percentage and time limits will be before you begin.)*

KEY: 4 = Satisfactory   0 = Unsatisfactory   NA = this step is not counted

PROCEDURE STEPS	SELF	PARTNER	INSTRUCTOR
1. Obtain the following the information before dialing: patient's name, age, sex, nature of medical condition, type of service the physician is requesting, any special instructions or requests the physician may have, your location, and any special information for access.	☐	☐	☐
2. Dial 911 or other EMS number.	☐	☐	☐
3. Calmly provide the dispatcher with the above information.	☐	☐	☐
4. Answer the dispatcher's questions calmly and professionally.	☐	☐	☐
5. Follow the dispatcher's instructions, if applicable.	☐	☐	☐
6. End the call as per dispatcher instructions.	☐	☐	☐
7. Complete the task within 10 minutes.	☐	☐	☐
8. **AFF** Explain how you would respond to a family member who is getting in the way of performing this task.	☐	☐	☐

_____

_____

_____

_____

CALCULATION

Total Possible Points: _____

Total Points Earned: _____ Multiplied by 100 = _____ Divided by Total Possible Points = _____ %

PASS   **FAIL**   **COMMENTS:**

☐   ☐

Student's signature _____ Date _____

Partner's signature _____ Date _____

Instructor's signature _____ Date _____

PSY PROCEDURE 5-3	Explain General Office Policies

Name: _____ Date: _____ Time: _____ Grade: _____

EQUIPMENT/SUPPLIES: Patient's chart, office brochure

STANDARDS: Given the needed equipment and a place to work, the student will perform this skill with _____%
accuracy in a total of _____ minutes. *(Your instructor will tell you what the percentage and time limits will be
before you begin.)*

KEY: 4 = Satisfactory   0 = Unsatisfactory   NA = this step is not counted

PROCEDURE STEPS	SELF	PARTNER	INSTRUCTOR
1. Assess the patient's level of understanding.	☐	☐	☐
2. Review important areas and highlight these in the office brochure.	☐	☐	☐
3. Ask the patient if he or she understands or has any questions.	☐	☐	☐
4. Give the patient the brochure to take home.	☐	☐	☐
5. Put in place a procedure for updating information and letting patients know of changes.	☐	☐	☐
6. **AFF** Explain how you would instruct a hearing-impaired patient about office procedures.	☐	☐	☐

CALCULATION

Total Possible Points: _____

Total Points Earned: _____ Multiplied by 100 = _____ Divided by Total Possible Points = _____ %

PASS   **FAIL**   **COMMENTS:**

☐   ☐

Student's signature _____ Date _____

Partner's signature _____ Date _____

Instructor's signature _____ Date _____

CHAPTER

6

Managing Appointments

Learning
Outcomes

Cognitive Domain

1. Spell and define the key terms
2. Describe the pros and cons of various types of appointment management systems for scheduling patient office visits, including manual and computerized scheduling
3. Describe scheduling guidelines
4. Explain guidelines for scheduling appointments for new patients, return visits, inpatient admissions, and outpatient procedures
5. Recognize office policies and protocols for handling appointments
6. Identify critical information required for scheduling patient admissions and/or procedures
7. Discuss referral process for patients in a managed care program
8. List three ways to remind patients about appointments
9. Describe how to triage patient emergencies, acutely ill patients, and walk-in patients
10. Describe how to handle late patients
11. Explain what to do if the physician is delayed
12. Describe how to handle patients who miss their appointments
13. Describe how to handle appointment cancellations made by the office or by the patient

Psychomotor Domain

1. Manage appointment schedule, using established priorities
   a. Schedule an appointment for a new patient (Procedure 6-1)
   b. Schedule an appointment for a return visit (Procedure 6-2)
2. Schedule patient admissions and/or procedures
   a. Schedule an appointment for a referral to an outpatient facility (Procedure 6-3)
   b. Arrange for admission to an inpatient facility (Procedure 6-4)
      • Verify eligibility for managed care services
      • Obtain precertification, including documentation
      • Apply third-party managed care policies and procedures
      • Apply third-party guidelines
3. Use office hardware and software to maintain office systems

Affective Domain

1. Implement time management principles to maintain effective office functions
2. Demonstrate empathy in communicating with patients, family, and staff
3. Demonstrate sensitivity in communicating with both providers and patients

4. Communicate in language the patient can understand regarding managed care and insurance plans
5. Demonstrate recognition of the patient's level of understanding in communications

ABHES Competencies

1. Schedule and manage appointments
2. Schedule inpatient and outpatient admissions
3. Be impartial and show empathy when dealing with patients

4. Apply third-party guidelines
5. Obtain managed care referrals and precertification
6. Apply computer application skills using a variety of different electronic programs including both practice management software and EMR software
7. Communicate on the recipient's level of comprehension
8. Serve as liaison between physician and others

Name: _____   Date: _____   Grade: _____

COG MULTIPLE CHOICE

1. If your medical office uses a manual system of scheduled appointments for patient office visits, you will need a(n):

   a. toolbar.

   b. appointment book.

   c. computer.

   d. buffer time.

   e. fixed schedule.

2. How much time should be blocked off each morning and afternoon to accommodate emergencies, late arrivals, and other delays?

   a. 5 to 10 minutes

   b. 10 to 20 minutes

   c. 15 to 30 minutes

   d. 45 minutes to 1 hour

   e. 1 to 2 hours

3. When scheduling an appointment, why should you ask the patient the reason he or she needs to see the doctor?

   a. To know the level of empathy to give the patient.

   b. To anticipate the time needed for the appointment.

   c. To confront the patient about his or her personal choices.

   d. To manipulate the patient's needs.

   e. To determine who should see the patient.

4. Which of the following is an advantage to clustering?

   a. Efficient use of employee's time

   b. Increased patient time for the physician

   c. Reduced staff costs for the office

   d. Shorter patient appointments

   e. Greater need for specialists in the office

5. In fixed scheduling, the length of time reserved for each appointment is determined by the:

   a. physician's personal schedule.

   b. number of hours open on a given day.

   c. reason for the patient's visit.

   d. type of insurance provider.

   e. patient's age.

6. Double booking works well when patients are being sent for diagnostic testing because:

   a. it gives each patient enough time to prepare for testing.

   b. it leaves time to see both patients without keeping either one waiting unnecessarily.

   c. the physician enjoys seeing two patients at one time.

   d. it challenges the medical practice's resources.

   e. it gives the physician more "downtime."

7. Which of the following is a disadvantage to open hours?

   a. Patients with emergencies cannot be seen quickly.

   b. Scheduling patients is a challenge.

   c. Effective time management is almost impossible.

   d. Walk-ins are encouraged.

   e. Patient charts aren't properly updated.

8. You should leave some time slots open during the schedule each day to:

   a. allow patients to make their own appointments online.

   b. make the schedule more well rounded.

   c. leave some time for personal responsibilities.

   d. provide the staff some flex time.

   e. make room for emergencies and delays.

9. Most return appointments are made:

   a. before the patient leaves the office.

   b. before the patient's appointment.

   c. after the patient leaves the office.

   d. during the patient's next visit.

   e. when the patient receives a mailed reminder.

10. Reminder cards should be mailed:

   a. the first day of every month.

   b. a week before the date of the appointment.

   c. the beginning of the year.

   d. with all billing statements.

   e. only when the patient requests one.

11. A condition that is abrupt in onset is described as:

   a. chronic.

   b. commonplace.

   c. lethal.

   d. acute.

   e. incurable.

12. Who is authorized to make the decision whether to see a walk-in patient or not?

   a. Medical assistant

   b. Emergency medical technician

   c. Provider

   d. Reception

   e. Nurse

13. If you reschedule an appointment, you should note the reason for the cancellation or rescheduling in:

   a. the patient's chart.

   b. the patient's immunization record.

   c. the patient's insurance card.

   d. the patient's billing form.

   e. the office's appointment book.

14. If you have to cancel on the day of an appointment because of a physician's illness:

   a. send the patient an apology letter.

   b. give the patient a detailed excuse.

   c. e-mail the patient a reminder.

   d. call the patient and explain.

   e. offer the patient a discount at his or her next appointment.

15. If you find that your schedule is chaotic nearly every day, then you should:

   a. evaluate the schedule over time.

   b. keep that information private.

   c. tell your supervisor that you would like a new job.

   d. stop the old schedule and make a new one.

   e. let the patients know that the schedule isn't working.

16. An instruction to transfer a patient's care to a specialist is a:

   a. precertification.

   b. consultation.

   c. transfer.

   d. referral.

   e. payback.

17. Established patients are:

   a. patients who are new to the practice.

   b. patients who have been to the practice before.

   c. patients who are over age 65 years.

   d. patients who are chronically ill.

   e. patients with insurance.

18. A flexible scheduling method that schedules patients for the first 30 minutes of an hour and leaves the second half of each hour open is called:

   a. clustering.

   b. wave scheduling system.

   c. streaming.

   d. fixed-schedule system.

   e. double booking.

19. A chronic problem is one that is:

　　a. not very serious.

　　b. occurring for a short period of time.

　　c. longstanding.

　　d. easily cured.

　　e. difficult to diagnose.

20. Which of the following is true of a constellation of symptoms?

　　a. It can only be assessed by a physician.

　　b. It is only an emergency if a patient is having a heart attack.

　　c. It means a patient is suffering from appendicitis.

　　d. It is a group of clinical signs indicating a particular disease.

　　e. It probably requires a call to emergency medical services.

21. When a patient calls with an emergency, your first responsibility is to:

　　a. determine if the patient has an appointment.

　　b. decide whether the problem can be treated in the office.

　　c. verify that the physician can see the patient.

　　d. identify the patient's constellation of symptoms.

22. What should you do if the physician decides not to see a walk-in patient?

　　a. Ask the patient to schedule an appointment to return later.

　　b. Explain that the physician is too busy.

　　c. Tell the patient to try a different medical office.

　　d. Tell the patient to go to the hospital.

23. When might you write a letter to a patient who has an appointment that you must cancel?

　　a. when you can't reach the patient by phone

　　b. when the physician leaves the office abruptly

　　c. when you do not have the patient's demographic information

　　d. when you want to use written communication

COG MATCHING　　　　　　　　　　　　　　　　　Grade: _____

Match the following key terms to their definitions.

Key Terms

24. _____ acute

25. _____ buffer

26. _____ chronic

27. _____ clustering

28. _____ constellation of symptoms

29. _____ consultation

30. _____ double booking

31. _____ matrix

Definitions

a. a group of clinical signs indicating a particular disease process

b. the practice of booking two patients for the same period with the same physician

c. term used in the medical field to indicate that something should be done immediately

d. a system for blocking off unavailable patient appointment times

e. a flexible scheduling method that allows time for procedures of varying lengths and the addition of unscheduled patients, as needed

f. referring to a longstanding medical problem

g. grouping patients with similar problems or needs

32. _____ precertification

33. _____ providers

34. _____ referral

35. _____ STAT

36. _____ streaming

37. _____ wave scheduling system

h. a method of allotting time for appointments based on the needs of the individual patient that helps minimize gaps in time and backups

i. extra time booked on the schedule to accommodate emergencies, walk-ins, and other demands on the provider's daily time schedule that are not considered direct patient care

j. health care workers who deliver medical care

k. referring to a medical problem with abrupt onset

l. request for assistance from one physician to another

m. approved documentation prior to referrals to specialists and other facilities

n. instructions to transfer a patient's care to a specialist

COG SHORT ANSWER

Grade: _____

38. List four advantages to clustering patients.

_____

_____

_____

_____

39. Name the three factors that can affect scheduling.

_____

_____

_____

_____

40. List the three ways to remind patients about appointments.

_____

_____

_____

_____

41. When calling another physician's office for an appointment for your patient, you'll need to provide certain information. List the seven pieces of information that you should provide to another physician's office.

_____

_____

_____

_____

42. List three items usually included in preadmission testing for surgery.

_____

_____

_____

_____

COG **TRUE OR FALSE?**   Grade: _____

Determine whether the following statements are true or false. If false, explain why.

43. Fixed scheduling is the most commonly used method.

_____

44. A medical office that operates with open hours for patient visits is open 24 hours a day, 7 days a week.

_____

45. Most appointments for new patients are made in person.

_____

46. Patients with medical emergencies need to be seen immediately.

_____

COG PSY ACTIVE LEARNING

Grade: _____

47. The appointment book below is divided into half-hour increments. The spaces below each time slot are empty. Fill in the appointment book with the following information: Dr. Brown has hospital rounds from 8:00 a.m. to 9:00 a.m. He has the following appointments: Cindy Wallis at 9:30 a.m.; Bill Waters at 10:00 a.m.; Rodney Kingston at 10:30 a.m.

8:00	8:30	9:00	9:30	10:00	10:30

Draw a line from the service to the appropriate time allotment.

Service	Estimated Time
48. blood pressure check	**a.** 5 minutes
49. complete physical exam	**b.** 10 minutes
50. dressing change	**c.** 15 minutes
51. recheck	**d.** 30 minutes
52. school physical	**e.** 1 hour

COG IDENTIFICATION

Grade: _____

Identify each type of scheduling system in the chart below.

Description	Type of Scheduling System
53. Several patients are scheduled for the first 30 minutes of each hour.	
54. Appointments are given based on the needs of individual patients.	
55. Each hour is divided into increments of 15, 30, 45, or 60 minutes for appointments depending on the reason for the visit.	
56. Patients are grouped according to needs or problems.	
57. Two patients are scheduled for the same period with the same physician.	

COG **PSY** **CORRECT OR INCORRECT?**   Grade: _____

Below are the steps for making a return appointment. Some of the steps are false or incomplete. Review each step and then decide if it is correct or incorrect. If incorrect, rewrite the statement to make it true and complete.

58. Carefully check your appointment book or screen before offering an appointment time. If a specific examination, test, or x-ray is to be performed on the return visit, avoid scheduling two patients for the same examination at the same time.

_____

59. Ask the patient when he or she would like to return.

_____

60. Write the patient's name and telephone number in the appointment book or enter the information in computer.

_____

61. Transfer the information to an appointment card that you will mail out to the patient at a later date.

_____

62. Double-check your book or screen to be sure there are no errors.

_____

63. End your conversation with a pleasant word and a smile.

_____

AFF **WHAT WOULD YOU DO?**   Grade: _____

64. An older adult patient walks into the medical office. His constellation of symptoms includes chest discomfort, shortness of breath, and nausea. He doesn't have an appointment. Explain what you would do.

_____

_____

_____

_____

65. Sometimes, a patient may neglect to keep an appointment. When this happens, you should call the patient. What should you do if you are unable to reach the patient by phone?

_____

_____

_____

_____

66. Maria has just called into the office to cancel her appointment for today. Explain what you should do.

_____

_____

_____

_____

67. If diagnostic testing requires preparation from the patient, what should you do?

_____

_____

_____

_____

AFF **PATIENT EDUCATION**   Grade: _____

68. Juan is consistently late for appointments. You've spoken with him several times. What should you do next? Explain what you will you say to him and the information you will provide him with.

_____

_____

_____

_____

AFF **CASE STUDY FOR CRITICAL THINKING A**   Grade: _____

You are the RMA at the front desk of a busy family practice. The success of the day depends on how smoothly the schedule runs. It is your responsibility to check patients in as they arrive. Your office uses a sign-in sheet. Mr. Simpson is always late for his appointments and today is no exception.

69. Regarding the sign-in sheet, what other methods could you use that would limit the potential for invasion of patient privacy?

   a. Have patients give their name to the receptionist as they arrive.

   b. Periodically walk through the waiting area to see who is there.

   c. Post a sign asking patients to whisper when they speak.

   d. Use a sign-in clipboard that has a sliding shield to prevent seeing other names.

70. You notice that patients typically wait 30 to 45 minutes past their scheduled appointment times because the physician is chronically behind schedule. How would you handle the situation? Circle the best answer.

   a. Tell the office manager to talk to him or you will find other employment.

   b. Ask the office manager to put the issue of running behind on the next office meeting agenda.

   c. Ask to speak with him or her in private and explain how his running behind affects the entire office.

   d. Tease him or her about running behind in front of the patients and employees.

71. Circle the best strategy to handle Mr. Simpson's chronic tardiness.

   a. Schedule him for the last appointment of the day.

   b. Dismiss him from the physician's care.

   c. Call his family and ask if they can get him there on time.

   d. Tell him that he is messing up your whole day and he MUST stop being late.

   e. Do not worry about it. No matter what you do, he will still be late.

PSY **PROCEDURE 6-1**   **Scheduling an Appointment for a New Patient**

Name: _____ Date: _____ Time: _____ Grade: _____

EQUIPMENT/ITEMS NEEDED: Patient's demographic information, patient's chief complaint, appointment book or computer with appointment software, information found in Activity #1

STANDARDS: Given the needed equipment and a place to work the student will perform this skill with _____ % accuracy in a total of _____ minutes. *(Your instructor will tell you what the percentage and time limits will be before you begin.)*

KEY: 4 = Satisfactory   0 = Unsatisfactory   NA = This step is not counted

PROCEDURE STEPS	SELF	PARTNER	INSTRUCTOR
1. Obtain as much information as possible from the patient, such as: • Full name and correct spelling • Mailing address (not all offices require this) • Day and evening telephone numbers • Reason for the visit • Name of the referring person	☐	☐	☐
2. Determine the patient's chief complaint or the reason for seeing the physician.	☐	☐	☐
3. Explain the payment policy of the practice. Instruct patients to bring all pertinent insurance information.	☐	☐	☐
4. Give concise directions if needed.	☐	☐	☐
5. Ask the patient if it is permissible to call at home or at work.	☐	☐	☐
6. Confirm the time and date of the appointment.	☐	☐	☐
7. Check your appointment book to be sure that you have placed the appointment on the correct day in the right time slot.	☐	☐	☐
8. If the patient was referred by another physician, call that physician's office before the appointment for copies of laboratory work, radiology, pathology reports, and so on. Give this information to the physician prior to the patient's appointment.	☐	☐	☐
9. **AFF** Explain how you would respond in a situation in which a patient does NOT give permission to phone him or her at work.	☐	☐	☐

CALCULATION

Total Possible Points: _____

Total Points Earned: _____ Multiplied by 100 = _____ Divided by Total Possible Points = _____ %

PASS   **FAIL**   **COMMENTS:**

☐   ☐

Student's signature _____ Date _____

Partner's signature _____ Date _____

Instructor's signature _____ Date _____

PSY PROCEDURE 6-2 | **Scheduling an Appointment for an Established Patient**

Name: _____ Date: _____ Time: _____ Grade: _____

EQUIPMENT: Appointment book or computer with appointment software, appointment card, information found in Activity #1

STANDARDS: Given the needed equipment and a place to work the student will perform this skill with _____% accuracy in a total of _____ minutes. *(Your instructor will tell you what the percentage and time limits will be before you begin.)*

KEY: 4 = Satisfactory 0 = Unsatisfactory NA = This step is not counted

PROCEDURE STEPS	SELF	PARTNER	INSTRUCTOR
1. Determine what will be done at the return visit. Check your appointment book or computer system before offering an appointment.	☐	☐	☐
2. Offer the patient a specific time and date. Avoid asking the patient when he or she would like to return, as this can cause indecision.	☐	☐	☐
3. Write the patient's name and telephone number in the appointment book or enter it in the computer.	☐	☐	☐
4. Transfer the pertinent information to an appointment card and give it to the patient. Repeat aloud the appointment day, date, and time to the patient as you hand over the card.	☐	☐	☐
5. Double-check your book or computer to be sure you have not made an error.	☐	☐	☐
6. End your conversation with a pleasant word and a smile.	☐	☐	☐
7. **AFF** Explain how you would respond to a patient who insists on coming for a return appointment at a time when their doctor is in surgery.	☐	☐	☐

CALCULATION

Total Possible Points: _____

Total Points Earned: _____ Multiplied by 100 = _____ Divided by Total Possible Points = _____ %

PASS   **FAIL**   **COMMENTS:**

☐   ☐

Student's signature _____ Date _____

Partner's signature _____ Date _____

Instructor's signature _____ Date _____

Name: _____ Date: _____ Time: _____ Grade: _____

EQUIPMENT: Patient's chart with demographic information; physician's order for services needed by the patient and reason for the services; patient's insurance card with referral information, referral form, and directions to office, information found in Activity #3

STANDARDS: Given the needed equipment and a place to work, the student will perform this skill with _____% accuracy in a total of _____ minutes. *(Your instructor will tell you what the percentage and time limits will be before you begin.)*

KEY: 4 = Satisfactory 0 = Unsatisfactory NA = This step is not counted

PROCEDURE STEPS	SELF	PARTNER	INSTRUCTOR
1. Make certain that the requirements of any third-party payers are met.	☐	☐	☐
2. Refer to the preferred provider list for the patient's insurance company. Allow the patient to choose a provider from the list.	☐	☐	☐
3. Have the following information available when you make the call: • Physician's name and telephone number • Patient's name, address, and telephone number • Reason for the call • Degree of urgency • Whether the patient is being sent for consultation or referral	☐	☐	☐
4. Record in the patient's chart the time and date of the call and the name of the person who received your call.	☐	☐	☐
5. Tell the person you are calling that you wish to be notified if your patient does not keep the appointment. If this occurs, be sure to tell your physician and enter this information in the patient's record.	☐	☐	☐
6. Write down the name, address, and telephone number of the doctor you are referring your patient to and include the date and time of the appointment. Give or mail this information to your patient. Be certain that the information is complete, accurate, and easy to read.	☐	☐	☐
7. If the patient is to call the referring physician to make the appointment, ask the patient to call you with the appointment date, then document this in the chart.	☐	☐	☐
8. **AFF** Explain how you would handle the following situation: There are two physicians listed for a certain specialty in a patient's managed care's preferred provider list. The patient asks you who she should choose.	☐	☐	☐

CALCULATION

Total Possible Points: _____

Total Points Earned: _____ Multiplied by 100 = _____ Divided by Total Possible Points = _____ %

PASS   **FAIL**   **COMMENTS:**

☐   ☐

Student's signature _____ Date _____

Partner's signature _____ Date _____

Instructor's signature _____ Date _____

PSY **PROCEDURE 6-4** | **Arranging for Admission to an Inpatient Facility**

Name: _____ Date: _____ Time: _____ Grade: _____

EQUIPMENT: Physician's order with diagnosis, patient's chart with demographic information, contact information for inpatient facility, information found in Activity #2

STANDARDS: Given the needed equipment and a place to work, the student will perform this skill with _____ % accuracy in a total of _____ minutes. *(Your instructor will tell you what the percentage and time limits will be before you begin.)*

KEY: 4 = Satisfactory   0 = Unsatisfactory   NA = This step is not counted

PROCEDURE STEPS	SELF	PARTNER	INSTRUCTOR
1. Determine the place patient and/or physician wants the admission arranged.	☐	☐	☐
2. Gather information for the other facility, including demographic and insurance information.	☐	☐	☐
3. Determine any precertification requirements. If needed, locate contact information on the back of the insurance card and call the insurance carrier to obtain a precertification number.	☐	☐	☐
4. Obtain from the physician the diagnosis and exact needs of the patient for an admission.	☐	☐	☐
5. Call the admissions department of the inpatient facility and give information from step 2.	☐	☐	☐
6. Obtain instructions for the patient and call or give the patient instructions and information.	☐	☐	☐
7. Provide the patient with the physician's orders for their hospital stay, including diet, medications, bed rest, etc.	☐	☐	☐
8. Document time, place, etc. in patient's chart, including any precertification requirements completed.	☐	☐	☐
9. **AFF** Explain how you would respond to a patient who is visibly shaken about finding out that he is being admitted to the hospital.	☐	☐	☐

CALCULATION

Total Possible Points: _____

Total Points Earned: _____ Multiplied by 100 = _____ Divided by Total Possible Points = _____ %

PASS   **FAIL**   **COMMENTS:**

☐   ☐

Student's signature _____ Date _____

Partner's signature _____ Date _____

Instructor's signature _____ Date _____

Activity #1: Scheduling New and Returning Patients

Place the patients on the appointment book page provided. In order to make this activity more realistic, imagine that the patients are calling the office in the order they are listed. You will need to determine the time needed for the visit and the urgency of the patient's problem in assigning slots. Refer to Box 6-1 in the textbook for suggested time allotment.

Set up the page and establish the matrix: Providers and availability:

Dr. Jones sees patients from 2:00 p.m. to 5:00 p.m. In surgery until 12:00.
Dr. Smith sees patients from 8:00 a.m. to 3:00 p.m. No lunch.
Dr. Stowe sees patients from 8:00 a.m. to 5:00 p.m. with lunch from 12:00-1:30 p.m.

Jessica Marshall, CMA (AAMA), can give injections and do blood pressure checks. Lunch 1:00-2:00 p.m. Use the lab column for patients who can see her.

Patient Name	Reason	Telephone #
1. Jeremy Cole	Stepped on rusty nail	570-7890
2. Cheryl Jennings (New)	Needs college physical	765-9087
3. Patty Cook	Sore throat	799-7225
4. Susan Stills	Woke up feeling dizzy	836-8765
5. Pamela Jones (New)	Wants to talk about weight reduction	765-0123
6. Steve Elliott	Hand laceration at work. (supv. called)	799-4391
7. Amy Quarrels	Vomiting and diarrhea × 3 days	571-5923
8. Layla Harris	Nosebleed that won't stop	799-0127
9. Sharon Morris	Needs refill on pain meds	836-2100
10. Jared Davis	Blood pressure check	792-8333
11. Ginger Parks	Knee injury last week, still swelling	791-4752
12. Landon Smythe	Coughing up blood	414-6787
13. Raymond Gray	Confused and foggy, per son	922-8641
14. Seth Etchison	Skin rash	266-0999
15. Raji Omar	Allergy injection	607-9125
16. Marilyn Easley	Shortness of breath and nausea	903-8957
17. Stephanie Lewis	Freq. urination and burning	792-1480
18. Shannon Mitchell	Pregnancy test	799-0731
19. Shantina Branch (New)	Kindergarten physical	792-4500
20. Lee Davis	Recheck on strep throat	799-4800

What might you do differently with the new patients?

_____

_____

_____

THURSDAY, APRIL 11

HOUR		Dr. Jones	Dr. Smith	Dr. Stowe	Lab
8	00				
8	15				
8	30				
8	45				
9	00				
9	15				
9	30				
9	45				
10	00				
10	15				
10	30				
10	45				
11	00				
11	15				
11	30				
11	45				
12	00				
12	15				
12	30				
12	45				
1	00				
1	15				
1	30				
1	45				
2	00				
2	15				
2	30				
2	45				
3	00				
3	15				
3	30				
3	45				
4	00				
4	15				
4	30				
4	45				
5	00				
5	15				
5	30				
5	45				
6	00				
6	15				
6	30				
6	45				
7	00				
NOTES					

Activity #2: Scheduling Inpatient Admission

You work for Dr. James Gibbs, whose office is at 102 South Hawthorne Road, Winston-Salem, NC 27103. The office phone number is 336-760-4216.

Stella Walker is a 42-year-old female patient with diabetes. She has Blue Cross Blue Shield of NC. Her date of birth is 5/6/64. Her subscriber ID# is 260-21-5612. Her group # is 26178. She is the policyholder.

Dr. Gibbs instructs you to arrange admission to Forsyth Medical Center for Stella Walker for tomorrow. Her admitting diagnosis is uncontrolled diabetes. Her insurance requires that you precertify her for this admission. The doctor gives you his written orders and instructs you to give them to the patient to hand carry to the hospital.

You call the insurance company using the phone number on the back of her insurance card. The insurance company gives you the precertification number 1238952-1 and tells you that she is certified to stay in the hospital for 3 days. She has a $100.00 co-pay for a hospital stay.

Complete the form provided.

Hospital Admission

Patient Name: _____

Patient Insurance Company:_____

Patient Date of Birth:_____

Patient Subscriber ID#:_____

Patient Group #:_____

Insurance Policy Holder:_____

Precertification #:_____

Reason for Admission:_____

_____

Admitting Physician Name and Address _____

_____

Approved Length of Stay:_____

In-Patient Co-Pay:_____

Activity #3: Scheduling an Outpatient Procedure

Using the information on the physician's order below, records the dates and times for appointments made for Grace Woods to have arthroscopy of the left knee and physical therapy at Miracle Rehabilitation before and after surgery. Read the information carefully!

Physician's Order:

Hinged knee brace fitting for use after surgery at Miracle Rehabilitation.

Left knee arthroscopy with medial meniscal repair. Follow up with me in office 5 days post op.

Physical Therapy at Miracle Rehabilitation for eight sessions beginning 1 week after surgery.

Date of surgery: _____

Date of Miracle Rehab appointment for fitting of brace: _____

Dates of Miracle Rehab physical therapy appointments: _____

_____

_____

Date of postoperative visit in your office: _____

Written Communications

Cognitive Domain

1. Spell and define the key terms
2. Recognize elements of fundamental writing skills
3. Discuss the basic guidelines for grammar, punctuation, and spelling in medical writing
4. Organize technical informaton and summaries
5. Discuss the 11 key components of a business letter
6. Describe the process of writing a memorandum
7. List the items that must be included in an agenda
8. Identify the items that must be included when typing minutes
9. Cite the various services available for sending written information
10. Discuss the various mailing options
11. Identify the types of incoming written communication seen in a physician's office
12. Explain the guidelines for opening and sorting mail
13. Discuss applications of electronic technology in effective communication

Psychomotor Domain

1. Compose a professional/business letter (Procedure 7-1)
2. Open and sort mail (Procedure 7-2)

Affective Domain

1. Use language/verbal skills that enable patient's understanding
2. Demonstrate empathy in communicating with patients, family, and staff
3. Demonstrate sensitivity appropriate to the message being delivered
4. Demonstrate recognition of the patient's level of understanding in communications

ABHES Competencies

1. Perform fundamental writing skills including correct grammar, spelling, and formatting techniques when writing prescriptions, documenting medical records, etc.
2. Apply electronic technology
3. Adapt communications to individual's ability to understand
4. Respond to and initiate written communications
5. Utilize electronic technology to receive, organize, prioritize, and transmit information
6. Use correct grammar, spelling, and formatting techniques in written word

Name: _____ Date: _____ Grade: _____

COG MULTIPLE CHOICE

Choose the letter preceding the correct answer.

1. In a letter, the word "Enc." indicates the presence of a(n):

a. summary.

b. abstract.

c. enclosure.

d. review.

e. invitation.

2. If you are instructed to write using the semiblock format, then you should:

a. indent the first line of each paragraph.

b. use left justification for everything.

c. use right justification for the date only.

d. write the recipient's full name in the salutation.

e. indent the first line of the first paragraph.

3. Which of the following items can be abbreviated in an inside address?

a. City

b. Town

c. Recipient's name

d. Business title

e. State

4. Which sentence is written correctly?

a. "We will have to do tests" said Doctor Mathis, "Then we will know what is wrong."

b. "We will have to do tests" said Doctor Mathis. "Then we will know what is wrong."

c. "We will have to do tests," said Doctor Mathis "Then we will know what is wrong."

d. "We will have to do tests", said Doctor Mathis "Then we will know what is wrong."

e. "We will have to do tests," said Doctor Mathis. "Then we will know what is wrong."

5. Which term should be capitalized?

a. morphine

b. fluoxetine

c. zithromax

d. antibiotic

e. catheter

6. If the fax machine is busy when sending an important fax, you should:

a. mail the document instead.

b. call the recipient and ask him to contact you when the machine is available.

c. ask a coworker to send the document.

d. make a note in the patient's chart.

e. wait with the document until you receive confirmation that it was sent.

7. Which sentence is written correctly?

a. The patient is 14 years old and is urinating 3 times more than normal.

b. The patient is 14 years old and is urinating three times more than normal.

c. The patient is fourteen years old and is urinating 3 times more than normal.

d. The patient is fourteen years old and is urinating three times more than normal.

e. The patient is fourteen years old and is urinating three times more than normally.

8. Which of the following always belongs on a fax cover sheet?

a. The number of pages, not including the cover sheet

b. A confidentiality statement

c. A summary of the content of the message

d. A summary of the content of the message, less confidential portions

e. The name of the patient discussed in the message

9. The USPS permit imprint program:

    a. guarantees overnight delivery.

    b. provides receipt of delivery.

    c. offers physicians cheaper postage.

    d. deducts the postage charges from a prepaid account.

    e. addresses envelopes for no additional charge.

10. Which USPS service will allow you to send a parcel overnight?

    a. Registered mail

    b. First-class mail

    c. Presorted mail

    d. Priority mail

    e. Express mail

11. Which is the best way to highlight a list of key points in a business letter?

    a. Use boldface text.

    b. Use a larger font.

    c. Use bulleted text.

    d. Use a highlighter.

    e. Use italicized text.

Scenario for questions 12-14: You are tasked with writing a letter to a patient on the basis of a chart from his last visit. Most important is a diagnosis listed as "HBV infection."

12. Which is an appropriate course of action?

    a. Including the words "HBV infection" in the letter

    b. Consulting the physician on the meaning of the term

    c. Omitting the diagnosis from the otherwise complete letter

    d. Guessing the meaning of the term and writing about that

    e. Asking the office manager what to do about the letter

13. Having learned that HBV means hepatitis B virus, you should:

    a. research HBV infection.

    b. give the patient your condolences.

    c. write a letter based on the physician's instructions.

    d. immediately schedule an appointment for the patient.

    e. ask the patient to visit the office to learn his or her condition.

14. Who might receive a memorandum you have written?

    a. A nurse in your office

    b. A drug sales representative

    c. An insurance agent

    d. An outside specialist

    e. A recently admitted patient

15. Which closing is written correctly?

    a. Best Regards

    b. Sincerely Yours,

    c. Best regards,

    d. Sincerely yours

    e. Best Regards,

16. The purpose of an agenda is to:

    a. summarize the opinions expressed at a meeting.

    b. provide a brief outline for topics to be discussed at a meeting.

    c. inform participants of any changes since the last meeting.

    d. remind group members about an upcoming meeting.

    e. communicate key issues that should be addressed at future meetings.

17. Correspondence that contains information about a patient should be marked:

    a. personal.

    b. confidential.

    c. urgent.

    d. classified.

    e. top secret.

18. Which of these should be included in minutes?

    a. Individuals' statements

    b. Your opinion of the vote

    c. Names of those voting against

    d. Names of those voting in favor

    e. Date and time of the next meeting

19. Which type of mail provides the greatest protection for valuables?

    a. Certified mail

    b. International mail

    c. Registered mail

    d. Standard mail

    e. First class mail

20. Among these, which type of mail should be handled first?

    a. Medication samples

    b. Professional journals

    c. Insurance information

    d. Patient correspondence

    e. Waiting room magazines

21. Which charting note is written correctly?

    a. Patient is a forty-four-year-old Hispanic man with two sprained fingers.

    b. Patient is a 44-year-old hispanic man with 2 sprained fingers.

    c. Patient is a 44-year-old Hispanic man with 2 sprained fingers.

    d. Patient is a 44-year-old hispanic man with two sprained fingers.

22. Which of these statements is both clear and concise?

    a. Mr. Jensen entered the office in the early evening complaining of stomach pain unlike any he had felt before.

    b. Mr. Jensen complained of severe stomach pain.

    c. Mr. Jensen came to the office complaining about pain.

    d. Mr. Jensen complained about stomach pain before leaving the office.

COG MATCHING   Grade: _____

Match the following key terms to their definitions.

Key Terms

23. _____ agenda

24. _____ annotation

25. _____ BiCaps/intercaps

26. _____ block

27. _____ enclosure

28. _____ font

Definitions

a. an informal intra-office communication, generally used to make brief announcements

b. a typographic style

c. a type of letter format in which the first sentence is indented

d. additional information intended to highlight key points in a document, typically written in margins

e. the process of reading a text to check grammatical and factual accuracy

29. _____ full block
30. _____ margin
31. _____ memorandum
32. _____ proofread
33. _____ salutation
34. _____ semiblock
35. _____ template
36. _____ transcription

f. a model used to ensure consistent format in writing

g. abbreviations, words, or phrases with unusual capitalization

h. a type of letter format in which all letter components are justified left

i. something that is included with a letter

j. the process of typing a dictated message

k. a brief outline of the topics discussed at a meeting

l. a type of letter format in which the date, subject line, closing, and signatures are justified right, and all other lines are justified left

m. the greeting of a letter

n. the blank space around the edges of a piece of paper that has been written on

SHORT ANSWER

Grade: _____

37. List the items that are usually included in the minutes of a business meeting.

_____

_____

_____

38. What three things must be included on every piece of mail before sending it?

_____

_____

_____

39. Why is an agenda useful for meetings? What does it include?

_____

_____

_____

40. What should you do after composing a piece of written communication? Why?

_____

_____

_____

AFF WHAT WOULD YOU DO?   Grade: _____

41. Suppose the physician told you to read his e-mails while he was on vacation. In doing so, you come across a personal piece of information that you know he would not want you to see. How would you handle it? Would you tell anyone that you saw it? Would you question the physician about it?

_____

_____

_____

PSY ACTIVE LEARNING   Grade: _____

42. Compose a letter from Dr. Joseph Cohen, 321 Gasthaus Lane, Germantown, PA 87641, to Mr. Ligero Delgado, 888 La Sala Boulevard, Germantown, PA 87642.

The letter should inform Mr. Delgado of the following:

- The results of the biopsy taken during his sigmoidoscopy were negative.
- While these initial results are encouraging, his medical complaints need to be investigated further. Dr. Cohen would like to refer Mr. Delgado to a specialist, Dr. Douloureux.
- Dr. Douloureux's practice is in Suite 100 of the Atroce Medical Center, 132 West Broadway, Germantown, PA 87642.
- With Mr. Delgado's consent, his records can be forwarded to Dr. Douloureux and an appointment will be arranged.

Prepare the letter on a sheet of letterhead if available. If this is not available to you, print the letter on a standard 8 1/2 × 11 white paper and attach to this sheet. Proof your unedited copy and, using proofreader's marks, indicate your corrections. Make the corrections and reprint a final copy. Ask your instructor to review both copies.

43. Write 10 sentences using terms from Box 7-3. Use some terms correctly and others incorrectly. Exchange your sentences with another student. Correct your peer's sentences.

44. Collect five pieces of mail that you have received at home. What method of affixing postage did they use? Go to your local USPS office. Obtain either a priority mail or express mail envelope. Correctly address the envelope.

COG CORRECT OR INCORRECT?   Grade: _____

Read the following sentences. If the sentence is free of errors, write "correct" on the line. If the sentence contains errors, circle the problem and explain how you would fix the sentence.

45. The patient has a cold and is bothered by the postnasal drip.

_____

46. The patient complained of constipation and has not had a bowl movement in 3 days.

_____

47. The patient, Mrs. Philips, sought weight-loss advise from the physician.

_____

48. The nurse applied antiseptic to the wounded elbow.

_____

COG IDENTIFICATION   Grade: _____

Review the list of terms below and place a check mark to indicate whether each term must always be capitalized.

Name	Always	Not Always
49. Streptococcus		
50. Tylenol		
51. Benadryl		
52. Diagnosis		
53. Analgesic		
54. Merck		
55. Antihistamine		
56. Tampax		

COG PSY ACTIVE LEARNING   Grade: _____

57. Dr. Bruce Mosley asks you to prepare a memorandum for distribution to the entire office. He hands you a note to use as the body of the memo. It reads as follows:

On May 9, Jerry Henderson, a representative of Conrad Insurance, will be visiting the office during the morning. Please extend him the utmost courtesy and introduce yourself if you have not yet met him. Jerry is a wonderful man who has been very helpful to our practice. I will be unavailable during the morning as a result of his visit. Please direct questions to Shelly or Dr. Garcia. Of course, I may be contacted in case of an emergency. Using the sample memorandum format in Figure 7-5 of your text, construct the memo.

COG IDENTIFICATION   Grade: _____

58. You have been asked to send a summary of a patient's recent visit to a specialist. Review the list of forms of written communication below and place a check mark to indicate whether it is an appropriate means of written communication.

Form	Appropriate	Not Appropriate
a. A formal letter labeled confidential		
b. An e-mail marked *urgent*		
c. A memorandum		
d. A fax with a confidentiality statement		
e. A memorandum labeled *urgent*		

59. You always take the minutes at the staff meeting, but you'll be on vacation during the next meeting. Identify and list for your coworker what information belongs in the minutes.

_____

_____

_____

60. Dr. Shadrick is at a week-long conference in another state. She needs a patient's complete history to present to the conference one day from now, but has forgotten it at the office. Name three suitable delivery options.

a. _____

b. _____

c. _____

61. Which of the following is/are good practice(s) in regard to handling mail? Place a check mark in the correct box below to answer "Yes" or "No."

Practice	Yes	No
a. Handling promotional materials last		
b. Opening mail addressed to a physician marked "confidential"		
c. Asking a physician or office manager about a piece of mail you are unsure about		
d. Leaving patient correspondence in an external mailbox		
e. Disposing of a physician's personal mail if he or she is away		
f. Informing a covering physician about mail requiring urgent attention		
g. Prioritizing patient care-related mail over pharmaceutical samples		

AFF　PSY　**WHAT WOULD YOU DO?**　　　　　　　　　　　　　Grade: _____

62. You are asked to open the mail today. There is a variety of material including several letters addressed to the physician marked "Urgent," "Confidential," and "Personal." Some of the other mail is from patients, but it is not marked in any unusual fashion. Other letters are from insurance companies with which your office is associated. There are also several advertisements and promotional mailings from medical supply companies, pharmaceutical companies, and insurance companies. In addition, there are pieces of mail that do not include a return address. Explain the procedure you would follow in dealing with this mail.

_____

_____

_____

_____

PSY　**PATIENT EDUCATION**　　　　　　　　　　　　　　　　Grade: _____

63. The office's policy is to mail a welcome letter to new patients. Make a list of information that should be included in this letter so the patient is prepared for her first visit.

_____

_____

_____

_____

AFF **CASE STUDY FOR CRITICAL THINKING**   Grade: _____

The office manager has asked you to compose a letter to every patient in the practice explaining why their physician will be out of the office for ten months. The physician is having extensive cosmetic surgery and is taking a medical leave of absence.

64. Your letter should _____ should not _____ include the reason for the absence.

65. Circle the more appropriate sentence for your letter from the two choices below:

   a. This letter is to tell you that Dr. Smith will not be here for the next ten months, effective October 1, 2012.

   b. This letter is to inform you that Dr. William Smith will be taking a ten-month leave of absence beginning October 1, 2012.

66. Circle the more appropriate sentence for your letter from the two choices below:

   a. We hope you will continue to receive medical care from our office. We have 12 other providers who will be available to handle your health care needs.

   b. Dr. Smith wants you to see one of our other many excellent providers in the interim.

PSY PROCEDURE 7-1   Composing a Business Letter

Name: _____   Date: _____   Time: _____   Grade: _____

EQUIPMENT/SUPPLIES: Computer with word processing software, 8 1/2 × 11 white paper, #10 sized envelope

STANDARDS: Given the needed equipment and a place to work, the student will perform this skill with _____ % accuracy in a total of _____ minutes. *(Your instructor will tell you what the percentage and time limits will be before you begin.)*

KEY: 4 = Satisfactory   0 = Unsatisfactory   NA = This step is not counted

PROCEDURE STEPS	SELF	PARTNER	INSTRUCTOR
1. Move cursor down 2 lines below the letterhead and enter today's date, flush right.	☐	☐	☐
2. Flush left, move cursor down 2 lines and enter the inside address using the name and address of the person to whom you are writing.	☐	☐	☐
3. Double space and type the salutation followed by a colon.	☐	☐	☐
4. Enter a reference line.	☐	☐	☐
5. Double space between paragraphs.	☐	☐	☐
6. Double space and flush right, enter the complimentary close.	☐	☐	☐
7. Move cursor down 4 spaces and enter the sender's name.	☐	☐	☐
8. Double space and enter initials of the sender in all caps.	☐	☐	☐
9. Enter a slash and your initials in lower case letters.	☐	☐	☐
10. Enter c: and names of those who get copies of the letter.	☐	☐	☐
11. Enter Enc: and the number and description of each enclosed sheet.	☐	☐	☐
12. Print on letterhead.	☐	☐	☐
13. Proofread the letter.	☐	☐	☐
14. Attach the letter to the patient's chart.	☐	☐	☐
15. Submit to the sender of the letter for review and signature.	☐	☐	☐
16. Make a copy of the letter for the patient's chart.	☐	☐	☐
17. Address envelopes using all caps and no punctuation.	☐	☐	☐
18. **AFF** Explain how you would respond in this situation: your physician receives the letter you prepared and asks you to insert a comma where you know a comma is not required.	☐	☐	☐

CALCULATION

Total Possible Points: _____

Total Points Earned: _____ Multiplied by 100 = _____ Divided by Total Possible Points = _____ %

PASS   **FAIL**   **COMMENTS:**

☐   ☐

Student's signature _____ Date _____

Partner's signature _____ Date _____

Instructor's signature _____ Date _____

PSY PROCEDURE 7-2   Opening and Sorting Incoming Mail

Name: _____ Date: _____ Time: _____ Grade: _____

EQUIPMENT/SUPPLIES: Letter opener, paper clips, directional tabs, date stamp

STANDARDS: Given the needed equipment and a place to work, the student will perform this skill with _____ % accuracy in a total of _____ minutes. *(Your instructor will tell you what the percentage and time limits will be before you begin.)*

KEY: 4 = Satisfactory   0 = Unsatisfactory   NA = This step is not counted

PROCEDURE STEPS	SELF	PARTNER	INSTRUCTOR
1. Gather the necessary equipment.	☐	☐	☐
2. Open all letters and check for enclosures.	☐	☐	☐
3. Paper clip enclosures to the letter.	☐	☐	☐
4. Date-stamp each item.	☐	☐	☐
5. Sort the mail into categories and deal with it appropriately. Generally, you should handle the following types of mail as noted: *Correspondence regarding a patient:* **a.** Use a paper clip to attach letters, test results, etc. to the patient's chart. **b.** Place the chart in a pile for the physician to review. *Payments and other checks:* **a.** Record promptly all insurance payments and checks and deposit them according to office policy. **b.** Account for all drug samples and appropriately log them into the sample book.	☐	☐	☐
6. Dispose of miscellaneous advertisements unless otherwise directed.	☐	☐	☐
7. Distribute the mail to the appropriate staff members. For example, mail might be for the physician, nurse manager, office manager, billing clerk, or other personnel.	☐	☐	☐
8. **AFF** Explain how you would handle a letter marked "Personal and Confidential."	☐	☐	☐

CALCULATION

Total Possible Points: _____

Total Points Earned: _____ Multiplied by 100 = _____ Divided by Total Possible Points = _____ %

PASS   **FAIL**   **COMMENTS:**

☐   ☐

Student's signature _____ Date _____

Partner's signature _____ Date _____

Instructor's signature _____ Date _____

Health Information Management and Protection

Cognitive Domain

1. Spell and define the key terms
2. Explain the requirements of the Health Insurance Portability and Accountability Act relating to the sharing and saving of personal and protected health information
3. Identify types of records common to the health care setting
4. Describe standard and electronic health record systems
5. Explain the process for releasing medical records to third-party payers and individual patients
6. Discuss principles of using an electronic medical record
7. Describe various types of content maintained in a patient's medical record
8. Identify systems for organizing medical records
9. Explain how to make an entry in a patient's medical record, using abbreviations when appropriate
10. Explain how to make a correction in a standard and electronic health record
11. Discuss pros and cons of various filing methods
12. Describe indexing rules
13. Discuss filing procedures
14. Identify both equipment and supplies needed for filing medical records
15. Explain the guidelines of sound policies for record retention
16. Describe the proper disposal of paper and electronic protected health information (PHI)
17. Explore issue of confidentiality as it applies to the medical assistant
18. Describe the implications of HIPAA for the medical assistant in various medical settings

Psychomotor Domain

1. Establish, organize, and maintain a patient's medical record (Procedure 8-1)
2. File a medical record (Procedure 8-2)
3. Maintain organization by filing

Affective Domain

1. Demonstrate sensitivity to patient rights
2. Demonstrate awarenesss of the consequences of not working within the legal scope of practice
3. Recognize the importance of local, state and federal legislation and regulations in the practice setting
4. Respond to issues of confidentiality
5. Apply HIPAA rules in regard to privacy/ release of information
6. Apply local, state and federal health care legislation and regulation appropriate to the medical assisting practice setting

ABHES Competencies

1. Perform basic clerical functions
2. Prepare and maintain medical records
3. Receive, organize, prioritize, and transmit information expediently
4. Apply electronic technology
5. Institute federal and state guidelines when releasing medical records or information
6. Efficiently maintain and understand different types of medical correspondence and medical reports

Name: _____   Date: _____   Grade: _____

COG MULTIPLE CHOICE

1. Who coordinates and oversees the various aspects of HIPAA compliance in a medical office?

   a. Medicaid and Medicare

   b. HIPAA officer

   c. Privacy officer

   d. Office manager

   e. Law enforcement

2. A release of records request must contain the patient's:

   a. next of kin.

   b. home phone number.

   c. original signature.

   d. medical history.

   e. date of birth.

3. Which is an example of protected health information?

   a. Published statistics by a credible source

   b. Insurance company's mailing address

   c. Physician's pager number

   d. First and last name associated with a diagnosis

   e. Poll published in a medical journal

4. If patients believe their rights have been denied or their health information isn't being protected, they can file a complaint with the:

   a. Journal of American Medical Assistants.

   b. American Medical Association.

   c. provider or insurer.

   d. medical assistant.

   e. state's attorney.

5. The only time an original record should be released is when the:

   a. patient asks for the record.

   b. patient is in critical condition.

   c. record is subpoenaed by the court of law.

   d. physician is being sued.

   e. patient terminates the relationship with the physician.

6. Do medical records have the same content if they are on paper or a computer disk?

   a. Yes

   b. No

   c. Sometimes

   d. Most of the time

   e. Never

7. Documentation of each patient encounter is called:

   a. consultation reports.

   b. medication administration.

   c. correspondence.

   d. narrative.

   e. progress notes.

8. Improved medication management is a feature of:

   a. SOAP.

   b. electronic health records.

   c. clearinghouses.

   d. PHI.

   e. workers' compensation.

9. To maintain security, a facility should:

   a. design a written confidentiality policy for employees to sign.

   b. provide public access to medical records.

   c. keep a record of all passwords and give a copy to each employee.

   d. keep doors unlocked during the evening hours only.

   e. have employees hide patient information from other coworkers.

10. Under source-oriented records, the most recent documents are placed on top of previous sheets, which is called:

    a. chronological order.

    b. reverse chronological order.

    c. alphabetical order.

    d. subject order.

    e. numeric order.

11. The acronym "SOAP" stands for:

    a. subjective-objective-adjustment-plan.

    b. subjective-objective-accounting-plan.

    c. subjective-objective-assessment-plan.

    d. subjective-objective-accounting-problem.

    e. subjective-objective-assessment-problem.

12. The acronym "POMR" stands for:

    a. presentation-oriented medical record.

    b. protection-oriented medical record.

    c. performance-oriented medical record.

    d. professional-oriented medical record.

    e. problem-oriented medical record.

13. Which of the following is contained in a POMR database?

    a. Marketing tools

    b. Field of interest

    c. Job description

    d. Review of systems

    e. Accounting review

14. Which of the following will reflect each encounter with the patient chronologically, whether by phone, by e-mail, or in person?

    a. Microfilm

    b. Narrative

    c. Progress notes

    d. Subject filing

    e. Flow sheet

15. Shingling is:

    a. printing replies to a patient's e-mail.

    b. recording laboratory results in the patient's chart.

    c. telephone or electronic communications with patients.

    d. taping the paper across the top to a regular-size sheet.

    e. filing records in chronological order.

16. How long are workers' compensation cases kept open after the last date of treatment for any follow-up care that may be required?

    a. 6 months

    b. 1 year

    c. 2 years

    d. 5 years

    e. 10 years

17. A cross-reference in numeric filing is called a(n):

    a. open file.

    b. locked file.

    c. straight digit file.

    d. master patient index.

    e. duplication index.

18. Security experts advise storing backup disks:

    a. in the office.

    b. offsite.

    c. at the physician's home.

    d. on every computer.

    e. at the library.

19. Drawer files are a type of:

   a. filing cabinet.

   b. storage container.

   c. computer system.

   d. shelving unit.

   e. subject filing.

20. The statute of limitations is:

   a. the end of a provider's ability to legally practice.

   b. the record retention system.

   c. a miniature photographic system.

   d. the legal time limit set for filing suit against an alleged wrongdoer.

   e. the number of records a storage system is able to hold.

COG MATCHING

Grade: _____

Match the following key terms to their definitions.

Key Terms

21. _____ alphabetic filing

22. _____ chief complaint

23. _____ chronological order

24. _____ clearinghouse

25. _____ covered entity

26. _____ cross-reference

27. _____ demographic data

28. _____ electronic health records (EHR)

29. _____ flow sheet

30. _____ medical history forms

31. _____ microfiche

32. _____ microfilm

33. _____ narrative

34. _____ numeric filing

35. _____ protected health information (PHI)

36. _____ present illness

37. _____ problem-oriented medical record (POMR)

38. _____ reverse chronological order

39. _____ SOAP

40. _____ subject filing

Definitions

a. information about patients that is recorded and stored on computer

b. photographs of records in a reduced size

c. a paragraph indicating the contact with the patient, what was done for the patient, and the outcome of any action

d. a specific account of the chief complaint, including time frames and characteristics

e. a common method of compiling information that lists each problem of the patient, usually at the beginning of the folder, and references each problem with a number throughout the folder

f. notation in a file indicating that a record is stored elsewhere and giving the reference; verification to another source; checking the tabular list against the alphabetic list in ICD-9 coding

g. entity that takes claims and other electronic data from providers, verifies the information, and forwards the proper forms to the payors for physicians

h. employer insurance for treatment of an employee's injury or illness related to the job

i. any information that can be linked to a specific person

j. items placed with oldest first

k. sheets of microfilm

l. arranging files according to their title, grouping similar subjects together

m. a style of charting that includes subjective, objective, assessment, and planning notes

n. arranging of names or titles according to the sequence of letters in the alphabet

o. health plan; health care clearinghouse; or health care provider who transmits any health information in electronic form in connection with a transaction covered under HIPAA

p. placing in order of time; usually the most recent is placed foremost

41. _____ workers' compensation

q. information relating to the statistical characteristics of populations

r. color-coded sheets that allow information to be recorded in graphic or tabular form for easy retrieval

s. arranging files by a numbered order

t. main reason for the visit to the medical office

u. record containing information about a patient's past and present health status

SHORT ANSWER   Grade: _____

42. List the four steps you should take to ensure that files are filed and retrieved quickly and efficiently.

_____

_____

_____

_____

43. Describe the difference between standard and electronic health record systems.

_____

_____

_____

_____

44. When documenting in a medical record or file, why should you use caution when using abbreviations?

_____

_____

_____

_____

45. How does a numeric filing system help a medical office meet HIPAA's privacy requirements?

_____

_____

_____

_____

46. Documentation is a large part of your job as a medical assistant. Legible, correct, and thorough documentation is necessary. List three instances, other than patient visits, when documentation is required.

_____

_____

_____

_____

47. When a health care provider's practice ends, either from retirement or death, what happens to the records?

_____

_____

_____

_____

48. Those who must abide by HIPAA are called "covered entities." List the three groups that are considered covered entities.

_____

_____

_____

_____

COG **PSY** **ACTIVE LEARNING**   Grade: _____

49. If you were opening a new medical facility, consider whether you would want staff members using abbreviations in patient records. Then create a list of 20 acceptable abbreviations that may be used in your new facility. Next create a "Do Not Use" list for abbreviations that may be confusing and should not be included in records. Visit the website for the Joint Commission at www.jointcommission.org and include all of those abbreviations in addition to five other abbreviations of your own choice.

50. Interview a fellow student with a hypothetical illness. Document the visit with the chief complaint and history of present illness.

51. The office you work in receives lab results on a printer throughout the day. Write an office policy for maintaining confidentiality with the PHI being transmitted electronically.

52. Your medical office uses an alphabetic filing system. Place the following names in the correct order to show how you would place each record in a filing system.

Brandon P. Snow	Kristen F. Darian-Lewes	Shante L. Dawes	Emil S. Faqir, Jr.
Shaunice L. DeBlase	Juan R. Ortiz	Kim Soo	Fernando P. Vasquez, D.O.

a. _____

b. _____

c. _____

d. _____

e. _____

f. _____

g. _____

h. _____

COG **IDENTIFICATION**   Grade: _____

53. HIPAA has privacy rules that protect your personal health information. Under HIPAA, covered entities must take certain safety measures to protect patients' information. Read the paragraph below. For each blank, there are two choices. Circle the correct word or phrase for each sentence.

Covered entities must designate a _____(a)_____ (HIPAA officer, privacy officer) to keep track of who has access to health information. They must also adopt written _____(b)_____ (privacy, health care) procedures. Under HIPAA, patients have the right to decide if they provide _____(c)_____ (permission, marketing) before their health information can be used or shared for certain purposes. They also have the right to get a _____(d)_____ (narrative, report) on when and why their health care information was shared for certain purposes.

COG PSY **IDENTIFICATION**

Grade: _____

The rules for releasing medical records and authorization are meant to protect patients' privacy rights. Read the questions below regarding the release of medical records and circle "Yes" or "No" for each question.

54. May an 18-year-old patient get copies of his or her own medical records? Yes No

55. May all minors seek treatment for sexually transmitted diseases and birth control without parental knowledge or consent? Yes No

56. When a patient requests copies of his or her own records, does the doctor make the decision about what to copy? Yes No

57. Must the authorization form give the patient the opportunity to limit the information released? Yes No

58. When a patient authorizes the release of information, may he request that the physician leave out information pertinent to the situation? Yes No

COG **FILL IN THE BLANKS**

Grade: _____

HIPAA requirements provide guidelines and suggestions for safe computer practices when storing or transferring patient information. The following is a list of guidelines that medical facilities are urged to follow. Complete each sentence with the appropriate word from the word bank below.

59. Store _____ in a bank safe-deposit box.

60. Change log-in _____ and passwords every 30 days.

61. Turn _____ away from areas where information may be seen by patients.

62. Use _____ with _____ other than letters.

63. Prepare a back-up _____ for use when the computer system is down.

Word Bank			
characters	plan	disks	information
codes	passwords	template	terminals
Note: Not all words will be used.			

MATCHING

Grade: _____

A standard medical record in an outpatient facility, known as a chart or file, contains clinical information as well as billing and insurance information. In the clinical section of the file, you will often find certain types of information. In the columns below, draw a diagonal line to match the clinical type of information with its correct description.

Name of Clinical Information	Description
64. Chief complaint	**a.** Documentation of each patient encounter
65. Family and personal history	**b.** Provider's opinion of the patient's problem
66. Progress notes	**c.** Symptoms that led the patient to seek the physician's care
67. Diagnosis or medical impression	**d.** Letters or memos generated in the facility and sent out
68. Correspondence pertaining to patient	**e.** Review of major illnesses of family members

TRUE OR FALSE?

Grade: _____

69. True or False? Determine whether the following statements are true or false. If false, explain why.

a. HIPAA allows patients to ask to see and get a copy of their health records.

_____

b. To maintain secure files, you should change log-in codes and passwords every 10 days.

_____

c. Medical history forms are commonly used to gather information from the patient before the visit with the physician.

_____

d. Before treating a patient for a possible workers' compensation case, you must first obtain verification from the employer unless the situation is life threatening.

_____

AFF **WHAT WOULD YOU DO?**   Grade: _____

70. A mother is accused of physically abusing her 16-year-old daughter, a patient with your facility. A police officer who has been asked to investigate visits the medical office and asks for the patient's medical records. What would you do?

_____

_____

_____

_____

71. You're in the medical office and you suddenly realize that you've forgotten to document a telephone conversation you had with a patient 2 days ago. What would you do?

_____

_____

_____

_____

AFF CASE STUDY FOR CRITICAL THINKING A

Grade: _____

You are tasked with creating the office policy for the retention of records for your facility.

72. Circle any appropriate actions from the list below.

    a. Research federal law that mandates how long you must keep records.

    b. Research the state legislature to determine the statute of limitations for your state.

    c. Make sure the time limit for retaining records includes inactive and closed files.

    d. Set the time limits for retaining children's records from their 18th birthday.

    e. Set the time limits for retaining the records of adults and children the same for ease of remembering.

    f. Have the policy approved by the physician and/or appropriate employee.

73. This task is not in your job description, and you feel that you are not qualified to set policy for the facility. Circle the appropriate actions from the list below.

    a. Tell your supervisor of your concerns and ask for his or her guidance.

    b. Consider this a great opportunity to show your employer your skills.

    c. Ask the attorney for the facility to create the policy for you.

    d. Ask the attorney not to tell your supervisor that he helped you.

    e. Do the task, but make sure everyone in the office knows who did it.

    f. Do the task without assistance and ask for a promotion and/or raise when finished.

74. What is the statute of limitations for patients to file malpractice or negligence suits in your state? _____

AFF **CASE STUDY FOR CRITICAL THINKING B** Grade: _____

Your mother's best friend is a patient in the office where you work. You have known her all of your life. She has just been seen for a suspicious lump in her breast. She is very nervous and calls you at home that night to see if you know the results of her test. You saw the stat biopsy report before you left work and you know that the lump is malignant. She was given an appointment in 2 days for the physician to give her the results.

75. Circle all appropriate actions from the list below.

    a. Tell her that it is not in your scope of practice to give patients results without specific instructions from a provider, even if they are friends.

    b. To minimize the time she must anxiously wait, try to move her appointment to tomorrow as soon as you get to work in the morning.

    c. Tell her that the report was not good and to bring someone with her to the visit.

    d. Call the physician at home to ask if you can tell her.

    e. Tell her that you do not know the results of the test, but even if you did you could not tell her.

    f. Call your mother, tell her the situation, and ask for her advice.

76. Let's say you tell the patient that you cannot give test results, and she replies, "I have a right to know what is wrong with me." Circle all of the appropriate responses below.

    a. Only a provider can give test results in my office unless they specifically direct an employee to do so.

    b. I am a professional, and I don't really care about your rights.

    c. I know you are my mother's friend, but I am a CMA, and I follow the rules.

    d. Giving you the results of your biopsy may have caused me to get fired. I'm not getting fired for you or anybody.

    e. You do have that right, but I do not have the right to tell you.

    f. Talk to the physician about it.

77. Why is it important for the physician to give test results such as the one in the case study?

_____

_____

_____

_____

PSY PROCEDURE 8-1   Establishing, Organizing, and Maintaining a Medical File

Name: _____ Date: _____ Time: _____ Grade: _____

EQUIPMENT/SUPPLIES: File folder; metal fasteners; hole punch; five divider sheets with tabs, title, year, and alphabetic or numeric labels

STANDARDS: Given the needed equipment and a place to work the student will perform this skill with _____% accuracy in a total of _____ minutes. *(Your instructor will tell you what the percentage and time limits will be before you begin.)*

KEY: 4 = Satisfactory   0 = Unsatisfactory   NA = this step is not counted

PROCEDURE STEPS	SELF	PARTNER	INSTRUCTOR
1. Place the label along the tabbed edge of the folder so that the title extends out beyond the folder itself. (Tabs can be either the length of the folder or tabbed in various positions, such as left, center, and right.)	☐	☐	☐
2. Place a year label along the top edge of the tab before the label with the title. This will be changed each year the patient has been seen. *Note:* Do not automatically replace these labels at the start of a new year; remove the old year and replace with a new one only when the patient comes in for the first visit of the new year.	☐	☐	☐
3. Place the appropriate alphabetic or numeric labels below the title.	☐	☐	☐
4. Apply any additional labels that your office may decide to use.	☐	☐	☐
5. Punch holes and insert demographic and financial information on the left side of the chart using top fasteners across the top.	☐	☐	☐
6. Make tabs for: Ex. H&P, Progress Notes, Medication Log, Correspondence, and Test Results.	☐	☐	☐
7. Place pages behind appropriate tabs.	☐	☐	☐
8. **AFF** Explain what you would do when you receive a revised copy correcting an error on a document already in a patient's chart.	☐	☐	☐

CALCULATION

Total Possible Points: _____

Total Points Earned: _____ Multiplied by 100 = _____ Divided by Total Possible Points = _____ %

PASS   **FAIL**   **COMMENTS:**

☐   ☐

Student's signature _____ Date _____

Partner's signature _____ Date _____

Instructor's signature _____ Date _____

PSY PROCEDURE 8-2 | Filing Medical Records

Name: _____ Date: _____ Time: _____ Grade: _____

EQUIPMENT/SUPPLIES: Simulated patient file folder, several single sheets to be filed in the chart, file cabinet with other file

STANDARDS: Given the needed equipment and a place to work the student will perform this skill with _____%
accuracy in a total of _____ minutes. *(Your instructor will tell you what the percentage and time limits will be before you begin.)*

KEY: 4 = Satisfactory 0 = Unsatisfactory NA = this step is not counted

PROCEDURE STEPS	SELF	PARTNER	INSTRUCTOR
1. Double check spelling of names on the chart and any single sheets to be placed in the folder.	☐	☐	☐
2. Condition any single sheets, etc.	☐	☐	☐
3. Place sheets behind proper tab in the chart.	☐	☐	☐
4. Remove guide.	☐	☐	☐
5. Place the folder between the two appropriate existing folders, taking care to place the folder between the two charts.	☐	☐	☐
6. Scan color coding to ensure none of the charts in that section are out of order.	☐	☐	☐
7. **AFF** Explain what you would do when you find a chart out of order. Should you bring it to the attention of your supervisor?	☐	☐	☐

_____
_____
_____
_____

CALCULATION

Total Possible Points: _____

Total Points Earned: _____ Multiplied by 100 = _____ Divided by Total Possible Points = _____ %

PASS **FAIL** **COMMENTS:**

☐ ☐

Student's signature _____ Date _____

Partner's signature _____ Date _____

Instructor's signature _____ Date _____

Electronic Applications in the Medical Office

Cognitive Domain

1. Spell and define the key words
2. Identify the basic computer components
3. Discuss the importance of routine maintenance of office equipment
4. Explain the basics of connecting to the Internet
5. Discuss the safety concerns for online searching
6. Describe how to use a search engine
7. List sites that can be used by professionals and sites geared for patients
8. Describe the benefits of an intranet and explain how it differs from the Internet
9. Describe the various types of clinical software that might be used in a physician's office
10. Describe the various types of administrative software that might be used in a physician's office
11. Discuss applications of electronic technology in effective communication
12. Describe the considerations for purchasing a computer
13. Describe various training options
14. Discuss the adoption of electronic health records
15. Describe the steps in making the transition from paper to electronic records
16. Discuss the ethics related to computer access

Affective Domain

1. Apply ethical behaviors, including honest/integrity in the performance of medical assisting practice

Psychomotor Domain

1. Care for and maintain computer hardware (Procedure 9-1)
2. Use the Internet to access information related to the medical office (Procedure 9-2)
3. Use office hardware and software to maintain office systems
4. Execute data management using electronic health care records such as the EMR
5. Use office hardware and software to maintain office systems

ABHES Competencies

1. Apply electronic technology
2. Receive, organize, prioritize, and transmit information expediently
3. Locate information and resources for patients and employers
4. Apply computer application skills using variety of different electronic programs including both practice management software and EMR software

Name: _____   Date: _____   Grade: _____

COG MULTIPLE CHOICE

1. Another name for a central processing unit is a:

   a. silicon chip.

   b. USB port.

   c. modem.

   d. microprocessor.

   e. handheld computer.

2. The purpose of a zip drive in a computer is to:

   a. scan information.

   b. delete information.

   c. store information.

   d. research information.

   e. translate information.

3. The acronym *DSL* stands for:

   a. data storage location.

   b. digital subscriber line.

   c. digital storage link.

   d. data saved/lost.

   e. digital software link.

4. In a physician's practice, the HIPAA officer:

   a. checks for security threats or gaps in electronic information.

   b. purchases new technological equipment.

   c. maintains computer equipment and fixes problems.

   d. trains staff in how to use computer equipment.

   e. monitors staff who may be misusing computer equipment.

Scenario for questions 5 and 6: A parent approaches you and asks how he can keep his 9-year-old daughter safe on the Internet.

5. Which of these actions would you recommend to the parent?

   a. Don't allow the daughter on the Internet after 7 p.m.

   b. Stand behind the daughter the entire time she is using the Internet.

   c. Don't permit the daughter to use the Internet until she is 10 years old.

   d. Add a filter to the daughter's computer to only allow safe sites as decided by the parent.

   e. Ask other parents for advice.

6. Which of these Web sites might be helpful to the parent?

   a. www.skyscape.com

   b. www.pdacortec.com

   c. www.ezclaim.com

   d. www.cyberpatrol.com

   e. www.nextgen.com

7. To protect your computer from a virus, you should:

   a. make sure that your computer is correctly shut down every time you use it.

   b. avoid opening any attachments from unknown Web sites.

   c. only download material from government Web sites.

   d. consult a computer technician before you use new software.

   e. only open one Web site at a time.

8. What is the advantage of encrypting an e-mail?

   a. It makes the e-mail arrive at its intended destination faster.

   b. It marks the e-mail as *urgent.*

   c. It scrambles the e-mail so that it cannot be read until it reaches the recipient.

   d. It translates the e-mail into another language.

   e. It informs the sender when the e-mail has been read by the recipient.

9. Which of these is an example of an inappropriate e-mail?

   a. "There will be a staff meeting on Wednesday at 9 a.m."

   b. "Please return Mrs. Jay's call: Her number is 608-223-3444."

   c. "If anyone has seen a lost pair of sunglasses, please return them to reception."

   d. "Mr. Orkley thinks he is having a stroke. Please advise."

   e. "Mrs. Jones called to confirm her appointment."

10. Which of the following is a peripheral?

    a. Zip drive

    b. Monitor

    c. Keyboard

    d. Internet

    e. Modem

11. Which of these would you most likely find on an intranet?

    a. Advice about health insurance

    b. Minutes from staff meetings

    c. Information about Medicare

    d. Descriptions of alternative treatments

    e. National guidelines on medical ethics

12. What is the difference between clinical and administrative software packages?

    a. Clinical software helps provide good medical care, whereas administrative software keeps the office efficient.

    b. Administrative software is designed to be used by medical assistants, whereas clinical software is used by physicians.

    c. Clinical software is cheaper than administrative software because it offers fewer technical features.

    d. Administrative software lasts longer than clinical software because it is of higher quality.

    e. Clinical software does not allow users to access it without a password, whereas anyone can use administrative software.

13. Which of these should you remember to do when paging a physician?

    a. Follow up the page with a phone call to make sure the physician got the message.

    b. Keep track of what time the message is sent and repage if there is no response.

    c. Document the fact that you sent a page to the physician.

    d. Contact the person who left the message to let him or her know you have paged the physician.

    e. E-mail the physician with a copy of the paged message.

14. You can use the Meeting Maker software program to:

    a. contact patients about appointment changes.

    b. coordinate internal meetings and calendars.

    c. print patient reminders for annual checkups.

    d. create slideshow presentations for meetings.

    e. page office staff when a meeting is about to start.

15. Which of these is an important consideration when purchasing a new computer for the office?

    a. Whether the computer's programs are HIPAA compliant

    b. Whether the computer will be delivered to the office

    c. The number of people who will be using the computer

    d. The amount of space the computer will take up in the office

    e. Which is the best-selling computer on the market

16. When assigning computer log-in passwords to staff, a physician should:

    a. make sure that everyone has the code for the hospital computers.

    b. give staff two log-in passwords: one for professional use and one for personal use.

    c. issue all new employees their own password.

    d. make sure that everyone has access to his or her e-mails, in case he or she is out of the office.

    e. use a standard log-in password for all the office computers.

17. It is a good idea to lock the hard drive when you are moving a computer to:

  a. prevent the zip drive from falling out.

  b. make sure that no information is erased.

  c. stop viruses from attacking the computer.

  d. protect the CPU and disk drives.

  e. avoid damaging the keyboard.

18. A modem is a(n):

  a. communication device that connects a computer to other computers, including the Internet.

  b. piece of software that enables the user to perform advanced administrative functions.

  c. name for the Internet.

  d. method of storing data on the computer.

  e. type of networking technology for local area networks.

19. Which of the following is true of an abstract found during a literary search?

  a. Abstracts are only found on government Web sites.

  b. Only physicians can access an abstract during a literary search.

  c. An abstract is a summary of a journal article.

  d. Most medical offices cannot afford to download an abstract.

  e. Abstracts can only be printed at a hospital library.

20. If a computer is exposed to static electricity, there is the potential risk of:

  a. electrical fire.

  b. memory loss.

  c. dust accumulation.

  d. slow Internet connection.

  e. viruses.

21. You have been asked to train new employees on how to use an administrative application. However, you do not have a lot of time or extra funding to spend on training. Circle the best option for training the new employees.

  a. Have them read the user manual.

  b. Have them call the help desk.

  c. Have them ask another colleague.

  d. Have them take a tutorial on the program.

  e. Hire experts from the software company.

22. When shopping for prescription management software, what is the minimum that a physician should be able to do with the program? Circle the correct answer.

  a. Find a patient name in a database, write the prescription, and download it to the pharmacy.

  b. Find a patient name in a database, check the prescription for contraindication, and download it to the pharmacy.

  c. Find a patient name in a database, write the prescription, and print it out for the patient.

  d. Find a medication in a database, write the prescription, and download the data to a handheld computer.

  e. Find a patient name in a database, write the prescription, download it to the pharmacy, and check that the medication is covered by insurance.

COG MATCHING   Grade: _____

Match the following key terms to their definitions.

Key Terms   **Definitions**

23. _____ cookies   **a.** a system that allows the computer to be connected to a cable or DSL system

24. _____ downloading   **b.** a private network of computers that share data

25. _____ encryption   **c.** a global system used to connect one computer to another

26. _____ Ethernet   **d.** tiny files left on your computer's hard drive by a Web site without your permission

27. _____ Internet   **e.** a dangerous invader that enters your computer through a source and can destroy
                                 your files, software programs, and possibly even the hard drive
28. _____ intranet
                             f. transferring information from an outside location to your computer's hard drive
29. _____ literary search
                             g. the process of scrambling e-mail messages so that they cannot be read until they
30. _____ search engine   reach the recipient

31. _____ surfing   **h.** the process of navigating Web sites

32. _____ virus   **i.** a program that allows you to find information on the Web related to specific terms

33. _____ virtual   **j.** a search that involves finding journal articles that present new facts or data about a
                                 given topic

                             k. simulated by your computer

COG SHORT ANSWER   Grade: _____

34. List three benefits of having appointment scheduling software in the office.

_____

_____

_____

_____

35. You receive an e-mail from a patient saying that his medication is working out well and is not causing any side effects. He will be in for his appointment next Tuesday. How do you document this information in the patient's medical record?

_____

_____

_____

_____

36. What are three benefits of using electronic health records instead of manual charts?

_____

_____

_____

_____

37. Mr. Jones requires special treatment that uses a laser machine. He makes an appointment for Thursday morning and takes time off work to attend. When he arrives at the facility, he is told that the machine is only available on Mondays and that the new receptionist was unaware of this fact when she made his appointment. How could an administrative software program have helped to prevent this situation?

_____

_____

_____

_____

_____

COG **PSY** **PATIENT EDUCATION**   Grade: _____

38. A patient has told you of his decision to start buying prescription medication on the Internet. What warnings/information should you give to him?

_____

_____

_____

_____

COG **PSY** ACTIVE LEARNING   Grade: _____

39. Perform research using the Internet to find information about a disease and possible treatments. Try using different key words to see which ones produce the most useful results. Make a list of the Web sites you have used and observe whether each one has the logo of a verification program such as the HON (Health on the Net) seal.

40. Use the PowerPoint program on the computer to turn your Internet research about a common disease into a presentation. Use the program to make handouts of your presentation for quick office reference. You can use the tutorial feature on the software if you are unsure how to perform certain functions.

41. Visit the Medicare Web site at www.medicare.gov. Find the part of the Web site that addresses FAQs, or frequently asked questions. Choose five of these questions that might be relevant to your patients and print the questions and answers. Then use presentation software to highlight these five questions in a presentation that you will give to your class.

COG IDENTIFICATION   Grade: _____

42. Your office has started converting many of your paper files into digital online files to save time. Recently, you have realized that accessing these records through your Internet service provider (ISP) is taking a very long time. Circle the solutions to this problem.

   a. Upgrade your office's ISP to cable.Q2

   b. Switch your Web browser.

   c. Switch your search engine.

   d. Upgrade your printer.

   e. Eliminate viruses with a virus scan.

   f. Upgrade your monitor.

   g. Upgrade your office's ISP to DSL.

43. A patient has asked you for information on how she can lower her cholesterol. You have decided to surf the Internet to find the latest information. Place a check in the "Yes" column for those key words that would lead to a faster, more efficient search. Place a check in the "No" column for those key words that would lead to a slower, less efficient search.

Key Words	Yes	No
a. cholesterol		
b. lowering cholesterol		
c. cholesterol diet		
d. How do people lower their cholesterol?		
e. cholesterol reduction		

44. A diabetic patient has been researching information on the disease. He has asked you to review a list of Web sites he has been reading. Place a check in the "Patient" box for sites that are more useful for patients. Place a check in the "Professional" box for sites that are more useful to physicians and medical assistants.

Web sites	Patient	Professional
a. www.mywebmd.com		
b. www.lancet.org		
c. www.jama.com		
d. www.healthfinder.gov		
e. www.tifaq.com		

COG PSY **PATIENT EDUCATION**   Grade: _____

45. A patient has expressed an interest in learning more about her food allergies on the Internet. You decide to give her advice on what to look out for when surfing. Place a check in the "Yes" column indicating that the statement is good advice. Place a check in the "No" column indicating that the statement is bad advice.

Key Words	Yes	No
a. Almost all testimonials can be trusted.		
b. Don't trust sites that claim to have secret formulas, medical miracles, or breakthroughs.		
c. Some treatments found online are best to not tell your physician about.		
d. No matter how professional the Web site, you cannot learn lifesaving skills on the Internet.		

TRUE OR FALSE?   Grade: _____

46. Determine whether the following statements are true or false. If false, explain why.

   a. The advanced search feature of a search engine should return more results.

   _____

   b. Internal job postings are often found on the Internet.

   _____

   c. The most popular program used to write presentations is PowerPoint.

   _____

   d. A computer system is divided into three areas: hardware, peripherals, and software.

   _____

Grade: _____

47. You perform most of the administrative tasks in a physician's office, and have been asked for your input concerning a new office computer. The physician asks you which administrative features you would find helpful in a new computer. List three administrative software programs that you would find useful and explain what functions they perform.

_____

_____

_____

_____

48. A patient tells you that her medicine has not been working properly and that she is thinking of researching alternative treatments on the Internet. What is the best advice you can give her?

_____

_____

_____

_____

49. One of your coworkers has a habit of getting up from her computer and leaving confidential patient information visible on the screen. She says that she sits too far away from patients for them to read anything on the screen, but you have seen several patients near the computer while your coworker is away from her desk. What do you say to her?

_____

_____

_____

_____

50. It is your first week working at a physician's office. You notice that the computer is dusty and in the morning sunlight. Disks are in a neat pile next to the uncovered computer. What steps would you take to maintain this computer?

_____

_____

_____

AFF CASE STUDY FOR CRITICAL THINKING   Grade: _____

You are teaching a new employee to use the computer system in the office where you work. Ginger is excited and enthusiastic about her new job. At every possible opportunity, Ginger checks her Facebook and Twitter pages. You know that this is against the office policy regarding accepted use of office computers.

51. Circle all appropriate actions from the list below.

   a. Beg the office manager to get someone else to train Ginger.

   b. Show her the policy in the office *Policies and Procedures Manual.*

   c. Tell her if she continues this practice she will get fired.

   d. Tell her that the IT department can and will track her use of the office computer.

   e. Suggest that she wait until she gets off work for personal computer use.

   f. Suggest that people should talk to each other the way they used to, face to face.

52. Circle the accurate statements from the list below. Businesses control personal use of their computers because:

   a. it reduces wear and tear on the computers.

   b. it is inefficient for employees to be doing personal things while at work.

   c. it is dishonest to use someone else's computer.

   d. it is unprofessional and unethical.

   e. you should never disobey the office rules, no matter what.

   f. they are not paying you to be on Facebook and Twitter.

   g. it is illegal.

53. You are teaching Ginger how to care for her computer. Why is it important to perform routine maintenance on the office computer? Circle all appropriate answers from the list below.

   a. It enhances the performance and prolongs the life of the equipment.

   b. It is a rule and you *always* follow the rules, no matter what.

   c. It shows that you are a clean person.

   d. It looks bad for the patients to see dust.

   e. It is in the office *Policy and Procedure Manual.*

PSY PROCEDURE 9-1 ▏ **Care for and Maintain Computer Hardware**

Name: _____ Date: _____ Time: _____ Grade: _____

EQUIPMENT/SUPPLIES: Computer CPU, monitor, keyboard, mouse, printer, duster, simulated warranties

STANDARDS: Given the needed equipment and a place to work the student will perform this skill with _____%
accuracy in a total of _____ minutes. *(Your instructor will tell you what the percentage and time limits will be
before you begin.)*

KEY: 4 = Satisfactory 0 = Unsatisfactory NA = this step is not counted

PROCEDURE STEPS	SELF	PARTNER	INSTRUCTOR
1. Place the monitor, keyboard, and printer in a cool, dry area out of direct sunlight.	☐	☐	☐
2. Place the computer desk on an antistatic floor mat or carpet.	☐	☐	☐
3. Clean the monitor screen with antistatic wipes.	☐	☐	☐
4. Use dust covers for the keyboard and the monitor when they are not in use.	☐	☐	☐
5. Lock the hard drive when moving the computer.	☐	☐	☐
6. Keep keyboard and mouse free of debris and liquids; dust and/or vacuum the keyboard.	☐	☐	☐
7. Create a file for maintenance and warranty contracts for the computer system.	☐	☐	☐
8. Handle data storage disks with special care.	☐	☐	☐
9. **AFF** If you were the office manager, explain how you would respond to an employee who continued to spill soft drinks on her keyboard.	☐	☐	☐

_____

_____

_____

_____

CALCULATION

Total Possible Points: _____

Total Points Earned: _____ Multiplied by 100 = _____ Divided by Total Possible Points = _____ %

PASS   **FAIL**   **COMMENTS:**

☐   ☐

Student's signature _____ Date _____

Partner's signature _____ Date _____

Instructor's signature _____ Date _____

PSY PROCEDURE 9-2   Searching on the Internet

Name: _____   Date: _____   Time: _____   Grade: _____

EQUIPMENT/SUPPLIES: Computer with Web browser software, modem, active Internet connection account

STANDARDS: Given the needed equipment and a place to work the student will perform this skill with _____% accuracy in a total of _____ minutes. *(Your instructor will tell you what the percentage and time limits will be before you begin.)*

KEY: 4 = Satisfactory   0 = Unsatisfactory   NA = this step is not counted

PROCEDURE STEPS	SELF	PARTNER	INSTRUCTOR
1. Connect computer to the Internet.	☐	☐	☐
2. Locate a search engine.	☐	☐	☐
3. Select two or three key words and type them at the appropriate place on the Web page.	☐	☐	☐
4. View the number of search results. If no sites are found, check spelling and retype or choose new key words.	☐	☐	☐
5. If the search produces a long list, do an advanced search and refine key words.	☐	☐	☐
6. Select an appropriate site and open its home page.	☐	☐	☐
7. If satisfied with the site's information, either download the material or bookmark the page. If unsatisfied with its information, either visit a site listed on the results page or return to the search engine.	☐	☐	☐
8. **AFF** You sit down to use your office computer to search for information with a patient when a coworker's Facebook page pops up. You are embarrassed at the unprofessionalism this displays in front of the patient. Explain how you would respond in this situation.	☐	☐	☐

CALCULATION

Total Possible Points: _____

Total Points Earned: _____ Multiplied by 100 = _____ Divided by Total Possible Points = _____ %

PASS   **FAIL**   **COMMENTS:**

☐   ☐

Student's signature _____ Date _____

Partner's signature _____ Date _____

Instructor's signature _____ Date _____

Medical Office Management, Safety, and Emergency Preparedness

Cognitive Domain

1. Spell and define the key terms
2. Describe what is meant by organizational structure
3. List seven responsibilities of the medical office manager
4. Explain the five staffing issues that a medical office manager will be responsible for handling
5. List the types of policies and procedures that should be included in a medical office's policy and procedures manual
6. List five types of promotional materials that a medical office may distribute
7. Discuss financial concerns that the medical office manager must be capable of addressing
8. Describe the duties regarding office maintenance, inventory, and service contracts
9. Discuss the need for continuing education
10. Describe liability, professional, personal injury and third-party insurance
11. List three services provided by most medical malpractice companies
12. List six guidelines for completing incident reports
13. List four regulatory agencies that require medical offices to have quality improvement programs
14. Describe the accreditation process of The Joint Commission
15. Describe the steps to developing a quality improvement program
16. Identify safety techniques that can be used to prevent accidents and maintain a safe work environment
17. Describe the importance of Material Safety Data Sheets (MSDS) in a health care setting
18. Identify safety signs, symbols, and labels
19. Describe fundamental principles for evacuation of a health care setting
20. Discuss fire safety issues in a health care environment
21. Discuss requirements for responding to hazardous material disposal
22. Identify principles of body mechanics and ergonomics
23. Discuss critical elements of an emergency plan for response to a natural disaster or other emergency
24. Identify emergency preparedness plans in your community
25. Discuss potential role(s) of the medical assistant in emergency preparedness
26. List and discuss legal and illegal interview questions
27. Discuss all levels of governmental legislation and regulation as they apply to medical assisting practice, including FDA and DEA regulations
28. Apply local, state and federal health care legislation and regulation appropriate to the medical assisting practice setting
29. Describe basic elements of first aid
30. Identify how the Americans with Disabilities Act (ADA) applies to the medical assisting profession

Psychomotor Domain

1. Create a policy and procedures manual (Procedure 10-1)
2. Perform an office inventory (Procedure 10-2)
3. Perform within scope of practice
4. Select appropriate barrier/personal protective equipment (PPE) for potentially infectious situations
5. Assist physician with patient care

6. Report relevant information to others succinctly and accurately
7. Evaluate the work environment to identify safe versus unsafe working conditions
8. Maintain a current list of community resources for emergency preparedness
9. Develop a personal (patient and employee) safety plan
10. Develop an environmental safety plan
11. Demonstrate proper use of the following equipment: eyewash, fire extinguishers, sharps disposal containers
12. Participate in a mock environmental exposure with documentation of steps taken
13. Explain the evacuation plan for a physician's office
14. Demonstrate methods of fire prevention in the health care setting
15. Complete an incident report
16. Incorporate the Patient's Bill of Rights into personal practice and medical office policies and procedures
17. Apply local, state and federal health care legislation and regulation appropriate to the medical assisting practice setting

Affective Domain

1. Recognize the effects of stress on all persons involved in emergency situations

2. Demonstrate self-awareness in responding to emergency situations
3. Apply active listening skills
4. Use appropriate body language and other nonverbal skills in communicating with patients, family, and staff
5. Recognize the importance of local, state and federal legislation and regulation in the practice setting

ABHES Competencies

1. Perform routine maintenance of administrative and clinical equipment
2. Maintain inventory, equipment and supplies
3. Maintain medical facility
4. Serve as liaison between physician and others
5. Interview effectively
6. Comprehend the current employment outlook for the medical assistant
7. Understand the importance of maintaining liability coverage once employed in the industry
8. Perform risk management procedures
9. Comply with federal, state and local health laws and regulations

Name: _____   Date: _____   Grade: _____

COG MULTIPLE CHOICE

Scenario for questions 1 and 2: It's your first day on the job as the medical office manager, so there's a lot you don't know yet about this office.

1. You want to know who's responsible for what in the office. Where is the best place to find that information?

   a. Payroll records

   b. The work schedule

   c. The chain-of-command chart

   d. The recent employee evaluations

   e. The bulletin board

2. You know the office is running low on paper and syringes. You're most likely to find out how to order supplies in:

   a. the QI plan.

   b. the service contracts folder.

   c. the operating budget.

   d. the policy and procedures manual.

   e. the communication notebook.

3. An MSDS is required to contain:

   a. general information about safety.

   b. a written hazard communication plan.

   c. information regarding hazardous chemicals found in a facility.

   d. the appropriate amount of bleach that can be stored in a medical office.

   e. a complete list of the hazardous materials in a facility.

4. The office keeps running out of tongue depressors. Which action should you take first?

   a. Establish a recycling program.

   b. Determine whether someone is stealing supplies.

   c. Review the system for keeping track of supplies.

   d. Tell the physicians not to use so many tongue depressors.

   e. Borrow some tongue depressors from the nearest medical office.

5. Which item should be in any job description?

   a. Age requirements

   b. Salary or hourly pay

   c. Physical requirements

   d. The preferred gender of the applicant

   e. Medical and dental benefits

6. Which task should you be expected to perform as medical office manager?

   a. Clean the waiting room

   b. Assign someone to make coffee

   c. Develop promotional pamphlets

   d. Assist with simple medical procedures

   e. Sign prescription refills

7. Which of the following is a medical office manager's responsibility?

   a. Completing all incident reports

   b. Teaching CPR

   c. Evaluating the physicians

   d. Hiring and firing employees

   e. Teaching employees about malpractice insurance

8. Which statement is true of an incident report about a patient?

   a. It should be mailed to the attorney of your choice.

   b. It should be written by a physician.

   c. It should be written within 24 hours of the incident.

   d. It should be written from the patient's point of view.

   e. It should be kept in the medical office.

9. Which action should be taken if an employee is stuck by a patient's needle?

   a. The patient should be informed.

   b. The physician should take disciplinary action against the employee.

   c. The employee should write an incident report.

   d. The employee should be kept away from patients.

   e. The employee should sign a form admitting liability.

10. Which of the following categories is part of a capital budget?

    a. Payroll

    b. Medical supplies

    c. Building maintenance

    d. Heating and air conditioning

    e. Electricity

11. Which item should be part of any medical office budget?

    a. Merit bonuses

    b. Billing service

    c. Continuing education

    d. Magazine subscriptions

    e. Children's play facility

12. Which agency licenses and monitors health care organizations and enforces regulations?

    a. CMS

    b. State health department

    c. The Joint Commission

    d. OSHA

    e. HCFA

13. General liability and medical malpractice insurance is for:

    a. all medical professionals.

    b. all physicians.

    c. physicians who perform risky procedures.

    d. medical professionals with high risk profiles.

    e. physicians and nurses.

14. The first step in creating a quality improvement plan is to:

    a. form a task force.

    b. identify the problem.

    c. establish a monitoring plan.

    d. assign an expected threshold.

    e. explore the problem.

15. Which of the following items should be included in an emergency kit?

    a. Alcohol wipes

    b. Syringe

    c. Penicillin

    d. Oscilloscope

    e. Sample containers

16. If you fill out an incident report, you should:

    a. keep a copy of the report.

    b. have a supervisor review it.

    c. give your title but not your name.

    d. fill out only the sections that apply.

    e. summarize what happened in the report.

17. The 2001 discovery of anthrax in an envelope to be delivered to a U.S. Congressman is an example of a(n):

    a. bioterrorist attack.

    b. epidemic.

    c. pandemic.

    d. ergonomics.

    e. ADF.

18. Which of the following is used to estimate expenditures and revenues?

    a. Budget

    b. Tracking file

    c. Expected threshold

    d. Financial statement

    e. Previous expenditures

19. Risk management is a(n):

a. process begun only after a sentinel event.

b. process intended to identify potential problems.

c. external process that deals with OSHA violations.

d. internal process that deals with recurring problems.

e. process undertaken by managers to reduce annual expenditure.

20. Which of the following is true of an expected threshold for a quality improvement program?

a. It is the expected percentage reduction in risk.

b. It is a way to measure the success of the program.

c. It should be set higher for more dangerous problems.

d. It should be set lower than you think you can achieve.

e. It should only be used for particularly severe problems.

21. General liability and medical malpractice insurance is needed:

a. only by employees in offices that use new medical procedures.

b. by physicians sued for malpractice, but not by nurses or office personnel.

c. to protect medical professionals from financial loss due to lawsuits or settlements.

d. because visitors who are hurt in the waiting room can sue unless an incident report is completed.

COG MATCHING   Grade: _____

Match the following key terms to their definitions.

Key Terms

22. _____ bioterrorism

23. _____ body mechanics

24. _____ budget

25. _____ compliance officer

26. _____ epidemic

27. _____ ergonomics

28. _____ expected threshold

29. _____ incident report

30. _____ job description

31. _____ mission statement

32. _____ organizational chart

33. _____ pandemic

34. _____ policy

35. _____ procedure

36. _____ quality improvement

37. _____ task force

Definitions

a. numerical goal for a given problem

b. statement of work-related responsibilities

c. series of steps required to perform a given task

d. written account of untoward patient, visitor, or staff event

e. description of the goals of the practice and whom it serves

f. statement regarding the organization's rules on a given topic

g. purposeful infliction of a dangerous agent into a populated area with intent to harm

h. financial planning tool used to estimate anticipated expenditures and revenues

i. staff member who ensures compliance with the rules and regulations of the office

j. implementation of practices that will help ensure high-quality patient care and service

k. flow sheet that allows staff to identify team members and see where they fit into the team

l. group of employees with different roles brought together to solve a problem

m. using the correct muscles and posture to complete a task safely and efficiently

n. the study of the fit between a worker and his/her physical work environment

o. a disease affecting many people in a specific geographic area

p. a disease infecting numerous people in many areas of the world at the same time

SHORT ANSWER

38. List three responsibilities of the office manager regarding service contractors.

_____

_____

_____

_____

39. List five types of promotional materials that a medical office might use.

_____

_____

_____

_____

40. List six items that should be included in employee fire safety training.

_____

_____

_____

_____

41. List the four basic requirements of the hazard communication standard.

_____

_____

_____

_____

42. List the four basic principles of proper body mechanics.

_____

_____

_____

_____

43. List five techniques used to reduce fatigue as you work.

_____

_____

_____

_____

COG IDENTIFICATION   Grade: _____

44. Below is a list of the steps for creating a quality improvement plan. Put the steps in logical order. Then explain the reason for each step.

Steps

Assign an expected threshold.
Document the entire process.
Establish a monitoring plan.
Explore the problem and propose solutions.
Form a task force.
Identify the problem.
Implement the solution.
Obtain feedback.

Step	Reason
1.	
2.	
3.	
4.	
5.	
6.	
7.	
8.	

COG YES OR NO?   Grade: _____

Answer "Yes," "No," or "Yes But" to the following questions about evaluating employees. If you answer "No" or "Yes But," be able to explain why.

	Yes	No	Yes But …
45. Are employee evaluations your responsibility as a medical office manager?			
46. Should new employees be evaluated annually?			
47. Should you coach new employees about how to do their jobs well?			
48. Can annual performance appraisals be done orally?			
49. Should you communicate with employees about performance problems when one of the physicians asks you to?			
50. Should you inform a good employee yearly that she or he is doing a good job?			

COG IDENTIFICATION   Grade: _____

51. Medical offices usually have an operating budget and a capital budget. Separate the following items into the two categories by checking the column for operating budget or capital budget.

Budget Item	Operating Budget	Capital Budget
a. payroll		
b. medical equipment		
c. office supplies		
d. Internet service		
e. medical supplies		
f. building maintenance		
g. telephone service		
h. electricity		
i. expensive furniture		
j. patient materials		
k. continuing education		

COG **PSY** ACTIVE LEARNING　　　　　　　　　　　　　　　　Grade: _____

52. When you complete your program of study, you would like to find a job as a medical office manager. Write the job description for your ideal job. Be sure to include all the essential elements, including a position summary, hours, location, and duties.

53. Your office manager has assigned you to a task force that will write a plan for fire prevention in your office. Your role in the group is to establish the headings for the plan. List five items that should be included.

_____

_____

_____

_____

54. The task force did such a good job with the last assignment, they are now asked to write the emergency action plan for your office as well. List the six items that should be included.

_____

_____

_____

_____

55. Working together with a partner, search the local classified ads for an open job as a medical office manager. Then prepare to role-play the interview process with your partner, taking turns acting as the interviewer and the interviewee. Make a list of questions that you would ask as both the interviewer and the interviewee. Switch places so you both get to experience the job interview process from each perspective.

_____

_____

_____

_____

COG IDENTIFICATION

Grade: _____

56. Circle all the following tasks that are the responsibility of the medical office manager.

    a. scheduling staff

    b. ordering supplies

    c. writing the budget

    d. keeping up to date on legal issues

    e. assisting with medical procedures

    f. cleaning the office and waiting room

    g. revising policy and procedures manuals

    h. presenting continuing education seminars

    i. developing HIPAA and OSHA regulations

    j. developing promotional pamphlets or newsletters

57. Inventory control is the responsibility of the office manager. On the checklist below, put an **M** beside the inventory tasks the manager should do and an **A** beside the things an assistant or other office staff member can do.

    _____ Receive supplies

    _____ Initial the packing slip

    _____ Develop a system to keep track of supplies

    _____ Determine the procedures for ordering supplies

    _____ Transfer supplies from packing boxes to supply shelves

    _____ Check the packing slip against the actual supply contents

    _____ Keep receipts or packing slips in a bills-pending file for payment

    _____ Develop a process to check that deliveries of supplies are complete and accurate

COG YES OR NO?   Grade: _____

58. Indicate by a check mark in the "Yes" or "No" column whether an item should be included in a medical office's policy and procedures manual.

Policy	Yes	No
a. a chain-of-command chart		
b. a list of employee benefits		
c. infection control guidelines		
d. the office operating budget		
e. annual employee evaluations		
f. procedures for bill collections		
g. copies of completed incident reports		
h. a description of the goals of the practice		
i. responsibilities and procedures for ordering supplies		
j. a list of responsibilities for the last employee to leave the office each day		

COG LISTING   Grade: _____

59. List six of the elements that should be included in any job description.

a. _____

b. _____

c. _____

d. _____

e. _____

f. _____

60. In addition to writing job descriptions and managing employee evaluations, list the three other staffing issues that are the responsibility of the medical office manager?

a. _____

b. _____

c. _____

61. List three services provided by most medical malpractice companies.

a. _____

b. _____

c. _____

COG **FALSE THEN TRUE**   Grade: _____

62. Each of the following statements about incident reports is false or incomplete. Rewrite each statement to make it true and complete.

   a. You should write up an incident report as the event was reported to you.

   _____

   b. The witness should summarize and explain the event.

   _____

   c. You should remain anonymous when you fill out a report.

   _____

   d. The form should be completed within 48 hours of the event.

   _____

   e. If a particular section of the report does not apply, it should be left blank.

   _____

   f. Keep a copy of the incident report for your own personal record.

   _____

   g. If the incident happened to a patient, put a copy of the report in the patient's chart.

   _____

   h. The report should be reviewed by a supervisor to make sure the office is not liable.

   _____

   i. Incident reports are written when negative events happen to patients or visitors.

   _____

COG **MATCHING**   Grade: _____

63. Below is a list of four regulatory agencies that require medical offices to have quality improvement programs. Draw a line between the two columns to match the regulatory agency with its description.

Agencies

1. CMS

2. OSHA

3. The Joint Commission

4. state health department

Descriptions

a. federal agency that regulates and runs Medicare and Medicaid

b. nonfederal agency to license and monitor health care organizations and enforce regulations

c. federal agency that enforces regulations to protect the health and welfare of patients and employees

d. agency that sets voluntary health care standards and evaluates a health care organization's implementation of those standards

COG WHICH IS WHICH?   Grade: _____

64. Explain how quality improvement programs and risk management work together in a medical office.

_____

_____

_____

_____

COG TRUE OR FALSE?   Grade: _____

65. Determine whether the following statements are true or false. If false, explain why.

a. Health care organizations are required to follow the regulations of the Joint Commission.

_____

b. Accreditation by The Joint Commission is valid for 5 years.

_____

c. If The Joint Commission's initial site review identifies unsatisfactory areas, the health care organization may later prove that corrections have been made by passing a focus survey.

_____

d. The health care organization should prepare for the Joint Commission survey by assessing its compliance with OSHA standards.

_____

Grade: _____

66. As you enter the office on the first day of your new job as the medical office manager, you notice a thick layer of dust on the plastic plants in the waiting room and see that the magazines are old and tattered. The staff greets you with enthusiasm, saying you are just what they need to deal with the patients' complaints about spending too much time waiting to be seen. Someone has left an incident report file on your desk. You look through it right away and learn that a needlestick has been reported almost every Wednesday evening for a month. What would you do first, and why?

_____

_____

_____

_____

67. You have a patient who lost her home and several pets to a recent tornado in your city. You know she is at risk for the development of a major psychiatric disorder. What are five ways to help this patient who has been exposed to trauma from natural or manmade disasters?

_____

_____

_____

_____

68. Mrs. Hadley, who is blind and walks with a cane, slipped on the wet floor near a leaky water cooler and fell, cutting her forearm. One of the nurses examined and treated her wound and apologized. Mrs. Hadley said it was no problem and left the office. The nurse told you she wasn't going to file an incident report because the wound was minor and Mrs. Hadley had accepted her apology. As the medical office manager, what should you do?

_____

_____

_____

_____

AFF **CASE STUDY FOR CRITICAL THINKING**   Grade: _____

You have been asked by your physician-employer to inspect the office for possible safety hazards. He wants a report of any negative findings by the end of the week.

69. Circle the most appropriate first step.

   a. Ask if you can assign a task force to help you.

   b. Design a form for checking off items as you inspect them.

   c. Tell him you are too busy with patients to take on such a large task.

   d. Call the local fire department to perform the inspection.

   e. Call the local OSHA representative to perform the inspection.

70. From the following list of actions, circle all that are appropriate.

   a. Check closets for the storage of flammable liquids.

   b. Check areas where oxygen is in use.

   c. Check to be sure all cylinders and tanks that contain flammable gases or liquids are uncapped and ready for use.

   d. Check to see that equipment and carts are on the right side of each hallway.

   e. Check the CMA schedule to be sure there is enough coverage to keep everyone safe.

PSY PROCEDURE 10-1 | Create a Procedures Manual

Name: _____ Date: _____ Time: _____ Grade: _____

EQUIPMENT/SUPPLIES: Word processor, three-ring binder, paper, choose any procedure approved by your instructor

STANDARDS: Given the needed equipment and a place to work the student will perform this skill with _____% accuracy in a total of _____ minutes. *(Your instructor will tell you what the percentage and time limits will be before you begin.)*

KEY: 4 = Satisfactory 0 = Unsatisfactory NA = this step is not counted

PROCEDURE STEPS	SELF	PARTNER	INSTRUCTOR
1. Check the latest information from key governmental agencies, local and state health departments, and health care organizations, such as OSHA, CDC, The Joint Commission, etc. to make sure that the policies and procedures being written comply with federal and state legislation and regulations.	☐	☐	☐
2. Gather product information; consult government agencies, if needed. Secure educational pamphlets.	☐	☐	☐
3. Title the procedure properly.	☐	☐	☐
4. Number the procedure appropriately.	☐	☐	☐
5. Define the overall purpose of the procedure in a sentence or two explaining the intent of the procedure.	☐	☐	☐
6. List all necessary equipment and forms. Include everything needed to complete the task.	☐	☐	☐
7. List each step with its rationale.	☐	☐	☐
8. Provide spaces for signatures.	☐	☐	☐
9. Record the date the procedure was written.	☐	☐	☐
10. **AFF** Describe how you would explain to employees why they were asked to work in a group to create a procedure manual.	☐	☐	☐

CALCULATION

Total Possible Points: _____

Total Points Earned: _____ Multiplied by 100 = _____ Divided by Total Possible Points = _____ %

PASS	FAIL	COMMENTS:
☐	☐	

Student's signature _____ Date _____

Partner's signature _____ Date _____

Instructor's signature _____ Date _____

PSY PROCEDURE 10-2 Perform an Office Inventory

Name: _____ Date: _____ Time: _____ Grade: _____

EQUIPMENT: Inventory form, reorder form

STANDARDS: Given the needed equipment and a place to work the student will perform this skill with _____%
accuracy in a total of _____ minutes. *(Your instructor will tell you what the percentage and time limits will be
before you begin.)*

KEY: 4 = Satisfactory   0 = Unsatisfactory   NA = this step is not counted

PROCEDURE STEPS	SELF	PARTNER	INSTRUCTOR
1. Using forms supplied by your instructor, count and record the amounts of specified supplies	☐	☐	☐
2. Record amount of each item.	☐	☐	☐
3. Compare amount on hand with amount needed.	☐	☐	☐
4. Complete reorder form based on these numbers.	☐	☐	☐
5. Submit reorder forms to office manager.	☐	☐	☐
6. Document your actions per the ordering procedure.	☐	☐	☐
7. AFF Explain how you would respond to an employee who continually takes a vacation day when the office plans to take inventory.	☐	☐	☐

CALCULATION

Total Possible Points: _____

Total Points Earned: _____ Multiplied by 100 = _____ Divided by Total Possible Points = _____ %

PASS   **FAIL**   **COMMENTS:**
☐   ☐

Student's signature _____ Date _____

Partner's signature _____ Date _____

Instructor's signature _____ Date _____

WORK PRODUCT 1   Grade: _____

USE METHODS OF QUALITY CONTROL

Louise Baggins, a 55-year-old patient, was visiting the physician for a physical exam. While waiting for her appointment, she asked you to direct her to the restroom. On her way into the restroom, she slipped and fell on a magazine that had fallen on the floor in the reception area. You did not see her fall, but she yelled out in pain after she fell. She was able to get up on her own but injured her wrist. Her wrist was immediately red, swollen, and painful to touch. Dr. Mikuski looked at her wrist and suggested she go to the hospital emergency room to have x-rays. You called an ambulance to transfer Mrs. Baggins to the hospital. Fill in the incident report below to document this event.

Workplace Requirements Program for Safety and Health

SUPERVISOR'S ACCIDENT REPORT FORM

This form is to be completed by the supervisor and forwarded to the Payroll Coordinator along with a copy of the North Carolina Industrial Commission Form 19 (Workers Compensation Form) within five days of the accident. All accidents involving serious bodily injury or death must be reported to the safety and health officer immediately.

ACCIDENT DATA

1. NAME OF EMPLOYEE:
or Patient

2. ADDRESS AND PHONE NO:

3. WORK DEPT. OR DIVISION: 4. SEX: ☐ MALE   ☐ FEMALE   5. DATE AND TIME OF INJURY:

6. NATURE OF INJURY: 7. PART OF BODY INJURED:

8. CAUSE OF INJURY: 9. LOCATION OF ACCIDENT:

10. OCCUPATION AND ACTIVITY OF PERSON AT TIME OF ACCIDENT: 11. STATUS OF JOB OR ACTIVITY: (CHOOSE ONE)

Halted

12. NAME AND PHONE NO. OF ACCIDENT WITNESS:

13. LIST UNSAFE ACT, IF ANY:

14. LIST UNSAFE PHYSICAL OR MECHANICAL CONDITION, IF ANY:

15. UNSAFE PERSONAL FACTOR:

16. LIST HAZARD CONTROLS IN EFFECT AT TIME OF INJURY DESIGNED TO PREVENT INJURY:

17. PERSONAL PROTECTIVE EQUIPMENT BEING USED AT TIME OF ACCIDENT:

GLOVES, SAFETY GLASSES, GOGGLES, FACE SHIELD, OTHER

18. BRIEF DESCRIPTION OF ACCIDENT:

19. CORRECTIVE ACTION TAKEN OR RECOMMENDED TO DEPARTMENT SAFETY COMMITTEE:

TREATMENT DATA

20. WAS INJURED TAKEN TO (CHOOSE ONE): Hospital

21. DIAGNOSIS AND TREATMENT, IF KNOWN:

22. ESTIMATED LOST WORKDAYS: _____   23. DATE OF REPORT:
(EXCLUDING DAY OF ACCIDENT)   Month   Day   Year

24. REPORT PREPARED BY:

25. SIGNATURE OF SUPERVISOR:

26. SIGNATURE OF AGENCY SAFETY AND HEALTH OFFICER:

WORK PRODUCT 2

USE METHODS OF QUALITY CONTROL

After Mrs. Baggins fell in the reception area (see Work Product 1), your supervisor asks you to review any other injuries in the reception area in the past 6 months. There are seven incident reports involving patient falls, and all of those occurred in some part of the reception area. Three patients slipped by the doorway on rainy days. Two more tripped on the corner of the doormat. The last two patients fell in the main lobby—one tripped over a children's toy, and the other slipped on a magazine, just like Mrs. Baggins did.

You are named to represent the medical assistants on a task force addressing these complaints. Assign an expected threshold using measurable, realistic goals. Explore the problem and propose solutions. Establish a QI monitoring plan explaining how data will be collected. Document the entire process and print the information to attach to this sheet. Using the blank memorandum below, write a memo to the staff with instructions to implement the solutions.

Memo

To:

From:

Date:

Re:

UNIT
THREE

Managing the Finances in the Practice

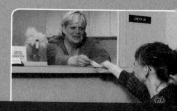

CHAPTER

11

Credit and Collections

Learning
Outcomes

Cognitive Domain

1. Spell and define the key terms
2. Discuss physician's fee schedules
3. Discuss forms of payment
4. Explain the legal considerations in extending credit
5. Discuss the legal implications of credit collection
6. Discuss procedures for collecting outstanding accounts
7. Describe the impact of both the Fair Debt Collection Act and the Federal Truth in Lending Act of 1968 as they apply to collections
8. Describe the concept of RBRVS
9. Define Diagnosis-Related Groups (DRGs)
10. Describe the implications of HIPAA for the medical assistant in various medical settings
11. Discuss all levels of government legislation and regulation as they apply to medical assisting practice, including FDA and DEA regulations

Psychomotor Domain

1. Evaluate and manage a patient account (Procedure 11-1)
2. Write a collection letter (Procedure 11-2)
3. Perform collection procedures

Affective Domain

1. Apply ethical behaviors, including honesty and integrity in performance of medical assisting practice
2. Demonstrate sensitivity and professionalism in handling accounts receivable activities with clients
3. Demonstrate sensitivity to patient rights
4. Recognize the importance of local, state, and federal legislation and regulations in the practice setting

ABHES Competencies

1. Perform billing and collection procedures
2. Use physician fee schedule

Name: _____   Date: _____   Grade: _____

COG MULTIPLE CHOICE

1. The total of all the charges posted to patients' accounts for the month of May is $16,000. The revenues the practice received for May total $12,000. What is the collection percentage for May?

   a. 5%

   b. 25%

   c. 75%

   d. 80%

   e. 133%

2. Interest that may be charged to a patient account is determined by:

   a. the physician.

   b. the patient.

   c. the insurance company.

   d. the law.

   e. the state.

3. In the UCR concept, the letters stand for:

   a. user, customer, and regulation.

   b. usual, competitive, and regular.

   c. usage, consumption, and return.

   d. usual, customary, and reasonable.

   e. usage, complaint, and rationale.

4. When credit cards are accepted by a medical practice, the medical practice generally agrees to pay the credit card company:

   a. 5.2%.

   b. 1.8%.

   c. 15%.

   d. 3.1%

   e. 25%.

5. Federal regulations require each medical office to describe its services and procedures and to give the procedure codes and prices by:

   a. giving a list to each patient at check in.

   b. offering the list to each patient at payment.

   c. posting a sign stating that a list is available.

   d. answering a patient's questions about billing.

   e. placing an ad in the newspaper describing the fees.

6. Physicians who chose to become participating providers with third-party payers usually do so in order to:

   a. charge higher fees.

   b. simplify fee schedules.

   c. build a solid patient base.

   d. reduce the time before payment.

   e. share a patient load with another physician.

7. It is a good and ethical business practice to:

   a. take payment in cash only.

   b. accept only patients who have insurance.

   c. refuse patients who have third-party payment plans.

   d. discuss fees with patients before they see a physician or nurse.

   e. charge the patient a small fee for paying with a credit card.

8. When dealing with a new patient, you should avoid:

   a. taking cash.

   b. taking a partial payment.

   c. taking a check with two picture IDs.

   d. taking co-payment with an insurance card.

   e. taking a payment by credit card.

9. Most fees for medical services:

   a. are paid by insurance companies.

   b. are paid by Medicare and Medicaid.

   c. are paid by patients who are private payers.

   d. are written off on the practice's federal taxes.

   e. are paid to the physician late.

10. When an insurance adjustment is made to a fee:

    a. the patient is charged less than the normal rate.

    b. the medical office receives more than its normal rate.

    c. the insurance carrier pays the adjustment rate.

    d. the insurance carrier's explanation of benefits shows how much the office may collect for the service.

    e. the difference between the physician's normal fee and the insurance carrier's allowed fee is written off.

11. Why would a medical office extend credit to a patient?

    a. To save money

    b. To accommodate the patient

    c. To postpone paying income tax

    d. To charge interest

    e. To make billing more cost effective

12. Why do many medical offices outsource their credit and billing functions?

    a. They don't want to ask their patients for money directly.

    b. They are not licensed to manage credit card transactions.

    c. Creating their own installment plans is too complicated legally.

    d. Managing patient accounts themselves costs about $5 per month per patient.

    e. Billing companies can manage the accounts more cost effectively.

13. It is illegal for a medical office to:

    a. use a collection agency.

    b. disclose fee information to patients who have insurance.

    c. deny credit to patients because they receive public assistance.

    d. charge patients interest, finance charges, or late fees on unpaid balances.

    e. change their established billing cycle

14. If you are attempting to collect a debt from a patient, you must:

    a. use reasonable self-restraint.

    b. call the patient only at home.

    c. hire a licensed bill collection agency.

    d. first take the patient to small claims court.

    e. wait one year before you can ask for payment.

15. When first attempting to collect a debt by telephone, you should:

    a. ask the patient to come in for a checkup.

    b. contact the patient before 8:00 a.m. or after 9:00 p.m.

    c. contact the patient only at his place of employment.

    d. leave a message explaining the situation on the answering machine.

    e. speak only to the patient or leave only your first name and number.

16. When you are collecting a debt from an estate, it is best to:

    a. send a final bill to the estate's executor.

    b. take the matter directly to small claims court.

    c. try to collect within a week of the patient's death.

    d. allow the family a month to mourn before asking for payment.

    e. ask a collection agency to contact the family.

17. If a billing cycle is to be changed, you are legally required to notify patients:

   a. 1 month before their payment is due.

   b. before the next scheduled appointment.

   c. 3 months prior to the billing change.

   d. after you approve the change with the insurance company.

   e. only if they have outstanding payments.

18. When you age an account, you:

   a. write off debts that have been outstanding longer than 120 days.

   b. send bills first to the patients who had the most recent procedures.

   c. organize patient accounts by how long they have been seeing the physician.

   d. calculate the time between the last bill and the date of the last payment.

   e. determine the time between the procedure and the date of the last payment.

19. A cancellation of an unpaid debt is called a(n):

   a. professional courtesy.

   b. co-payment.

   c. write-off.

   d. adjustment.

   e. credit.

20. Which collections method takes the least staff time?

   a. Using a collection agency

   b. Going to small claims court

   c. Billing the patient monthly until paid

   d. Scheduling all payments on the first of the month

   e. Reporting patients to the credit bureaus

COG MATCHING

Grade: _____

Match the following key terms to their definitions.

Key Terms

21. _____ adjustment

22. _____ aging schedule

23. _____ collections

24. _____ credit

25. _____ installment

26. _____ participating provider

27. _____ patient co-payment

28. _____ professional courtesy

29. _____ write-off

Definitions

a. change in a posted account

b. balance in one's favor on an account.

c. process of seeking payment for overdue bills

d. arrangement for a patient to pay on an installment plan

e. charging other health care professionals a reduced rate

f. cancellation of an unpaid debt.

g. a certain share of the bill that a managed care company usually requires the patient to pay

h. physician who agrees to participate with managed care companies and other third-party payers

i. record of a patient's name, balance, payments made, time of outstanding debt, and relevant comments

Grade: _____

30. Fee setting also considers RBRVS, by which fees are adjusted for geographical differences. What does RBRVS stand for?

_____

_____

_____

_____

31. There should be a sign posted in the office, where patients can see it, giving information about procedure fees. What should be on the sign?

_____

_____

_____

_____

32. Which third-party payers affect fee schedules if the physicians in your office are participating providers, and how many fee schedules might there be?

_____

_____

_____

_____

33. How many times should you contact patients asking them to pay overdue bills? Why?

_____

_____

_____

34. How often should you ask the patient for his or her insurance card, and what should you do with it when you get it?

_____

_____

_____

_____

35. What are the three most common ways of collecting overdue accounts?

_____

_____

_____

_____

36. What are some of the negative aspects of extending credit to patients? Consider costs, patient attitudes, and legal requirements in your answer.

_____

_____

_____

_____

COG ACTIVE LEARNING

Grade: _____

37. Use the Internet to research the three major credit bureaus and find out how to check a new patient's credit history. Specifically, find out what's available to help you decide how to handle payment from people without traditional credit histories. This group includes college students, young adults, recent immigrants, traditional housewives, and people who choose not to use credit cards.

38. Many people feel uncomfortable asking other people for money. However, you need to feel comfortable discussing finance and account information with patients. Working with a partner, role-play a scenario in which a patient has an overdue account that the medical assistant must address. Take turns playing the parts of the medical assistant and the patient to understand both perspectives.

39. In recent years, the government has called into question the practice of professional courtesy extended to other health care professionals. Perform research online or talk to health care professionals to find out more about the issues surrounding professional courtesy. Then write a viewpoint paper arguing for or against the practice of professional courtesy.

COG **FALSE THEN TRUE**   Grade: _____

40. All the statements below are false or inaccurate. Rewrite each statement so that it accurately reflects the consumer protection laws regarding credit collection.

a. You cannot contact a patient directly about an unpaid bill.

_____

b. You should not try to contact a debtor before 9:00 a.m. or after 5:00 p.m.

_____

c. You have every right to call debtors at work.

_____

d. You should keep calling a patient about a debt after turning the case over to a collection agency, in order to increase your chances of recovering the money.

_____

e. It's okay to use abusive language to intimidate a debtor, as long as you don't give false or misleading information.

_____

f. If a patient dies and the estate can't meet all of his or her debts, the probate court will pay the medical bills first.

_____

COG **SHORT ANSWER**   Grade: _____

41. List three situations in which calling a patient to collect an overdue payment may be least helpful.

_____

_____

_____

_____

42. What should be in a mailing that asks a patient to settle an overdue account?

_____

_____

_____

43. What is a good way to use a patient's visit as an opportunity to try to collect payment on an overdue bill?

_____

_____

_____

_____

44. What should you say and not say if you call a patient to collect on a bill and you are asked to leave a message?

_____

_____

_____

_____

COG TRUE OR FALSE?   Grade: _____

45. Determine whether the following statements are true or false. If false, explain why.

a. A physician's fee schedule takes into consideration the costs of operating the office, such as rent, utilities, malpractice insurance, and salaries.

_____

b. If a patient has insurance, you must charge him the insurance carrier's allowed fee for a procedure.

_____

c. To maintain good relations with patients, you should be vague and polite when you ask them to pay their bills.

_____

d. You should monitor the activity on a patient's credit account in order to keep the collection ratio low.

_____

46. You have several patients who have long-standing debts. They don't come into the office anymore, and they don't respond to your telephone calls or letters. You outsourced your overdue billing to a collections agency but these longtime patients have told you that they have been very upset by the "nastiness" of the collections people who contacted them.

    You spoke with a collections agency representative who assured you his employees were doing nothing illegal or inappropriate. You have considered changing collection agencies; but this one's rates are better, and they did collect the debts. What would you do?

    _____

    _____

    _____

    _____

47. Mrs. Sanchez is seeing Dr. Roland for the first time and has asked you to explain the physician's fees. How would you explain to Mrs. Sanchez how Dr. Roland establishes the fees he charges his patients?

    _____

    _____

    _____

    _____

AFF **CASE STUDY FOR CRITICAL THINKING**   Grade: _____

Mr. Green has been a patient with your practice for more than 20 years and has always paid his co-payment or bill before he left the office. Recently, however, he has not been paying anything at all, and his outstanding bill is 60 days past due. You have called his home and left several phone messages, but you still haven't heard from him.

48. What should you do? Circle all appropriate actions from the following list.

   a. Send him a letter demanding that he pay his balance immediately.

   b. Flag his account for the credit manager to speak with him about his bill when he comes in for a visit.

   c. Send a letter asking him to please call the office. State in the letter that you are worried about him.

   d. Flag his record to warn anyone making an appointment for him that he is not to be seen until he pays on his bill.

   e. Terminate the physician-patient contract in writing.

49. A coworker tells you that the patient is very rich. She says that he is just getting old and can't keep up with his bills any longer. Circle all appropriate actions in the list below.

   a. Tell the coworker to mind her own business.

   b. Do not consider this gossip in your dealings with the patient.

   c. Contact the patient's next of kin and tell them that he needs help.

   d. Send the patient a letter telling him you know he has the funds to pay his bill.

   e. Do nothing until you reach the patient.

   f. Do not mention this new information when you do speak with him.

PSY PROCEDURE 11-1 | **Evaluate and Manage a Patient's Account**

Name: _____ Date: _____ Time: _____ Grade: _____

EQUIPMENT: Simulation including scenario; sample patient ledger card with transactions; yellow, blue, and red stickers (yellow for accounts 30 days past due; blue for accounts 60 days past due; red for accounts 90 days past due). See Work Product 1.

STANDARDS: Given the needed equipment and a place to work the student will perform this skill with _____% accuracy in a total of _____ minutes. *(Your instructor will tell you what the percentage and time limits will be before you begin.)*

KEY: 4 = Satisfactory   0 = Unsatisfactory   NA = This step is not counted

PROCEDURE STEPS	SELF	PARTNER	INSTRUCTOR
1. Review the patient's account history to determine the "age" of the account. If payment has not been made between 30 and 59 days from today's date, the account is 40 days past due, and so on.	☐	☐	☐
2. Flag the account for appropriate action. Place a yellow flag (sticker) on accounts that are 30 days old. Place a blue flag on accounts that are 60 days old. Place a red flag on accounts that are 90 days old.	☐	☐	☐
3. Set aside accounts that have had no payment in 91 days or longer.	☐	☐	☐
4. Make copies of the ledger cards.	☐	☐	☐
5. Sort the copies by category: 30, 60, 90 days.	☐	☐	☐
6. Write or stamp the copies with the appropriate message.	☐	☐	☐
7. Mail the statements to the patients.	☐	☐	☐
8. Follow through with the collection process by continually reviewing past due accounts.	☐	☐	☐
9. **AFF** When you call a patient with a seriously past due account, he informs you that he has not paid because his wife passed away and he cannot hardly get through the day. Explain how you would respond.	☐	☐	☐

CALCULATION

Total Possible Points: _____

Total Points Earned: _____ Multiplied by 100 = _____ Divided by Total Possible Points = _____ %

PASS   **FAIL**   **COMMENTS:**

☐   ☐

Student's signature _____ Date _____

Partner's signature _____ Date _____

Instructor's signature _____ Date _____

PSY PROCEDURE 11-2 | **Composing a Collection Letter**

Name: _____ Date: _____ Time: _____ Grade: _____

EQUIPMENT: Ledger cards generated in Procedure 11-1, word processor, stationery with letterhead

STANDARDS: Given the needed equipment and a place to work the student will perform this skill with ____% accuracy in a total of ____ minutes. *(Your instructor will tell you what the percentage and time limits will be before you begin.)*

KEY: 4 = Satisfactory   0 = Unsatisfactory   NA = This step is not counted

PROCEDURE STEPS	SELF	PARTNER	INSTRUCTOR
1. Review the patients' accounts and sort the accounts by age.	☐	☐	☐
2. Design a rough draft of a form letter that can be used for collections.	☐	☐	☐
3. In the first paragraph, tell the patient why you are writing.	☐	☐	☐
4. Inform the patient of the action you expect. For example: "To avoid further action, please pay $50.00 on this account by Friday, May 1, 20__."	☐	☐	☐
5. Proofread the rough draft for errors, clarity, accuracy, and retype.	☐	☐	☐
6. Take the collection letter to a supervisor or physician for approval.	☐	☐	☐
7. Fill in the appropriate amounts and dates on each letter. Ask for at least half of the account balance within a 2-week period.	☐	☐	☐
8. Print, sign, and mail the letter.	☐	☐	☐
9. **AFF** You are helping a coworker get her collections letters in the mail. You notice several errors in the letters. Explain how you would respond.	☐	☐	☐

_____

_____

_____

_____

CALCULATION

Total Possible Points: _____

Total Points Earned: _____ Multiplied by 100 = _____ Divided by Total Possible Points = _____ %

PASS   **FAIL**   **COMMENTS:**
☐   ☐

Student's signature _____ Date _____

Partner's signature _____ Date _____

Instructor's signature _____ Date _____

WORK PRODUCT 1

Grade: _____

PERFORM ACCOUNTS RECEIVABLE PROCEDURES

Your office's billing cycle posts bills on the first of every month. Review the list of outstanding payments and organize in the Aging of Accounts Receivable Report below.

- Oliver Santino visited the office on April 27 for a physical and blood work. The bill was $250.
- Warren Gates visited the office on May 8. His bill was $55.
- Tamara Jones visited the office on June 18 for a physical. The cost for the physical was $125, with an additional $55 for lab work.
- Amir Shell visited the office on June 25 for a physical exam and chest x-rays. The bill was $315.
- Nora Stevenson visited the office on July 9 to have a wound sutured. The bill was $100.

Below is an aging schedule as of August 30, 2012. Fill in the information for these patients. You may enter an account number of 000-00-0000 for all patients.

Aging of Accounts Receivable Report: August 30, 2012

Patient Name	Account Number	Due Date	Amount

Accounts 30 Days Past Due:

Accounts 60 Days Past Due:

Accounts 90 Days Past Due:

Accounts 120 Days or More Past Due:

Total Overdue Accounts Receivable _____

WORK PRODUCT 2

Grade: _____

PERFORM BILLING AND COLLECTION PROCEDURES

Caroline Cusick has an outstanding balance of $415 due to the medical office Pediatric Associates, 1415 San Juan Way, Santa Cruz, CA 95060. Write a collection letter to the patient to tell her about her overdue account. Her contact information is as follows: Caroline Cusick, 24 Beach Street, Santa Cruz, CA 95060. Print the letter and attach to this sheet.

Accounting Responsibilities

Cognitive Domain

1. Spell and define the key terms
2. Explain the concept of the pegboard bookkeeping system
3. Describe the components of the pegboard system
4. Identify and discuss the special features of the pegboard daysheet
5. Describe the functions of a computer accounting system
6. List the uses and components of computer accounting reports
7. Explain banking services, including types of accounts and fees
8. Describe the accounting cycle
9. Describe the components of a record-keeping system
10. Explain the process of ordering supplies and paying invoices
11. Explain basic booking computations
12. Differentiate between bookkeeping and accounting
13. Describe banking procedures
14. Discuss predations for accepting checks
15. Compare types of endorsement
16. Differentiate between accounts payable and accounts receivable
17. Compare manual and computerized bookkeeping systems used in ambulatory health care
18. Describe common periodic financial reports
19. Explain billing and payment options
20. Identify procedure for preparing patient accounts
21. Discuss types of adjustments that may be made to a patient's account

Psychomotor Domain

1. Prepare a bank deposit (Procedure 12-9)
2. Perform accounts receivable procedures, including:
   a. Post entries on a daysheet (Procedures 12-1, 12-2)
   b. Perform billing procedures
   c. Perform collection procedures
   d. Post adjustments (Procedure 12-5)
   e. Process a credit balance (Procedure 12-3)
   f. Process refunds (Procedure 12-4)
   g. Post non-sufficient fund (NSF) checks (Procedure 12-7)
   h. Post collection agency payments (Procedure 12-6)
3. Balance a daysheet (Procedure 12-8)
4. Reconcile a bank statement (Procedure 12-10)
5. Maintain a petty cash account (Procedure 12-11)
6. Order supplies (Procedure 12-12)
7. Write a check (Procedure 12-13)

Affective Domain

1. Apply ethical behaviors, including honesty and integrity in performance of medical assisting practice
2. Apply local, state and federal health care legislation and regulation appropriate to the medical assisting practice setting
3. Demonstrate sensitivity and professionalism in handling accounts receivable activities with clients

ABHES Competencies

1. Prepare and reconcile a bank statement and deposit record
2. Post entries on a daysheet
3. Perform billing and collection procedures
4. Perform accounts receivable procedures
5. Use physician fee schedule
6. Establish and maintain a petty cash fund
7. Post adjustments
8. Process credit balance
9. Process refunds
10. Post non-sufficient funds (NSF)
11. Post collection agency payments
12. Use manual or computerized bookkeeping systems

Name: _____   Date: _____   Grade: _____

COG MULTIPLE CHOICE

1. The best place to put petty cash is:

 a. in the same drawer as the other cash and checks.

 b. in a separate, secured drawer.

 c. in an envelope stored in the staff room.

 d. in the physician's office.

 e. in a locked supply cabinet.

2. Which of the following information is found on a patient's ledger card?

 a. Date of birth

 b. Social Security number

 c. Blood type

 d. Insurance information

 e. Marital status

3. The purpose of the posting proofs section is to:

 a. enter the day's totals and balance the daysheet.

 b. update and maintain a patient's financial record.

 c. make note of any credit the patient has on file.

 d. make note of any debit the patient has on file.

 e. allow for any adjustments that need to be made.

4. Which of the following might you purchase using petty cash?

 a. Cotton swabs

 b. Thermometer covers

 c. Office supplies

 d. Non-latex gloves

 e. New x-ray machine

Scenario for questions 5 and 6: A new patient comes in and gives you his insurance card. The patient's insurance allows $160.00 for a routine checkup. Of this, insurance will pay 75% of his bill. The actual price of the checkup is $160.00.

5. How much will the patient need to pay?

 a. $0

 b. $40.00

 c. $120.00

 d. $75.00

 e. $160.00

6. How much will the insurance company pay?

 a. $120.00

 b. $40.00

 c. $160.00

 d. $32.00

 e. $0

7. A check register is used to:

 a. hold checks until they are ready for deposit.

 b. create a checklist of daily office duties.

 c. make a list of payments the office is still owed.

 d. record all checks that go in and out of the office.

 e. remind patients when their payments are due.

8. Ideally if you are using a pegboard accounting system, what is the best way to organize your ledgers?

 a. File all ledgers alphabetically in a single tray.

 b. Alphabetically file paid ledgers in one tray and ledgers with outstanding balances in another.

 c. Numerically file paid ledgers in the front of the tray and ledgers with outstanding balances in the back.

 d. Alphabetically file paid ledgers into the patient's folders and ledgers with outstanding balances in a tray.

 e. file all ledgers into the patient's files.

9. Accounts receivable is:

 a. a record of all monies due to the practice.

 b. the people the practice owes money to.

 c. the transactions transferred from a different office.

 d. any outstanding inventory bills.

 e. a list of patients who have paid in the last month.

CHAPTER 12 • Accounting Responsibilities 187

10. It is unsafe to use credit card account numbers on purchases made:

    a. over the phone.

    b. by fax.

    c. through e-mail.

    d. from a catalog.

    e. in person.

11. When you have a deposit that includes cash, what is the only way you should get it to the bank?

    a. Deliver it by hand.

    b. Deliver it into a depository.

    c. Send it by mail with enough postage.

    d. Deliver checks by mail and cash by hand.

    e. Do not accept cash as payment.

12. Which of the following is a benefit of paying bills by computer?

    a. You do not need to keep a record of paying your bills.

    b. Entering data into the computer is quick and easy.

    c. Information can be "memorized" and stored.

    d. You can divide columns into groups of expenses (rent, paychecks, etc.).

    e. You can easily correct any errors.

13. Most medical offices generally use:

    a. standard business checks.

    b. certified checks.

    c. traveler's checks.

    d. money orders.

    e. cash deposits.

14. What is a quick way to find order numbers when making a purchase?

    a. Check the packing slip of a previous order.

    b. Find a previous bill for any item numbers.

    c. Check past purchase orders for their order numbers.

    d. Call the supplier for a list of item numbers.

    e. Look at the supplier's Web site.

15. Summation reports are:

    a. lists of all the clients who entered the office.

    b. reports that track all expenses and income.

    c. computer reports that compile all daily totals.

    d. lists that analyze an office's activities.

    e. reports the IRS sends an office being audited.

16. Why is the adjustment column so important?

    a. It assists you in deciding the discount percentage.

    b. It records all transactions a patient has made in your office.

    c. It allows you to add discounts and credit to change the total.

    d. It keeps track of any changes a patient has in health care.

    e. It keeps track of bounced checks.

17. Which of the following is NOT an important reason for performing an office inventory of equipment and supplies?

    a. It will help you know when to order new supplies and/or equipment.

    b. It will help you calculate how much money you will need to spend on new equipment.

    c. It will alert you of any misuse/theft of supplies or equipment.

    d. The information will be needed for tax purposes.

    e. It will help you see if you will have excess supplies to share with employees.

18. In a bookkeeping system, things of value relating to the practice are called:

    a. assets.

    b. liabilities.

    c. debits.

    d. credits.

    e. audits.

19. The amount of capital the physician has invested in the practice is referred to as:

a. assets.

b. credits.

c. equity.

d. liabilities.

e. invoices.

20. Overpayments under $5 are generally:

a. sent back to the patient.

b. placed in petty cash.

c. left on the account as a credit.

d. deposited in a special overpayment account.

e. mailed to the insurance company.

COG MATCHING

Grade: _____

Match the following key terms to their definitions.

Key Terms

21. _____ accounting cycle

22. _____ accounts payable

23. _____ adjustment

24. _____ audit

25. _____ balance

26. _____ bookkeeping

27. _____ charge slip

28. _____ check register

29. _____ check stub

30. _____ credit

31. _____ daysheet

32. _____ debit

33. _____ encounter form

34. _____ Internal Revenue Service (IRS)

35. _____ invoice

36. _____ liabilities

37. _____ ledger card

Definitions

a. a preprinted three-part form that can be placed on a daysheet to record the patient's charges and payments along with other information in an encounter form

b. a charge or money owed to an account

c. a record of all money owed to the business

d. a document that accompanies a supply order and lists the enclosed items

e. any report that provides a summary of activities, such as a payroll report or profit-and-loss statement

f. a daily business record of charges and payments

g. a statement of income and expenditures; shows whether in a given period a business made or lost money and how much

h. statement of debt owed; a bill

i. a review of an account

j. a consecutive 12-month period for financial record keeping following either a fiscal year or the calendar year

k. a balance in one's favor on an account; a promise to pay a bill at a later date; record of payment received

l. listing financial transactions in a ledger

m. a continuous record of business transactions with debits and credits

n. change in a posted account

o. a federal agency that regulates and enforces various taxes

p. amount of money a bank or business charges for a check written on an account with insufficient funds

q. amounts of money the practice owes

r. organized and accurate record-keeping system of financial transactions

s. a document that lists required items to be purchased

38. _____ packing slip

39. _____ posting

40. _____ profit-and-loss statement

41. _____ purchase order

42. _____ returned check fee

43. _____ service charge

44. _____ summation report

t. preprinted patient statement that lists codes for basic office charges and has sections to record charges incurred in an office visit, the patient's current balance, and next appointment

u. that which is left over after the additions and subtractions have been made to an account

v. piece of paper that indicates to whom a check was issued, in what amount, and on what date

w. a document used to record the checks that have been written

x. a charge by a bank for various services

COG SHORT ANSWER   Grade: _____

45. What are banking services?

_____

_____

_____

_____

46. Why is correction fluid not used in a medical office, and what is the proper procedure to correct a mistake?

_____

_____

_____

_____

47. What are four steps you can take if an item you ordered was not delivered?

_____

_____

_____

48. List four items that should be readily available in case your office is audited.

_____

_____

_____

_____

49. What is a returned check fee?

_____

_____

_____

_____

50. Why might you run a trial daily report before you run a final daily report?

_____

_____

_____

_____

51. The office you are working in has recently updated its bookkeeping system from pegboard to computer. Now, the physician wants to utilize all the capabilities the new system offers. One particular function that interests her is the computer accounting reports. List the different types of reports and briefly describe their uses.

_____

_____

_____

_____

COG **PSY** **ACTIVE LEARNING** Grade: _____

52. During a staff meeting, the issue of ordering supplies comes up. The office has been buying small quantities of all supplies, causing some items to quickly run out, while others are stockpiled in disuse. The head physician wants to figure out a way to spend the budget more efficiently, and asks you to be in charge of the next order. What steps can you take to determine which items you will order in the office's next purchase? How can you further improve the office's expenditure?

_____

_____

_____

_____

53. Your office currently is using a checking account at a local bank. However, the physician you work for is thinking about changing over to a money market account, because he has heard the interest is much better in a money market account. He knows about an offer through another bank that will waive the minimum balance of $500 for 3 months. What important information should you look into before you give him your opinion? Discuss the differences between a checking account and a money market account, and include the advantages and disadvantages to switching accounts.

_____

_____

_____

_____

COG **IDENTIFICATION** Grade: _____

54. There are several advantages of a computerized system over a manual system. Read the selection below, and circle the functions that are computerized accounting functions only.

  a. Entries are recorded in a patient's file.

  b. Quickly create invoices and receipts.

  c. Calculation of each transaction is made, as well as a total at the end of the day.

  d. Performs bookkeeping, making appointments, and generating office reports.

  e. Daily activities are recorded.

  f. Bill reminders are placed to keep track of expenses.

55. A medical office is just starting up, and one of the first things the bookkeeper needs to do is find a bank. Fill in the chart below with descriptions of checking, savings, and money market accounts.

Checking Account	Savings Account	Money Market Account

56. The office you are working in has an accounting cycle that begins in June. Describe what the accounting cycle is, and what kind of year your office follows.

_____

_____

_____

_____

57. The office manager ordered a new endorsement stamp from the bank. In the meantime, you need to deposit a check for Rinku Banjere, MD, into account number 123-4567-890. Endorse the check below for deposit.

ENDORSE HERE

_____

_____

_____

DO NOT SIGN/WRITE/STAMP BELOW THIS LINE
FOR FINANCIAL INSTITUTION USE ONLY*

PSY **WHAT WOULD YOU DO?**

Grade: _____

58. A patient's check has been returned for insufficient funds. The patient asks you to send it back through the bank. What would you do?

_____

_____

_____

_____

59. Explain the process of ordering supplies and paying invoices.

_____

_____

_____

_____

COG **TRUE OR FALSE?**

Grade: _____

Determine whether the following statements are true or false. If false, explain why.

60. Once you have entered a patient transaction on the daysheet, you give the ledger to the patient as a receipt.

_____

61. As long as your bookkeeping records are accurate and the figures balance, you do not need to save receipts.

_____

62. You should always compare the prices and quality of office supplies when you are placing an order.

_____

63. Audits are performed in the office yearly by the IRS.

_____

64. Packing slips are used by the manufacturer and can be destroyed upon opening a package of supplies.

_____

COG PATIENT EDUCATION

Grade: _____

65. Your patient is a young woman who does not understand what happens to the difference between what a physician charges and what her insurance company will pay. In her case, the physician's charge is $100, but insurance only allows for $80. The insurance company will pay for 75% of the cost. How much will the patient pay? Explain to her how this works, and how the charge is determined.

_____

_____

_____

_____

AFF CASE STUDY FOR CRITICAL THINKING

Grade: _____

You have been working at a small, one-physician practice for about 2 weeks. You share the front office with the office manager, who has been working there for 20 years. She goes on vacation and in the course of covering some of her duties, you discover suspicious entries in the accounts payable records. You wonder if she is paying her own bills out of the office account.

66. What should you do? Choose all appropriate actions from the list below.

 a. Nothing, she is your boss and you are new here.

 b. Ask your coworkers for advice.

 c. Question her about what you found when she returns.

 d. Tell the physician immediately.

 e. Tell the physician's wife of your suspicions.

 f. Keep it to yourself; it is none of your business.

 g. Post the situation on Facebook and ask for advice.

 h. Investigate further while she is away by going over all of the check entries.

PSY **PROCEDURE 12-1**   **Post Charges on a Daysheet**

Name: _____ Date: _____ Time: _____ Grade: _____

EQUIPMENT/SUPPLIES: Pen, pegboard, calculator, daysheet, encounter forms, ledger cards, previous day's balance, list of patients and charges, fee schedule

STANDARDS: Given the needed equipment and a place to work the student will perform this skill with _____% accuracy in a total of _____ minutes. *(Your instructor will tell you what the percentage and time limits will be before you begin.)*

KEY: 4 = Satisfactory   0 = Unsatisfactory   NA = This step is not counted

PROCEDURE STEPS	SELF	PARTNER	INSTRUCTOR
1. Place a new daysheet on the pegboard and record the totals from the previous daysheet.	☐	☐	☐
2. Align the patient's ledger card with the first available line on the daysheet.	☐	☐	☐
3. Place the receipt to align with the appropriate line on the ledger card.	☐	☐	☐
4. Record the number of the receipt in the appropriate column.	☐	☐	☐
5. Write the patient's name on the receipt.	☐	☐	☐
6. Record any existing balance the patient owes in the previous balance column of the daysheet.	☐	☐	☐
7. Record a brief description of the charge in the description line.	☐	☐	☐
8. Record the total charges in the charge column. Press hard so that the marks go through to the ledger card and the daysheet.	☐	☐	☐
9. Add the total charges to the previous balance and record in the current balance column.	☐	☐	☐
10. Return the ledger card to appropriate storage.	☐	☐	☐

CALCULATION

Total Possible Points: _____

Total Points Earned: _____ Multiplied by 100 = _____ Divided by Total Possible Points = _____ %

PASS   **FAIL**   **COMMENTS:**

☐   ☐

Student's signature _____ Date _____

Partner's signature _____ Date _____

Instructor's signature _____ Date _____

PSY PROCEDURE 12-2 Post Payments on a Daysheet

Name: _____ Date: _____ Time: _____ Grade: _____

EQUIPMENT/SUPPLIES: Pen, pegboard, calculator, daysheet, encounter forms, ledger cards, previous day's balance, list of patients and charges, fee schedule

COMPUTER AND MEDICAL OFFICE SOFTWARE: Follow the software requirements for posting credits to patient accounts.

STANDARDS: Given the needed equipment and a place to work the student will perform this skill with _____% accuracy in a total of _____ minutes. *(Your instructor will tell you what the percentage and time limits will be before you begin.)*

KEY: 4 = Satisfactory   0 = Unsatisfactory   NA =This step is not counted

PROCEDURE STEPS	SELF	PARTNER	INSTRUCTOR
1. Place a new daysheet on the pegboard and record the totals from the previous daysheet.	☐	☐	☐
2. Align the patient's ledger card with the first available line on the daysheet.	☐	☐	☐
3. Place receipt to align with the appropriate line on the ledger card.	☐	☐	☐
4. Record the number of the receipt in the appropriate column.	☐	☐	☐
5. Write the patient's name on the receipt.	☐	☐	☐
6. Record any existing balance the patient owes in the previous balance column of the daysheet.	☐	☐	☐
7. Record the source and type of the payment in the description line.	☐	☐	☐
8. Record appropriate adjustments in adjustment column.	☐	☐	☐
9. Record the total payment in the payment column. Press hard so that marks go through to the ledger card and the daysheet.	☐	☐	☐
10. Subtract the payment and adjustments from the outstanding/ previous balance, and record the current balance.	☐	☐	☐
11. Return the ledger card to appropriate storage.	☐	☐	☐

CALCULATION

Total Possible Points: _____

Total Points Earned: _____ Multiplied by 100 = _____ Divided by Total Possible Points = _____ %

PASS   **FAIL**   **COMMENTS:**

☐   ☐

Student's signature _____ Date _____

Partner's signature _____ Date _____

Instructor's signature _____ Date _____

PSY PROCEDURE 12-3 **Process a Credit Balance**

Name: _____   Date: _____   Time: _____   Grade: _____

EQUIPMENT/SUPPLIES: Pen, pegboard, calculator, daysheet, ledger card

STANDARDS: Given the needed equipment and a place to work the student will perform this skill with _____% accuracy in a total of _____ minutes. *(Your instructor will tell you what the percentage and time limits will be before you begin.)*

KEY: 4 = Satisfactory   0 = Unsatisfactory   NA =This step is not counted

PROCEDURE STEPS	SELF	PARTNER	INSTRUCTOR
1. Determine the reason for the credit balance.	☐	☐	☐
2. Place brackets around the balance indicating that it is a negative number.	☐	☐	☐
3. Write a refund check and follow the steps in Procedure 12-7.	☐	☐	☐

CALCULATION

Total Possible Points: _____

Total Points Earned: _____ Multiplied by 100 = _____ Divided by Total Possible Points = _____ %

PASS   **FAIL**   **COMMENTS:**

☐   ☐

Student's signature _____ Date _____

Partner's signature _____ Date _____

Instructor's signature _____ Date _____

PSY PROCEDURE 12-4 **Process Refunds**

Name: _____ Date: _____ Time: _____ Grade: _____

EQUIPMENT/SUPPLIES: Pen, pegboard, calculator, daysheet, ledger card, checkbook, check register, word processor letterhead, envelope, postage, copy machine, patient's chart, refund file

STANDARDS: Given the needed equipment and a place to work the student will perform this skill with _____% accuracy in a total of _____ minutes. *(Your instructor will tell you what the percentage and time limits will be before you begin.)*

KEY: 4 = Satisfactory   0 = Unsatisfactory   NA =This step is not counted

PROCEDURE STEPS	SELF	PARTNER	INSTRUCTOR
1. Determine who gets the refund, the patient or the insurance company.	☐	☐	☐
2. Pull patient's ledger card and place on current daysheet aligned with the first available line.	☐	☐	☐
3. Post the amount of the refund in the adjustment column in brackets indicating it is a debit, not a credit, adjustment.	☐	☐	☐
4. Write "Refund to Patient" or "Refund to _____" (name of insurance company) in the description column.	☐	☐	☐
5. Write a check for the credit amount made out to the appropriate party.	☐	☐	☐
6. Record the amount and name of payee in the check register.	☐	☐	☐
7. Mail check with letter of explanation to patient or insurance company.	☐	☐	☐
8. Place copy of check and copy of letter in the patient's record or in refund file.	☐	☐	☐
9. Return the patient's ledger card to its storage area.	☐	☐	☐

CALCULATION

Total Possible Points: _____

Total Points Earned: _____ Multiplied by 100 = _____ Divided by Total Possible Points = _____ %

PASS   FAIL   COMMENTS:

☐   ☐

Student's signature _____ Date _____

Partner's signature _____ Date _____

Instructor's signature _____ Date _____

PSY PROCEDURE 12-5 Post Adjustments to a Daysheet

Name: _____ Date: _____ Time: _____ Grade: _____

EQUIPMENT/SUPPLIES: Pen, pegboard, calculator, daysheet, encounter forms, ledger cards, previous day's balance, list of patients and charges, fee schedule

COMPUTER AND MEDICAL OFFICE SOFTWARE: Follow the software requirements for posting credits to patient accounts.

STANDARDS: Given the needed equipment and a place to work the student will perform this skill with _____% accuracy in a total of _____ minutes. *(Your instructor will tell you what the percentage and time limits will be before you begin.)*

KEY: 4 = Satisfactory   0 = Unsatisfactory   NA =This step is not counted

PROCEDURE STEPS	SELF	PARTNER	INSTRUCTOR
1. Pull patient's ledger card and place on current daysheet aligned with the first available line.	☐	☐	☐
2. Post the amount to be written off in the adjustment column in brackets indicating it is a debit, not a credit, adjustment.	☐	☐	☐
3. Subtract the adjustment from the outstanding/previous balance, and record in the current balance column.	☐	☐	☐
4. Return the ledger card to appropriate storage.	☐	☐	☐

CALCULATION

Total Possible Points: _____

Total Points Earned: _____ Multiplied by 100 = _____ Divided by Total Possible Points = _____ %

PASS   **FAIL**   **COMMENTS:**

☐   ☐

Student's signature _____ Date _____

Partner's signature _____ Date _____

Instructor's signature _____ Date _____

PSY PROCEDURE 12-6 | **Post Collection Agency Payments**

Name: _____ Date: _____ Time: _____ Grade: _____

EQUIPMENT/SUPPLIES: Pen, pegboard, calculator, daysheet, patient's ledger card

STANDARDS: Given the needed equipment and a place to work the student will perform this skill with _____% accuracy in a total of _____ minutes. *(Your instructor will tell you what the percentage and time limits will be before you begin.)*

KEY: 4 = Satisfactory   0 = Unsatisfactory   NA =This step is not counted

PROCEDURE STEPS	SELF	PARTNER	INSTRUCTOR
1. Review check stub or report from the collection agency explaining the amounts to be applied to the accounts.	☐	☐	☐
2. Pull the patients' ledger cards.	☐	☐	☐
3. Post the amount to be applied in the payment column for each patient.	☐	☐	☐
4. Adjust off the amount representing the percentage of the payment charged by the collection agency.	☐	☐	☐

CALCULATION

Total Possible Points: _____

Total Points Earned: _____ Multiplied by 100 = _____ Divided by Total Possible Points = _____ %

PASS   **FAIL**   **COMMENTS:**

☐   ☐

Student's signature _____ Date _____

Partner's signature _____ Date _____

Instructor's signature _____ Date _____

PSY PROCEDURE 12-7   Process NSF Checks

Name: _____ Date: _____ Time: _____ Grade: _____

EQUIPMENT/SUPPLIES: Pen, pegboard, calculator, daysheet, patient's ledger card

STANDARDS: Given the needed equipment and a place to work the student will perform this skill with _____% accuracy in a total of _____ minutes. *(Your instructor will tell you what the percentage and time limits will be before you begin.)*

KEY: 4 = Satisfactory   0 = Unsatisfactory   NA =This step is not counted

PROCEDURE STEPS	SELF	PARTNER	INSTRUCTOR
1. Pull patient's ledger card and place on current daysheet aligned with the first available line.	☐	☐	☐
2. Write the amount of the check in the payment column in brackets indicating it is a debit, not a credit, adjustment.	☐	☐	☐
3. Write "Check Returned For Nonsufficient Funds" in the description column.	☐	☐	☐
4. Post a returned check charge with an appropriate explanation in the charge column.	☐	☐	☐
5. Write "Bank Fee for Returned Check" in the description column.	☐	☐	☐
6. Call the patient to advise him of the returned check and the fee.	☐	☐	☐
7. Construct a proper letter of explanation and a copy of the ledger card and mail to patient.	☐	☐	☐
8. Place a copy of the letter and the check in the patient's file.	☐	☐	☐
9. Make arrangements for the patient to pay cash.	☐	☐	☐
10. Flag the patient's account as a credit risk for future transactions.	☐	☐	☐
11. Return the patient's ledger card to its storage area.	☐	☐	☐
12. **AFF** You see a patient whose check was returned for nonsufficient funds out at a soccer game. He whispers to you to keep quiet about the bad check. Explain how you would respond.	☐	☐	☐

CALCULATION

Total Possible Points: _____

Total Points Earned: _____ Multiplied by 100 = _____ Divided by Total Possible Points = _____ %

PASS   **FAIL**   **COMMENTS:**

☐   ☐

Student's signature _____ Date _____

Partner's signature _____ Date _____

Instructor's signature _____ Date _____

PSY PROCEDURE 12-8 Balance a Daysheet

Name: _____ Date: _____ Time: _____ Grade: _____

EQUIPMENT/SUPPLIES: Daysheet with totals brought forward, simulated exercise, calculator, pen

STANDARDS: Given the needed equipment and a place to work the student will perform this skill with _____% accuracy in a total of _____ minutes. *(Your instructor will tell you what the percentage and time limits will be before you begin.)*

KEY: 4 = Satisfactory   0 = Unsatisfactory   NA = This step is not counted

PROCEDURE STEPS	SELF	PARTNER	INSTRUCTOR
1. Be sure the totals from the previous daysheet are recorded in the column for previous totals.	☐	☐	☐
2. Total the charge column and place that number in the proper blank.	☐	☐	☐
3. Total the payment column and place that number in the proper blank.	☐	☐	☐
4. Total the adjustment column and place that number in the proper blank.	☐	☐	☐
5. Total the current balance column and place that number in the proper blank.	☐	☐	☐
6. Total the previous balance column and place that number in the proper blank.	☐	☐	☐
7. Add today's totals to the previous totals.	☐	☐	☐
8. Take the grand total of the previous balances, add the grand total of the charges, and subtract the grand total of the payments and adjustments. This number must equal the grand total of the current balance.	☐	☐	☐
9. If the numbers do not match, calculate your totals again, and continue looking for errors until the numbers match. This will prove that the daysheet is balanced, and there are no errors.	☐	☐	☐
10. Record the totals of the columns in the proper space on the next daysheet. You will be prepared for balancing the new daysheet.	☐	☐	☐

CALCULATION

Total Possible Points: _____

Total Points Earned: _____ Multiplied by 100 = _____ Divided by Total Possible Points = _____ %

PASS   **FAIL**   **COMMENTS:**

☐   ☐

Student's signature _____ Date _____

Partner's signature _____ Date _____

Instructor's signature _____ Date _____

PSY PROCEDURE 12-9 Complete a Bank Deposit Slip and Make a Deposit

Name: _____ Date: _____ Time: _____ Grade: _____

EQUIPMENT/SUPPLIES: Calculator with tape, currency, coins, checks for deposit, deposit slip, endorsement stamp, deposit envelope

STANDARDS: Given the needed equipment and a place to work the student will perform this skill with _____% accuracy in a total of _____ minutes. *(Your instructor will tell you what the percentage and time limits will be before you begin.)*

KEY: 4 = Satisfactory 0 = Unsatisfactory NA = This step is not counted

PROCEDURE STEPS	SELF	PARTNER	INSTRUCTOR
1. Arrange bills face up and sort with the largest denomination on top.	☐	☐	☐
2. Record the total in the cash block on the deposit slip	☐	☐	☐
3. Endorse the back of each check with "For Deposit Only."	☐	☐	☐
4. Record the amount of each check beside an identifying number on the deposit slip.	☐	☐	☐
5. Total and record the amounts of checks in the total of checks line on the deposit slip.	☐	☐	☐
6. Total and record the amount of cash and the amount of checks.	☐	☐	☐
7. Record the total amount of the deposit in the office checkbook register.	☐	☐	☐
8. Make a copy of both sides of the deposit slip for office records.	☐	☐	☐
9. Place the cash, checks, and the completed deposit slip in an envelope or bank bag for transporting to the bank for deposit.	☐	☐	☐

CALCULATION

Total Possible Points: _____

Total Points Earned: _____ Multiplied by 100 = _____ Divided by Total Possible Points = _____ %

PASS **FAIL** **COMMENTS:**

☐ ☐

Student's signature _____ Date _____

Partner's signature _____ Date _____

Instructor's signature _____ Date _____

PSY PROCEDURE 12-10 | **Reconcile a Bank Statement**

Name: _____ Date: _____ Time: _____ Grade: _____

EQUIPMENT/SUPPLIES: Simulated bank statement, reconciliation worksheet, calculator, pen

STANDARDS: Given the needed equipment and a place to work the student will perform this skill with _____% accuracy in a total of _____ minutes. *(Your instructor will tell you what the percentage and time limits will be before you begin.)*

KEY: 4 = Satisfactory   0 = Unsatisfactory   NA =This step is not counted

PROCEDURE STEPS	SELF	PARTNER	INSTRUCTOR
1. Compare the opening balance on the new statement with the closing balance on the previous statement.	☐	☐	☐
2. List the bank balance in the appropriate space on the reconciliation worksheet.	☐	☐	☐
3. Compare the check entries on the statement with the entries in the check register.	☐	☐	☐
4. Determine if there are any outstanding checks.	☐	☐	☐
5. Total outstanding checks.	☐	☐	☐
6. Subtract from the checkbook balance items such as withdrawals, automatic payments, or service charges that appeared on the statement but not in the checkbook.	☐	☐	☐
7. Add to the bank statement balance any deposits not shown on the bank statement.	☐	☐	☐
8. Make sure balance in the checkbook and the bank statement agree.	☐	☐	☐

CALCULATION

Total Possible Points: _____

Total Points Earned: _____ Multiplied by 100 = _____ Divided by Total Possible Points = _____ %

PASS   **FAIL**   **COMMENTS:**

☐   ☐

Student's signature _____ Date _____

Partner's signature _____ Date _____

Instructor's signature _____ Date _____

Name: _____ Date: _____ Time: _____ Grade: _____

EQUIPMENT/SUPPLIES: Cash box, play money, checkbook, simulated receipts, and/or vouchers representing expenditures

STANDARDS: Given the needed equipment and a place to work the student will perform this skill with _____% accuracy in a total of _____ minutes. *(Your instructor will tell you what the percentage and time limits will be before you begin.)*

KEY: 4 = Satisfactory 0 = Unsatisfactory NA =This step is not counted

PROCEDURE STEPS	SELF	PARTNER	INSTRUCTOR
1. Count the money remaining in the box.	☐	☐	☐
2. Total the amounts of all vouchers in the petty cash box and determine the amount of expenditures.	☐	☐	☐
3. Subtract the amount of receipts from the original amount in petty cash, to equal the amount of cash remaining in the box.	☐	☐	☐
4. Balance the cash against the receipts.	☐	☐	☐
5. Write a check only for the amount that was used.	☐	☐	☐
6. Record totals on the memo line of the check stub.	☐	☐	☐
7. Sort and record all vouchers to the appropriate accounts.	☐	☐	☐
8. File the list of vouchers and attached receipts.	☐	☐	☐
9. Place cash in petty cash fund.	☐	☐	☐
10. **AFF** A co-worker asks to borrow money from petty cash for bus fair home. She promises to pay it back tomorrow. Explain how you would respond.	☐	☐	☐

CALCULATION

Total Possible Points: _____

Total Points Earned: _____ Multiplied by 100 = _____ Divided by Total Possible Points = _____ %

PASS **FAIL** **COMMENTS:**

☐ ☐

Student's signature _____ Date _____

Partner's signature _____ Date _____

Instructor's signature _____ Date _____

PSY PROCEDURE 12-12 Order Supplies

Name: _____ Date: _____ Time: _____ Grade: _____

EQUIPMENT/SUPPLIES: 5 × 7 index cards, file box with divider cards, computer with Internet (optional), medical supply catalogues

STANDARDS: Given the needed equipment and a place to work the student will perform this skill with _____% accuracy in a total of _____ minutes. *(Your instructor will tell you what the percentage and time limits will be before you begin.)*

KEY: 4 = Satisfactory   0 = Unsatisfactory   NA = This step is not counted

PROCEDURE STEPS	SELF	PARTNER	INSTRUCTOR
1. Create a list of supplies to be ordered that is based on inventory done by employees.	☐	☐	☐
2. Create an index card for each supply on the list including the name of the supply in the top left corner, the name and contact information of vendor(s), and product identification number.	☐	☐	☐
3. File the index cards in the file box with divider cards alphabetically or by product type.	☐	☐	☐
4. Record the current price of the item and how the item is supplied.	☐	☐	☐
5. Record the reorder point.	☐	☐	☐

CALCULATION

Total Possible Points: _____

Total Points Earned: _____ Multiplied by 100 = _____ Divided by Total Possible Points = _____ %

PASS   **FAIL**   **COMMENTS:**

☐   ☐

Student's signature _____ Date _____

Partner's signature _____ Date _____

Instructor's signature _____ Date _____

PSY **PROCEDURE 12-13** Write a Check

Name: _____ Date: _____ Time: _____ Grade: _____

EQUIPMENT/SUPPLIES: Simulated page of checks from checkbook, scenario giving amount of check, check register

STANDARDS: Given the needed equipment and a place to work the student will perform this skill with _____%
accuracy in a total of _____ minutes. *(Your instructor will tell you what the percentage and time limits will be
before you begin.)*

KEY: 4 = Satisfactory   0 = Unsatisfactory   NA =This step is not counted

PROCEDURE STEPS	SELF	PARTNER	INSTRUCTOR
1. Fill out the check register with the following information:	☐	☐	☐
a. check number			
b. date			
c. payee information			
d. amount			
e. previous balance			
f. new balance			
2. Enter date on check.	☐	☐	☐
3. Enter payee on check.	☐	☐	☐
4. Enter the amount of check using numerals.	☐	☐	☐
5. Write out the amount of the check beginning as far left as possible and make a straight line to fill in space between dollars and cents.	☐	☐	☐
6. Record cents as a fraction with 100 as the denominator.	☐	☐	☐
7. Obtain appropriate signature(s).	☐	☐	☐
8. Proofread for accuracy.	☐	☐	☐

CALCULATION

Total Possible Points: _____

Total Points Earned: _____ Multiplied by 100 = _____ Divided by Total Possible Points = _____ %

PASS   **FAIL**   **COMMENTS:**

☐   ☐

Student's signature _____ Date _____

Partner's signature _____ Date _____

Instructor's signature _____ Date _____

WORK PRODUCT 1   Grade: _____

Perform an Inventory of Supplies

When you are working in a medical office, you may need to keep an inventory of all supplies. The inventory will help you decide when to order new supplies. It will also help you calculate how much money you will need to spend on supplies. Supplies are those items that are consumed quickly and need to be reordered on a regular basis.

If you are currently working in a medical office, use the form below to take an inventory of the supplies in the office. If you do not have access to a medical office, complete an inventory of the supplies in your kitchen or bathroom at home.

Third Street
Physician's Office, Inc.
123 Main Street
Baltimore, MD 21201
410-895-6214

Supply Inventory

Item Description	Item Number or Code	Number Needed in Stock	Number Currently in Stock	Date Ordered	Number Ordered	Unit Price	Total	Actual Delivery Date

WORK PRODUCT 2

Grade: _____

Perform an Inventory of Equipment

When you are working in a medical office, you may need to keep an inventory of all equipment. The inventory will help you decide when to order new equipment. It will also help you calculate how much money you will need to spend on new equipment. Equipment includes items that can be used over and over and generally last many years.

If you are currently working in a medical office, use the form below to take an inventory of the equipment in the office. If you do not have access to a medical office, complete an inventory of the equipment in your kitchen or bathroom at home.

**Third Street
Physician's Office, Inc.**
123 Main Street
Baltimore, MD 21201
410-895-6214

Equipment Inventory

Item Description	Item Number or Code	Purchase Date	Condition	Comments	Expected New Purchase Date	Cost if Purchased This Year

WORK PRODUCT 3

Grade: _____

Process a Credit Balance

Mr. Juan Rodriguez has switched to a different insurance company. His co-pay with his old carrier was $35 per visit. His new co-pay is $20 per visit. However, there was a billing oversight and Mr. Rodriguez paid his old co-pay. Process Mr. Rodriguez's credit balance on the daysheet.

CREDITS

Date	Description	Charges	Payments	Adjustments	Current Balance	Previous Balance	NAME

Totals This Page

Totals Previous Page

Month-To-Date Totals

WORK PRODUCT 4

Grade: _____

Process a Refund

Mr. Rodriguez has a credit balance of $15 on his account. You need to mail him a refund check. Post this transaction on the daysheet.

CREDITS

Date	Description	Charges	Payments	Adjustments	Current Balance	Previous Balance	NAME

Totals This Page
Totals Previous Page
Month-To-Date Totals

WORK PRODUCT 5

Grade: _____

Post Adjustments

Mr. Rodriguez visits your office for an x-ray of his knee. Your office normally charges $225 for a knee x-ray. However, your physician is a participating provider for Mr. Rodriguez's insurance carrier. His insurance pays your office only $175 for a knee x-ray. Post the proper adjustment on the daysheet.

CREDITS

Date	Description	Charges	Payments	Adjustments	Current Balance	Previous Balance	NAME

Totals This Page
Totals Previous Page
Month-To-Date Totals

WORK PRODUCT 6

Grade: _____

Post NSF Checks

You have just received a check that was returned for nonsufficient funds. The check was written by Martha Montgomery for $750. Post the proper information on the daysheet.

			CREDITS				
Date	Description	Charges	Payments	Adjust ments	Current Balance	Previous Balance	NAME

Totals This Page
Totals Previous Page
Month-To-Date Totals

WORK PRODUCT 7

Grade: _____

Post Collection Agency Payments

You receive a check for $787.50 and the following statement from your collection agency.

Jones & Jones Collections

Account:d. Larsen, MD

Debtor	Amount Collected	Fee	Balance
Martha Montgomery	$750.00	$187.50	$562.50
Johan Johansen	$300.00	$75.00	$225.00
		Total	$787.50

Post the payments to the daysheet.

CREDITS

Date	Description	Charges	Payments	Adjust ments	Current Balance	Previous Balance	NAME

Totals This Page
Totals Previous Page
Month-To-Date Totals

WORK PRODUCT 8

Grade: _____

Posting Payments from Medicare

On a blank daysheet provided, post the following Medicare payments. You will need to calculate the adjustments by subtracting the amount allowed from the amount charged. The patient's previous balance will be the amount charged back on the date of service.

Keep in mind that on an actual MEOB, the CPT-4 codes would be used instead of OV, x-ray, etc.

MEDICARE EXPLANATION OF BENEFITS

Name	Charges	Date of Service	Amount Allowed	Amount Paid to Provider	Patient's Responsibility
Smith, John	OV 40.00	3-2-xx	18.00	14.40	3.60
Jones, Anne Total:	OV 100.00 Lab 50.00 150.00	3-2-xx	65.00 50.00 115.00	52.00 40.00 92.00	13.00 10.00 23.00
Stevens, Sally Total:	OV 150.00 X-ray 200.00 350.00	3-2-xx	120.00 160.00 280.00	96.00 128.00 224.00	24.00 32.00 56.00
Reynolds, Susan	Consult 300.00	3-2-xx	250.00	200.00	50.00

CREDITS

Date	Description	Charges	Payments	Adjustments	Current Balance	Previous Balance	NAME

Totals This Page
Totals Previous Page
Month-To-Date Totals

WORK PRODUCT 9

Grade: _____

Putting It All Together

On a blank daysheet provided, complete 1–8.
Post the following transactions on the daysheet provided. Use today's date.

1. Stanley Gleber came in and paid $25.00 in cash on his account. His previous balance is $100.00.

2. Lisa Moore sent a check in the mail for $100.00 to be paid on her account, which carries a balance of $500.00.

3. Elaine Newman came in and handed you a check she received from Blue Cross Blue Shield for $700.00 to be paid on her account, which has a balance of $900.00. The explanation attached to the check indicates it is for surgery she had on 3-1-09. Your physician does NOT participate with Blue Cross Blue Shield. Post the payment with an appropriate description. Will there be an adjustment?

4. Madeline Bell saw the doctor and brings out an encounter form with a charge for an office visit at $50.00 and lab at $150.00. Post her charges. She does not pay today. Her previous balance was zero.

5. Post the collection agency payment for John Simms. His account with a balance of $250.00 was turned over to Equifax on 03/01/12. They collected the entire amount. You receive a check from Equifax. They charge 30% of what they collect, so the check is for 200.00. His balance was not written off when turned over to Equifax, so his previous balance should be 250.00.

6. Hazel Wilbourne paid her charges of $200.00 in full at her last visit. Now you receive a check from Aetna for that visit. The check is for $130.00. Your physician participates with this insurance company, which means he agrees to accept what they pay. In other words, you will not bill the patient for the difference. Post the check to Ms. Wilbourne's account.

7. Ms. Wilbourne now has a credit balance. You will need to send her a check from the office account as a refund. Post the appropriate entry for this transaction. In accounting, a credit balance is put in angle brackets: <200.00>.

8. Calculate and record each column total. Make sure the columns balance by starting with your previous balance, adding the charges, subtracting the payments and adjustments, and this should give you the total of your current balance column. Remember, brackets in accounting mean that you do the opposite when adding your columns, so instead of adding a credit balance when totaling, you will subtract it.

Date	Description	Charges	Payments	Adjustments	Current Balance	Previous Balance	NAME

Totals This Page
Totals Previous Page
Month-To-Date Totals

WORK PRODUCT 10

Grade: _____

Prepare a Bank Deposit

Prepare a bank deposit for the following:

- check for $750 from Martin Montgomery
- check for $35 from Rita Gonzalez
- $125 cash

Use fictitious demographic information for the account holder on the deposit slip.

Newtown Bank, N.A.		DEPOSIT	ITEMS DEPOSITED	DOLLARS	CENTS
			Currency		.
			Coin		.
			Checks 1		.
Name and account number will be verified when presented.			2		.
Name		Date			
Address			3		.
			4		.
			Sub Total		.
Signature	Sign here only if cash is received from deposit		Less Cash		.
Store Number (Commercial Accounts Only)	Account Number (For CAP Accounts, use 10-digit number.)		Total Deposit $		

Health Insurance and Reimbursement

Cognitive Domain

1. Spell and define the key terms
2. Identify types of insurance plans
3. Discuss workers' compensation as it applies to patients
4. Identify models of managed care
5. Describe procedures for implementing both managed care and insurance plans
6. Discuss utilization review principles
7. Discuss referral process for patients in a managed care program
8. Describe how guidelines are used in processing an insurance claim
9. Compare processes for filing insurance claims both manually and electronically
10. Describe guidelines for third-party claims
11. Discuss types of physician fee schedules
12. Describe the concept of resource-based relative value scale (RBRVS)
13. Define diagnosis-related groups (DRGs)
14. Name two legal issues affecting claims submissions

Psychomotor Domain

1. Complete a CMS-1500 claim form (Procedure 13-1)
2. Apply both managed care policies and procedures

3. Apply third-party guidelines
4. Complete insurance claim forms
5. Obtain precertification, including documentation
6. Verify eligibility for managed care services

Affective Domain

1. Demonstrate assertive communication with managed care and/or insurance providers
2. Demonstrate sensitivity in communicating with both providers and patients
3. Communicate in language the patient can understand regarding managed care and insurance plans
4. Apply ethical behaviors, including honesty/integrity in performance of medical assisting practice

ABHES Competencies

1. Prepare and submit insurance claims
2. Serve as liaison between physician and others
3. Comply with federal, state and local health laws and regulations

Name: _____   Date: _____   Grade: _____

COG MULTIPLE CHOICE

1. Which of the following is frequently not covered in group health benefits packages?

   a. Birth control

   b. Childhood immunizations

   c. Routine diagnostic care

   d. Treatment for substance abuse

   e. Regular physical examinations

2. Any payment for medical services that is not paid by the patient or physician is said to be paid by a(n):

   a. second-party payer.

   b. first-party payer.

   c. insurance party payer.

   d. third-party payer.

   e. health care party payer.

3. The criteria a patient must meet for a group benefit plan to provide coverage are called:

   a. eligibility requirements.

   b. patient requirements.

   c. benefit plan requirements.

   d. physical requirements.

   e. insurance requirements.

4. Eligibility for a dependent requires that he or she is:

   a. unmarried.

   b. employed.

   c. living with the employee.

   d. younger than 18.

   e. an excellent student.

5. Whom should you contact about the eligibility of a patient for the health benefits plan?

   a. Claims administrator

   b. Claims investigator

   c. Insurance salesperson

   d. Insurance reviewer

   e. Claims insurer

Scenario for questions 6 and 7: Aziz pays premiums directly to the insurance company, and the insurance company reimburses him for eligible medical expenses.

6. What type of insurance does Aziz have?

   a. Individual health benefits

   b. Public health benefits

   c. Managed care

   d. PPO

   e. HMO

7. Which of the following is likely true of Aziz's insurance?

   a. The insurance is provided by his employer.

   b. Money can be put aside into accounts used for medical expenses.

   c. There are certain restrictions for some illnesses and injuries.

   d. All providers are under contract with the insurer.

   e. There are two levels of benefits in the health plan.

8. An optional health benefits program offered to persons signing up for Social Security benefits is:

   a. Medicare Part A.

   b. Medicare Part B.

   c. Medicaid.

   d. TRICARE/CHAMPVA.

   e. HMO.

9. After the deductible has been met, what percentage of the approved charges does Medicare reimburse to the physician?

   a. 0

   b. 20

   c. 75

   d. 80

   e. 100

10. Which benefits program bases eligibility on a patient's eligibility for other state programs such as welfare assistance?

    a. Workers' Compensation

    b. Medicare

    c. Medicaid

    d. TRICARE/CHAMPVA

    e. Social Security

11. Which of the following is a medical expense that Medicaid provides 100% coverage for?

    a. Family planning

    b. Colorectal screening

    c. Bone density testing

    d. Pap smears

    e. Mammograms

12. In a traditional insurance plan:

    a. the covered patient may seek care from any provider.

    b. the insurer has no relationship with the provider.

    c. a patient can be admitted to a hospital only if that admission has been certified by the insurer.

    d. there is no third-party payer.

    e. the patient cannot be billed for the deductible.

13. Which of the following is a plan typically developed by hospitals and physicians to attract patients?

    a. HMO

    b. PPO

    c. HSA

    d. TPA

    e. UCR

14. Which of the following is true about both HMOs and PPOs?

    a. Both allow patients to see any physician of their choice and receive benefits.

    b. Both contract directly with participating providers, hospitals, and physicians.

    c. Both offer benefits at two levels, commonly referred to as *in-network* and *out-of-network.*

    d. Both are not risk-bearing and do not have any financial involvement in the health plan.

    e. Both incorporate independent practice associations.

15. Which of the following is a government-sponsored health benefits plan?

    a. TRICARE/CHAMPVA

    b. HMO

    c. HSA

    d. PPO

    e. PHO

16. If a provider is unethical, you should:

    a. correct the issue yourself.

    b. immediately stop working for the provider.

    c. comply with all requests to misrepresent medical records but report the physician.

    d. do whatever the physician asks to avoid confrontation.

    e. explain that you are legally bound to truthful billing, and report the physician.

17. A patient's ID card:

    a. contains the information needed to file a claim on it.

    b. should be updated at least once every 2 years.

    c. must be cleared before an emergency can be treated.

    d. is updated and sent to Medicaid patients bimonthly.

    e. is not useful for determining if the patient is a dependent.

18. What information is needed to fill out a CMS-1500 claim form?

    a. A copy of the patient's chart

    b. Location where patient will be recovering

    c. Diagnostic codes from encounter form

    d. Copies of hospitalization paperwork

    e. Physician's record and degree

19. Claims that are submitted electronically:

    a. violate HIPAA standards.

    b. contain fewer errors than those that are mailed.

    c. require approval from the patient.

    d. increase costs for Medicare patients.

    e. reduce the reimbursement cycle.

20. Normally, coverage has an amount below which services are not reimbursable. This is referred to as the:

    a. deductible.

    b. coinsurance.

    c. balance billing.

    d. benefits.

    e. claim.

21. Which is true about how a managed care system is different from a traditional insurance coverage system?

    a. They usually are less costly.

    b. They cost more but have more benefits.

    c. They cost the same but have more benefits.

    d. You can only use network physicians.

COG MATCHING

Grade: _____

Match the following key terms to their definitions.

Key Terms

22. _____ assignment of benefits

23. _____ balance billing

24. _____ capitation

25. _____ carrier

26. _____ claims administrator

27. _____ co-insurance

28. _____ coordination of benefits

29. _____ co-payments

30. _____ crossover claim

31. _____ deductible

32. _____ dependent

33. _____ eligibility

34. _____ explanation of benefits (EOB)

Definitions

a. an individual who manages the third-party reimbursement policies for a medical practice

b. the part of the payment for a service that a patient must pay

c. the determination of an insured's right to receive benefits from a third-party payer based on criteria such as payment of premiums

d. spouse, children, and sometimes other individuals designated by the insured who are covered under a health care plan

e. the transfer of the patient's legal right to collect third-party benefits to the provider of the services

f. a company that assumes the risk of an insurance company

g. a group of physicians and specialists that conducts a review of a disputed case and makes a final recommendation

h. an organization that provides a wide range of services through a contract with a specified group at a predetermined payment

i. billing the patients for the difference between the physician's charges and the Medicare-approved charges

j. an organization of nongroup physicians developed to allow independent physicians to compete with prepaid group practices

k. a coalition of physicians and a hospital contracting with large employers, insurance carriers, and other benefits groups to provide discounted health services

35. _____ fee-for-service

36. _____ fee schedule

37. _____ group member

38. _____ healthcare savings account (HSA)

39. _____ health maintenance organization (HMO)

40. _____ independent practice association (IPA)

41. _____ managed care

42. _____ Medicare

43. _____ peer review organization

44. _____ physician hospital organization

45. _____ preferred provider organization (PPO)

46. _____ usual, customary, and reasonable (UCR)

47. _____ utilization review

l. an established set of fees charged for specific services and paid by the patient or insurance carrier

m. the practice of third-party payers to control costs by requiring physicians to adhere to specific rules as a condition of payment

n. the method of designating the order in multiple-carriers pay benefits to avoid duplication of payment

o. a statement from an insurance carrier that outlines which services are being paid

p. a government-sponsored health benefits package that provides insurance for the elderly

q. a claim that moves over automatically from one coverage to another for payment

r. a policyholder who is covered by a group insurance carrier

s. a type of health benefit program whose purpose is to contract with providers, then lease this network of contracted providers to health care plans

t. an employee benefit that allows individuals to save money through payroll deduction to accounts that can be used only for medical care

u. a list of pre-established fee allowances set for specific services performed by a provider

v. a managed care plan that pays a certain amount to a provider over a specific time for caring for the patients in the plan, regardless of what or how many services are performed

w. the basis of a physician's fee schedule for the normal cost of the same service or procedure in a similar geographic area and under the same or similar circumstances

x. the agreed-upon amount paid to the provider by a policyholder

y. an analysis of individual cases by a committee to make sure services and procedures being billed to a third-party payer are medically necessary

z. the amount paid by the patient before the carrier begins paying

COG SHORT ANSWER   Grade: _____

48. What does the acronym DRG represent? How are DRGs used?

_____

_____

_____

49. What does the acronym RBRVS represent? Briefly explain RBRVS.

_____

_____

_____

50. What is a third-party payer?

_____

_____

_____

51. Elaine is 22 years old and is still eligible as a dependent. What could be a possible reason for this?

_____

_____

_____

52. Why do managed care programs require approved referrals?

_____

_____

_____

53. What does a gatekeeper physician do?

_____

_____

_____

54. A new patient comes to your office, and he hands you his insurance card. What information can you find on the back of his identification card?

_____

_____

_____

55. What form do you fill out to submit an insurance claim?

_____

_____

_____

56. When is a physician required to file a patient's claim or to extend credit?

_____

_____

_____

57. Why is it important to check the Explanation of Benefits?

_____

_____

_____

58. What is a preexisting condition?

_____

_____

_____

COG PSY ACTIVE LEARNING

Grade: _____

59. Interview three people about their health insurance. Ask them what they like about their service. What do they dislike? Compile a list of their comments to discuss with the class.

60. Visit the Web site for Medicare at http://www.medicare.gov. Locate their Frequently Asked Questions page. Read over the questions, and choose five that you believe are the most likely to be asked in a medical office. Design a pamphlet for your office that addresses these five questions.

61. Although a large percentage of Americans have some sort of health insurance, there are still many people who go without. Research online and in medical journals to see what solutions the government and health care companies are devising to reduce the number of uninsured Americans, and to provide better, cheaper, and more widespread health care. Choose one solution, and write a letter to the editor of a local newspaper explaining your position.

COG IDENTIFICATION

Grade: _____

62. Jim works for a company that offers an employee benefit whereby money is taken out of his paycheck and put toward medical care expenses. What is the name of this practice?

_____

_____

63. Determine which of the following are characteristics of Medicare or Medicaid. Place a check mark in the appropriate column below.

	Medicare	Medicaid
a. Provides coverage for low-income or indigent persons of all ages		
b. In a crossover claim, this is the primary coverage		
c. Implemented on a state or local level		
d. Physician reimbursement is considerably less than other insurances		
e. Patients receive a new ID card each month		
f. Program is broken down into part A and part B		
g. Provides coverage for persons suffering from end-stage renal disease		

64. Read each person's health insurance scenario and then match it with the correct type of health insurance plan.

Scenario

a. Sandra was recently let go from her job and is unemployed. _____

b. Thomas has a plan that has less generous coverage and may limit or eliminate benefits for certain illnesses or injuries. _____

c. Mario just started a new job and signed up for health insurance at work. _____

Health Insurance Plan

1. group

2. individual health

3. government

PSY **WHAT WOULD YOU DO?**

Grade: _____

65. Claims are sometimes denied, and it is your responsibility to take corrective actions. Read the scenarios below, and briefly state what action you should take.

a. Services are not covered by the plan._____

b. Coding is deemed inappropriate for services provided._____

c. Data is incomplete._____

d. Patient cannot be identified as a covered person._____

e. The patient is no longer covered by the plan._____

66. Kairi is a dependent, and both of her parents have health care plans. There are no specific instructions about which plan is primary, so how do you choose which plan to use?

_____

_____

_____

_____

67. Describe the two main characteristics of primary and secondary insurance below.

Primary Insurance	Secondary Insurance

COG **TRUE OR FALSE?**

68. Determine if the statements below are true or false. If false, explain why.

a. Approximately 80% of Americans are enrolled in health benefits plans of one sort or another.

_____

b. A network of providers that make up the PHO may have no financial obligation to subscribers.

_____

c. In managed care, a patient is not usually required to use network providers to receive full coverage.

_____

d. An HMO requires the patient to pay the provider directly, then reimburses the patient.

_____

PSY **WHAT WOULD YOU DO?**

69. Mrs. Smith is moving out of the area and is seeing Dr. Jones, her primary care physician, for the last time. After the move, Mrs. Smith will have to choose a new physician. Mrs. Smith has the choice of an HMO or a PPO. Mrs. Smith asks you to explain the difference. How would you teach Mrs. Smith about the differences between an HMO and a PPO?

_____

_____

_____

_____

70. Mandy's primary care physician is included under her health plan. However, she has recently been experiencing chest pains, and her physician refers her to a cardiologist. What would you to do to help make sure the specialist's visit is covered?

_____

_____

_____

AFF **CASE STUDY FOR CRITICAL THINKING**   Grade: _____

You are tasked with arranging a referral for Mrs. Williams. She has Blue Cross Blue Shield of VA. She needs a carpal tunnel release. She insists that her insurance will pay, but when you call for preauthorization, you are told her policy is no longer in effect. She did not pay her premium last month, and the policy was cancelled. Apparently she has not been notified.

71. Word for word, what would you say to her?

_____

_____

_____

_____

72. Circle all appropriate contacts below that you could suggest to Mrs. Williams.

    a. The Yellow Pages

    b. The local Department of Social Services

    c. An attorney

    d. Another physician. She probably will not be able to pay.

    e. A free clinic

    f. Her employer

    g. The phone number on the back of her insurance card

PSY PROCEDURE 13-1 Completing a CMS-1500 Claim Form

Name: _____ Date: _____ Time: _____ Grade: _____

EQUIPMENT: Case scenario (see work product), completed encounter form, blank CMS-1500 Claim Form, pen

STANDARDS: Given the needed equipment and a place to work the student will perform this skill with _____% accuracy in a total of _____ minutes. *(Your instructor will tell you what the percentage and time limits will be before you begin.)*

KEY: 4 = Satisfactory   0 = Unsatisfactory   NA = This step is not counted

PROCEDURE STEPS	SELF	PARTNER	INSTRUCTOR
1. Using the information provided in the case scenario, complete the demographic information in lines 1 through 11d.	☐	☐	☐
2. Insert "SOF" (signature on file) on lines 12 and 13. Check to be sure there is a current signature on file in the chart and that it is specifically for the third-party payer being filed.	☐	☐	☐
3. If the services being filed are for a hospital stay, insert information in lines 16, 18, and 32.	☐	☐	☐
4. If the services are related to an injury, insert the date of the accident in line 14.	☐	☐	☐
5. Insert dates of service.	☐	☐	☐
6. Using the encounter form, place the CPT code listed for each service and procedure checked off in column D of lines 21–24 on the form.	☐	☐	☐
7. Place the diagnostic codes indicated on the encounter form in lines 21 (1–4). List the reason for the encounter on line 21.1 and any other diagnoses listed on the encounter form that relate to the services or procedures.	☐	☐	☐
8. Reference the codes placed in lines 21 (1–4) to each line listing a different CPT code by placing the corresponding one-digit in line 24, column e.	☐	☐	☐
9. **AFF** You notice that Mr. Dishman has no signature on file, but the box on line 12 of his claim form says he does. Explain how you would respond.	☐	☐	☐

CALCULATION

Total Possible Points: _____

Total Points Earned: _____ Multiplied by 100 = _____ Divided by Total Possible Points = _____ %

PASS   **FAIL**   **COMMENTS:**
☐   ☐

Student's signature _____ Date _____

Partner's signature _____ Date _____

Instructor's signature _____ Date _____

WORK PRODUCT 1

Grade: _____

COMPLETE INSURANCE CLAIM FORMS

Jackson Dishman is a 58-year-old man who is seen in the office for acute abdominal pain. Complete the CMS-1500 form using the information provided below:

297-01-2222
Jackson W. Dishman   Group #68735
123 Smith Avenue
Winston-Salem NC 27103   Date of Birth: 06-01-49

He is charged for an office visit, which carries the CPT code 99213 and costs $150.00. The doctor has the CMA do a radiologic examination, abdomen; complete acute abdomen series (the CPT code 774022); and the charge for the x-rays is $250.00. The x-rays are normal. He pays nothing today. The physician sends Mr. Dishman home with a diagnosis of acute abdominal pain (IDC-9 code is 789.0). He is to return in 2 days unless the pain becomes unbearable.

PLEASE
DO NOT
STAPLE
IN THIS
AREA

HEALTH INSURANCE CLAIM FORM

| | PICA | | | | | PICA | | |

1. MEDICARE   MEDICAID   CHAMPUS   CHAMPVA   GROUP HEALTH PLAN   FECA BLK LUNG   OTHER   1a. INSURED'S I.D. NUMBER   (FOR PROGRAM IN ITEM 1)

☐ (Medicare #)   ☐ (Medicaid #)   ☐ (Sponsor's SSN)   ☐ (VA File #)   ☐ (SSN or ID)   ☐ (SSN)   ☐ (ID)

2. PATIENT'S NAME (Last Name, First Name, Middle Initial)   3. PATIENT'S BIRTH DATE MM DD YY   SEX   M ☐ F ☐   4. INSURED'S NAME (Last Name, First Name, Middle Initial)

5. PATIENT'S ADDRESS (No., Street)   6. PATIENT RELATIONSHIP TO INSURED   Self ☐ Spouse ☐ Child ☐ Other ☐   7. INSURED'S ADDRESS (No., Street)

CITY   STATE   8. PATIENT STATUS   Single ☐ Married ☐ Other ☐   CITY   STATE

ZIP CODE   TELEPHONE (Include Area Code) ( )   Employed ☐ Full-Time Student ☐ Part-Time Student ☐   ZIP CODE   TELEPHONE (INCLUDE AREA CODE) ( )

9. OTHER INSURED'S NAME (Last Name, First Name, Middle Initial)   10. IS PATIENT'S CONDITION RELATED TO: 11. INSURED'S POLICY GROUP OR FECA NUMBER

a. OTHER INSURED'S POLICY OR GROUP NUMBER   a. EMPLOYMENT? (CURRENT OR PREVIOUS) ☐ YES ☐ NO   a. INSURED'S DATE OF BIRTH MM DD YY   SEX   M ☐ F ☐

b. OTHER INSURED'S DATE OF BIRTH MM DD YY   SEX   M ☐ F ☐   b. AUTO ACCIDENT?   PLACE (State) ☐ YES ☐ NO   b. EMPLOYER'S NAME OR SCHOOL NAME

c. EMPLOYER'S NAME OR SCHOOL NAME   c. OTHER ACCIDENT? ☐ YES ☐ NO   c. INSURANCE PLAN NAME OR PROGRAM NAME

d. INSURANCE PLAN NAME OR PROGRAM NAME   10d. RESERVED FOR LOCAL USE   d. IS THERE ANOTHER HEALTH BENEFIT PLAN? ☐ YES ☐ NO *If yes*, return to and complete item 9 a-d.

READ BACK OF FORM BEFORE COMPLETING & SIGNING THIS FORM.
12. PATIENT'S OR AUTHORIZED PERSON'S SIGNATURE I authorize the release of any medical or other information necessary to process this claim. I also request payment of government benefits either to myself or to the party who accepts assignment below.

SIGNED _____   DATE _____

13. INSURED'S OR AUTHORIZED PERSON'S SIGNATURE I authorize payment of medical benefits to the undersigned physician or supplier for services described below.

SIGNED _____

14. DATE OF CURRENT: MM DD YY ◄ ILLNESS (First symptom) OR INJURY (Accident) OR PREGNANCY(LMP)   15. IF PATIENT HAS HAD SAME OR SIMILAR ILLNESS. GIVE FIRST DATE MM DD YY   16. DATES PATIENT UNABLE TO WORK IN CURRENT OCCUPATION FROM MM DD YY TO MM DD YY

17. NAME OF REFERRING PHYSICIAN OR OTHER SOURCE   17a. I.D. NUMBER OF REFERRING PHYSICIAN   18. HOSPITALIZATION DATES RELATED TO CURRENT SERVICES FROM MM DD YY TO MM DD YY

19. RESERVED FOR LOCAL USE   20. OUTSIDE LAB? ☐ YES ☐ NO $ CHARGES

21. DIAGNOSIS OR NATURE OF ILLNESS OR INJURY. (RELATE ITEMS 1,2,3 OR 4 TO ITEM 24E BY LINE)
1. L___ . ___   3. L___ . ___
2. L___ . ___   4. L___ . ___

22. MEDICAID RESUBMISSION CODE   ORIGINAL REF. NO.

23. PRIOR AUTHORIZATION NUMBER

24. A. DATE(S) OF SERVICE						B. Place of Service	C. Type of Service	D. PROCEDURES, SERVICES, OR SUPPLIES (Explain Unusual Circumstances) CPT/HCPCS	MODIFIER	E. DIAGNOSIS CODE	F. $ CHARGES	G. DAYS OR UNITS	H. EPSDT Family Plan	I. EMG	J. COB	K. RESERVED FOR LOCAL USE
From MM	DD	YY	To MM	DD	YY											
1																
2																
3																
4																
5																
6																

25. FEDERAL TAX I.D. NUMBER   SSN ☐ EIN ☐   26. PATIENT'S ACCOUNT NO.   27. ACCEPT ASSIGNMENT? (For govt. claims, see back) ☐ YES ☐ NO   28. TOTAL CHARGE $ 29. AMOUNT PAID $ 30. BALANCE DUE $

31. SIGNATURE OF PHYSICIAN OR SUPPLIER INCLUDING DEGREES OR CREDENTIALS (I certify that the statements on the reverse apply to this bill and are made a part thereof.)

SIGNED _____   DATE _____

32. NAME AND ADDRESS OF FACILITY WHERE SERVICES WERE RENDERED (If other than home or office)

33. PHYSICIAN'S, SUPPLIER'S BILLING NAME, ADDRESS, ZIP CODE & PHONE #

PIN# _____   GRP# _____

(APPROVED BY AMA COUNCIL ON MEDICAL SERVICE 8/88)   *PLEASE PRINT OR TYPE*   APPROVED OMB-0938-0008 FORM CMS-1500 (12-90), FORM RRB-1500,
APPROVED OMB-1215-0055 FORM OWCP-1500,   APPROVED OMB-0720-0001 (CHAMPUS)

CARRIER

PATIENT AND INSURED INFORMATION

PHYSICIAN OR SUPPLIER INFORMATION

Diagnostic Coding

Cognitive Domain

1. Spell and define the key terms
2. Describe the relationship between coding and reimbursement
3. Name and describe the coding system used to describe diseases, injuries, and other reasons for encounters with a medical provider
4. Explain the format of the ICD-9-CM
5. Give four examples of ways E codes are used
6. Describe how to use the most current diagnostic coding classification system
7. Describe the ICD-10-CM/PCS version and its differences from ICD-9

Psychomotor Domain

1. Perform diagnostic coding (Procedure 14-1)
2. Apply third-party guidelines

Affective Domain

1. Work with physician to achieve the maximum reimbursement

ABHES Competencies

1. Apply third-party guidelines
2. Perform diagnostic and procedural coding
3. Comply with federal, state, and local health laws and regulations

Name: _____   Date: _____   Grade: _____

COG MULTIPLE CHOICE

1. Which most accurately states the purpose of coding?

   a. Coding assists patients in accessing insurance databases.

   b. Coding determines the reimbursement of medical fees.

   c. Coding is used to track a physician's payments.

   d. Coding is used to index patients' claims forms.

   e. Coding identifies patients in a database.

2. A patient signs an advance beneficiary notice (ABN) to:

   a. consent to medically necessary procedures.

   b. assign payment to Medicare.

   c. accept responsibility for payment.

   d. assign responsibility for payment to a beneficiary.

   e. consent to a medically unnecessary procedure.

3. The content of the ICD-9-CM is a(n):

   a. classification of diseases and list of procedures.

   b. statistical grouping of trends in diseases.

   c. clinical modification of codes used by hospitals.

   d. ninth volume in an index of diseases.

   e. international document for monitoring coding.

4. Which is true of Volume 3 of the ICD-9-CM?

   a. It is organized by location on the patient's body.

   b. It is used to code mostly outpatient procedures.

   c. It is an alphabetical listing of diseases.

   d. It is used by hospitals to report procedures and services.

   e. It is an index of Volumes 1 and 2.

5. Physicians' services are reported:

   a. on the UB-04.

   b. on the CMS-1500.

   c. on the uniform bill.

   d. on the advance beneficiary notice.

   e. on bills from health institutions.

6. Which of these would be considered inpatient coding?

   a. Hospital same-day surgery

   b. Hour-long testing in a hospital CAT scan

   c. Treatment in the emergency room

   d. Observation status in a hospital

   e. Meals and testing during a hospital stay

7. In Volume 1 of the ICD-9-CM, chapters are grouped:

   a. by alphabetic ordering of diseases and injuries.

   b. alphabetically by eponym.

   c. by location in the body.

   d. by etiology and anatomic system.

   e. by surgical specialty.

8. The fourth and fifth digits in a code indicate the:

   a. anatomical location where a procedure was performed.

   b. number of times a test was executed.

   c. higher definitions of a code.

   d. code for the patient's general disease.

   e. traumatic origins of a disease (i.e., injury, deliberate violence).

9. A V-code might indicate a(n):

   a. immunization.

   b. poisoning.

   c. accident.

   d. diagnosis.

   e. treatment.

10. V-codes are used:

   a. for outpatient coding.

   b. when reimbursement is not needed.

   c. when a patient is not sick.

   d. to indicate testing for HIV.

   e. for infectious diseases.

11. What is the purpose of E-codes?

    a. They code for immunizations and other preventive procedures.

    b. They are used to code medical testing before a diagnosis.

    c. They assist insurance companies in making reimbursements.

    d. They indicate why a patient has an injury or poisoning.

    e. They indicate if a procedure was inpatient or outpatient.

12. Which of the following agencies are least interested in E-codes?

    a. Insurance underwriters

    b. Insurance claim providers

    c. National safety programs

    d. Public health agencies

    e. Workers' compensation lawyers

13. How is Volume 2 of the ICD-9-CM different from Volume 1?

    a. Volume 2 contains diagnostic terms that are not used in Volume 1.

    b. Volume 2 is organized into 17 chapters rather than 3 sections.

    c. Volume 2 does not contain E-codes, but Volume 1 does.

    d. Volume 2 contains hospital coding to cross-reference with Volume 1.

    e. Volume 2 provides information about the fourth and fifth digits of a code.

14. After finding a code in Volume 2, you should:

    a. record the code on the CMS-1500.

    b. consult Volume 3 for subordinate terms.

    c. cross-reference the code with Volume 1.

    d. indicate if the code is inpatient or outpatient.

    e. record the code on the UB-04.

15. Volume 3 of the ICD-9-CM is organized:

    a. by disease.

    b. by anatomy.

    c. into 17 chapters.

    d. into three sections.

    e. by surgical specialty.

16. One example of an eponym is:

    a. Crohn disease.

    b. bacterial meningitis.

    c. influenza virus.

    d. pruritus.

    e. pneumonia.

17. What is the first step to locating a diagnostic code?

    a. Determine where the diagnosis occurs in the body.

    b. Choose the main term within the diagnostic statement.

    c. Begin looking up the diagnosis in Volume 1 of the ICD-9-CM.

    d. Consult the CMS-1500 for reimbursement codes.

    e. Use Volume 3 of the ICD-9-CM to find the disease.

18. Which code is listed first on a CMS-1500?

    a. A reasonable second opinion

    b. Relevant laboratory work

    c. Diagnostic tests

    d. The symptoms of an illness

    e. The primary diagnosis

19. How do you code for late effects?

    a. Code for the treatment of the disease that causes late effects.

    b. Code for the disease that is causing the current condition.

    c. First code for the current condition, and then list the cause.

    d. Only code for the current condition.

    e. Only code for the cause of the current condition.

20. You should not code for a brain tumor:

    a. when the patient comes in for an MRI.

    b. after the tumor is confirmed on an MRI.

    c. when the diagnosed patient comes in for treatment.

    d. any time after the patient has been diagnosed.

    e. when the patient seeks specialist care.

COG MATCHING

Grade: _____

Match the following key terms to their definitions.

Key Terms

21. _____ advance beneficiary notice

22. _____ audits

23. _____ conventions

24. _____ cross-reference

25. _____ E-codes

26. _____ eponym

27. _____ etiology

28. _____ inpatient

29. _____ International Classification of Diseases, Ninth Revision, Clinical Modification

30. _____ late effects

31. _____ main terms

32. _____ medical necessity

33. _____ outpatient

34. _____ primary diagnosis

35. _____ service

36. _____ specificity

37. _____ V-codes

Definitions

a. codes indicating the external causes of injuries and poisoning

b. conditions that result from another condition

c. general notes, symbols, typeface, format, and punctuation that direct and guide a coder to the most accurate ICD-9 code

d. the condition or chief complaint that brings a person to a medical facility for treatment

e. a procedure or service that would have been performed by any reasonable physician under the same or similar circumstances

f. a document that informs covered patients that Medicare may not cover a certain service and the patient will be responsible for the bill

g. a word based on or derived from a person's name

h. codes assigned to patients who receive service but have no illness, injury, or disorder

i. the billable tasks performed by a physician

j. refers to a medical setting in which patients are admitted for diagnostic, radiographic, or treatment purposes

k. an investigation performed by government, managed health care companies, and health care organizations to determine compliance and to detect fraud

l. a system for transforming verbal descriptions of disease, injuries, conditions, and procedures to numeric codes

m. refers to the cause of disease

n. refers to a medical setting in which patients receive care but are not admitted

o. verification against another source

p. relating to a definite result

q. words in a multiple-word diagnosis that a coder should locate in the alphabetic listing

COG SHORT ANSWER   Grade: _____

38. Why is the third volume of the ICD-9-CM not used at a hospital's emergency department?

_____

_____

_____

_____

39. What is the title of the new edition of the ICD manuals? When will the new codes go into effect?

_____

_____

_____

_____

40. You are reading a patient's chart and notice that it is marked with an E-code. However, the patient has experienced no physical injuries. Why might an E-code be used in this situation?

_____

_____

_____

_____

41. You ask a veteran medical assistant for advice on coding, especially how to go about finding a diagnosis with more than one word. Her response is, "Find the condition, not the location." What does she mean by this?

_____

_____

_____

_____

42. What is listed first in the diagnosis section of the CMS-1500? What does it represent?

_____

_____

_____

_____

43. If a construction worker falls from a ladder and suffers an ankle fracture, what supplemental code is used?

_____

_____

_____

_____

44. When would you use the V-code for laboratory examination?

_____

_____

_____

_____

45. What should you do after finding a seemingly appropriate code in the alphabetic listing of Volume 1 of the ICD-9-CM?

_____

_____

_____

_____

46. If you do not know the medical terminology for a diagnosis for a common problem, what would be a good first plan of action?

_____

_____

_____

_____

47. What is the purpose of the fourth and fifth digits often appended to categories?

_____

_____

_____

_____

COG **PSY** **ACTIVE LEARNING**   Grade: _____

48. A reasonable and capable physician believes that a patient needs a chest x-ray to rule out pneumonia. Does the procedure meet the grounds for medical necessity? Why? Why not?

_____

_____

_____

_____

49. A patient comes in complaining of chest pain. When you enter the codes for this patient encounter, you code that the patient has "acute myocardial infarction." Why would it be better to code this encounter "chest pain rule out myocardial infarction"?

_____

_____

_____

_____

50. George Cregan has been seen by the physician for controlled non–insulin-dependent type 2 diabetes mellitus for about 10 years. While being seen for a routine check of his blood sugar, he complains of numbness and tingling in his left lower leg and foot. An x-ray of both legs is performed because poor circulation in the extremities can be a complication of diabetes. The x-ray confirms the diagnosis of peripheral neuropathy. Which ICD-9 code should be listed with the office visit? Which code indicates the reason for the x-ray? Which code should be placed on the CMA-1500 first as the primary diagnosis or reason for the visit?

_____

_____

51. In the ICD-9-CM, burns are listed in the range 940–949, a subset of 800–999—Injury and Poisoning. However, if you look for the code for sunburn, you will not find it there. Find the code for sunburn and explain why it does not belong in the range 940–949. You do not need to know exactly why, but consider the diagnoses that appear in 940–949 and how sunburn compares with them.

_____

_____

_____

_____

Determine the main term for the following multiple-word diagnoses.

Diagnosis	Main Term
52. chronic fatigue syndrome	
53. severe acute respiratory syndrome	
54. hemorrhagic encephalitis	
55. acute fulminating multiple sclerosis	
56. fractured left tibia	
57. breast cyst	

COG IDENTIFICATION

Grade: _____

58. Review the list of circumstances below and place a check mark to indicate whether a patient would be forced, given the circumstance, to sign an ABN. All of the patients below are covered by Medicare.

Circumstance	ABN	No ABN
a. The patient wishes to receive an immunization not covered by Medicare.		
b. The patient is undergoing a regularly scheduled checkup.		
c. The patient demands to be tested for an illness that the physician considers an impossibility.		
d. The patient has a badly sprained ankle and wishes to be treated.		
e. The patient is undergoing x-ray imaging per order of a physician.		

59. When it comes to coding, it makes a difference if the patient is seen in an inpatient or outpatient facility. Review the list of places below. Place an **I** next to those places that are considered "Inpatient" and an **O** next to those places that are considered "Outpatient."

a. _____ Hospital clinic

b. _____ Health care provider's office

c. _____ Hospital for less than 24 hours

d. _____ Hospital for 24 hours or more

e. _____ Hospital emergency room

60. Circle the main terms where you will find obstetric conditions.

| delivery | fetus | pregnancy | labor |
| baby | obstetrics | puerperal | gestational |

COG **TRUE OR FALSE?**   Grade: _____

True or False? Determine whether the following statements are true or false. If false, explain why.

61. Only the first three numbers of a code are necessary.

_____

62. One should never code directly from the alphabetic index.

_____

63. The main term describes a condition, not an aspect of anatomy.

_____

64. In the outpatient setting, coders list conditions after the patient's testing is complete.

_____

AFF **WHAT WOULD YOU DO?**   Grade: _____

65. A patient calls complaining of pain and swelling in the right hand since awakening this morning. The patient comes in, sees the doctor, and returns to the front desk with an encounter form that states his diagnosis is "gout." In order to make this diagnosis, the physician would need to know the patient's uric acid level. You know that the patient just had blood drawn for the test. It is a test that must be sent to an outside lab. Do you still code today's visit as "gout"? What would you do?

_____

_____

_____

_____

66. A patient is concerned that her insurance provider will not cover her visit because the diagnosis is for a very minor ailment. She requests that you mark her CMA-1500 with a more severe disorder that demands similar treatment. How would you deal with this situation? What would you tell the patient? How might you involve the physician?

_____

_____

_____

_____

67. A patient entered the office complaining of chest pains. After examination, the physician decided to send him to a specialist in order to rule out the possibility of angina pectoris. Which code should be placed on the CMA-1500 first as the primary diagnosis or reason for the visit? Why?

_____

_____

_____

_____

AFF **CASE STUDY FOR CRITICAL THINKING**   Grade: _____

Your physician-employer works with you closely to choose the most appropriate codes. He tells you that he would like for you to code patients who have B_{12} injections with "pernicious anemia." You ask if these patients should have a lab work to substantiate that diagnosis, and he says, "don't worry about that."

68. What would you say to him?

_____

_____

_____

_____

69. What would be the possible consequences of such an action?

_____

_____

_____

_____

70. Which of these is an unethical act? Explain why.

  a. Coding multiple conditions on the same CMS-1500

_____

_____

_____

  b. Coding an unsupported diagnosis in order to make a service appear medically necessary

_____

_____

_____

  c. Using a V-code to better explain the reason for a patient's visit

_____

_____

_____

  d. Using ICD-9-CM search software to more easily access the codes contained in the ICD-9-CM

_____

_____

_____

PSY PROCEDURE 14-1 **Locating a Diagnostic Code**

Name: _____ Date: _____ Time: _____ Grade: _____

EQUIPMENT: Diagnosis, ICD-9-CM, Volumes 1 and 2 codebook, medical dictionary.

STANDARDS: Given the needed equipment and a place to work the student will perform this skill with _____%
accuracy in a total of _____ minutes. *(Your instructor will tell you what the percentage and time limits will be
before you begin.)*

KEY: 4 = Satisfactory   0 = Unsatisfactory   NA = this step is not counted

PROCEDURE STEPS	SELF	PARTNER	INSTRUCTOR
1. Using the diagnosis "chronic rheumatoid arthritis," choose the main term within the diagnostic statement. If necessary, look up the word(s) in your dictionary.	☐	☐	☐
2. Locate the main term in Volume 2.	☐	☐	☐
3. Refer to all notes and conventions under the main term.	☐	☐	☐
4. Find the appropriate indented subordinate term.	☐	☐	☐
5. Follow any relevant instructions, such as "see also."	☐	☐	☐
6. Confirm the selected code by cross-referencing to Volume 1. Make sure you have added any fourth or fifth digits necessary.	☐	☐	☐
7. Assign the code.	☐	☐	☐
8. **AFF** Your office manager instructs you to assign a diagnosis code to a claim for a patient that you know does not have the diagnosis. Explain how you would respond.	☐	☐	☐

_____

_____

_____

_____

CALCULATION

Total Possible Points: _____

Total Points Earned: _____ Multiplied by 100 = _____ Divided by Total Possible Points = _____ %

PASS   **FAIL**   **COMMENTS:**

☐   ☐

Student's signature _____ Date _____

Partner's signature _____ Date _____

Instructor's signature _____ Date _____

WORK PRODUCT 1

Grade: _____

Underline the main term in these diagnoses with more than one word. Using a current ICD-9-CM book, then code the diagnoses:

1. sick sinus syndrome
2. congestive heart failure with malignant hypertension
3. bilateral stenosis of carotid artery
4. aspiration pneumonia
5. massive blood transfusion thrombocytopenia
6. acute rheumatic endocarditis
7. acute viral conjunctivitis with hemorrhage
8. *E. coli* intestinal infection
9. postgastrectomy diarrhea
10. congenital syphilitic osteomyelitis

WORK PRODUCT 2

Grade: _____

Determine the diseases associated with the following ICD-9-CM codes:

1. 555.9

   _____

2. 676.54

   _____

3. 314.01

   _____

4. 726.71

   _____

5. 722.93

   _____

WORK PRODUCT 3

Grade: _____

Determine the E-codes for the following:

1. Injured when hot air balloon crashed

_____

2. Skin frozen, contact with dry ice

_____

3. Bicyclist injured by train

_____

4. Injured by fireworks

_____

5. Hand slashed by circular saw

_____

WORK PRODUCT 4

Grade: _____

Code Sequencing

Kayla Moore, age 38 years, is seen in the clinic today. She has a few chronic conditions but is seen today for fluttering in her chest. Because she is here, and it is time for her regular diabetes checkup, the doctor orders a test to check on her blood sugar. Because Ms. Moore is a breast cancer survivor, in addition she was given a mammogram. Her physician also prescribed a tetanus booster as well, because she has been renovating an old stable and has suffered several small skin punctures over the past few weeks. Her encounter form indicates the following charges:

- an EKG to monitor a previously diagnosed arrhythmia
- fasting blood sugar for known diabetes
- mammogram
- tetanus booster

List the diagnoses in the proper order to be placed on line #21 of the CMS-1500 form.

21.

1._____   3._____

2._____   4._____

Outpatient Procedural Coding

Cognitive Domain

1. Spell and define the key terms
2. Explain the Healthcare Common Procedure Coding System (HCPCS), levels I and II
3. Explain the format of level I, Current Procedural Terminology (CPT-4) and its use
4. Describe the relationship between coding and reimbursement
5. Describe how to use the most current procedure coding system
6. Define upcoding and why it should be avoided
7. Describe how to uses the most current HCPCS coding
8. Describe the concept of RBRVS
9. Discuss all levels of governmental legislation and regulation as they apply to medical assisting practice, including FDA and DEA regulations
10. Define both medical terms and abbreviations related to all body systems

Psychomotor Domain

1. Perform procedural coding (Procedure 15-1)
2. Apply third-party guidelines

Affective Domain

1. Work with physician to achieve the maximum reimbursement
2. Demonstrate assertive communication with managed care and/or insurance providers
3. Apply ethical behaviors, including honesty/integrity in performance of medical assisting practice

ABHES Competencies

1. Apply third-party guidelines
2. Perform diagnostic and procedural coding
3. Comply with federal, state, and local health laws and regulations

Name: _____   Date: _____   Grade: _____

COG MULTIPLE CHOICE

1. In the case of an unlisted code, the medical assistant should:

   a. notify the AMA so that a new code is issued.

   b. submit a copy of the procedure report with the claim.

   c. obtain authorization from the AMA to proceed with the procedure.

   d. include the code that fits the most and add a note to explain the differences.

   e. not charge the patient for the procedure.

2. Which kind of information appears in a special report?

   a. Type of medicine prescribed

   b. Patient history

   c. Allergic reactions

   d. Possible procedural risks

   e. Equipment necessary for the treatment

3. On a medical record, the key components contained in E/M codes indicate:

   a. the scope and result of a medical visit.

   b. the duties of a physician toward his patients.

   c. the definition and description of a performed procedure.

   d. the services that a medical assistant may perform.

   e. the charges that are owed to the insurance company.

4. Time becomes a key component in a medical record when:

   a. the visit lasts more than 1 hour.

   b. more than half of the visit is spent counseling.

   c. the physician decides for a series of regular visits.

   d. the visit lasts longer than it was initially established.

   e. the patient is constantly late for his or her appointments.

5. When assigning a level of medical decision making, you should consider the:

   a. medication the patient is on.

   b. available coding for the procedure.

   c. patient's symptoms during the visit.

   d. insurance coverage allowed to the patient.

   e. patient's medical history.

6. In the anesthesia section, the physical status modifier indicates the patient's:

   a. medical history.

   b. conditions after surgery.

   c. good health before surgery.

   d. reactions to past anesthesia.

   e. condition prior to the administration of anesthesia.

7. Which of the following is included in a surgical package?

   a. General anesthesia

   b. Hospitalization time

   c. Complications related to the surgery

   d. Prescriptions given after the operation

   e. Uncomplicated follow-up care

8. How are procedures organized in the subsections of the surgery section of the CPT-4?

   a. By invasiveness

   b. By location and type

   c. In alphabetical order

   d. In order of difficulty of procedure

   e. By average recurrence of procedure

9. Which is the first digit that appears on radiology codes?

   a. 1

   b. 6

   c. 7

   d. 8

   e. 9

10. Diagnostic-related groups (DRGs) are a group of:

    a. codes pertaining to one particular treatment.

    b. inpatients sharing a similar medical history.

    c. modifiers attached to a single procedural form.

    d. physicians agreeing on a procedure for a particular medical condition.

    e. inpatients sharing similar diagnoses, treatment, and length of hospital stay.

11. The resource-based relative value scale (RBRVS) gives information on the:

    a. difficulty level of a particular surgical operation.

    b. maximum fee that physicians can charge for a procedure.

    c. reimbursement given to physicians for Medicare services.

    d. average fee asked by physicians for emergency procedures.

    e. minimum amount of time the physician should spend with a patient.

12. The Medicare allowed charge is calculated by:

    a. adding the RVU and the national conversion factor.

    b. dividing the RVU by the national conversion factor.

    c. multiplying the RVU by the national conversion factor.

    d. subtracting the RVU from the national conversion factor.

    e. finding the average between the RVU and the national conversion factor.

13. Upcoding is:

    a. billing more than the proper fee for a service.

    b. correcting an erroneous code in medical records.

    c. auditing claims retroactively for suspected fraud.

    d. comparing the documentation in the record with the codes received.

    e. researching new codes online.

14. Who has jurisdiction over a fraudulent medical practice?

    a. CMS

    b. AMA

    c. Medicare

    d. U.S. Attorney General

    e. State's supreme court

15. The purpose of the Level II HCPCS codes is to:

    a. decode different types of code modifiers.

    b. attribute a code to every step of a medical procedure.

    c. list the practices eligible for reimbursement by Medicare.

    d. identify services, supplies, and equipment not identified by CPT codes.

    e. provide coding information for various types of anesthesia.

16. Which of these sections is included in the HCPCS Level I code listing?

    a. Orthotics

    b. Injections

    c. Vision care

    d. Dental services

    e. Pathology and laboratory

17. How is a consultation different from a referral?

    a. A consultation is needed when the patient wants to change physicians.

    b. A consultation is needed when the physician asks for the opinion of another provider.

    c. A consultation is needed when the patient is transferred to another physician for treatment.

    d. A consultation is needed when the physician needs a team of doctors to carry out a procedure.

    e. A consultation is needed before the physician can submit insurance claims.

18. Which of the following is contained in Appendix B in the CPT-4?

    a. Legislation against medical fraud

    b. Detailed explanation of the modifiers

    c. Revisions made since the last editions

    d. Explanation on how to file for reimbursement

    e. Examples concerning the Evaluation and Management sections

19. Drug screening is considered *quantitative* when checking:

 a. for the amount of illegal drugs in the blood.

 b. for the presence of illegal drugs in the blood.

 c. for the proper level of therapeutic drugs in the blood.

 d. that the therapeutic drug is not interacting with other medications.

 e. that the drug is not causing an allergic reaction.

20. Which place requires the use of an emergency department service code?

 a. Private clinic

 b. Nursing home

 c. Physician's office

 d. 24-hour pharmacy

 e. Mental health center

21. How many numbers do E/M codes have?

 a. Two

 b. Five

 c. Six

 d. Seven

 e. Ten

COG MATCHING   Grade: _____

Match the following key terms to their definitions.

Key Terms

22. _____ Current Procedural Terminology

23. _____ descriptor

24. _____ diagnostic-related group

25. _____ Health Care Common Procedure Coding System

26. _____ key component

27. _____ modifiers

28. _____ outlier

29. _____ procedure

30. _____ resource-based relative value scale

31. _____ upcoding

Definitions

a. a patient whose hospital stay is longer than amount allowed by the DRG

b. categories used to determine hospital and physician reimbursement for Medicare patients' inpatient services

c. a value scale designed to decrease Medicare Part B costs and establish national standards for coding and payment

d. billing more than the proper fee for a service by selecting a code that is higher on the coding scale

e. description of a service listed with its code number

f. numbers or letters added to a code to clarify the service or procedure provided

g. a comprehensive listing of medical terms and codes for the uniform coding of procedures and services that are provided by physicians

h. a medical service or test that is coded for reimbursement

i. a standardized coding system that is used primarily to identify products, supplies, and services

j. the criteria or factors on which the selection of CPT-4 evaluation and management is based

COG SHORT ANSWER   Grade: _____

32. What role do modifiers play in coding?

_____

_____

_____

_____

33. When would you use 99 as the first numbers in your modifier?

_____

_____

_____

_____

34. What is the goal of the RBRVS?

_____

_____

_____

_____

35. How does coding play a part in reimbursement?

_____

_____

_____

_____

36. What are DRGs, and how are they used to determine Medicare payments?

_____

_____

_____

_____

37. List three ways to reduce the likelihood of a Medicare audit of your office.

_____

_____

_____

_____

38. Name four factors that go into radiology coding.

_____

_____

_____

_____

39. Why is it important to check the components of a surgery package with a third-party payer?

_____

_____

_____

_____

40. A patient experiences complications after an appendectomy and has to be hospitalized for several days. Will the time spent in the hospital be coded as part of a surgery package or separately?

_____

_____

_____

COG PSY **ACTIVE LEARNING**   Grade: _____

Using a current CPT book, assign the appropriate CPT code for the following:

41. occult blood in stool, two simultaneous guaiac tests

_____

42. blood ethanol levels

_____

43. transurethral resection of prostate

_____

44. flexible sigmoidoscopy for biopsy

_____

45. radiation therapy requiring general anesthesia

_____

46. hair transplant, 21 punch grafts

_____

47. breast reduction, left

_____

48. open repair of left Dupuytren contracture

_____

49. partial removal left turbinate

_____

50. newborn clamp circumcision

_____

COG PSY IDENTIFICATION

Grade: _____

What digit would be the first digit of the following codes?

51. routine prothrombin time

_____

52. ultrasound guidance for amniocentesis

_____

53. well-child check

_____

54. EKG

_____

55. removal of skin tags

_____

COG TRUE OR FALSE?

Grade: _____

Determine whether the following statements are true or false. If false, explain why.

56. It is permissible to leave out modifiers if a note is made on the patient's sheet.

_____

57. When time spent with a patient is more than 50% of the typical time for the visit, time becomes the deciding factor in choosing a code.

_____

58. The number of tests you perform is the final number in the coding.

_____

59. The amount of time a physician spends with a patient has no effect on the coding for that exam.

_____

COG IDENTIFICATION   Grade: _____

60. Fill in the chart below to show the difference between Level I HPCS and Level II.

Level I	Level II

61. What are the six major sections of the CPT-4?

a. _____

b. _____

c. _____

d. _____

e. _____

f. _____

62. Define the seven components of the E/M codes.

Component	Definition
a. history	
b. physician examination	
c. medical decision making	
d. counseling	
e. coordination of care	
f. nature of presenting problem	
g. time	

PSY **WHAT WOULD YOU DO?** Grade: _____

63. Read the scenario below. Then, highlight or underline the medical decision-making section.
    Anikka was seen today for a followup on her broken wrist. The cast was removed 2 weeks ago, and she said she is still unable to achieve full range of movement in her wrist without pain. On exam, her wrist appeared swollen, and she mentioned tenderness. X-ray revealed slight fracture in carpals. Dr. Levy splinted the wrist, and referred her to an orthopedic surgeon for possible surgery. I spoke with Anikka, instructing her to avoid exerting her wrist and to keep it splinted until she has seen the surgeon. Dr. Levy suggested aspirin for pain.

64. Now, read the same scenario again. Circle the history section.
    Anikka was seen today for a followup on her broken wrist. The cast was removed 2 weeks ago, and she said she is still unable to achieve full range of movement in her wrist without pain. On exam, her wrist appeared swollen, and she mentioned tenderness. X-ray revealed slight fracture in carpals. Dr. Levy splinted the wrist, and referred her to an orthopedic surgeon for possible surgery. I spoke with Anikka, instructing her to avoid exerting her wrist and to keep it splinted until she has seen the surgeon. Dr. Levy suggested aspirin for pain.

65. Read the scenario below.
    Mr. Ekko presents today for removal of stitches from calf wound. Upon inspection, wound seems to have healed well, but scar tissue is still slightly inflamed. I prescribed antibacterial cream for him to apply twice a day, and instructed him to still keep the area bandaged. I told him to let us know if the swelling has not gone down within a week, and to come in if it gets any worse.

    Circle the correct level of medical decision making involved.

    Straightforward   Low complexity

    Moderate complexity   High complexity

COG **IDENTIFICATION** Grade: _____

Fill in the medical terminology chart below about the CPT subcategory on repair, revision, or reconstruction.

Suffix	Meaning
66. -pexy	
	67. surgical repair
68. -rrhaphy	

CASE STUDY FOR CRITICAL THINKING   Grade: _____

69. A patient will be undergoing surgery to remove her gallbladder. Her insurance company labels this sort of operation as an outpatient surgery. She lives alone with no assistance after surgery. She wants to stay in the hospital overnight. The patient asks if you can do anything in the coding of the procedure to make her insurance company pay for a night in the hospital. What do you say to her? Can you do anything to code this information on the claim form for more reimbursement?

_____

_____

_____

_____

Name: _____ Date: _____ Time: _____ Grade: _____

EQUIPMENT: CPT-4 codebook, patient chart, scenario (Work Product 1)

STANDARDS Given the needed equipment and a place to work the student will perform this skill with _____% accuracy in a total of _____ minutes. *(Your instructor will tell you what the percentage and time limits will be before you begin.)*

KEY: 4 = Satisfactory   0 = Unsatisfactory   NA = This step is not counted

PROCEDURE STEPS	SELF	PARTNER	INSTRUCTOR
1. Identify the exact procedure performed.	☐	☐	☐
2. Obtain the documentation of the procedure in the patient's chart.	☐	☐	☐
3. Choose the proper codebook.	☐	☐	☐
4. Using the alphabetic index, locate the procedure.	☐	☐	☐
5. Locate the code or range of codes given in the tabular section.	☐	☐	☐
6. Read the descriptors to find the one that most closely describes the procedure.	☐	☐	☐
7. Check the section guidelines for any special circumstances.	☐	☐	☐
8. Review the documentation to be sure it justifies the code.	☐	☐	☐
9. Determine if any modifiers are needed.	☐	☐	☐
10. Select the code and place it in the appropriate field of the CMS-1500 form.	☐	☐	☐
11. **AFF** Your physician is helping you find a code in the CPT-4 codebook. He chooses a code based on what the surgery entailed, but the operative report does not support what he says he did. Explain how you would advise the physician to correct the problem and proceed.	☐	☐	☐

_____

_____

_____

_____

CALCULATION

Total Possible Points: _____

Total Points Earned: _____ Multiplied by 100 = _____ Divided by Total Possible Points = _____ %

PASS   **FAIL**   **COMMENTS:**

☐   ☐

Student's signature _____ Date _____

Partner's signature _____ Date _____

Instructor's signature _____ Date _____

WORK PRODUCT 1

Grade: _____

Perform Procedural Coding

Kayla Moore, age 38 years, has just completed a general physical. Her examination consisted of the following:

- an EKG to monitor a previously diagnosed arrhythmia
- urine collection to test for diabetes
- blood sampling to test cholesterol levels

Because Ms. Moore is a breast cancer survivor, in addition to the routine examination, she was given a mammogram. Her physician prescribed a tetanus booster as well, because she has been renovating an old stable and has suffered several small skin punctures over the past few weeks.

Complete the CMS-1500 form with the proper procedural coding for the patient's visit. Use the same personal patient information you used for Work Product 1 in Chapter 14 to fill in all essential details when completing the CMS-1500.

PLEASE
DO NOT
STAPLE
IN THIS
AREA

CARRIER

| | PICA | | | **HEALTH INSURANCE CLAIM FORM** | PICA | |

HEALTH INSURANCE CLAIM FORM

| 1. MEDICARE | MEDICAID | CHAMPUS | CHAMPVA | GROUP HEALTH PLAN | FECA BLK LUNG | OTHER | 1a. INSURED'S I.D. NUMBER (FOR PROGRAM IN ITEM 1) |
| (Medicare #) | (Medicaid #) | (Sponsor's SSN) | (VA File #) | (SSN or ID) | (SSN) | (ID) | |

2. PATIENT'S NAME (Last Name, First Name, Middle Initial)

3. PATIENT'S BIRTH DATE MM DD YY   SEX   M ☐   F ☐

4. INSURED'S NAME (Last Name, First Name, Middle Initial)

5. PATIENT'S ADDRESS (No., Street)

6. PATIENT RELATIONSHIP TO INSURED
Self ☐   Spouse ☐   Child ☐   Other ☐

7. INSURED'S ADDRESS (No., Street)

CITY   STATE

8. PATIENT STATUS
Single ☐   Married ☐   Other ☐
Employed ☐   Full-Time Student ☐   Part-Time Student ☐

CITY   STATE

ZIP CODE   TELEPHONE (Include Area Code)
(   )

ZIP CODE   TELEPHONE (INCLUDE AREA CODE)
(   )

9. OTHER INSURED'S NAME (Last Name, First Name, Middle Initial)

10. IS PATIENT'S CONDITION RELATED TO:

11. INSURED'S POLICY GROUP OR FECA NUMBER

a. OTHER INSURED'S POLICY OR GROUP NUMBER

a. EMPLOYMENT? (CURRENT OR PREVIOUS)
☐ YES   ☐ NO

a. INSURED'S DATE OF BIRTH MM DD YY   SEX   M ☐   F ☐

b. OTHER INSURED'S DATE OF BIRTH MM DD YY   SEX M ☐   F ☐

b. AUTO ACCIDENT?   PLACE (State)
☐ YES   ☐ NO

b. EMPLOYER'S NAME OR SCHOOL NAME

c. EMPLOYER'S NAME OR SCHOOL NAME

c. OTHER ACCIDENT?
☐ YES   ☐ NO

c. INSURANCE PLAN NAME OR PROGRAM NAME

d. INSURANCE PLAN NAME OR PROGRAM NAME

10d. RESERVED FOR LOCAL USE

d. IS THERE ANOTHER HEALTH BENEFIT PLAN?
☐ YES   ☐ NO   If yes, return to and complete item 9 a-d.

READ BACK OF FORM BEFORE COMPLETING & SIGNING THIS FORM.
12. PATIENT'S OR AUTHORIZED PERSON'S SIGNATURE I authorize the release of any medical or other information necessary to process this claim. I also request payment of government benefits either to myself or to the party who accepts assignment below.

SIGNED _____   DATE _____

13. INSURED'S OR AUTHORIZED PERSON'S SIGNATURE I authorize payment of medical benefits to the undersigned physician or supplier for services described below.

SIGNED _____

14. DATE OF CURRENT: MM DD YY   ILLNESS (First symptom) OR INJURY (Accident) OR PREGNANCY(LMP)

15. IF PATIENT HAS HAD SAME OR SIMILAR ILLNESS. GIVE FIRST DATE MM DD YY

16. DATES PATIENT UNABLE TO WORK IN CURRENT OCCUPATION MM DD YY   FROM   TO   MM DD YY

17. NAME OF REFERRING PHYSICIAN OR OTHER SOURCE

17a. I.D. NUMBER OF REFERRING PHYSICIAN

18. HOSPITALIZATION DATES RELATED TO CURRENT SERVICES MM DD YY   FROM   TO   MM DD YY

19. RESERVED FOR LOCAL USE

20. OUTSIDE LAB? $ CHARGES
☐ YES   ☐ NO

21. DIAGNOSIS OR NATURE OF ILLNESS OR INJURY. (RELATE ITEMS 1,2,3 OR 4 TO ITEM 24E BY LINE)
1. |___.__   3. |___.__
2. |___.__   4. |___.__

22. MEDICAID RESUBMISSION CODE   ORIGINAL REF. NO.

23. PRIOR AUTHORIZATION NUMBER

24. A DATE(S) OF SERVICE						B Place of Service	C Type of Service	D PROCEDURES, SERVICES, OR SUPPLIES (Explain Unusual Circumstances) CPT/HCPCS | MODIFIER	E DIAGNOSIS CODE	F $ CHARGES	G DAYS OR UNITS	H EPSDT Family Plan	I EMG	J COB	K RESERVED FOR LOCAL USE
From MM	DD	YY	To MM	DD	YY										
1															
2															
3															
4															
5															
6															

25. FEDERAL TAX I.D. NUMBER   SSN ☐ EIN ☐

26. PATIENT'S ACCOUNT NO.

27. ACCEPT ASSIGNMENT? (For govt. claims, see back)
☐ YES   ☐ NO

28. TOTAL CHARGE $

29. AMOUNT PAID $

30. BALANCE DUE $

31. SIGNATURE OF PHYSICIAN OR SUPPLIER INCLUDING DEGREES OR CREDENTIALS (I certify that the statements on the reverse apply to this bill and are made a part thereof.)

SIGNED _____   DATE _____

32. NAME AND ADDRESS OF FACILITY WHERE SERVICES WERE RENDERED (If other than home or office)

33. PHYSICIAN'S, SUPPLIER'S BILLING NAME, ADDRESS, ZIP CODE & PHONE #

PIN#   GRP#

(APPROVED BY AMA COUNCIL ON MEDICAL SERVICE 8/88)   **PLEASE PRINT OR TYPE**   APPROVED OMB-0938-0008 FORM CMS-1500 (12-90), FORM RRB-1500, APPROVED OMB-1215-0055 FORM OWCP-1500, APPROVED OMB-0720-0001 (CHAMPUS)

PATIENT AND INSURED INFORMATION

PHYSICIAN OR SUPPLIER INFORMATION

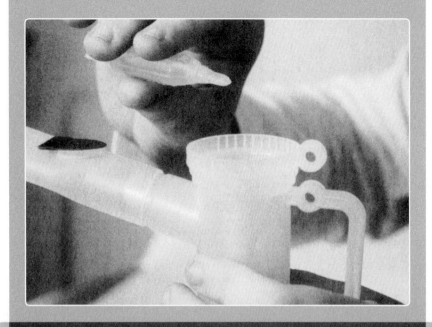

PART

III

The Clinical Medical Assistant

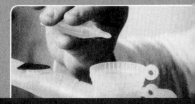

CHAPTER

16

Nutrition and Wellness

Learning
Outcomes

Cognitive Domain

1. Spell and define the key terms
2. Describe the normal function of the digestive system
3. Analyze charts, graphs, and/or tables in the interpretation of health care results
4. Name all of the essential nutrients
5. Discuss the body's basal metabolic rate and its importance in weight management
6. Explain how to use the food pyramid and MyPlate guides to promote healthy food choices
7. Read and explain the information on food labels
8. Describe special therapeutic diets and the patients who need them
9. List the components of physical fitness
10. Discuss suggestions for a healthy lifestyle
11. Explain the importance of disease prevention
12. List and describe the effects of the substances most commonly abused
13. Recognize the dangers of substance abuse

Psychomotor Domain

1. Teach a patient how to read food labels (Procedure 16-1)
2. Instruct patients according to their needs to promote health maintainence and disease prevention
3. Document patient education
4. Perform within scope of practice

Affective Domain

1. Apply critical thinking skills in performing patient assessment and care

2. Use language/verbal skills that enable patients' understanding
3. Demonstrate respect for diversity in approaching patients and families
4. Apply active listening skills
5. Demonstrate empathy in communicating with patients, family, and staff
6. Use appropriate body language and other nonverbal skills in communicating with patients, family, and staff
7. Demonstrate awareness of the territorial boundaries of the person with whom you are communicating
8. Demonstrate sensitivity appropriate to the message being delivered
9. Demonstrate recognition of the patient's level of understanding communications
10. Recognize and protect personal boundaries in communicating with others
11. Demonstrate respect for individual diversity, incorporating awareness of one's own biases in areas including gender, race, religion, age, and economic status

ABHES Competencies

1. Comprehend and explain to the patient the importance of diet and nutrition
2. Effectively convey and educate patients regarding the proper diet and nutrition guidelines
3. Identify categories of patients that require special diets or diet modifications
4. Document accurately

Name: _____   Date: _____   Grade: _____

COG MULTIPLE CHOICE

Circle the letter preceding the correct answer.

1. The nutrient that cushions and protects body organs and sustains normal body temperature is:

   a. carbohydrate.

   b. fat.

   c. mineral.

   d. protein.

   e. vitamin.

2. The purpose of a therapeutic diet is to:

   a. treat an underlying condition or disease.

   b. enjoy foods that put a person in a good mood.

   c. experiment with foods not normally allowed on other diets.

   d. eat foods the person likes but only in moderation.

   e. replace medications.

3. Which of the following is true about the effects of drugs or alcohol on a developing fetus?

   a. They have no effect on the developing fetus.

   b. They could cause the baby to be addicted to the substance after birth.

   c. Drugs could cause the brain to stop developing, but alcohol has no effect.

   d. They can harm the fetus only if the mother harms herself while using them.

   e. They could make the fetus hyper in the womb but cause no long-term effects after birth.

4. Which of the following statements about cholesterol is true?

   a. A diet high in fat but low in cholesterol is healthy.

   b. Cholesterol is found only in animal products.

   c. Cholesterol is found in fresh fruits and vegetables.

   d. Since the body cannot produce cholesterol it must be part of the diet.

   e. Adults should consume at least 350 mg of dietary cholesterol each day.

5. Which of the following would leave a person vulnerable to a disease?

   a. Keeping your immunizations up-to-date

   b. Washing your hands after using the bathroom

   c. Wearing insect repellent when outside in the summer

   d. Using someone else's antibiotics because he or she didn't finish them

   e. Washing cutting boards with soap and water after cutting uncooked chicken

6. Although alcohol intoxication may give a person a euphoric feeling, alcohol is a depressant. What does that mean?

   a. It gives the person a sad and gloomy feeling.

   b. It causes the person to suffer from depression.

   c. It causes increased heart rate and sleeplessness.

   d. It speeds up the functioning of the central nervous system.

   e. It causes a lack of coordination and impaired brain function.

7. The following statement about exercise is true:

   a. It induces stress.

   b. It suppresses the production of endorphins.

   c. It is effective if done for at least 40 minutes.

   d. It reduces the risk of developing certain diseases.

   e. Aerobic activities are most effective before target heart rate is reached.

8. Basal metabolic rate is:

   a. the constructive phase of metabolism.

   b. the destructive phase of metabolism.

   c. the baseline metabolic rate that is considered normal for the average adult.

   d. the amount of energy used in a unit of time to maintain vital functions by a fasting, resting person.

   e. the combination of the calories a person can consume and how long it takes to burn those calories.

9. A person who follows a lacto-ovo-vegetarian diet eats:

    a. vegetables only.

    b. vegetables and milk and cheese.

    c. vegetables and milk, eggs, and cheese.

    d. vegetables and milk, eggs, and poultry.

    e. vegetables and milk, eggs, and seafood.

10. Which of the following foods is a good source of fiber?

    a. Fish

    b. Milk

    c. Butter

    d. Chicken

    e. Vegetables

11. The five basic food groups include:

    a. dairy, vitamins, produce, meat, and grains.

    b. carbohydrates, fiber, vegetables, fruits, and meat.

    c. oils, lipids, refined sugars, whole grains, and dairy.

    d. grains, vegetables, milk, fruits, and meat and beans.

    e. proteins, carbohydrates, lipids, cholesterol, and minerals.

12. An overweight teenager asks you to suggest a cardiovascular exercise. Which of the following could you suggest?

    a. Yoga

    b. Sit-ups

    c. Stretching

    d. Lifting weights

    e. Jumping rope

13. Which vitamin is important for pregnant women because it reduces the risk of neural tube defects?

    a. Calcium

    b. Folate

    c. Mercury

    d. Potassium

    e. Zinc

14. To determine the correct number of daily servings from each food group, you need to know your:

    a. resting heart rate.

    b. height and weight.

    c. age and gender.

    d. waist measurement and target heart rate.

    e. level of physical activity and blood type.

15. How are refined grains different from whole grains?

    a. Refined grains are full of fiber.

    b. Whole grains lack fiber and iron.

    c. Whole grains are made with the entire grain kernel.

    d. Refined grains contain nutrients like carbohydrates and proteins.

    e. Refined grains are darker in color because they have more nutrients.

16. Water-soluble vitamins should be consumed:

    a. once a week.

    b. once a month.

    c. twice a week.

    d. daily.

    e. twice a month.

17. Pregnant women are advised to eat no more than one can of tuna per week because of the:

    a. iron content.

    b. lead content.

    c. mercury content.

    d. zinc content.

    e. calcium content.

18. How are substances such as cocaine and marijuana different from alcohol and nicotine?

    a. Alcohol and nicotine are legal; marijuana and cocaine are illegal.

    b. Cocaine and marijuana will not cause sudden death; alcohol and nicotine will cause sudden death.

    c. Alcohol and nicotine do not harm the body; marijuana and cocaine do harm the body.

    d. Cocaine and marijuana are used by people with health problems; alcohol and nicotine are not.

    e. Alcohol and nicotine are not additive drugs; marijuana and cocaine are addictive drugs.

19. Which of the following drugs damages blood vessels, decreases heart strength, and causes several types of cancer?

    a. Caffeine

    b. Nicotine

    c. Hashish

    d. Mescaline

    e. Phencyclidine

20. Why does inhaling marijuana smoke cause more damage to a person's body than tobacco smoke?

    a. Marijuana smoke is inhaled as unfiltered smoke, so users take in more cancer-causing agents and do more damage to the respiratory system than with regular filtered tobacco smoke.

    b. Marijuana smoke is thicker and more odorous.

    c. Marijuana smoke is inhaled as filtered smoke, so users take in less cancer-causing agents and do more damage to the respiratory system than with regular filtered tobacco smoke.

    d. Marijuana smoke is inhaled more quickly than tobacco smoke.

    e. Marijuana plants are grown in more toxic environments than tobacco plants.

COG MATCHING

Grade: _____

Match the essential nutrient with its description by placing the letter preceding the description of its function on the line next to the name of the nutrient.

Nutrients

21. _____ carbohydrates

22. _____ proteins

23. _____ fats

24. _____ vitamins

25. _____ minerals

Description

a. cushion and protect body organs and sustain normal body temperature

b. chemical substances that provide the body with energy

c. inorganic substances used in the formation of hard and soft body tissue

d. organic substances that enhance the breakdown of other nutrients in the body

e. substances that contain amino acids and help to build and repair tissue

COG MATCHING

Grade: _____

Match the following terms to the correct definitions. Place the letter preceding the term on the line next to the sentence that best describes its definition.

Key Terms

26. _____ anabolism

27. _____ anencephaly

28. _____ basal metabolic rate

29. _____ body mass index

30. _____ calorie

31. _____ catabolism

32. _____ dental cavities

33. _____ endorphins

34. _____ essential amino acids

35. _____ euphoria

36. _____ homeostasis

37. _____ metabolism

38. _____ minerals

39. _____ spina bifida

40. _____ lipoprotein

Definitions

a. inorganic substances used in the formation of hard and soft body tissue

b. a process in which larger molecules break down into smaller molecules

c. a neural tube defect that causes an incomplete closure of a fetus' spine during early pregnancy

d. a neural tube defect that affects the fetus' brain during early pregnancy

e. a good feeling

f. maintaining a constant internal environment by balancing positive and negative feedback

g. a process in which smaller molecules are converted into larger molecules as food is absorbed into the bloodstream

h. the amount of energy used in a unit of time to maintain vital function by a fasting, resting subject

i. transports cholesterol between the liver and arterial walls

j. the sum of chemical processes that result in growth, energy production, elimination of waste, and body functions performed as digested nutrients are distributed

k. areas of decay in the teeth

l. pain-relieving substance released naturally from the brain

m. an individual's ratio of fat to lean body mass

n. proteins that come from your diet because the body does not produce them

o. the amount of energy used by the body

COG IDENTIFICATION

Grade: _____

41. Indicate whether the following vitamins are fat-soluble or water-soluble by writing FS (fat-soluble) or WS (water-soluble) on the line preceding the name of the vitamin.

a. _____ Vitamin A

b. _____ Vitamin B-complex

c. _____ Vitamin C

d. _____ Vitamin D

e. _____ Vitamin E

f. _____ Vitamin K

g. _____ Thiamin

h. _____ Riboflavin

i. _____ Niacin

j. _____ Folic acid

COG COMPLETION

Grade: _____

42. Calculate the maximum heart rate and target heart rate for the individuals below based on their ages and desired intensity.

Person	Age	Maximum Heart Rate	Desired Intensity	Target Heart Rate
a. Tara	25		80%	
b. Yolanda	45		65%	
c. Hilel	37		75%	
d. Marco	18		90%	

43. Review the food pyramid in your textbook and answer the following questions based on a 2,000-calorie diet.

a. How much food from the grains category should be eaten in a day? _____

b. How many vegetables should be eaten in a day? _____

c. How much fruit should be eaten in a day? _____

d. How much milk should be consumed in a day? _____

e. How much from the meat and beans category should be consumed in a day? _____

44. Answer the following questions based on the food label (Figure 16-4) in your textbook.

a. How many servings are in this can of vegetables? _____

b. What is the serving size? _____

c. How many calories are from fat per serving? _____

d. What is the least amount of sugar you would consume if you ate 1 cup of this vegetable? _____

e. What is the percentage of sodium in one serving? _____

COG SHORT ANSWER   Grade: _____

45. Explain what BMI stands for and describe how it is calculated.

_____

_____

_____

_____

46. Explain the three basic ways the body expends energy.

a. Basal metabolic rate:

_____

_____

_____

_____

b. Levels of physical activity:

_____

_____

_____

_____

c. Thermic effect of food:

_____

_____

_____

_____

47. What is the best defense against illness?

_____

_____

_____

_____

48. List three techniques that can help lessen stress.

_____

_____

_____

_____

49. Drugs can be classified as stimulants and/or depressants that cause various effects on the body. Read each symptom below and place a check in the appropriate column.

Symptom	Depressant	Stimulant	Both
a. Poor fetal health			
b. Increased heart rate			
c. Psychological and physical dependence			
d. Increased pulse rate			
e. Slow respiratory rate			
f. Sleeplessness and anxiety			
g. Decreased activities of the central nervous system			

50. There are two phases in the process of metabolism: anabolism and catabolism. Indicate on the line provided whether the statement about metabolism describes anabolism (A) or catabolism (C).

a. _____ Constructive phase.

b. _____ Amino acids are converted into proteins.

c. _____ Destructive phase.

d. _____ Smaller molecules are converted into larger molecules.

e. _____ Larger molecules are converted into smaller molecules.

f. _____ Breakdown fats to use for energy.

g. _____ Complex carbohydrates, such as starch, are converted into simple sugars.

51. Look at the list of foods and indicate on the line whether the food contains a good fat (G) or bad fat (B). Place the letter G on the line if the item is "good" and B if the item is "bad."

a. _____ Salmon

b. _____ Olive oil

c. _____ Hamburger

d. _____ Margarine

e. _____ Crackers

f. _____ Soybean oil

g. _____ Nuts

h. _____ Cookies

i. _____ Steak

j. _____ Sunflower oil

COG AFF CASE STUDY FOR CRITICAL THINKING   Grade: _____

1. While conducting a patient interview, your patient, a 20-year-old college student, is concerned about gaining weight. She says she eats the same foods as her roommate, but her roommate does not gain weight, and she has put on 25 pounds since starting school. The roommate has told your patient that she can eat more food because she has a "high" metabolism rate. The patient is not sure what this means. How will you answer your patient? Would you recommend a reduced fat and/or calorie diet? Why or why not?

_____

_____

_____

_____

2. When educating a patient on the difference between whole grains and refined grains, what would you tell your patient?

_____

_____

_____

3. Mr. Consuelo is the president of a large manufacturing company. He is seeing Dr. Smith for frequent headaches. Dr. Smith has diagnosed the headaches as stress-induced and has recommended that Mr. Consuelo develop some coping mechanisms to reduce the stress in his life. As Mr. Consuelo leaves the office, he asks you about ways he can comply with Dr. Smith's recommendation to decrease the stress in his life. What strategies can you offer this patient?

    _____

    _____

    _____

    _____

4. Marco is 53 years old and has been smoking since he was 13. He says he would like to try and quit smoking, but he doesn't think it's worth it because the damage is probably already done. What would you say to him?

    _____

    _____

    _____

    _____

5. The physician asks you to explain the DASH diet to a patient with high blood pressure. How would you explain this diet including the basic dietary guidelines to a patient who speaks very little English?

    _____

    _____

    _____

    _____

6. Angelo, a 22-year-old man, comes to the office for a checkup. While interviewing him, he tells you that he drinks a lot on the weekends, but it's "no big deal." What three things could you say to Angelo that may help him understand that excessive alcohol is a big deal?

    _____

    _____

    _____

    _____

7. Dr. Mercer has given Joe, an overweight patient, clearance to start exercising. He told him to include workouts that will target each of the components of physical fitness. Joe feels overwhelmed. When talking to Joe, describe how you would explain the three components of physical fitness and how each one will help his body and health.

_____

_____

_____

_____

8. Your patient Carolyn is working with a nutritionist to improve her health. The nutritionist told her it is okay to take vitamins C and B every day, however she indicated that Carolyn should not take vitamin E every day. During her office visit, Carolyn asks you why she should not take vitamin E every day because she thought it was necessary to take all vitamins every day. What would you say to Carolyn?

_____

_____

_____

_____

9. A patient is upset because he has been placed on a special therapeutic diet because of his high blood pressure. He doesn't understand why he needs to stop eating some of his favorite foods, and he is worried he will not be successful with changing his diet. How can you encourage him to follow the physicians order to improve his health?

_____

_____

_____

_____

10. Your 17-year-old patient comes in to the physician's office because he has a bad cough. This is the second time this winter that he has seen the physician for respiratory problems. When you review the patient's chart, you see that he had asthma when he was younger. You ask the patient if he smokes and he says that he does occasionally with his friends, but also indicates that he is "not a smoker" because he's not addicted to nicotine. He also notes that he would prefer that his parents not know that he smokes, even occasionally. What should you say to this patient about his breathing issues? Would it be appropriate to tell his parents? Why or why not?

_____

_____

_____

_____

PSY PROCEDURE 16-1 | **Teach a Patient How to Read Food Labels**

Name: _____ Date: _____ Time: _____ Grade: _____

EQUIPMENT/SUPPLIES: Two boxes of the same item, one low calorie or "lite," the other regular; measuring cup; two bowls

STANDARDS: Given the needed equipment and a place to work the student will perform this skill with _____% accuracy in a total of _____ minutes. *(Your instructor will tell you what the percentage and time limits will be before you begin.)*

KEY: 4 = Satisfactory   0 = Unsatisfactory   NA = This step is not counted

PROCEDURE STEPS	SELF	PARTNER	INSTRUCTOR
1. Identify the patient.	☐	☐	☐
2. Introduce yourself and explain the procedure.	☐	☐	☐
3. Have the patient look at the labels comparing the two.	☐	☐	☐
4. Ask the patient to pour out a normal serving.	☐	☐	☐
5. Measure the exact serving size printed on the label.	☐	☐	☐
6. Compare the two. Discuss the difference, if any.	☐	☐	☐
7. Explain to the patient the sections of the label: serving size and servings per package.	☐	☐	☐
8. Explain column for amount in serving.	☐	☐	☐
9. Explain column for percent daily value (formerly RDA).	☐	☐	☐
10. Explain calories and calories from fat.	☐	☐	☐
11. Have the patient calculate the percentage of fat calories and compare with the label.	☐	☐	☐
12. Read down the label and discuss each nutrient, pointing out the amounts and percentages.	☐	☐	☐
13. Have the patient compare the two labels and tell you how many total carbohydrates are in each label, sugars, protein, etc.	☐	☐	☐
14. **AFF** Explain how to respond to a patient who has religious or personal beliefs against eating specific food groups, such as meats.	☐	☐	☐
15. Ask the patient if she has any questions.	☐	☐	☐
16. Document the instruction in the patient record.	☐	☐	☐

CALCULATION

Total Possible Points: _____

Total Points Earned: _____ Multiplied by 100 = _____ Divided by Total Possible Points = _____ %

PASS   **FAIL**   **COMMENTS:**

☐   ☐

Student's signature _____ Date _____

Partner's signature _____ Date _____

Instructor's signature _____ Date _____

Medical Asepsis and Infection Control

Cognitive Domain

1. Spell and define key terms
2. Describe the infection cycle, including the infectious agent, reservoir, susceptible host, means of transmission, portals of entry, and portals of exit
3. List major types of infectious agents
4. Compare different methods of controlling the growth of microorganisms
5. Discuss infection control procedures
6. List the various ways microbes are transmitted
7. Differentiate between medical and surgical asepsis used in ambulatory care settings, identifying when each is appropriate
8. Compare the effectiveness in reducing or destroying microorganisms using the various levels of infection control
9. Identify personal safety precautions as established by the Occupational Safety and Health Administration (OSHA)
10. Match types and uses of personal protective equipment (PPE)
11. Describe standard precautions, including transmission-based precautions, purpose, and activities regulated
12. Discuss the application of standard precautions with regard to all body fluids, secretions, and excretions; blood; nonintact skin; and mucous membranes
13. List the required components of an exposure control plan

14. Explain the facts pertaining to the transmission and prevention of the hepatitis B virus and the human immunodeficiency virus in the medical office
15. Identify the role of the Centers for Disease Control (CDC) regulations in health care settings

Psychomotor Domain

1. Participate in training on standard precautions
2. Perform a medical aseptic handwashing procedure (Procedure 17-1)
3. Remove contaminated gloves (Procedure 17-2)
4. Clean and decontaminate biohazardous spills (Procedure 17-3)
5. Apply local, state, and federal health care legislation and regulation appropriate to the medical assisting practice setting
6. Select appropriate barrier/PPE for potentially infectious situations

Affective Domain

1. Explain the rationale for performance of a procedure to the patient
2. Apply critical thinking skills in performing patient assessment and care

ABHES Competencies

1. Apply principles of aseptic techniques and infection control
2. Use standard precautions
3. Dispose of biohazardous materials

Name: _____   Date: _____   Grade: _____

COG MULTIPLE CHOICE

Circle the letter preceding the correct answer.

Scenario for Questions 1 through 3: Susan enters the examination room, where a patient is being seen for flu-like symptoms. While Susan takes the patient's blood pressure, the patient suddenly coughs near her face. Three days later Susan has the same signs and symptoms as the patient.

1. Which of the following terms best describes the patient in the infection cycle?

   a. Reservoir host

   b. Disease portal

   c. Pathogen portal

   d. Susceptible host

   e. Disease transmitter

2. Which of the following procedures could Susan have performed that might have helped to minimize contracting the patient's disease?

   a. Ask the patient to look the other way while coughing.

   b. Put on a facemask before entering the exam room.

   c. Run out of the room right after the patient coughed.

   d. Wash her face right after the coughing episode.

   e. Sterilize the examination room.

3. What type of transmission process occurred during Susan's contact with the patient?

   a. Direct

   b. Vector

   c. Viable

   d. Manual

   e. Indirect

4. *Clostridium tetani* causes tetanus. Because it does not require oxygen to survive, this microbe is an example of an:

   a. anoxic bacteria.

   b. aerobic bacteria.

   c. anaerobic bacteria.

   d. anaerolytic bacteria.

   e. aerosolized bacteria.

5. Which of the following groups of conditions best favors microbial growth?

   a. Cold, light, and dry

   b. Dry, dark, and warm

   c. Dark, moist, and cool

   d. Warm, moist, and light

   e. Moist, warm, and dark

6. *Escherichia coli* is normally found in the intestinal tract. *E. coli* can be transmitted to the urinary tract, causing an infection. When in the urinary tract, *E. coli* is an example of:

   a. viral flora.

   b. normal flora.

   c. resident flora.

   d. resistant flora.

   e. transient flora.

7. Which of the following practices is most important for maintaining medical asepsis?

   a. Airing out examination rooms after each patient

   b. Receiving all available vaccinations on an annual basis

   c. Wearing gloves before and after handling medical tools

   d. Wearing a gown if you are concerned about bodily fluids

   e. Washing your hands before and after each patient contact

8. To minimize infection, an endoscope should be:

   a. rinsed.

   b. sanitized.

   c. sterilized.

   d. disinfected.

   e. germicided.

9. At which temperature do most pathogenic microorganisms thrive?

   a. Below 32°F

   b. Above 212°F

   c. Around body temperature

   d. Around room temperature

   e. At any temperature

10. What level of disinfection would be appropriate to use when cleaning a speculum?

   a. None

   b. Low

   c. Intermediate

   d. High

   e. Sterilization

11. Which of the following job responsibilities has the highest risk exposure in the group?

   a. Measuring a patient's body temperature

   b. Covering a urine-filled specimen jar

   c. Drawing blood for lab analysis

   d. Auscultating a blood pressure

   e. Irrigating a patient's ear for excess earwax.

12. OSHA is responsible for:

   a. certifying all medical doctors.

   b. vaccinating school-age children.

   c. ensuring the safety of all workers.

   d. analyzing medical laboratory samples.

   e. caring for people with contagious diseases.

13. Jeremy approaches you and says that he just accidentally stuck himself with a needle while drawing a blood sample from a patient. He points to his thumb, where you can see a puncture. There is no bleeding. Which of the following actions should you take *first*?

   a. Direct Jeremy to wash his hands with soap and water.

   b. Lance the puncture with a scalpel to induce bleeding.

   c. Help him complete an exposure report right away.

   d. Call the physician in the office to ask for advice.

   e. Drive him to an occupational health clinic.

14. One example of PPE includes:

   a. name tag.

   b. stethoscope.

   c. face shield.

   d. scrub pants.

   e. syringe.

15. A patient arrives at the urgent care center complaining of nausea. As you begin to assess her, she begins to vomit bright red blood. Which of the following sets of PPE would be *most* appropriate to wear in this circumstance?

   a. Gown, gloves, and booties

   b. Eyewear, gown, and uniform

   c. Face shield and safety glasses

   d. Gloves, face shield, and gown

   e. Face shield, gown, and booties

16. Which of the following statements is *true* regarding hepatitis B virus (HBV)?

   a. HBV dies quickly outside the host body.

   b. There are no effective treatments for HBV.

   c. There is no vaccine protection against HBV.

   d. HBV is transmitted through blood contact, such as a needle puncture.

   e. It is easier to contract human immunodeficiency virus (HIV) than HBV.

17. Which of the following is *not* part of the body's natural defenses against disease?

   a. Plasma in blood

   b. Mucus in the nose

   c. Lysozyme in tears

   d. Saliva in the mouth

   e. Acid in the stomach

18. A vial of blood fell on the floor, glass broke, and the contents spilled on the floor. Proper cleaning of this spill includes:

    a. depositing the blood-soaked towels into a biohazard container.

    b. pouring hot water carefully onto the spill to avoid any splash.

    c. notifying the physician.

    d. allowing the blood to dry before cleaning.

    e. trying to piece the vial back together.

19. If a biohazard container becomes contaminated on the outside, you should:

    a. fill out a biohazard report form.

    b. immediately wash the surface in a sink.

    c. dispose of the container in a trash facility outside.

    d. place the container inside another approved container.

    e. call the biohazard removal company as soon as possible.

20. You should change your gloves *after*:

    a. touching a patient's saliva.

    b. measuring a patient's weight.

    c. auscultating a blood pressure.

    d. palpating a patient's abdomen.

    e. taking a patient's temperature.

COG MATCHING   Grade: _____

Match each key term with its description.

Key Terms

21. _____ aerobe

22. _____ asymptomatic

23. _____ disinfection

24. _____ germicide

25. _____ immunization

26. _____ microorganisms

27. _____ pathogens

28. _____ resistance

29. _____ spore

30. _____ sanitation

31. _____ standard precautions

32. _____ virulent

Definitions

a. the killing or rendering inert of most, but not all, pathogenic microorganisms

b. disease-causing microorganisms

c. bacterial life form that resists destruction by heat, drying, or chemicals

d. highly pathogenic and disease-producing; describes a microorganism

e. chemical that kills most pathogenic microorganisms; disinfectant

f. maintenance of a healthful, disease-free environment

g. microscopic living organisms

h. usual steps to prevent injury or disease

i. without any symptoms

j. body's immune response to prevent infections by invading pathogenic microorganisms

k. microorganism that requires oxygen to live and reproduce

l. act or process of rendering an individual immune to specific disease

COG IDENTIFICATION

33. Indicate whether the following microorganisms are resident or transient flora by writing RF (resident flora) or TF (transient flora) on the line preceding the name of the microbe and its location on or in the body.

    a. _____ Escherichia coli (large intestine)

    b. _____ Staphylococcus aureus (subcutaneous tissue)

    c. _____ Escherichia coli (peritoneum)

    d. _____ Staphylococcus aureus (epidermis; skin)

    e. _____ Helicobacter pylori (digestive tract)

34. Indicate whether the following situations could be a direct or indirect mode of disease transmission by writing D (direct) or I (indirect) on the line preceding the situation.

    a. _____ Shaking hands with someone

    b. _____ Getting a mosquito bite

    c. _____ Cleaning up a broken blood tube on the floor without gloves

    d. _____ Sneezing

    e. _____ Removing a tick from your leg

    f. _____ Sharing a soda with a friend using the same straw

35. What should a medical assistant wear when facing specific types of bodily fluids? Place a check mark on the line under each of the types of PPE you would use based on the patient's presentation.

Patient Presentation	Gloves	Protective Eyewear	Mask	Gown
a. Abdominal pain, vomiting				
b. Abdominal pain				
c. Headache, coughing				
d. Confusion				
e. Fever, nonproductive cough				
f. Generalized weakness				

COG **SHORT ANSWER**

Grade: _____

36. Your body is in a constant state of war—battling pathogens that are intent on getting into your body to grow and reproduce. Fortunately, your body has a variety of mechanisms to fight off pathogens. For each of the body structures below, explain how it fights the pathogens to protect the body.

   a. Nose cilia: _____

   b. Mucus: _____

   c. Skin: _____

   d. Urination: _____

   e. Tears: _____

   f. Saliva: _____

   g. Stomach: _____

37. A nondisposable vaginal speculum has just been used by the physician on a patient. After the exam is over and the patient leaves, how do you prepare this equipment for the next patient?

   _____

   _____

   _____

   _____

   _____

38. Name four factors that affect the disinfection process.

   _____

   _____

   _____

   _____

39. You accidentally stick yourself with a bloody needle. After washing the site, describe what you should do next.

   _____

   _____

   _____

   _____

COG TRUE OR FALSE?   Grade: _____

40. Indicate whether the statements are true or false by placing the letter T (true) or F (false) on the line preceding the statement.

   a. _____ Adhering to "clean technique," or medical asepsis, ensures that an object or area is free from all microorganisms.

   b. _____ Sterilization is the highest level of infection control.

   c. _____ Low-level disinfection destroys bacteria, but not viruses.

   d. _____ There are three levels of disinfection: minor, moderate, and severe.

   e. _____ Handwashing is a form of surgical or sterile asepsis.

COG AFF CASE STUDIES FOR CRITICAL THINKING   Grade: _____

1. Mei Lin is a clinical medical assistant who works in an outpatient clinic. Today she arrives at work with a minor cold. Over the course of an hour, she sees four patients. She draws a blood sample from one patient and retrieves a urine sample from another patient. During the hour she sneezes three times. She is preparing to leave for her lunch break. How many times should she have washed her hands during this time period?

_____

_____

_____

_____

2. Your patient is a 24-year-old female who has been diagnosed with bacterial pneumonia. The physician has ordered antibiotic therapy and bedrest. When leaving the office, she tells you that she is concerned about the fact that she has a 7-month-old baby at home. What information could you give her to clearly explain what steps she can take to avoid transmitting her illness to her child?

_____

_____

_____

_____

3. An established patient in your office is a 38-year-old female with AIDS. One of your coworkers, Steve, is afraid of interacting with this patient and has made disparaging remarks about her in the back office. You worry that Steve's attitude will affect patient care and you decide to talk to him privately. What points will you make? Should you also talk with your supervisor about Steve? Why, or why not?

_____

_____

_____

_____

4. The test results for 15-year-old Ashley Lewis come in and show that she is positive for hepatitis C. Her mother phones and asks you for the results. Is it appropriate for you to give her mother the test results? Why, or why not? How would you handle this call?

_____

_____

_____

_____

5. A middle-aged male comes into the medical office with a low-grade fever and productive cough that has lasted several weeks. The physician orders a chest x-ray to aid in diagnosis. After the patient leaves to get his chest x-ray, you begin to clean the room for the next patient. What level of disinfection will you use? What product(s) will you use? Provide detailed information about your actions, including dilution instructions, if appropriate.

_____

_____

_____

_____

6. You work in a pediatrician's office and have been working extra hours to save for a new, more reliable vehicle. Between work and school, you are tired and rundown. This morning, you woke up with a sore throat and headache. The last thing you want to do is call in sick because you need the money and you want your supervisor to think you are reliable. What should you do? Explain your answer.

_____

_____

_____

_____

PSY PROCEDURE 17-1 | Perform Medical Aseptic Handwashing

Name: _____ Date: _____ Time: _____ Grade: _____

EQUIPMENT/SUPPLIES: Liquid soap, disposable paper towels, an orangewood manicure stick, a waste can

STANDARDS: Given the needed equipment and a place to work the student will perform this skill with _____% accuracy in a total of _____ minutes. *(Your instructor will tell you what the percentage and time limits will be before you begin.)*

KEY: 4 = Satisfactory 0 = Unsatisfactory NA = this step is not counted

PROCEDURE STEPS	SELF	PARTNER	INSTRUCTOR
1. Remove all rings and wristwatch.	☐	☐	☐
2. Stand close to the sink without touching it.	☐	☐	☐
3. Turn on the faucet and adjust the temperature of the water to warm.	☐	☐	☐
4. Wet hands and wrists, apply soap, and work into a lather.	☐	☐	☐
5. Rub palms together and rub soap between your fingers at least 10 times.	☐	☐	☐
6. Scrub one palm with fingertips, work soap under nails, and then reverse hands.	☐	☐	☐
7. Rinse hands and wrists under warm running water.	☐	☐	☐
8. Hold hands lower than elbows and avoid touching the inside of the sink.	☐	☐	☐
9. Using the orangewood stick, clean under each nail on both hands.	☐	☐	☐
10. Reapply liquid soap and rewash hands and wrists.	☐	☐	☐
11. Rinse hands again while holding hands lower than the wrists and elbows.	☐	☐	☐
12. Use a dry paper towel to dry your hands and wrists gently.	☐	☐	☐
13. Use a dry paper towel to turn off the faucets and discard the paper towel.	☐	☐	☐

CALCULATION

Total Possible Points: _____

Total Points Earned: _____ Multiplied by 100 = _____ Divided by Total Possible Points = _____ %

PASS **FAIL** **COMMENTS:**
☐ ☐

Student's signature _____ Date _____

Partner's signature _____ Date _____

Instructor's signature _____ Date _____

PSY PROCEDURE 17-2 | Remove Contaminated Gloves

Name: _____ Date: _____ Time: _____ Grade: _____

EQUIPMENT/SUPPLIES: Clean examination gloves; biohazard waste container

STANDARDS: Given the needed equipment and a place to work the student will perform this skill with _____% accuracy in a total of _____ minutes. *(Your instructor will tell you what the percentage and time limits will be before you begin.)*

KEY: 4 = Satisfactory 0 = Unsatisfactory NA = this step is not counted

PROCEDURE STEPS	SELF	PARTNER	INSTRUCTOR
1. Choose the appropriate size gloves and apply one glove to each hand.	☐	☐	☐
2. After "contaminating" gloves, grasp the glove palm of the nondominant hand with fingers of the dominant hand.	☐	☐	☐
3. Pull the glove away from the nondominant hand.	☐	☐	☐
4. Slide the nondominant hand out of the contaminated glove while rolling the contaminated glove into the palm of the gloved dominant hand.	☐	☐	☐
5. Hold the soiled glove in the palm of your gloved hand. a. Slip ungloved fingers under the cuff of the gloved hand. b. Stretch the glove of the dominant hand up and away from your hand while turning it inside out with the nondominant hand glove balled up inside.	☐	☐	☐
6. Discard both gloves as one unit into a biohazard waste receptacle.	☐	☐	☐
7. Wash your hands.	☐	☐	☐

CALCULATION

Total Possible Points: _____

Total Points Earned: _____ Multiplied by 100 = _____ Divided by Total Possible Points = _____ %

PASS   **FAIL**   **COMMENTS:**

☐   ☐

Student's signature _____ Date _____

Partner's signature _____ Date _____

Instructor's signature _____ Date _____

PSY PROCEDURE 17-3 | Cleaning Biohazardous Spills

Name: _____ Date: _____ Time: _____ Grade: _____

EQUIPMENT/SUPPLIES: Commercially prepared germicide *or* 1:10 bleach solution, gloves, bag, protective eyewear (goggles or mask and face shield), disposable shoe coverings, disposable gown or apron made of plastic or other material that is impervious to soaking up contaminated fluids

STANDARDS: Given the needed equipment and a place to work the student will perform this skill with _____% accuracy in a total of _____ minutes. *(Your instructor will tell you what the percentage and time limits will be before you begin.)*

KEY: 4 = Satisfactory   0 = Unsatisfactory   NA = this step is not counted

PROCEDURE STEPS	SELF	PARTNER	INSTRUCTOR
1. Put on gloves.	☐	☐	☐
2. Wear protective eyewear, gown or apron, and shoe covers if splashing is anticipated.	☐	☐	☐
3. Apply chemical absorbent to the spill.	☐	☐	☐
4. Clean up the spill using disposable paper towels.	☐	☐	☐
5. Dispose of paper towels and absorbent material in a biohazard waste bag.	☐	☐	☐
6. Further decontaminate using a commercial germicide or bleach solution: **a.** Wipe with disposable paper towels. **b.** Discard the towels used for decontamination in a biohazard bag.	☐	☐	☐
7. With gloves on, remove the protective eyewear and discard or disinfect.	☐	☐	☐
8. Remove the gown/apron and shoe coverings and place in biohazard bag.	☐	☐	☐
9. Place the biohazard bag in an appropriate waste receptacle.	☐	☐	☐
10. Remove contaminated gloves and wash hands thoroughly.	☐	☐	☐

CALCULATION

Total Possible Points: _____

Total Points Earned: _____ Multiplied by 100 = _____ Divided by Total Possible Points = _____ %

PASS   **FAIL**   **COMMENTS:**

☐   ☐

Student's signature _____ Date _____

Partner's signature _____ Date _____

Instructor's signature _____ Date _____

18 Medical History and Patient Assessment

Cognitive Domain

1. Spell and define key terms
2. Recognize communication barriers
3. Identify techniques for overcoming communication barriers
4. Give examples of the type of information included in each section of the patient history
5. Identify guidelines for conducting a patient interview using principles of verbal and nonverbal communication
6. Differentiate between subjective and objective information
7. Discuss open-ended and closed-ended questions and explain when to use each type during the patient interview

Psychomotor Domain

1. Obtain and record a patient history (Procedure 18-1)
2. Practice within the standard of care for a medical assistant
3. Use reflection, restatement, and clarification techniques to obtain a patient history
4. Use medical terminology, pronouncing medical terms correctly, to communicate information, patient history, data and observations
5. Apply local, state, and federal health care legislation and regulation appropriate to the medical assisting practice setting
6. Accurately document a chief complaint and present illness (Procedure 18-2)

Affective Domain

1. Demonstrate empathy in communicating with patients, family, and staff
2. Apply active listening skills
3. Use appropriate body language and other nonverbal skills in communicating with patients, family, and staff
4. Demonstrate sensitivity to patients' rights
5. Demonstrate awareness of the territorial boundaries of the person with whom you are communicating
6. Demonstrate sensitivity appropriate to the message being delivered
7. Demonstrate recognition of the patient's level of understanding communications
8. Recognize and protect personal boundaries in communicating with others
9. Demonstrate respect for individual diversity, incorporating awareness of one's own biases in areas including gender, race, religion, age, and economic status
10. Apply critical thinking skills in performing patient assessment and care

ABHES Competencies

1. Be impartial and show empathy when dealing with patients
2. Interview effectively
3. Recognize and respond to verbal and nonverbal communication
4. Obtain chief complaint, recording patient history

Name: _____ Date: _____ Grade: _____

COG MULTIPLE CHOICE

Circle the letter preceding the correct answer.

1. The best place to interview a patient is:

　a. over the phone.

　b. at the patient's home.

　c. in the reception area.

　d. in an examination room.

　e. in the physician's office.

2. Which of the following would appear in the past history (PH) section of a patient's medical history?

　a. Hospitalizations

　b. Chief complaint

　c. Insurance carrier

　d. Review of systems

　e. Deaths in immediate family

3. You are collecting the medical history of a patient. The patient discloses that her brother, sister, paternal grandfather, and paternal aunt are overweight. For this patient, obesity is considered to be:

　a. familial.

　b. historic.

　c. hereditary.

　d. homeopathic.

　e. demographic.

4. Under HIPAA, who may access a patient's medical records?

　a. Any health care provider

　b. The patient's family and friends

　c. Anyone who fills out the proper forms

　d. Only the patient's primary care physician

　e. Only health care providers directly involved in the patient's care

5. During an interview, your patient tells you that she drinks alcohol four to five times a week. This information should be included in the:

　a. chief complaint.

　b. past history.

　c. present illness.

　d. social history.

　e. family history.

6. Which of the following is included in the patient's present illness (PI)?

　a. Self-care activities

　b. Hereditary diseases

　c. Signs and symptoms

　d. Preventative medicine

　e. Name, address, and phone number

7. Who completes the patient's medical history form?

　a. The patient only

　b. The patient's insurance provider

　c. The patient's immediate family

　d. The patient, the medical assistant, and the physician

　e. The patient's former physician or primary care provider

8. A homeopathic remedy for a headache could be a(n):

　a. prescription painkiller.

　b. extended period of rest.

　c. 1,000 mg dose of acetaminophen.

　d. icepack on the forehead for 10 minutes.

　e. small dose of an agent that causes headache.

9. An open-ended question is one that:

   a. determines the patient's level of pain.

   b. determines where something happened.

   c. is rhetorical and does not require an answer.

   d. can be answered with a "yes" or a "no" response.

   e. requires the responder to answer using more than one word.

10. One sign of illness might be:

    a. coughing.

    b. headache.

    c. dizziness.

    d. nausea.

    e. muscle pain.

11. Which of the following is a closed-ended question?

    a. "What is the reason for your appointment today?"

    b. "Tell me what makes the pain worse?"

    c. "Does the pain leave and return throughout the day?"

    d. "How would you describe the pain you are feeling?"

    e. "What have you done to help eliminate the pain?"

12. At the beginning of an interview, you can establish a trusting, professional relationship with the patient by:

    a. thoroughly introducing yourself.

    b. listing the physician's credentials.

    c. observing the patient's signs of illness.

    d. conducting the review of systems (ROS).

    e. disclosing the patient's weight in private.

13. If you suspect that the patient you are assessing is the victim of abuse, you should:

    a. report your suspicions to the local police station.

    b. record your suspicion of abuse in the patient's chief complaint (CC).

    c. ask the patient if he or she is being abused with a closed-ended question.

    d. document the objective signs and notify the physician of your suspicions.

    e. review the patient's medical history for signs of an abusive spouse or parent.

14. Which of the following is included in the identifying database of a patient's medical history?

    a. The patient's emergency contact

    b. The patient's Social Security number

    c. The patient's reason for visiting the office

    d. The patient's signs and symptoms of illness

    e. The patient's family's addresses

15. One example of a symptom of an illness is:

    a. rash.

    b. cough.

    c. nausea.

    d. vomiting.

    e. wheezing.

16. The patient's PI includes which of the following:

    a. social history.

    b. family history.

    c. chronology of the illness.

    d. demographic information.

    e. history of hospitalizations.

17. Before you proceed with a patient interview, you should obtain:

    a. signs and symptoms.

    b. social and family history.

    c. the duration of pain and self-treatment information.

    d. the chief complaint and patient's present illness.

    e. the location of pain and self-treatment information.

18. Which of the following is a poor interview technique?

    a. Asking open-ended questions

    b. Noting observable information

    c. Suggesting expected symptoms

    d. Introducing yourself to the patient

    e. Reading through the patient's medical history beforehand

19. You think that a patient has a disease that was passed down from her parents. Where could you look to find information on the patient's parents?

   a. Medical history forms

   b. History of self-treatment

   c. Demographic information

   d. Notes during the patient interview

   e. Chief complaints from previous visits

20. While obtaining a patient's present illness, you need to find out:

   a. where she lives.

   b. the chief complaint.

   c. if she smokes tobacco.

   d. the severity of the pain.

   e. any hereditary disease(s) she has.

COG MATCHING   Grade: _____

Match each key term with its definition.

Key Terms

21. _____ assessment

22. _____ chief complaint

23. _____ demographic

24. _____ familial

25. _____ hereditary

26. _____ homeopathic

27. _____ medical history

28. _____ over the counter

29. _____ signs

30. _____ symptoms

Definitions

a. relating to the statistical characteristics of populations

b. subjective indications of disease or bodily dysfunction as sensed by the patient

c. process of gathering information about a patient and the presenting condition

d. a record containing information about a patient's past and present health status

e. traits or disorders that are passed from parent to offspring

f. objective indications of disease or bodily dysfunction as observed or measured by the health care professional

g. the main reason for a patient's visit to the medical office

h. medications and natural drugs that are available without a prescription

i. traits that tend to occur often within a particular family

j. describing a type of alternative medicine in which patients are treated with small doses of substances that produce similar symptoms and use the body's own healing abilities

COG IDENTIFICATION

Grade: _____

31. Indicate whether the following patient interview questions during a patient assessment are helpful or not helpful by writing H (helpful) or NH (not helpful) on the line preceding the question.

   a. _____ "Do you feel pain?"

   b. _____ "How often does the pain occur?"

   c. _____ "What were you doing when the pain started?"

   d. _____ "Have you taken ibuprofen for the pain?"

   e. _____ "Does lying down lessen the pain you feel?"

32. Two types of home remedies are over-the-counter medications and homeopathic medications. Determine whether the items below are over-the-counter or homeopathic medications by writing OTC (over-the-counter) or H (homeopathic) on the line next to the item.

   a. _____ 1,000 mg of acetaminophen to relieve the pain of a sprained ankle

   b. _____ A small dose of mercury to treat symptoms similar to mercury poisoning

   c. _____ Ingesting ipecacuanha, a root that causes vomiting, in order to treat vomiting

   d. _____ A cooling topical ointment applied to skin afflicted by sunburn

33. As a medical assistant, you will have many responsibilities. Place a check mark on the line next to the actions that you may perform as a medical assistant.

   a. _____ Documenting the patient's chief complaint (CC)

   b. _____ Assessing the patient's present illness (PI) during a patient interview

   c. _____ Going over the medical file to the patient's family and friends

   d. _____ Reviewing the patient's medical history before interviewing the patient

   e. _____ Recording judgments based on the patient's appearance in the patient's record

   f. _____ Advising patient which over-the-counter or homeopathic treatments to use

COG COMPLETION

Grade: _____

34. Using any available resources, find information about influenza. On the lines below, list three signs and three symptoms that a patient may have influenza (or the flu).

Signs	Symptoms
a.	a.
b.	b.
c.	c.

35. The section of the patient history that reviews each body system and invites the patient to share any information that he or she may have forgotten to mention earlier is called _____.

36. The _____ section covers the health status of the patient's immediate family members.

37. Information needed for administrative purposes, such as the patient's name, address, and telephone number, is included in the _____ section.

38. Important information about the patient's lifestyle is documented in the _____ section.

39. The section of the patient history that focuses on the patient's prior health status is called _____.

COG SHORT ANSWER   Grade: _____

40. What is the purpose of gathering a patient's social history?

_____

_____

_____

_____

41. When are closed-ended questions appropriate during a patient interview? Give one example of an appropriate closed-ended question.

_____

_____

_____

_____

42. During a patient interview, you learn that the patient is an extreme sports enthusiast and works in a coal mine. Where should you record this information in the patient's medical history forms?

_____

_____

_____

43. Why is the reception area a poor place to interview a patient? What would be a better location for interviewing a patient?

_____

_____

_____

_____

44. What are two ways in which a patient's medical history is gathered in the medical office?

_____

_____

_____

_____

45. What should you say to the patient when introducing yourself? Why is a thorough introduction important?

_____

_____

_____

_____

COG **TRUE OR FALSE?**   Grade: _____

Indicate whether the statements are true or false by placing the letter T (true) or F (false) on the line preceding the statement.

46. _____ Unlike OTC medications, homeopathic medications are only available by prescription.

47. _____ Nausea is a sign of food poisoning.

48. _____ It is always the patient's responsibility to fill out his medical history completely and accurately.

49. _____ The chief complaint is always a description of a patient's signs and symptoms.

50. _____ Obtaining a urine specimen from the patient may be part of the chief complaint.

51. _____ It is appropriate to assist an older adult who cannot hold a pen due to arthritis with filling out the medical history form.

52. _____ Entries made in the patient record should be signed and dated.

53. _____ It is the responsibility of the receptionist to make sure the demographic information is complete.

AFF **COG** **CASE STUDIES FOR CRITICAL THINKING**   Grade: _____

1. You are interviewing a patient, Mr. Gibson. You learn that Mr. Gibson is a 55-year-old male. He is starting a new job as a childcare provider and needs to submit a physical examination to his new place of employment. Mr. Gibson's father died of colon cancer when he was 60 years old, and Mr. Gibson's wife is a smoker. Mr. Gibson says he feels healthy and has not had any health-related problems in the last few years. What should you record as the chief complaint in Mr. Gibson's medical record?

_____

_____

_____

_____

2. Mrs. Frank is a returning patient at Dr. Mohammad's office. She is 89 years old and needs the assistance of a wheelchair. What are some important considerations that you should make when showing Mrs. Frank to an exam room, gathering her medical history, and performing a patient assessment? How would those considerations change if the patient was a 2-year-old child?

_____

_____

_____

_____

3. Your patient is a 49-year-old female who speaks very little English. She is a returning patient, so her medical history is already on file at the office. You have called a coworker who can act as a translator, but he will not arrive at the office for an hour. Meanwhile, the patient is clearly uncomfortable. She appears sweaty and lethargic. She leans on you as you escort her to an examination room. Describe how you can determine the patient's chief complaint and present illness so that you and the physician can begin to help her.

_____

_____

_____

_____

4. Alicia, a medical assistant in Dr. Howard's office, has recorded the following in a patient assessment:

"CC: Pt. c/o fatigue, depressed mood, and inability to stay asleep at night. Has taken Tylenol PM for two nights with "no effect" on sleep. Has not eaten for 2 days because of lack of appetite, which is likely caused by his depression. Face pale, skin clammy."

Was there anything in this documentation that should not have been recorded? Explain your answer.

5. Giles is a medical assistant in Dr. Yardley's office. Giles enters the examination room to interview a patient. Giles notices that the patient is lying on the examination table, holding his abdomen. He is holding a black trash bin that contains a small amount of his vomit. The patient is flushed and sweating. Before even speaking to the patient, Giles has realized some of the patient's signs and symptoms of illness. Explain the significance of signs and symptoms and then fill in this patient's signs and symptoms in the chart below.

Signs	Symptoms
a.	a.
b.	b.
c.	c.

6. There are two patients waiting in examination rooms to see the physician. Patient A is a new patient, and Patient B is coming into the office for a complete physical examination. When sorting these patients to determine who should be taken back to the exam room first, what factors should be considered?

_____

_____

_____

_____

7. What are your ethical and legal responsibilities as a medical assistant concerning a patient's medical history records?

_____

_____

_____

_____

8. Your patient is a 17-year-old male. His symptoms are shortness of breath and fatigue. During the interview, you learn that his father and older brother are obese. You also learn that both of his grandfathers died of complications resulting from heart disease. Although this patient is not overweight, he tells you that he does not have time to exercise but would like to avoid gaining weight, especially when he enters college this fall. What changes does the patient needs to make in his lifestyle in order to improve his health and avoid obesity and heart disease? Should you make suggestions for the members of his family who are obese? Why or why not?

_____

_____

_____

_____

9. Ms. Butler, 20 years old, received a pregnancy test during a visit to the physician's office. A week later, Mr. Gordon, a 25-year-old male, comes into the office demanding to see the results of Ms. Butler's test. He tells you that he is her boyfriend and that if Ms. Butler is pregnant, he deserves to know. What would you say to Mr. Gordon?

_____

_____

_____

_____

10. On your way to the exam room, you notice a coworker weighing another patient on the scales located in the hallway. As the patient steps onto the scale, your coworker moves the weights on the scale and then reads the patient's weight out loud. The patient appears embarrassed. What would you say, if anything, to your coworker? Why or why not?

_____

_____

_____

_____

PSY PROCEDURE 18-1 | **Obtain and Record a Patient History**

Name: _____ Date: _____ Time: _____ Grade: _____

EQUIPMENT/SUPPLIES: Medical history form or questionnaire, black or blue pen

STANDARDS: Given the needed equipment and a place to work the student will perform this skill with _____% accuracy in a total of _____ minutes. *(Your instructor will tell you what the percentage and time limits will be before you begin.)*

KEY: 4 = Satisfactory   0 = Unsatisfactory   NA = This step is not counted

PROCEDURE STEPS	SELF	PARTNER	INSTRUCTOR
1. Gather the supplies.	☐	☐	☐
2. Review the medical history form for completeness.	☐	☐	☐
3. If the form is partially completed or if the patient could not complete any of the form, take the patient to a private area or the examination room and assist him or her with completing the form.	☐	☐	☐
4. Sit across from the patient at eye level and maintain eye contact.	☐	☐	☐
5. Introduce yourself and explain the purpose of the interview.	☐	☐	☐
6. Ask the appropriate questions and document the patient's responses.	☐	☐	☐
7. Listen actively by looking at the patient from time to time while he or she is speaking.	☐	☐	☐
8. Avoid projecting a judgmental attitude with words or actions.	☐	☐	☐
9. **AFF** Explain how to respond to a patient who does not speak English.	☐	☐	☐
10. Explain to the patient what to expect during examinations or procedures at that visit.	☐	☐	☐
11. Thank the patient for cooperating during the interview and offer to answer any questions.	☐	☐	☐

CALCULATION

Total Possible Points: _____

Total Points Earned: _____ Multiplied by 100 = _____ Divided by Total Possible Points = _____ %

PASS	FAIL	COMMENTS:
☐	☐	

Student's signature _____ Date _____

Partner's signature _____ Date _____

Instructor's signature _____ Date _____

PSY PROCEDURE 18-2 Document a Chief Complaint and Present Illness

Name: _____ Date: _____ Time: _____ Grade: _____

EQUIPMENT/SUPPLIES: Patient medical record including a cumulative problem list or progress notes form, black or blue ink pen

STANDARDS: Given the needed equipment and a place to work the student will perform this skill with _____% accuracy in a total of _____ minutes. *(Your instructor will tell you what the percentage and time limits will be before you begin.)*

KEY: 4 = Satisfactory 0 = Unsatisfactory NA = This step is not counted

PROCEDURE STEPS	SELF	PARTNER	INSTRUCTOR
1. Gather the supplies including the medical record containing the cumulative problem list or progress note form.	☐	☐	☐
2. Review the new or established patient's medical history form.	☐	☐	☐
3. Greet and identify the patient while escorting him or her to the examination room. Close the door.	☐	☐	☐
4. Use open-ended questions to find out why the patient is seeking medical care; maintain eye contact.	☐	☐	☐
5. Determine the PI using open-ended and closed-ended questions.	☐	☐	☐
6. **AFF** Explain how to respond to a patient who has dementia.	☐	☐	☐
7. Document the CC and PI correctly on the cumulative problem list or progress report form.	☐	☐	☐
8. Thank the patient for cooperating and explain that the physician will soon be in to examine the patient.	☐	☐	☐

CALCULATION

Total Possible Points: _____

Total Points Earned: _____ Multiplied by 100 = _____ Divided by Total Possible Points = _____ %

PASS   **FAIL**   **COMMENTS:**

☐   ☐

Student's signature _____ Date _____

Partner's signature _____ Date _____

Instructor's signature _____ Date _____

19 Anthropometric Measurements and Vital Signs

Cognitive Domain

1. Spell and define key terms
2. Explain the procedures for measuring a patient's height and weight
3. Identify and describe the types of thermometers
4. Compare the procedures for measuring a patient's temperature using the oral, rectal, axillary, and tympanic methods
5. List the fever process, including the stages of fever
6. Describe the procedure for measuring a patient's pulse and respiratory rates
7. Identify the various sites on the body used for palpating a pulse
8. Define Korotkoff sounds and the five phases of blood pressure
9. Identify factors that may influence the blood pressure
10. Explain the factors to consider when choosing the correct blood pressure cuff size
11. Discuss implications for disease and disability when homeostasis is not maintained

Psychomotor Domain

1. Measure and record a patient's weight (Procedure 19-1)
2. Measure and record a patient's height (Procedure 19-2)

4. Measure and record a patient's oral temperature using a glass mercury thermometer (Procedure 19-3)
5. Measure and record a patient's rectal temperature (Procedure 19-4)
6. Measure and record a patient's axillary temperature (Procedure 19-5)
7. Measure and record a patient's temperature using an electronic thermometer(Procedure 19-6)
8. Measure and record a patient's temperature using a tympanic thermometer (Procedure 19-7)
9. Measure and record a patient's temperature using a temporal artery thermometer (Procedure 19-8)
10. Measure and record a patient's radial pulse (Procedure 19-9)
11. Measure and record a patient's respirations (Procedure 19-10)
12. Measure and record a patient's blood pressure (Procedure 19-11)
13. Obtain vital signs
14. Document accurately in the patient record
15. Practice standard precautions

Affective Domain

1. Apply critical thinking skills in performing patient assessment and care
2. Demonstrate respect for diversity in approaching patients and families

3. Explain rationale for performance of a procedure to the patient
4. Apply active listening skills
5. Demonstrate empathy in communicating with patients, family, and staff
6. Use appropriate body language and other nonverbal skills in communicating with patients, family, and staff
7. Demonstrate awareness of the territorial boundaries of the person with whom you are communicating
8. Demonstrate sensitivity appropriate to the message being delivered
9. Demonstrate recognition of the patient's level of understanding communications
10. Recognize and protect personal boundaries in communicating with others
11. Demonstrate respect for individual diversity, incorporating awareness of one's own biases in areas including gender, race, religion, age, and economic status

ABHES Competencies

1. Take vital signs
2. Document accurately

Name: _____   Date: _____   Grade: _____

COG MULTIPLE CHOICE

Circle the letter preceding the correct answer.

1. Anthropometric measurements:

   a. include vital signs.

   b. include height and weight.

   c. don't include height in adults.

   d. are taken only at the first visit.

   e. are used only as baseline information.

2. What are the cardinal signs?

   a. Height and weight

   b. Baseline measurements

   c. Pulse, respiration, and blood pressure

   d. Pulse, respiration, blood pressure, and temperature

   e. Temperature, pulse, blood pressure, respiration, and cardiac output

3. When you greet a patient, what should you always do before taking any measurements?

   a. Put on gloves.

   b. Identify the patient.

   c. Get a family history.

   d. Get a medical history.

   e. Determine whether the patient speaks English.

4. After getting an accurate weight measurement, what is the next thing you should do?

   a. Remove the paper towel.

   b. Write down the measurement.

   c. Assist the patient off the scale.

   d. Tell the patient his or her weight.

   e. Convert the measurement to kilograms.

5. If the balance bar of a balance beam scale points to the midpoint when the large counterweight is at 100, and the small counterweight is 2 lines to the right of the mark for 30, what is the patient's weight?

   a. 32 pounds

   b. 73 pounds

   c. 128 pounds

   d. 132 pounds

   e. 264 pounds

6. To get an accurate height measurement, you should:

   a. wash your hands and put down a paper towel.

   b. have the patient stand barefoot with heels together.

   c. have the patient face the ruler and look straight ahead.

   d. put the measuring bar on the patient's hair and deduct an inch.

   e. record the measurement before helping the patient off the scale.

7. An axillary temperature would be a good measurement to take when:

   a. the patient is very talkative.

   b. there are no more disposable plastic sheaths.

   c. the office is so full that there is little privacy.

   d. the patient is wearing many layers of clothing.

   e. you need to know the temperature as quickly as possible.

8. One difference between using electronic thermometers and using glass thermometers is the:

   a. use of gloves for rectal measurements.

   b. use of a disposable cover for the thermometer.

   c. color code for oral and rectal measurements.

   d. wait time before the thermometer is removed.

   e. receptacle for disposable covers after measurements.

9. The three stages of fever are:

   a. abrupt onset, course, and lysis.

   b. onset, various course, and lysis.

   c. onset, sustained fever, and crisis.

   d. abrupt or gradual onset, course, and resolution.

   e. onset, fluctuating course, and abrupt resolution.

10. Which method would you use to take a brachial pulse?

    a. Palpation alone

    b. Auscultation alone

    c. Palpation and/or auscultation

    d. Palpation and/or use of a Doppler unit

    e. Auscultation and/or use of a Doppler unit

11. Which method would you use to take an apical pulse?

    a. Palpation alone

    b. Auscultation alone

    c. Palpation and/or auscultation

    d. Palpation and/or use of a Doppler unit

    e. Auscultation and/or use of a Doppler unit

12. Which statement is true of a respiratory rate?

    a. It increases when a patient is lying down.

    b. It is the number of expirations in 60 seconds.

    c. It is the number of complete inspirations per minute.

    d. It should be taken while the patient is not aware of it.

    e. It is the number of inspirations and expirations in 30 seconds.

13. Abnormal breathing may be characterized by:

    a. inhalations that are medium and rhythmic.

    b. inhalations and exhalations that are regular and consistent.

    c. air moving in and out heard with a stethoscope.

    d. breathing that is shallow or wheezing.

    e. a rate of 16 to 20.

14. Hyperpnea is:

    a. no respiration.

    b. shallow respirations.

    c. abnormally deep, gasping breaths.

    d. inability to breathe while lying down.

    e. a respiratory rate that is too high for oxygen demand.

15. The Korotkoff sound that signals systolic blood pressure is:

    a. faint tapping.

    b. soft swishing.

    c. soft tapping that becomes faint.

    d. rhythmic, sharp, distinct tapping.

    e. sharp tapping that becomes soft swishing.

16. Which group of factors is likely to affect blood pressure?

    a. Age, exercise, occupation

    b. Activity, stress, tobacco use

    c. Alcohol, education, prescriptions

    d. Body position, height, history of heart conditions

    e. Dietary habits, wealth, family history of heart disease

17. Which blood pressure cuff is the correct size?

    a. One that has the Velcro in places that match up

    b. One with a length that wraps three times around the arm

    c. One with a width that goes halfway around the upper arm

    d. One with a width that wraps all the way around the lower arm

    e. One with a length that wraps one and a half times around the arm

18. Which measurement is a normal axillary temperature?

    a. 36.4°C

    b. 37.0°C

    c. 37.6°C

    d. 98.6°F

    e. 99.6°F

19. A tympanic thermometer measures temperature:

   a. in the ear.

   b. in the mouth.

   c. under the armpit.

   d. on the temple.

   e. in the rectum.

20. Diaphoresis is:

   a. sweating.

   b. constant fever.

   c. elevated blood pressure.

   d. needing to sit upright to breathe.

   e. blood pressure that drops upon standing.

COG MATCHING

Grade: _____

Match each key term with its definition.

Key Terms

21. _____ afebrile

22. _____ anthropometric

23. _____ apnea

24. _____ baseline

25. _____ calibrated

26. _____ cardiac cycle

27. _____ cardinal signs

28. _____ diastole

29. _____ diaphoresis

30. _____ dyspnea

31. _____ febrile

32. _____ hyperpnea

33. _____ hyperpyrexia

34. _____ hypertension

35. _____ hyperventilation

36. _____ hypopnea

37. _____ intermittent

38. _____ orthopnea

39. _____ palpation

40. _____ postural hypotension

41. _____ pyrexia

42. _____ relapsing fever

43. _____ remittent fever

44. _____ sphygmomanometer

45. _____ sustained fever

46. _____ systolev

Definitions

a. profuse sweating

b. fever that is fluctuating

c. no respiration

d. fever that is constant

e. shallow respirations

f. occurring at intervals

g. elevated blood pressure

h. pertaining to measurements of the human body

i. difficult or labored breathing

j. device used to measure blood pressure

k. abnormally deep, gasping breaths

l. phase in which the heart contracts

m. having a temperature above normal

n. original or initial measure with which other measurements will be compared

o. having a temperature within normal limits

p. extremely high temperature, from 105° to 106°F

q. marked in units of measurement

r. phase in which the heart pauses briefly to rest and refill

s. fever of 102°F or higher rectally or 101°F or higher orally

t. act of pressing an artery against an underlying firm surface

u. sudden drop in blood pressure upon standing

v. fever returning after an extended period of normal readings

w. respiratory rate that greatly exceeds the body's oxygen demand

x. period from the beginning of one heartbeat to the beginning of the next

y. inability to breathe lying down

z. measurements of vital signs

COG IDENTIFICATION

47. Place a check mark on the line next to each factor that can affect blood pressure.

    a. _____ Activity

    b. _____ Age

    c. _____ Alcohol use

    d. _____ Arteriosclerosis

    e. _____ Atherosclerosis

    f. _____ Body position

    g. _____ Dietary habits

    h. _____ Economic status

    i. _____ Education

    j. _____ Exercise

    k. _____ Family history of heart conditions

    l. _____ General health of the patient

    m. _____ Height

    n. _____ History of heart conditions

    o. _____ Medications

    p. _____ Occupation

    q. _____ Stress

    r. _____ Tobacco use

Grade: _____

48. Indicate whether the following measurements are anthropometric, cardinal signs, performed at the first office visit (baseline), or performed at every office visit. Place a check mark in the appropriate column. Measurements may have more than one check mark.

	Anthropometric	Baseline (First Time)	Every Time	Cardinal Sign	Medical Assistant
a. Blood pressure					
b. Cardiac output					
c. Height					
d. Pulse rate					
e. Respiratory rate					
f. Temperature					
g. Weight					

49. The steps for weighing a patient with a balance beam scale are listed below, but they are not in the correct order. Starting with the number one (1), number the steps in the correct order.

_____ Record the weight.

_____ Memorize the weight.

_____ Help the patient off the scale.

_____ Help the patient onto the scale.

_____ Be sure the counterweights are both at zero.

_____ Be sure the counterweights are both at zero.

_____ Slide the larger counterweight toward zero until it rests securely in a notch.

_____ Slide the smaller counterweight toward zero until the balance bar is exactly at the midpoint.

_____ Slide the larger counterweight away from zero until the balance bar moves below the midpoint.

_____ Slide the smaller counterweight away from zero until the balance bar moves below the midpoint.

_____ Add the readings from the two counterweight bars, counting each line after the smaller counterweight as 1/4 pound.

50. For each step listed in measuring a patient's height, circle the correct word or phrase from the two options given in parentheses.

a. Wash your hands if the height is measured at (a different time from/the same time as) the weight.

b. The patient should (remove/wear) shoes.

c. The patient should stand straight with heels (a hand's width apart/together).

d. The patient's eyes should be looking (at the floor/straight ahead).

e. A better measurement is usually taken with the patient's (back/front) to the ruler.

f. Position the measuring bar perpendicular to the (ruler/top of the head).

g. Slowly lower the measuring bar until it touches the patient's (hair/head).

h. Measure at the (point of movement/top of the ruler).

i. A measurement of 66 inches should be recorded as (5 feet, 6 inches/66 inches).

COG **SHORT ANSWER**   Grade: _____

51. What does the hypothalamus do when it senses that the body is too warm?

_____

_____

_____

_____

52. What happens when the body temperature is too cool?

_____

_____

_____

_____

53. What factors aside from illness affect body temperature?

_____

_____

_____

_____

54. List and describe the three stages of fever. Include the variations in the time and their related terms.

_____

_____

_____

_____

55. If the patient has 19 full inspirations and 18 full expirations in 1 minute, what is the patient's respiratory rate?

_____

_____

_____

_____

56. At which sound is the systolic blood pressure recorded?

_____

_____

_____

_____

57. At which sound is the diastolic blood pressure recorded?

_____

_____

_____

_____

COG **TRUE OR FALSE?**   Grade: _____

58. Indicate whether the statements are true or false by placing the letter T (true) or F (false) on the line preceding the statement.

a. _____ The weight scale should be kept in the waiting room for ease of access.

b. _____ An axillary temperature can be taken with either an oral or a rectal thermometer.

c. _____ In pediatric offices, temperatures are almost always taken rectally.

d. _____ If a glass mercury thermometer breaks, you should soak up the mercury immediately with tissues and put them in the trash before the mercury sinks into any surfaces.

CASE STUDIES FOR CRITICAL THINKING   Grade: _____

1. Ms. Green arrived at the office late for her appointment, frantic and explaining that her alarm clock had not gone off. She discovered that her car was almost out of gas, and she had to stop to refuel. Once she got to the clinic, she could not find a parking place in the lot and she had to park two blocks away. How would you expect this to affect her vital signs? Explain why.

_____

_____

_____

_____

2. A patient comes into the office complaining of fever and chills. While taking her vital signs, you notice that her skin feels very warm. When you take her temperature, you find that her oral temperature is 105°F. What should you do?

_____

_____

_____

_____

3. Mr. Juarez, the father of a 6-month-old baby and a 4-year-old child, would like to purchase a thermometer. He is not sure which one to buy and isn't familiar with how to use the different kinds of thermometers. He also isn't aware of the possible variations that may occur in readings. How would you explain the various types of thermometers and temperature readings to him? What would you recommend and why?

_____

_____

_____

_____

4. Mrs. Chin has come into the office complaining of pain in her right foot. You take her vital signs, which are normal, and you help her remove her shoes so that the doctor can examine both feet. You notice a difference in appearance between her two feet, and it occurs to you to check her femoral, popliteal, posterior tibial, and dorsalis pedis pulses. What are you looking for, and what should you look for next?

_____

_____

_____

_____

5. You've noticed that whenever you try to take Mr. Kimble's respiration rate, he always breathes in when you do and breathes out when you do. You're concerned that you're not assessing Mr. Kimble's breathing accurately, and you know that he has had asthma on occasion. What can you do to get an accurate reading?

_____

_____

_____

_____

PSY PROCEDURE 19-1 | **Measure and Record a Patient's Weight**

Name: _____ Date: _____ Time: _____ Grade: _____

EQUIPMENT/SUPPLIES: Calibrated balance beam scale, digital scale or dial scale; paper towel

STANDARDS: Given the needed equipment and a place to work the student will perform this skill with _____% accuracy in a total of _____ minutes. *(Your instructor will tell you what the percentage and time limits will be before you begin.)*

KEY: 4 = Satisfactory   0 = Unsatisfactory   NA = This step is not counted

PROCEDURE STEPS	SELF	PARTNER	INSTRUCTOR
1. Wash your hands.	☐	☐	☐
2. Ensure that the scale is properly balanced at zero.	☐	☐	☐
3. Escort the patient to the scale and place a paper towel on the scale.	☐	☐	☐
4. Have the patient remove shoes, heavy coats, or jackets.	☐	☐	☐
5. Assist the patient onto the scale facing forward.	☐	☐	☐
6. Ask patient to stand still, without touching or holding on to anything if possible.	☐	☐	☐
7. Weigh the patient.	☐	☐	☐
8. Return the bars on the top and bottom to zero.	☐	☐	☐
9. Assist the patient from the scale if necessary and discard the paper towel.	☐	☐	☐
10. Record the patient's weight.	☐	☐	☐
11. **AFF** Explain how to respond to a patient who is visually impaired.	☐	☐	☐

CALCULATION

Total Possible Points: _____

Total Points Earned: _____ Multiplied by 100 = _____ Divided by Total Possible Points = _____ %

PASS   **FAIL**   **COMMENTS:**

☐   ☐

Student's signature _____ Date _____

Partner's signature _____ Date _____

Instructor's signature _____ Date _____

PSY PROCEDURE 19-2 | Measure and Record a Patient's Height

Name: _____ Date: _____ Time: _____ Grade: _____

EQUIPMENT/SUPPLIES: A scale with a ruler

STANDARDS: Given the needed equipment and a place to work the student will perform this skill with _____% accuracy in a total of _____ minutes. *(Your instructor will tell you what the percentage and time limits will be before you begin.)*

KEY: 4 = Satisfactory   0 = Unsatisfactory   NA = This step is not counted

PROCEDURE STEPS	SELF	PARTNER	INSTRUCTOR
1. Wash your hands.	☐	☐	☐
2. Have the patient remove his or her shoes and stand straight and erect on the scale, heels together, and eyes straight ahead.	☐	☐	☐
3. With the measuring bar perpendicular to the ruler, slowly lower until it firmly touches patient's head.	☐	☐	☐
4. Read the measurement at the point of movement on the ruler.	☐	☐	☐
5. Assist the patient from the scale.	☐	☐	☐
6. Record the height measurements in the medical record. The height may be recorded with the weight measurement.	☐	☐	☐
7. **AFF** Explain how to respond to a patient who has dementia.	☐	☐	☐

_____

_____

_____

_____

CALCULATION

Total Possible Points: _____

Total Points Earned: _____ Multiplied by 100 = _____ Divided by Total Possible Points = _____ %

PASS   **FAIL**   **COMMENTS:**

☐   ☐

Student's signature _____ Date _____

Partner's signature _____ Date _____

Instructor's signature _____ Date _____

Measure and Record a Patient's Oral Temperature Using a Glass Thermometer

Name: _____ Date: _____ Time: _____ Grade: _____

EQUIPMENT/SUPPLIES: Glass oral thermometer, tissues or cotton balls, disposable plastic sheath, gloves, biohazard waste container, cool soapy water, disinfectant solution

STANDARDS: Given the needed equipment and a place to work the student will perform this skill with _____% accuracy in a total of _____ minutes. *(Your instructor will tell you what the percentage and time limits will be before you begin.)*

KEY: 4 = Satisfactory 0 = Unsatisfactory NA = This step is not counted

PROCEDURE STEPS	SELF	PARTNER	INSTRUCTOR
1. Wash your hands and assemble the necessary supplies.	☐	☐	☐
2. Dry the thermometer if it has been stored in disinfectant.	☐	☐	☐
3. Carefully check the thermometer for chips or cracks.	☐	☐	☐
4. Check the level of the chemical in the thermometer.	☐	☐	☐
5. If the chemical level is above 94°F, carefully shake down thermometer.	☐	☐	☐
6. Insert the thermometer into the plastic sheath.	☐	☐	☐
7. Greet and identify the patient.	☐	☐	☐
8. Explain the procedure and ask about any eating, drinking hot or cold fluids, gum chewing, or smoking.	☐	☐	☐
9. Place the thermometer under the patient's tongue.	☐	☐	☐
10. Tell the patient to keep his or her mouth and lips closed but caution against biting down on the glass stem.	☐	☐	☐
11. Leave the thermometer in place for 3 to 5 minutes.	☐	☐	☐
12. At the appropriate time, remove the thermometer from the patient's mouth while wearing gloves.	☐	☐	☐
13. Remove the sheath by holding the very edge of the sheath with your thumb and forefinger.	☐	☐	☐
14. Discard the sheath into a biohazard waste container.	☐	☐	☐
15. Hold the thermometer horizontal at eye level and note the level of chemical in the column.	☐	☐	☐
16. Record the patient's temperature.	☐	☐	☐
17. **AFF** Explain how to respond to a patient who speaks English as a second language.	☐	☐	☐

_____
_____
_____

CALCULATION

Total Possible Points: _____

Total Points Earned: _____ Multiplied by 100 = _____ Divided by Total Possible Points = _____ %

PASS	**FAIL**	**COMMENTS:**
☐	☐	

Student's signature _____ Date _____

Partner's signature _____ Date _____

Instructor's signature _____ Date _____

Name: _____ Date: _____ Time: _____ Grade: _____

EQUIPMENT/SUPPLIES: Glass mercury rectal thermometer, tissues or cotton balls, disposable plastic sheaths, surgical lubricant, biohazard waste container, cool soapy water, disinfectant solution, gloves

STANDARDS: Given the needed equipment and a place to work the student will perform this skill with _____% accuracy in a total of _____ minutes. *(Your instructor will tell you what the percentage and time limits will be before you begin.)*

KEY: 4 = Satisfactory 0 = Unsatisfactory NA = This step is not counted

PROCEDURE STEPS	SELF	PARTNER	INSTRUCTOR
1. Wash your hands and assemble the necessary supplies.	☐	☐	☐
2. Dry the thermometer if it has been stored in disinfectant.	☐	☐	☐
3. Carefully check the thermometer for chips or cracks.	☐	☐	☐
4. Check the level of the mercury in the thermometer.	☐	☐	☐
5. If the mercury level is above 94°F, carefully shake down.	☐	☐	☐
6. Insert the thermometer into the plastic sheath.	☐	☐	☐
7. Spread lubricant onto a tissue and then from the tissue onto the sheath of the thermometer.	☐	☐	☐
8. Greet and identify the patient and explain the procedure.	☐	☐	☐
9. Ensure patient privacy by placing the patient in a side-lying position facing the examination room door. Drape appropriately.	☐	☐	☐
10. Apply gloves and view the anus by lifting the top buttock with your non-dominant hand.	☐	☐	☐
11. Gently insert thermometer past the sphincter muscle.	☐	☐	☐
12. Release the upper buttock and hold the thermometer in place with your dominant hand for 3 minutes.	☐	☐	☐
13. After 3 minutes, remove the thermometer and the sheath.	☐	☐	☐
14. Discard the sheath into a biohazard waste container.	☐	☐	☐
15. Note the reading with the thermometer horizontal at eye level.	☐	☐	☐
16. Give the patient a tissue to wipe away excess lubricant.	☐	☐	☐
17. Assist with dressing if necessary.	☐	☐	☐
18. Record the procedure and mark the letter *R* next to the reading.	☐	☐	☐
19. **AFF** Explain how to respond to a patient who is developmentally challenged.	☐	☐	☐

_____

_____

_____

_____

CALCULATION

Total Possible Points: _____

Total Points Earned: _____ Multiplied by 100 = _____ Divided by Total Possible Points = _____ %

PASS　　　**FAIL**　　　　　　**COMMENTS:**

☐　　　　☐

Student's signature _____ Date _____

Partner's signature _____ Date _____

Instructor's signature _____ Date _____

PSY PROCEDURE 19-5 Measure and Record an Axillary Temperature

Name: _____ Date: _____ Time: _____ Grade: _____

EQUIPMENT/SUPPLIES: Glass (oral or rectal) thermometer or electronic thermometer, tissues or cotton balls, disposable plastic sheaths, biohazard waste container, cool soapy water, disinfectant solution

STANDARDS: Given the needed equipment and a place to work the student will perform this skill with _____% accuracy in a total of _____ minutes. *(Your instructor will tell you what the percentage and time limits will be before you begin.)*

KEY: 4 = Satisfactory   0 = Unsatisfactory   NA = This step is not counted

PROCEDURE STEPS	SELF	PARTNER	INSTRUCTOR
1. Wash your hands.	☐	☐	☐
2. Dry the glass thermometer if it has been stored in disinfectant. Obtain the electronic thermometer if this type is used.	☐	☐	☐
3. Carefully check the glass thermometer for chips or cracks or make sure the electronic thermometer is charged.	☐	☐	☐
4. Check the level of the chemical in the glass thermometer if used and shake down if the level is above 94°F.	☐	☐	☐
5. Insert the thermometer into a plastic sheath.	☐	☐	☐
6. Uncover the patient's axilla, exposing as little of the upper body as possible.	☐	☐	☐
7. Place the bulb or end of the thermometer well into the axilla.	☐	☐	☐
8. Bring the patient's arm down, crossing the forearm over the chest.	☐	☐	☐
9. Leave the thermometer in place for 10 minutes (glass) or until the thermometer signals that a temperature has been recorded.	☐	☐	☐
10. Remove the thermometer from the patient's axilla.	☐	☐	☐
11. Remove and discard the sheath into a biohazard waste container.	☐	☐	☐
12. Hold the glass thermometer horizontal at eye level and note the level of chemical. If electronic, note the digital reading.	☐	☐	☐
13. Record the procedure and mark a letter *A* next to the reading, indicating that an axillary temperature was taken.	☐	☐	☐
14. **AFF** Explain how to respond to a patient who is from a different (older) generation.	☐	☐	☐

CALCULATION

Total Possible Points: _____

Total Points Earned: _____ Multiplied by 100 = _____ Divided by Total Possible Points = _____ %

PASS   **FAIL**   **COMMENTS:**

☐   ☐

Student's signature _____ Date _____

Partner's signature _____ Date _____

Instructor's signature _____ Date _____

PSY PROCEDURE 19-6   Measure and Record a Patient's Temperature Using an Electronic Thermometer

Name: _____   Date: _____   Time: _____   Grade: _____

EQUIPMENT/SUPPLIES: Electronic thermometer with oral or rectal probe, lubricant and gloves for rectal temperatures, disposable probe covers, biohazard waste container

STANDARDS: Given the needed equipment and a place to work the student will perform this skill with _____% accuracy in a total of _____ minutes. *(Your instructor will tell you what the percentage and time limits will be before you begin.)*

KEY: 4 = Satisfactory   0 = Unsatisfactory   NA = This step is not counted

PROCEDURE STEPS	SELF	PARTNER	INSTRUCTOR
1. Wash your hands and assemble the necessary supplies.	☐	☐	☐
2. Greet and identify the patient and explain the procedure.	☐	☐	☐
3. Choose the method (oral, axillary, or rectal) most appropriate for the patient.	☐	☐	☐
4. Insert the probe into a probe cover.	☐	☐	☐
5. Position the thermometer into the patient depending on the route used.	☐	☐	☐
6. Wait for the electronic thermometer unit to "beep."	☐	☐	☐
7. Remove the probe and note the reading on the digital display screen on the unit.	☐	☐	☐
8. Discard the probe cover into a biohazard waste container.	☐	☐	☐
9. Record the procedure result.	☐	☐	☐
10. **AFF** Explain how to respond to a patient who is hearing impaired.	☐	☐	☐
11. Return the unit and probe to the charging base.	☐	☐	☐

CALCULATION

Total Possible Points: _____

Total Points Earned: _____ Multiplied by 100 = _____ Divided by Total Possible Points = _____ %

PASS　　　　**FAIL**　　　　　　**COMMENTS:**

☐　　　　　☐

Student's signature _____ Date _____

Partner's signature _____ Date _____

Instructor's signature _____ Date _____

PSY PROCEDURE 19-7 **Measure and Record a Patient's Temperature Using a Tympanic Thermometer**

Name: _____ Date: _____ Time: _____ Grade: _____

EQUIPMENT/SUPPLIES: Tympanic thermometer, disposable probe covers, biohazard waste container

STANDARDS: Given the needed equipment and a place to work the student will perform this skill with _____% accuracy in a total of _____ minutes. *(Your instructor will tell you what the percentage and time limits will be before you begin.)*

KEY: 4 = Satisfactory   0 = Unsatisfactory   NA = This step is not counted

PROCEDURE STEPS	SELF	PARTNER	INSTRUCTOR
1. Wash your hands and assemble the necessary supplies.	☐	☐	☐
2. Greet and identify the patient and explain the procedure.	☐	☐	☐
3. Insert the ear probe into a probe cover.	☐	☐	☐
4. Place the end of the ear probe into the patient's ear after retracting the pinna correctly to straighten the ear canal.	☐	☐	☐
5. Press the button on the thermometer. Watch the digital display.	☐	☐	☐
6. Remove the probe at the "beep" or other thermometer signal.	☐	☐	☐
7. Discard the probe cover into a biohazard waste container.	☐	☐	☐
8. Record the procedure result.	☐	☐	☐
9. **AFF** Explain how to respond to a patient who is deaf.	☐	☐	☐
10. Return the unit and probe to the charging base.	☐	☐	☐

CALCULATION

Total Possible Points: _____

Total Points Earned: _____ Multiplied by 100 = _____ Divided by Total Possible Points = _____ %

PASS   **FAIL**   **COMMENTS:**

☐   ☐

Student's signature _____ Date _____

Partner's signature _____ Date _____

Instructor's signature _____ Date _____

Measure and Record a Patient's Temperature Using a Temporal Artery Thermometer

Name: _____ Date: _____ Time: _____ Grade: _____

EQUIPMENT/SUPPLIES: Temporal artery thermometer, antiseptic wipes

STANDARDS: Given the needed equipment and a place to work the student will perform this skill with _____% accuracy in a total of _____ minutes. *(Your instructor will tell you what the percentage and time limits will be before you begin.)*

KEY: 4 = Satisfactory 0 = Unsatisfactory NA = This step is not counted

PROCEDURE STEPS	SELF	PARTNER	INSTRUCTOR
1. Wash your hands and assemble the necessary supplies.	☐	☐	☐
2. Greet and identify the patient and explain the procedure.	☐	☐	☐
3. Place the flat end of the temporal thermometer against the patient's forehead.	☐	☐	☐
4. Depress the "on" button and slide the thermometer across the forehead, stopping at the temporal artery.	☐	☐	☐
5. Release the "on" button and remove the thermometer from the skin.	☐	☐	☐
6. Read the temperature on the digital display screen.	☐	☐	☐
7. Record the procedure result.	☐	☐	☐
8. **AFF** Explain how to respond to a patient who is visually impaired.	☐	☐	☐
9. Return the unit to the charging base.	☐	☐	☐

CALCULATION

Total Possible Points: _____

Total Points Earned: _____ Multiplied by 100 = _____ Divided by Total Possible Points = _____ %

PASS **FAIL** **COMMENTS:**

☐ ☐

Student's signature _____ Date _____

Partner's signature _____ Date _____

Instructor's signature _____ Date _____

PSY PROCEDURE 19-9 | **Measure and Record a Patient's Radial Pulse**

Name: _____ Date: _____ Time: _____ Grade: _____

EQUIPMENT/SUPPLIES: A watch with a sweeping second hand

STANDARDS: Given the needed equipment and a place to work the student will perform this skill with _____% accuracy in a total of _____ minutes. *(Your instructor will tell you what the percentage and time limits will be before you begin.)*

KEY: 4 = Satisfactory　　　　0 = Unsatisfactory　　　　NA = This step is not counted

PROCEDURE STEPS	SELF	PARTNER	INSTRUCTOR
1. Wash your hands.	☐	☐	☐
2. Greet and identify the patient and explain the procedure.	☐	☐	☐
3. Position the patient with the arm relaxed and supported.	☐	☐	☐
4. Locate the radial artery.	☐	☐	☐
5. If the pulse is regular, count the pulse for 30 seconds (irregular, count 60 seconds).	☐	☐	☐
6. Multiply the number of pulsations in 30 seconds by 2.	☐	☐	☐
7. Record the rate in the patient's medical record with the other vital signs.	☐	☐	☐
8. Also, note the rhythm if irregular and the volume if thready or bounding.	☐	☐	☐
9. **AFF** Explain how to respond to a patient who is developmentally challenged.	☐	☐	☐

CALCULATION

Total Possible Points: _____

Total Points Earned: _____ Multiplied by 100 = _____ Divided by Total Possible Points = _____ %

PASS　　**FAIL**　　　　**COMMENTS:**

☐　　　☐

Student's signature _____ Date _____

Partner's signature _____ Date _____

Instructor's signature _____ Date _____

PSY PROCEDURE 19-10 **Measure and Record a Patient's Respirations**

Name: _____ Date: _____ Time: _____ Grade: _____

EQUIPMENT/SUPPLIES: A watch with a sweeping second hand

STANDARDS: Given the needed equipment and a place to work the student will perform this skill with _____%
accuracy in a total of _____ minutes. *(Your instructor will tell you what the percentage and time limits will be
before you begin.)*

KEY: 4 = Satisfactory   0 = Unsatisfactory   NA = This step is not counted

PROCEDURE STEPS	SELF	PARTNER	INSTRUCTOR
1. Wash your hands.	☐	☐	☐
2. Greet and identify the patient and explain the procedure.	☐	☐	☐
3. Observe watch second hand and count a rise and fall of the chest as one respiration.	☐	☐	☐
4. For a regular breathing pattern count for 30 seconds and multiply by 2 (irregular for 60 seconds).	☐	☐	☐
5. Record the respiratory rate.	☐	☐	☐
6. Note the rhythm if irregular and any unusual or abnormal sounds such as wheezing.	☐	☐	☐
7. **AFF** Explain how to respond to a patient who has dementia.	☐	☐	☐

_____

_____

_____

_____

CALCULATION

Total Possible Points: _____

Total Points Earned: _____ Multiplied by 100 = _____ Divided by Total Possible Points = _____ %

PASS   **FAIL**   **COMMENTS:**

☐   ☐

Student's signature _____ Date _____

Partner's signature _____ Date _____

Instructor's signature _____ Date _____

PSY PROCEDURE 19-11　Measure and Record a Patient's Blood Pressure

Name: _____　Date: _____　Time: _____　Grade: _____

EQUIPMENT/SUPPLIES: Sphygmomanometer, stethoscope

STANDARDS: Given the needed equipment and a place to work the student will perform this skill with _____%
accuracy in a total of _____ minutes. *(Your instructor will tell you what the percentage and time limits will be
before you begin.)*

KEY:　　　　4 = Satisfactory　　　　0 = Unsatisfactory　　　　NA = This step is not counted

PROCEDURE STEPS	SELF	PARTNER	INSTRUCTOR
1. Wash your hands.	☐	☐	☐
2. Greet and identify the patient and explain the procedure.	☐	☐	☐
3. Position the patient with upper arm supported and level with the patient's heart.	☐	☐	☐
4. Expose the patient's upper arm.	☐	☐	☐
5. Palpate the brachial pulse in the antecubital area.	☐	☐	☐
6. Center the deflated cuff directly over the brachial artery.	☐	☐	☐
7. Lower edge of the cuff should be 1 to 2 inches above the antecubital area.	☐	☐	☐
8. Wrap the cuff smoothly and snugly around the arm, secure with the Velcro edges.	☐	☐	☐
9. Turn the screw clockwise to tighten. Do not tighten it too tightly for easy release.	☐	☐	☐
10. Palpate the brachial pulse. Inflate the cuff.	☐	☐	☐
11. Note the point or number on the dial or mercury column at which the brachial pulse disappears.	☐	☐	☐
12. Deflate the cuff by turning the valve counterclockwise.	☐	☐	☐
13. Wait at least 30 seconds before reinflating the cuff.	☐	☐	☐
14. Place the stethoscope earpieces into your ear canals with the openings pointed slightly forward.	☐	☐	☐
15. Stand about 3 feet from the manometer with the gauge at eye level.	☐	☐	☐
16. Place the diaphragm of the stethoscope against the brachial artery and hold in place.	☐	☐	☐
17. Close the valve and inflate the cuff.	☐	☐	☐
18. Pump the valve bulb to about 30 mm Hg above the number noted during step 11.	☐	☐	☐
19. Once the cuff is inflated to proper level, release air at a rate of about 2–4 mm Hg per second.	☐	☐	☐

20. Note the point on the gauge at which you hear the first clear tapping sound.	☐	☐	☐
21. Maintaining control of the valve screw, continue to deflate the cuff.	☐	☐	☐
22. When you hear the last sound, note the reading and quickly deflate the cuff.	☐	☐	☐
23. Remove the cuff and press the air from the bladder of the cuff.	☐	☐	☐
24. If this is the first recording or the first time the patient has been into the office, the physician may also want a reading in the other arm or in a position other than sitting.	☐	☐	☐
25. Record the reading with the systolic over the diastolic pressure (note which arm was used or any position other than sitting).	☐	☐	☐
26. **AFF** Explain how to respond to a patient who is from a different culture.	☐	☐	☐

_____

_____

_____

_____

CALCULATION

Total Possible Points: _____

Total Points Earned: _____ Multiplied by 100 = _____ Divided by Total Possible Points = _____ %

PASS   **FAIL**   **COMMENTS:**

☐   ☐

Student's signature _____ Date _____

Partner's signature _____ Date _____

Instructor's signature _____ Date _____

Cognitive Domain

1. Spell and define the key terms
2. Identify and state the use of the basic and specialized instruments and supplies used in the physical examination
3. Describe the four methods used to examine the patient
4. State your responsibilities before, during, and after the physical examination
5. List the basic sequence of the physical examination
6. Describe the normal function of each body system

Psychomotor Domain

1. Assist with the adult physical examination (Procedure 20-1)
2. Assist the physician with patient care
3. Practice standard precautions
4. Document accurately in the patient record
5. Practice within the standard of care for a medical assistant

Affective Domain

1. Apply critical thinking skills in performing patient assessment and care
2. Demonstrate awareness of diversity in providing patient care
3. Explain rationale for performance of a procedure to the patient

4. Apply active listening skills
5. Demonstrate sensitivity to patients' rights
6. Demonstrate empathy in communicating with patients, family, and staff
7. Use appropriate body language and other nonverbal skills in communicating with patients, family, and staff
8. Demonstrate awareness of the territorial boundaries of the person with whom you are communicating
9. Demonstrate sensitivity appropriate to the message being delivered
10. Demonstrate recognition of the patient's level of understanding communications
11. Recognize and protect personal boundaries in communicating with others
12. Demonstrate respect for individual diversity, incorporating awareness of one's own biases in areas including gender, race, religion, age, and economic status

ABHES Competencies

1. Prepare and maintain examination and treatment area
2. Prepare patient for examinations and treatments
3. Assist physician with routine and specialty examinations and treatments

Name: _____   Date: _____   Grade: _____

cog MULTIPLE CHOICE

Circle the letter preceding the correct answer.

1. Which of these instruments would a physician use to examine a patient's throat?

   a. Stethoscope

   b. Laryngeal mirror

   c. Percussion hammer

   d. Ayre spatula

   e. Tuning fork

2. The purpose of a regular physical examination is to:

   a. identify a disease or condition based on patient symptoms.

   b. compare symptoms of several diseases that the patient may exhibit.

   c. look for late warning signs of disease.

   d. maintain the patient's health and prevent disease.

   e. ensure the patient is maintaining a healthy diet and exercise regime.

3. Which of the following tasks would be performed by a medical assistant?

   a. Collecting specimens for diagnostic testing

   b. Diagnosing a patient

   c. Prescribing treatment for a patient

   d. Performing a physical examination

   e. Testing a patient's reflexes

4. Which of the following statements is true about physical examinations?

   a. Patients aged 20–40 should have a physical examination every year.

   b. It is not necessary to have a physical examination until you are over age 40 years.

   c. Women should have physical examinations more frequently than men.

   d. Patients ages 20–40 years should have a physical examination every 1–3 years.

   e. Patients over the age 60 years should have a physical examination every 6 months.

5. In which information-gathering technique might a physician use his or her sense of smell?

   a. Palpation

   b. Percussion

   c. Inspection

   d. Auscultation

   e. Visualization

6. If a physician notices asymmetry in a patient's features, it means that the patient:

   a. is normal and has nothing wrong.

   b. has features that are of unequal size or shape.

   c. has features that are abnormally large.

   d. will need immediate surgery.

   e. has perfectly even features.

7. Which part of the body can be auscultated?

   a. Lungs

   b. Legs

   c. Spine

   d. Feet

   e. Ears

8. The best position in which to place a female patient for a genital and rectum examination is the:

   a. Sims position.

   b. Fowler position.

   c. lithotomy position.

   d. Trendelenburg position.

   e. prone position.

9. A patient may be asked to walk around during a physical examination in order to:

   a. raise the pulse rate.

   b. observe gait and coordination.

   c. loosen the muscles in the legs.

   d. assess posture.

   e. demonstrate balance.

10. Women over age 40 years should receive mammograms every:

    a. 6 months.

    b. 2 years.

    c. 5 years.

    d. 1 year.

    e. 3 months.

11. How would a physician use a tuning fork to test a patient's hearing?

    a. By striking the prongs against the patient's leg and holding the handle in front of the patient's ear

    b. By holding the prongs behind the patient's ear and tapping the handle against their head

    c. By striking the prongs against the hand and holding the handle against the skull near the patient's ear

    d. By repeatedly tapping the prongs against the skull near the patient's ear

    e. By tapping the prongs on the table and inserting the handle into the patient's ear

12. Which of these may be an early warning sign of cancer?

    a. Obvious change in a wart or mole

    b. Dizziness or fainting spells

    c. Loss of appetite

    d. Inability to focus attention

    e. Sudden weight gain

13. How would a physician most likely be able to diagnose a hernia?

    a. Inspection

    b. Percussion

    c. Auscultation

    d. Palpation

    e. Visualization

Scenario for questions 14-16: A patient arrives for her physical checkup. While you are obtaining the patient's history, she mentions to you that she is taking several over-the-counter medications.

14. What is the correct procedure?

    a. Tell the physician immediately.

    b. Tell the patient that it will not affect her physical examination.

    c. Make a note of the medications the patient is taking in her medical record.

    d. Ask the patient to reschedule the physical examination when she has stopped taking the medications for at least a week.

    e. Prepare the necessary materials for a blood test.

15. During the patient's physical examination, the physician asks you to hand her the instruments needed to examine the patient's eyes. You should give her a(n):

    a. otoscope and penlight.

    b. stethoscope and speculum.

    c. ophthalmoscope and penlight.

    d. laryngoscope and gloves.

    e. anoscope and speculum.

16. Once the examination is over, you escort the patient to the front desk. After she has left the office, what do you do with her medical record?

    a. Check that the data has been accurately documented and release it to the billing department.

    b. Check that the data has been accurately documented and file the medical report under the patient's name.

    c. Pass the medical report on to the physician to check for any errors.

    d. Give the medical report directly to the billing department to maintain confidentiality.

    e. File the medical report under the patient's name for easy retrieval.

17. What is the difference between an otoscope and an audioscope?

   a. An otoscope is used to screen patients for hearing loss, whereas an audioscope is used to assess the internal structures of the ear.

   b. An audioscope is used to screen patients for hearing loss, whereas an otoscope is used to assess the internal structures of the ear.

   c. An otoscope is made of stainless steel, whereas an audioscope is made of plastic.

   d. An audioscope is made of plastic, whereas an otoscope is made of stainless steel.

   e. An otoscope is an older version of an audioscope and is not used much anymore.

18. A baseline examination is a(n):

   a. examination to determine the cause of an illness.

   b. full medical examination for people over age 50 years.

   c. initial examination to give physicians information about the patient.

   d. examination based on the patient's symptoms.

   e. examination of the abdominal regions of the patient.

19. Which of the following materials should be stored in a room away from the examination room?

   a. Gloves

   b. Tongue depressors

   c. Tape measure

   d. Cotton tipped applicators

   e. Syringes

20. What does the "P" stand for in PERRLA?

   a. Position

   b. Protrusion

   c. Posture

   d. Pupil

   e. Perception

COG MATCHING

Match each key term with its definition.

Key Terms

21. _____ auscultation

22. _____ Babinski reflex

23. _____ bimanual

24. _____ bruit

25. _____ cerumen

26. _____ extraocular

27. _____ hernia

28. _____ occult

29. _____ Papanicolaou (Pap) test

30. _____ PERRLA

31. _____ range of motion (ROM)

32. _____ sclera

33. _____ speculum

34. _____ transillumination

35. _____ tympanic membrane

36. _____ clinical diagnosis

37. _____ differential diagnosis

38. _____ gait

39. _____ lubricant

40. _____ manipulation

41. _____ nasal septum

42. _____ rectovaginal

43. _____ peripheral

Definitions

a. an instrument used for examining body cavities

b. thin, semitransparent membrane in the middle ear that transmits vibrations

c. a reflex noted by the extension of the great toe and abduction of the other toes

d. a test in which cells from the cervix are examined microscopically for abnormalities

e. an examination performed with both hands

f. the extent of movement in the joints

g. abnormal sound or murmur in the blood vessels

h. white fibrous tissue covering the eye

i. passage of light through body tissues for the purpose of examination

j. blood present in stool that is not visibly apparent

k. a diagnosis based only on a patient's symptoms

l. act of listening to the sounds within the body to evaluate the heart, lungs, intestines, or fetal heart tones

m. an acronym that means pupils are equal, round, and reactive to light and accommodation

n. earwax

o. a protrusion of an organ through a weakened muscle wall

p. outside of the eye

q. a diagnosis made by comparing symptoms of several diseases

r. the passive movement of the joints to determine the extent of movement

s. pertaining to the rectum and vagina

t. equality in size and shape or position of parts on opposite sides of the body

u. a water-soluble agent that reduces friction

v. device for applying local treatments and tests

w. inequality in size and shape on opposite sides of the body

x. pertaining to or situated away from the center

y. partition dividing the nostrils

z. a manner of walking

44. _____ applicator

45. _____ symmetry

46. _____ asymmetry

COG MATCHING   Grade: _____

Match each physical examination technique with its description by placing the letter preceding the definition on the line next to the correct basic examination technique.

Techniques

47. _____ inspection

48. _____ palpation

49. _____ percussion

50. _____ auscultation

Descriptions

a. touching or moving body areas with fingers or hands

b. looking at areas of the body to observe physical features

c. listening to the sounds of the body

d. tapping the body with the hand or an instrument to produce sounds

COG MATCHING   Grade: _____

Match each medical instrument with its description by placing the letter preceding the definition on the line next to the correct instrument.

Instruments

51. _____ tuning fork

52. _____ ophthalmoscope

53. _____ anoscope

54. _____ stethoscope

55. _____ laryngeal mirror

56. _____ headlight

Descriptions

a. an instrument used for listening to body sounds and taking blood pressure

b. an instrument used to examine the interior structures of the eyes

c. an instrument with two prongs used to test hearing

d. a light attached to a headband that provides direct light on the area being examined

e. an instrument used to examine areas of the patient's throat and larynx

f. a short stainless steel or plastic speculum used to inspect the anal canal

COG IDENTIFICATION

Grade: _____

Anticipating what the physician will need during a patient examination is a skill that the competent medical assistant must develop. Indicate which of the following instruments would the physician most likely ask for to examine the patient in each situation. Place a check mark on the line next to the possible instrument (more than one instrument may apply).

57. A patient comes into the physician's office complaining of ringing in her ears.

  a. _____ percussion hammer

  b. _____ tuning fork

  c. _____ laryngeal mirror

  d. _____ otoscope

  e. _____ ophthalmoscope

58. A male patient complains of weakness in his legs.

  a. _____ percussion hammer

  b. _____ tuning fork

  c. _____ laryngeal mirror

  d. _____ otoscope

  e. _____ ophthalmoscope

59. A young female patient complains of a headache and fever.

  a. _____ percussion hammer

  b. _____ tuning fork

  c. _____ laryngeal mirror

  d. _____ otoscope

  e. _____ ophthalmoscope

60. Listed below are the body areas inspected by the physician during a physical examination, but they are not in the correct order. Starting with the number one (1), number the body areas in the correct order in which they are examined.

_____ Eyes and ears

_____ Legs

_____ Head and neck

_____ Chest, breasts, and abdomen

_____ Nose and sinuses

_____ Reflexes

_____ Posture, gait, balance, and strength

_____ Mouth and throat

_____ Genitalia and rectum

61. Place a check mark on the line next to each factor that may be a warning sign for cancer. Check all that apply.

_____ an itchy rash on the arms and legs

_____ a nagging cough or hoarse voice

_____ unusual bleeding or discharge

_____ stiffness in joints

_____ a sore that will not heal

_____ frequent upper respiratory infections

_____ pain in any body area

62. As a medical assistant, you will be required to assist the physician before, during, and after physical examinations. Read the list of tasks below and place a letter on the line preceding the task indicating whether you would perform the task before (B), during (D), or after (A) the examination.

  a. _____ Escort the patient to the front desk.

  b. _____ Obtain a urine specimen from the patient, if required.

  c. _____ Adjust the drape on the patient to expose the necessary body part.

  d. _____ Ask the patient about medication used on a regular basis.

  e. _____ Check the patient's medical record to ensure all the information has been accurately documented.

  f. _____ Place the patient's chart outside the examining room door.

  g. _____ Offer reassurance to the patient and check for signs of anxiety.

63. A patient calls the physician's office and explains that her daughter cries continuously, has been vomiting regularly, and stumbles a lot. Which of these do you recommend and why?

a. Tell her that it is probably a bug and to keep her child home from school for a couple of days.

_____

_____

_____

_____

b. Advise that she keep an eye on the child and inform the physician if there is any change.

_____

_____

_____

_____

c. Tell her to have the child examined immediately.

_____

_____

_____

_____

64. A patient comes into the physician's office with an open wound. When obtaining the patient's medical records, you discover that he last had a tetanus booster 4 years ago. What is the correct procedure and why?

a. Recommend the patient has another tetanus booster.

_____

_____

_____

b. Tell the patient he does not need immunizing for another 6 years.

_____

_____

_____

_____

c. Tell the patient he should have a booster if he is traveling abroad.

_____

_____

_____

_____

65. Dr. O'Brien tells you that a patient's eardrum is infected. What are the symptoms that could have led Dr. O'Brien to this diagnosis?

_____

_____

_____

_____

66. As a medical assistant, you are responsible for checking each examination room at the beginning of the day to make sure that it is ready for patients. List three things that need to be done to ensure that a room is ready.

_____

_____

_____

_____

COG TRUE OR FALSE?

Grade: _____

Indicate whether the statements are true or false by placing the letter T (true) or F (false) on the line preceding the statement.

67. _____ A normal tympanic membrane will be light pink and curve slightly outward.

68. _____ Patients should have a baseline electrocardiogram (ECG) when they turn age 60 years.

69. _____ The instruments used to examine the rectum and colon are all one standard size.

70. _____ The medical assistant is responsible for preparing the examination room, preparing the patient, assisting the physician, and cleaning the equipment and examination room.

COG AFF CASE STUDIES FOR CRITICAL THINKING

Grade: _____

1. A 19-year-old patient has never had a Pap smear before and does not understand what the test is for, or what is going to happen during the procedure. The physician asks you to explain the process to her in simple terms. List some key aspects of a Pap smear and explain the purpose of the procedure to this patient in a way that she will understand.

_____

_____

_____

_____

2. Alicia is assisting a male physician with performing a gynecological examination. Midway through the examination, she is paged to assist another medical procedure. Explain what she should do and why.

_____

_____

_____

3. Your patient is a 35-year-old male who has a long family history of cancer. The patient is terrified of developing cancer and has been to see the physician several times for minor false alarms. Prepare an information sheet for the patient, explaining the early warning signs of cancer. What else can you do to alleviate the fear in this patient?

_____

_____

_____

_____

4. You are assisting with the physical examination of a 55-year-old male. When the physician begins to prepare for the rectal examination, the patient refuses and says that it is unnecessary and that he is fine. What would be the most appropriate thing to do at this point?

_____

_____

_____

_____

5. At the beginning of the day, you are preparing the examination rooms with a fellow medical assistant. You are both in a hurry because the first patients are arriving and the physicians are waiting for you to finish. Your fellow medical assistant suggests that you don't need to check the batteries in the equipment because everything worked well yesterday. What would you do or say?

_____

_____

_____

_____

6. While you are escorting a patient to the front desk, the patient asks you whether an over-the-counter medication will affect her prescribed treatment. You are familiar with both drugs. What is the correct response?

_____

_____

_____

_____

7. You are assisting a physician during a genital and pelvic examination on a female disabled patient who cannot be placed into the lithotomy position. What is the correct course of action?

_____

_____

_____

_____

PSY PROCEDURE 20-1 Assisting with the Adult Physical Examination

Name: _____ Date: _____ Time: _____ Grade: _____

EQUIPMENT/SUPPLIES: A variety of basic instruments and supplies including a stethoscope, ophthalmoscope, otoscope, penlight, tuning fork, nasal speculum, tongue blade, percussion hammer, gloves, and patient gowning and draping supplies

STANDARDS: Given the needed equipment and a place to work the student will perform this skill with _____%
accuracy in a total of _____ minutes. *(Your instructor will tell you what the percentage and time limits will be before you begin.)*

KEY: 4 = Satisfactory   0 = Unsatisfactory   NA = This step is not counted

PROCEDURE STEPS	SELF	PARTNER	INSTRUCTOR
1. Wash your hands.	☐	☐	☐
2. Prepare the examination room and assemble the equipment.	☐	☐	☐
3. Greet the patient by name and escort him or her to the examining room.	☐	☐	☐
4. Explain the procedure.	☐	☐	☐
5. Obtain and record the medical history and chief complaint.	☐	☐	☐
6. Take and record the vital signs, height, weight, and visual acuity.	☐	☐	☐
7. If anticipated, instruct the patient to obtain a urine specimen and escort him or her to the bathroom.	☐	☐	☐
8. When patient has returned, instruct him or her to disrobe. Leave the room unless the patient needs assistance.	☐	☐	☐
9. **AFF** Explain how to respond to a patient who has cultural or religious beliefs and is uncomfortable about disrobing.	☐	☐	☐
10. Assist patient into a sitting position on the edge of the examination table. Cover the lap and legs with a drape.	☐	☐	☐
11. Place the patient's medical record outside the examination room door. Notify the physician that the patient is ready.	☐	☐	☐
12. Assist the physician during the examination by:	☐	☐	☐
a. handing him or her the instruments needed for the examination.			
b. positioning the patient appropriately.			

13. Help the patient return to a sitting position.	☐	☐	☐
14. Perform any follow-up procedures or treatments.	☐	☐	☐
15. Leave the room while the patient dresses unless assistance is needed.	☐	☐	☐
16. Return to the examination room after the patient has dressed to: 　**a.** answer questions. 　**b.** reinforce instructions. 　**c.** provide patient education.	☐	☐	☐
17. Escort the patient to the front desk.	☐	☐	☐
18. Properly clean or dispose of all used equipment and supplies.	☐	☐	☐
19. Clean the room with a disinfectant and prepare for the next patient.	☐	☐	☐
20. Wash your hands. 　**a.** Record any instructions that were ordered for the patient. 　**b.** Note if any specimens were obtained. 　**c.** Indicate the results of the test or note the laboratory where the specimens are being sent for testing.	☐	☐	☐

CALCULATION

Total Possible Points: _____

Total Points Earned: _____ Multiplied by 100 = _____ Divided by Total Possible Points = _____ %

PASS　　　**FAIL**　　　　　**COMMENTS:**

　☐　　　　　☐

Student's signature _____ Date _____

Partner's signature _____ Date _____

Instructor's signature _____ Date _____

Sterilization and Surgical Instruments

Learning Outcomes

Cognitive Domain

1. Spell and define the key terms
2. Differentiate between medical and surgical asepsis used in ambulatory care settings, identifying when each is appropriate
3. Describe several methods of sterilization
4. Categorize surgical instruments based on use and identify each by its characteristics
5. Identify surgical instruments specific to designated specialties
6. State the difference between reusable and disposable instruments
7. Explain how to handle and store instruments, equipment, and supplies
8. Describe the necessity and steps for maintaining documents and records of maintenance for instruments and equipment

Psychomotor Domain

1. Sanitize equipment and instruments (Procedure 21-1)
2. Prepare items for autoclaving
3. Properly wrap instruments for autoclaving (Procedure 21-2)
4. Perform sterilization technique and operate an autoclave (Procedure 21-3)
5. Perform sterilization procedures
6. Practice standard precautions

Affective Domain

1. Apply ethical behaviors, including honesty/integrity in peformance of medical assisting practice

ABHES Competencies

1. Wrap items for autoclaving
2. Practice quality control
3. Use standard precautions
4. Perform sterilization techniques

Name: _____   Date: _____   Grade: _____

COG **MULTIPLE CHOICE**

Circle the letter preceding the correct answer:

1. A sterile field is defined as an area:

   a. where the autoclave is kept.

   b. that is free of all microorganisms.

   c. where sterilized instruments are stored.

   d. that has been cleaned with a chemical disinfectant.

   e. in which only sanitized equipment can be used.

2. Instruments that are sterilized in the autoclave maintain their sterility for:

   a. 15 days.

   b. 20 days.

   c. 25 days.

   d. 30 days.

   e. 35 days.

3. Autoclave tape indicates that an object:

   a. has not been sterilized.

   b. contains a specific type of microorganism.

   c. has been exposed to steam in the autoclave.

   d. needs to be placed on its side in the autoclave.

   e. did not reach the proper pressure and temperature in the autoclave.

4. Material used to wrap items that are being sterilized in the autoclave must be:

   a. permeable to steam but not contaminants.

   b. permeable to distilled water but not tap water.

   c. permeable to heat but not formaldehyde.

   d. permeable to ethylene oxide but not pathogens.

   e. permeable to contaminants but not microorganisms.

5. Which of the following should be included in an equipment record?

   a. Expiration date

   b. Date of purchase

   c. Physician's name

   d. The office's address

   e. Date of last sterilization

6. Which of the following should be included in a sterilization record?

   a. Location of the item

   b. Number of items in the load

   c. Method of sterilization used

   d. Reason for the service request

   e. Results of the sterilization indicator

7. One instrument commonly used in urology is a(n):

   a. curet.

   b. tonometer.

   c. urethral sound.

   d. sigmoidoscope.

   e. uterine dilator.

8. Forceps are used to:

   a. cut sutures.

   b. dissect tissue.

   c. make incisions.

   d. guide instruments.

   e. compress or join tissue.

9. All packs containing bowls or containers should be placed in the autoclave:

    a. upright.

    b. under a cloth.

    c. on their sides.

    d. stacked on top of each other.

    e. with their sterilization indicators facing up.

10. Consult the material safety data sheet (MSDS) before:

    a. handling a chemical spill.

    b. reading a sterilization indicator.

    c. sterilizing an instrument in the autoclave.

    d. requesting service for a piece of equipment.

    e. disposing of a disposable scalpel handle and blade.

11. Why does the autoclave use pressure in the sterilization process?

    a. Pathogens and microorganisms thrive in low-pressure environments.

    b. High pressure makes the wrapping permeable to steam and not contaminants.

    c. Pressure must be applied to distilled water in order to release sterilizing agents.

    d. High pressure prevents microorganisms from penetrating the objects being sterilized.

    e. High pressure allows the steam to reach the high temperatures needed for sterilization.

12. Which of the following instruments are used to hold sterile drapes in place during surgical procedures?

    a. Directors

    b. Serrations

    c. Towel clamps

    d. Curved scissors

    e. Alligator biopsies

13. Notched mechanisms that hold the tips of the forceps together tightly are called:

    a. springs.

    b. sutures.

    c. ratchets.

    d. serrations.

    e. clamps.

14. After use, scalpel blades should be:

    a. sterilized in the autoclave.

    b. discarded in a sharps container.

    c. reattached to a scalpel handle.

    d. processed in a laboratory.

    e. wrapped in cotton muslin.

15. The instrument used to hold open layers of tissue to expose the areas underneath during a surgical procedure is a:

    a. retractor.

    b. scalpel.

    c. director.

    d. clamp.

    e. forceps.

16. Ratcheted instruments should be stored:

    a. open.

    b. closed.

    c. hanging.

    d. standing.

    e. upside down.

17. Medical asepsis is intended to prevent the spread of microbes from:

    a. one patient to another.

    b. the autoclave to the patient.

    c. the instruments to the physician.

    d. the inside to the outside of the body.

    e. the physician to the medical assistant.

18. A punch biopsy is used to:

    a. diagnose glaucoma.

    b. dissect delicate tissues.

    c. explore bladder depths.

    d. remove tissue for microscopic study.

    e. guide an instrument during a procedure.

19. The best way to test the effectiveness of an autoclave is to use:

    a. thermometers.

    b. wax pellets.

    c. autoclave tape.

    d. color indicators.

    e. strips with heat-resistant spores.

20. Which is a step in operating the autoclave?

    a. Stacking items on top of each other

    b. Filling the reservoir tank with tap water

    c. Filling the reservoir a little past the fill line

    d. Removing items from the autoclave the moment they are done

    e. Setting the timer after the correct temperature has been reached

COG MATCHING

Grade: _____

Match each key term with its definition.

Key Terms

21. _____ autoclave
22. _____ disinfection
23. _____ ethylene oxide
24. _____ forceps
25. _____ hemostat
26. _____ needle holder
27. _____ obturator
28. _____ ratchet
29. _____ sanitation
30. _____ sanitize
31. _____ scalpel
32. _____ scissors
33. _____ serration
34. _____ sound
35. _____ sterilization

Definitions

a. surgical instrument used to grasp, hold, compress, pull, or join tissue, equipment, or supplies

b. a long instrument used to explore or dilate body cavities

c. a gas used to sterilize surgical instruments and other supplies

d. appliance used to sterilize medical instruments with steam under pressure

e. a surgical instrument with slender jaws that is used to grasp blood vessels

f. groove, either straight or crisscross, etched or cut into the blade or tip of an instrument to improve its bite or grasp

g. a notched mechanism that clicks into position to maintain tension on the opposing blades or tips of the instrument

h. killing or rendering inert most but not all pathogenic microorganisms

i. to reduce the number of microorganisms on a surface by use of low-level disinfectant practices

j. a sharp instrument composed of two opposing cutting blades, held together by a central pin on which the blades pivot

k. a type of forceps that is used to hold and pass suture through tissue

l. a small pointed knife with a convex edge for surgical procedures

m. a process, act, or technique for destroying microorganisms using heat, water, chemicals, or gases

n. the maintenance of a healthful, disease-free environment

o. a smooth, rounded, removable inner portion of a hollow tube that allows for easier insertion

COG MATCHING

Grade: _____

Match each instrument with its description.

Instruments

36. _____ forceps
37. _____ scissors
38. _____ scalpels
39. _____ clamps
40. _____ retractors

Descriptions

a. dissect delicate tissue

b. hold sterile drapes in place

c. grasp tissue for dissection

d. make an incision

e. transfer sterile supplies

f. cut off a bandage

g. excise tissue

h. hold open layers of tissue

COG IDENTIFICATION
Grade: _____

41. Complete this table, which identifies four types of scissors and their use.

Type	Use
bandage scissors	**a.**
b.	dissect superficial and delicate tissues
straight scissors	**c.**
d.	remove sutures

42. Complete the chart below by identifying one instrument used in each specialty.

Specialty	Instrument
Obstetrics, gynecology	**a.**
Orthopedics	**b.**
Urology	**c.**
Proctology	**d.**
Otology, rhinology	**e.**
Ophthalmology	**f.**
Dermatology	**g.**

43. Complete this table, which describes the most effective method of sterilizing various instruments and materials.

Method of sterilization	Most effective for
a.	minor surgical instruments surgical storage trays and containers bowls for holding sterile equipment
b.	instruments or equipment subject to water damage
c.	instruments or equipment subject to heat damage

COG SHORT ANSWER
Grade: _____

44. Describe the process by which an autoclave sterilizes instruments.

_____

_____

_____

_____

45. What is the purpose of sterilization indicators? What factors may alter the results of a sterilization indicator?

_____

_____

_____

_____

46. What components must be properly set in order for the autoclave to work effectively?

_____

_____

_____

_____

47. List the guidelines that you should follow when handling and storing sharp instruments.

_____

_____

_____

_____

48. What is the purpose of autoclave tape?

_____

_____

_____

_____

49. Which method of sterilization is more effective: boiling water or the autoclave? Why?

_____

_____

_____

50. Compare the qualities of medical asepsis and surgical asepsis.

_____

_____

_____

_____

COG TRUE OR FALSE?   Grade: _____

Indicate whether the statements are true or false by placing the letter T (true) or F (false) on the line preceding the statement.

51. _____ Equipment must be sanitized before it is sterilized.

52. _____ Autoclave indicator tape is 100% effective in indicating whether a package is sterile.

53. _____ It is the medical assistant's responsibility to maintain complete and accurate records of sterilized equipment.

54. _____ The handle and blade of a reusable steel scalpel may be reused after being properly sterilized.

COG AFF CASE STUDIES FOR CRITICAL THINKING   Grade: _____

1. You are one of two medical assistants working in a small office that specializes in ophthalmology. There is one examination room. The office sees about 50 patients a week, with an average of 3 patients a week needing minor ophthalmologic procedures. The physician has asked you to order new instruments for the office for the next month. What are two of the instruments that you will order? What factors will you need to consider when placing the order?

_____

_____

_____

_____

2. Your medical office has one autoclave along with two pairs of sterilized suture scissors and adequate numbers of other instruments. In the morning, the physician uses one pair of suture scissors to perform a minor procedure. He tosses the scissors into a sink when he is finished, damaging the instrument. At noon, the autoclave suddenly malfunctions, and you put in a service request to repair it. In the afternoon, a patient comes into the office complaining that her sutures are painful. The physician decides that he must remove them right away. Right before the procedure begins, the physician drops the only sterile pair of suture scissors in the office before he can use them. Describe two possible plans of action you can take to help the patient who is still in pain.

_____

_____

_____

_____

3. The physician has just completed a procedure in which he used a disposable scalpel. How should you dispose of this instrument and why? Would it be appropriate to autoclave this scalpel to save money? Why or why not?

_____

_____

_____

_____

4. Your patient is about to undergo a minor office surgery and is concerned because she once received a facial piercing that led to a massive infection due to improperly sterilized instruments. Now, she is worried about the cleanliness of your office. How would you explain the precautions your office takes to ensure that all instruments and equipment are safe and sterile in a language that the patient can understand?

_____

_____

_____

_____

5. A package arrives at your office and you and your coworker are unable to open it. After looking around the immediate area, your coworker leaves the room and comes back with a pair of sterile operating scissors to open the package. Should you allow your coworker to use the scissors to open the package? What reason would you give your coworker for allowing or not allowing him or her to use the scissors?

_____

_____

_____

6. Your office uses formaldehyde to sterilize some instruments. While transporting the instruments soaking in formaldehyde, you accidentally spill the formaldehyde. You are in a hurry and consider leaving the small amount of chemical on the floor until later. Would this be an appropriate action to take? Why or why not? How would you clean up this spill?

_____

_____

_____

_____

PSY PROCEDURE 21-1 | **Sanitize Equipment and Instruments**

Name: _____ Date: _____ Time: _____ Grade: _____

EQUIPMENT/SUPPLIES: Instruments or equipment to be sanitized, gloves, eye protection, impervious gown, soap and water, small hand-held scrub brush

STANDARDS: Given the needed equipment and a place to work the student will perform this skill with _____%
accuracy in a total of _____ minutes. *(Your instructor will tell you what the percentage and time limits will be before you begin.)*

KEY: 4 = Satisfactory   0 = Unsatisfactory   NA = This step is not counted

PROCEDURE STEPS	SELF	PARTNER	INSTRUCTOR
1. Put on gloves, gown, and eye protection.	☐	☐	☐
2. For equipment that requires assembly, take removable sections apart.	☐	☐	☐
3. Check the operation and integrity of the equipment.	☐	☐	☐
4. Rinse the instrument with cool water.	☐	☐	☐
5. Force streams of soapy water through any tubular or grooved instruments.	☐	☐	☐
6. Use a hot, soapy solution to dissolve fats or lubricants left on the surface.	☐	☐	☐

7. Soak 5 to 10 minutes.
   a. Use friction (brush or gauze) to wipe down the instruments.
   b. Check jaws or scissors/forceps to ensure that all debris has been removed.
	☐	☐	☐

8. Rinse well.	☐	☐	☐
9. Dry well before autoclaving if sterilizing or soaking in disinfecting solution.	☐	☐	☐
10. Items (brushes, gauze, solution) used in sanitation process must be disinfected or discarded.	☐	☐	☐

CALCULATION

Total Possible Points: _____

Total Points Earned: _____ Multiplied by 100 = _____ Divided by Total Possible Points = _____ %

PASS   **FAIL**   **COMMENTS:**

☐   ☐

Student's signature _____ Date _____

Partner's signature _____ Date _____

Instructor's signature _____ Date _____

PSY PROCEDURE 21-2 **Properly Wrap Instruments for Autoclaving**

Name: _____   Date: _____   Time: _____   Grade: _____

EQUIPMENT/SUPPLIES: Sanitized and wrapped instruments or equipment, distilled water, autoclave operating manual

STANDARDS: Given the needed equipment and a place to work the student will perform this skill with _____%
accuracy in a total of _____ minutes. *(Your instructor will tell you what the percentage and time limits will be
before you begin.)*

KEY: 4 = Satisfactory   0 = Unsatisfactory   NA = This step is not counted

PROCEDURE STEPS	SELF	PARTNER	INSTRUCTOR
1. Assemble the equipment and supplies.	☐	☐	☐
2. Check the instruments being wrapped for working order.	☐	☐	☐
3. Obtain correct material for wrapping instruments to be autoclaved.	☐	☐	☐
4. Tear off 1 to 2 pieces of autoclave tape. On one piece, label the contents of the pack, the date, and your initials.	☐	☐	☐

5. Lay the wrap diagonally on a flat, clean, dry surface.
 	
   a. Place instrument in the center, with ratchets or handles in open position.
 	
   b. Include a sterilization indicator.
	☐	☐	☐

6. Fold the first flap up at the bottom of the diagonal wrap. Fold back the corner to make a tab.	☐	☐	☐
7. Fold left corner of the wrap toward the center. Fold back the corner to make a tab.	☐	☐	☐
8. Fold right corner of the wrap toward the center. Fold back the corner to make a tab.	☐	☐	☐
9. Fold the top corner down, making the tab tuck under the material.	☐	☐	☐
10. Secure the package with labeled autoclave tape.	☐	☐	☐

CALCULATION

Total Possible Points: _____

Total Points Earned: _____ Multiplied by 100 = _____ Divided by Total Possible Points = _____ %

PASS   **FAIL**   **COMMENTS:**

☐   ☐

Student's signature _____ Date _____

Partner's signature _____ Date _____

Instructor's signature _____ Date _____

PSY PROCEDURE 21-3   Perform Sterilization Technique and Operate an Autoclave

Name: _____   Date: _____   Time: _____   Grade: _____

EQUIPMENT/SUPPLIES: Sanitized and wrapped instruments or equipment, distilled water, autoclave operating manual

STANDARDS: Given the needed equipment and a place to work the student will perform this skill with _____%
accuracy in a total of _____ minutes. *(Your instructor will tell you what the percentage and time limits will be
before you begin.)*

KEY: 4 = Satisfactory   0 = Unsatisfactory   NA = This step is not counted

PROCEDURE STEPS	SELF	PARTNER	INSTRUCTOR
1. Assemble the equipment including the wrapped articles. Refer to the manufacturer's manual for information specific to the model of autoclave you are using.	☐	☐	☐
2. Check the water level of the autoclave reservoir and add more if needed.	☐	☐	☐
3. Add water to the internal chamber of the autoclave to the fill line.	☐	☐	☐

4. Load the autoclave:
  a. Place trays and packs on their sides, 1 to 3 inches from each other.
  b. Put containers on the sides with the lids off.
  c. In mixed loads, place hard objects on bottom shelf and softer packs on top racks.
	☐	☐	☐

5. Read the instructions, which should be available and close to the machine.
  a. Close the door and secure or lock it.
  b. Turn the machine on.
  c. When the gauge reaches the temperature required for the contents of the load (usually 250°F), set the timer.
  d. When the timer indicates that the cycle is over, vent the chamber.
  e. After pressure has been released to a safe level, crack the door of the autoclave.
	☐	☐	☐

6. When the load has cooled, remove the items.	☐	☐	☐
7. Check the separately wrapped sterilization indicator, if used, for proper sterilization.	☐	☐	☐
8. Store the items in a clean, dry, dust-free area for 30 days.	☐	☐	☐
9. Clean the autoclave following the manufacturer's directions.	☐	☐	☐
10. Rinse the machine thoroughly and allow it to dry.	☐	☐	☐

CALCULATION

Total Possible Points: _____

Total Points Earned: _____ Multiplied by 100 = _____ Divided by Total Possible Points = _____ %

PASS   **FAIL**   **COMMENTS:**

☐   ☐

Student's signature _____ Date _____

Partner's signature _____ Date _____

Instructor's signature _____ Date _____

22 Assisting with Minor Office Surgery

Cognitive Domain

1. Spell and define key terms
2. List your responsibilities before, during, and after minor office surgery
3. Identify the guidelines for preparing and maintaining sterility of the field and surgical equipment during a minor office procedure
4. State your responsibility in relation to informed consent and patient preparation
5. Explain the purpose of local anesthetics and list three commonly used in the medical office
6. Describe the types of needles and sutures and the uses of each
7. Describe the various methods of skin closure used in the medical office
8. Explain your responsibility during surgical specimen collection
9. List the types of laser surgery and electrosurgery used in the medical office and explain the precautions for each
10. Describe the guidelines for applying a sterile dressing
11. Describe implications for treatment related to pathology

Psychomotor Domain

1. Practice standard precautions
2. Open sterile surgical packs (Procedure 22-1)
3. Use sterile transfer forceps (Procedure 22-2)
4. Add sterile solution to a sterile field (Procedure 22-3)
5. Prepare a patient for procedures and/or treatments
6. Document accurately in the patient record
7. Perform skin preparation and hair removal (Procedure 22-4)
8. Apply sterile gloves (Procedure 22-5)
9. Apply a sterile dressing (Procedure 22-6)
10. Change an existing sterile dressing (Procedure 22-7)

11. Assist physician with patient care
12. Assist with excisional surgery (Procedure 22-8)
13. Assist with incision and drainage (Procedure 22-9)
14. Remove sutures (Procedure 22-10)
15. Remove staples (Procedure 22-11)

Affective Domain

1. Apply ethical behaviors, including honesty/integrity in peformance of medical assisting practice
2. Apply critical thinking skills in performing patient assessment and care
3. Demonstrate empathy in communicating with patients, family, and staff
4. Apply active listening skills
5. Use appropriate body language and other nonverbal skills in communicating with patients, family, and staff
6. Demonstrate awareness of the territorial boundaries of the person with whom you are communicating
7. Demonstrate sensitivity appropriate to the message being delivered
8. Demonstrate recognition of the patient's level of understanding in communications
9. Recognize and protect personal boundaries in communicating with others
10. Demonstrate respect for individual diversity, incorporating awareness of one's own biases in areas including gender, race, religion, age, and economic status

ABHES Competencies

1. Prepare patients for examinations and treatments
2. Assist physician with minor office surgical procedures
3. Dispose of biohazardous materials
4. Use standard precautions
5. Document accurately

Name: _____   Date: _____   Grade: _____

COG **MULTIPLE CHOICE**

Circle the letter preceding the correct answer.

1. Which of the following statements is true about working in a sterile field?

   a. Sterile packages should be kept damp.

   b. Your back must be kept to the sterile field at all times.

   c. A 3-inch border around the field is considered contaminated.

   d. All sterile items should be held above waist level.

   e. Cover your mouth when coughing near the sterile field.

2. Why is a fenestrated drape helpful during surgery?

   a. It is made of lightweight fabric.

   b. It has an opening to expose the operative site.

   c. It can be used as a blanket to keep the patient warm.

   d. It does not need to be sterilized before surgery.

   e. It allows for easy cleanup after the surgery.

3. Epinephrine is added to local anesthetics during surgery to:

   a. ensure sterilization.

   b. protect the tips of the fingers.

   c. lengthen the anesthetic's effectiveness.

   d. prevent vasoconstriction.

   e. create rapid absorption.

4. Which needles are used most frequently in the medical office?

   a. Curved swaged needles

   b. Traumatic needles

   c. Straight needles

   d. Domestic needles

   e. Keith needles

5. A preservative is added to specimen containers to be sent to a pathologist to:

   a. help the pathologist see the specimen.

   b. delay decomposition.

   c. identify the patient.

   d. make the specimen grow.

   e. prevent contamination.

6. Which type of electrosurgery destroys tissue with controlled electric sparks?

   a. Electrocautery

   b. Electrodesiccation

   c. Electrosection

   d. Fulguration

   e. Electrophysiology

7. Why is it important to know if a patient has a pacemaker before performing electrosurgery?

   a. Metal implants can become very hot and malfunction during the procedure.

   b. The electrical charge can cause the electrosurgical device to malfunction.

   c. The patient needs to sign a separate consent form if he has any heart problems.

   d. The patient can receive an electrical shock from the equipment.

   e. The implants may counteract the electrosurgery results.

Scenario for questions 8 and 9: A female patient returns to the office to have sutures removed from her forearm. When you remove the dressing, you notice that there is a small amount of clear drainage.

8. The patient's drainage is:

 a. purulent.

 b. sanguineous.

 c. serous.

 d. copious.

 e. serosanguineous.

9. Before you remove the patient's sutures, you should:

 a. apply a local anesthetic to numb the area.

 b. offer the patient pain medication to reduce discomfort.

 c. place an ice pack on the patient's forearm.

 d. advise the patient that she should feel pulling sensation but not pain.

 e. gently tug on the ends of the suture to make sure they are secure.

10. Which of the following is characteristic of healing by primary intention?

 a. Clean incision

 b. Gaping, irregular wound

 c. Increased granulation

 d. Wide scar

 e. Indirect edge joining

11. What happens during phase II of wound healing?

 a. Fibroblasts build scar tissue to guard the area.

 b. The scab dries and pulls the edges of the wound together.

 c. Circulation increases and brings white blood cells to the area.

 d. Serum and red blood cells form a fibrin to plug the wound.

 e. An antiseptic sterilizes the area from possible contamination.

12. How must the physician care for an abscess in order for it to heal properly?

 a. Drain the infected material from the site.

 b. Suture the site closed.

 c. Cover the site with a sterile dressing.

 d. Perform cryosurgery to remove the site.

 e. Perform a skin graft to cover the site.

13. Which of the following items should be added to the label on a specimen container?

 a. The contents of the container

 b. The office number

 c. The patient's age

 d. The patient's gender

 e. The date

14. Which of the following is true about laser surgery?

 a. The Argon laser is the only laser used for coagulation.

 b. Colored filters allow the physician to see the path of the laser.

 c. Most lasers are used simply as markers for surgery.

 d. Laser incisions generally bleed more than regular incisions.

 e. Everyone in the room must wear goggles to protect his or her eyes.

15. What is the best way to prepare a patient for surgery?

 a. Remind the patient of procedures by calling a few days before the surgery.

 b. Tell the patient all the instructions on the visit before the surgery.

 c. Send the patient home with written instructions on what to do.

 d. Instruct the patient to call the day of the procedure for instructions.

 e. Have the patient tell a second person about what she needs to do.

16. Which of the following supplies must be added at the time of setup for a surgery?

    a. Liquids in open containers

    b. Sterile transfer forceps

    c. Peel-back envelopes

    d. Sterile gloves

    e. Fenestrated drape

17. Absorbable sutures are most frequently used:

    a. in medical offices for wound sutures.

    b. in hospitals for deep-tissue surgery.

    c. in hospitals for surface-tissue surgery.

    d. when patients are young and heal easily.

    e. whenever a wound needs to be sutured.

18. Which of the following might contaminate a sterile dressing?

    a. A patient accidentally bumps into another person.

    b. The wound still has sutures underneath.

    c. The weather outside has been rainy and damp.

    d. The patient adjusted the dressing at home.

    e. The patient has had a cold for the past week.

19. A child came in with a slight cut on his leg, but there is little tension on the skin and the cut is clean. The physician believes the wound will heal on its own, with time, and wants to approximate the edges of the wound so that it will heal with minimum scarring. Which of the following would be best used to close the child's wound?

    a. Adhesive skin closures

    b. Fine absorptive sutures

    c. Traumatic sutures

    d. Staples

    e. Nothing

20. The last step in any surgical procedure is to:

    a. assist the patient to leave.

    b. instruct the patient on postoperative procedures.

    c. remove all biohazardous materials.

    d. wash your hands.

    e. record the procedure.

COG MATCHING

Place the letter preceding the definition on the line next to the term.

Key Terms

21. _____ approximate
22. _____ atraumatic
23. _____ bandage
24. _____ cautery
25. _____ coagulate
26. _____ cryosurgery
27. _____ dehiscence
28. _____ dressing
29. _____ electrode
30. _____ fulgurate
31. _____ keratosis
32. _____ lentigines
33. _____ preservative
34. _____ purulent
35. _____ swaged needle
36. _____ traumatic

Definitions

a. separation or opening of the edges of a wound

b. a medium for conducting or detecting electrical current

c. tissue surfaces that are as close together as possible

d. a covering applied directly to a wound to apply pressure, support, absorb secretions, protect from trauma, slow or stop bleeding, or hide disfigurement

e. a means or device that destroys tissue using an electric current, freezing, or burning

f. causing or relating to tissue damage

g. a swaged type of needle that does not require threading

h. to destroy tissue by electrodesiccation

i. a soft material applied to a body part to immobilize the body part or control bleeding

j. to change from a liquid to a solid or semisolid mass

k. brown skin macules occurring after exposure to the sun; freckles

l. drainage from a wound that is white, green, or yellow, signaling an infection

m. a metal needle fused to suture material

n. a skin condition characterized by overgrowth and thickening

o. a substance that delays decomposition

p. surgery in which abnormal tissue is removed by freezing

COG MATCHING

Place the letter preceding the description on the line next to the procedure.

Procedures

37. _____ electrocautery
38. _____ electrodesiccation
39. _____ electrosection
40. _____ fulguration

Descriptions

a. destroys tissue with controlled electric sparks

b. causes quick coagulation of small blood vessels with the heat created by the electric current

c. is used for incision or excision of tissue

d. dries and separates tissue with an electric current

COG IDENTIFICATION

Grade: _____

41. As a medical assistant, you may be called on to assist a physician with minor office surgery. Review the list of tasks below and determine which tasks you are responsible for as a medical assistant. Place a check in the "Yes" column for those duties you will assist with as a medical assistant, and place a check in the "No" column for those tasks that you would not be able to perform.

Task	Yes	No
a. Remind the patient of the physician's presurgery instructions, such as fasting.		
b. Prepare the treatment room, including the supplies and equipment.		
c. Obtain the informed consent document from the patient.		
d. Inject the patient with local anesthesia if necessary.		
e. Choose the size of the suture to be used to close the wound.		
f. Apply a dressing or bandage to the wound.		
g. Instruct the patient about postoperative wound care.		
h. Prescribe pain medication for the patient to take at home.		
i. Prepare lab paperwork for any specimens that must be sent out to the lab.		
j. Clean and sterilize the room for the next patient.		

42. A patient comes into the physician's office with a large wound on his leg. The physician asks you to assist with minor surgery to care for the wound. Because you must help maintain a sterile field before and during the procedure, review the list of actions below and indicate whether sterility (S) was maintained or if there has been any possible contamination (C).

   a. _____ The sterile package was moist before the surgery started.

   b. _____ The physician spills a few drops of sterile water onto the sterile field.

   c. _____ You hold the sterile items for the physician above waist level.

   d. _____ The physician rests the sterile items in the middle of the sterile field.

   e. _____ You ask the physician a question over the sterile field.

   f. _____ The physician leaves the room and places a drape over the field.

   g. _____ The physician passes soiled gauze over the sterile field and asks you
   to dispose of them properly.

43. As a medical assistant, you may be responsible for preparing and maintaining sterile packs. Determine if the packs listed below are appropriately sterilized (S) or if they need to be repackaged (R) and sterilized again.

   a. _____ No moisture is present on the pack.

   b. _____ The package was sterilized onsite 15 days ago.

   c. _____ The wrapper is ripped down one side.

   d. _____ The sterilization indicator has changed color.

   e. _____ An item from the package fell out onto the floor when you picked it up.

44. Which of the following information must be stated on the informed consent document? Circle the letter preceding all items that apply.

    a. The name of the procedure

    b. The tools used in the procedure

    c. The purpose of the procedure

    d. The expected results

    e. The patient's Social Security number

    f. Possible side effects

    g. The length of the procedure

    h. Potential risks and complications

    i. The date of the follow-up appointment

45. Listed below are the steps that a medical assistant should take to clean the examination room and prepare it for the next patient after a minor office surgical procedure. However, the steps below are not listed in the correct order. Review the steps and then place a number on the line next to each step to show the correct order in which they should occur with number 1 being the first step taken.

    a. _____ Put on gloves.

    b. _____ Remove papers and sheets from the table and discard properly.

    c. _____ Replace the table sheet paper for the next patient.

    d. _____ Wipe down the examination table, surgical stand, sink, counter, and other surfaces used during the procedure with a disinfectant and allow them to dry.

COG **SHORT ANSWER**   Grade: _____

46. List the three ways in which you may add the contents of peel-back packages to a sterile field.

    a. _____

    b. _____

    c. _____

47. Name four anesthetics that are commonly used in a medical office.

    a. _____

    b. _____

    c. _____

    d. _____

48. Name three ways in which needles can be classified.

    a. _____

    b. _____

    c. _____

COG TRUE OR FALSE?

Grade: _____

Indicate whether the statements are true or false by placing the letter T (true) or F (false) on the line preceding the statement.

49. _____ Anesthesia with epinephrine is approved for use on the tips of the fingers, toes, nose, and penis.

50. _____ Atraumatic needles need to be threaded by the physician before they can be used.

51. _____ Nonabsorbable sutures must be removed after healing.

52. _____ All metal must be removed from a patient before electrosurgery.

COG AFF CASE STUDIES FOR CRITICAL THINKING

Grade: _____

1. The physician asks you to position a patient for surgery in the lithotomy position. You know that the physician has to meet with another patient before he will come into the room to perform the surgery. What can you do to keep the patient comfortable before the physician is ready to begin? List three things you can do, and explain why they are important.

_____

_____

_____

_____

2. There is a delay in the office, and all of the appointments are running 30 minutes late. The patients are becoming upset, and the office manager said that you should work quickly to try to get back on schedule. You assist the physician with the removal of a small wart from a patient's neck. After the surgery is completed, you need to meet with a new patient to go over the new patient interview and paperwork. But it's also your job to label the specimen and complete the paperwork to send it to the lab. It's almost lunchtime, and you know the lab won't get to it right away. Which task should you complete first—meeting with the patient or preparing the specimen for the lab? Explain your answer.

_____

_____

_____

_____

3. Dante is a clinical medical assistant who is assisting a physician with minor office surgery. Dr. Yan asks him to prepare the local anesthesia. Dante chooses the anesthetic and draws the medication into a syringe. Next, he places the filled syringe on the sterile tray. Were these actions appropriate? Why or why not? Should Dr. Yan put on sterile gloves before or after she administers the anesthesia? Explain your answer.

_____

_____

_____

_____

4. A homeless patient comes into the urgent care office with a cut on his chin. Which size suture would the physician likely want for this procedure in order to reduce the size of the scar—a size 3 suture or a size 23-0 suture? The patient seems confused and smells of alcohol. How would you handle this situation before, during, and after the procedure?

_____

_____

_____

_____

5. Ghani is a clinical medical assistant. On Monday, he assisted the physician while she sutured a deep wound on a 7-year-old boy's leg. A few hours after the surgery, the mother brings the boy back to the office because she is concerned the site is infected. When Ghani inspects the sterile dressing, he notes that there is a moderate amount of pink drainage. What does this drainage indicate about the healing process? Is the mother's concern legitimate? How would you respond to her?

_____

_____

_____

_____

6. Your patient is a 79-year-old female who has had a large mole excised from her forearm. The cyst is being sent out for pathology to rule out skin cancer. You give her extra bandages so she can change the dressing herself and explain that the physician wants to see her back in the office in 1 week. She is very hard of hearing and lives alone. What instructions would you need to explain to the patient about caring for the wound? How would you handle this situation?

_____

_____

_____

7. Your patient is a 13-year-old boy who received staples for a wound he got in a biking accident. While you are removing the staples, he asks why staples are being used, and not stitches. Explain the difference between sutures and staples, and when it is more appropriate to use each.

_____

_____

_____

_____

8. A 15-year-old patient has a mole on her face that needs to be removed. She feels anxious about having to wear a large dressing to cover the wound on her face while it heals. In addition, she is nervous about the possibilities of scarring and she is worried that the mole is cancerous. How would you handle this situation? What would you say to her to ease her mind before and after the procedure?

_____

_____

_____

_____

9. You are working with another medical assistant to prepare a sterile field for surgery. You are almost finished setting up the sterile field when your coworker sneezes over the sterile field. She says that it's only allergies and that she's not contagious, so the field isn't contaminated. She assures you that you don't need to start your work over again. How would you handle this situation? What would you say to your coworker? What should you do next?

_____

_____

_____

_____

PSY PROCEDURE 22-1 | Opening Sterile Surgical Packs

Name: _____ Date: _____ Time: _____ Grade: _____

EQUIPMENT/SUPPLIES: Surgical pack, surgical or Mayo stand

STANDARDS: Given the needed equipment and a place to work the student will perform this skill with _____% accuracy in a total of _____ minutes. *(Your instructor will tell you what the percentage and time limits will be before you begin.)*

KEY: 4 = Satisfactory   0 = Unsatisfactory   NA = This step is not counted

PROCEDURE STEPS	SELF	PARTNER	INSTRUCTOR
1. Verify the surgical procedure to be performed and gather supplies.	☐	☐	☐
2. Check the label for contents and the expiration date.	☐	☐	☐
3. Check the package for tears or areas of moisture.	☐	☐	☐
4. Place the package, with the label facing up on the Mayo or surgical stand.	☐	☐	☐
5. Wash your hands.	☐	☐	☐
6. Without tearing the wrapper, carefully remove the sealing tape.	☐	☐	☐
7. Open the first flap: pull it up, out, and away; let it fall over the far side of the table.	☐	☐	☐
8. Open the side flaps in a similar manner. Do not touch the sterile inner surface.	☐	☐	☐
9. Pull the remaining flap down and toward you.	☐	☐	☐
10. Repeat steps 4 through 6 for packages with a second or inside wrapper.	☐	☐	☐
11. If you must leave the area after opening the field, cover the tray with a sterile drape.	☐	☐	☐

CALCULATION

Total Possible Points: _____

Total Points Earned: _____ Multiplied by 100 = _____ Divided by Total Possible Points = _____ %

PASS   **FAIL**   **COMMENTS:**

☐   ☐

Student's signature _____ Date _____

Partner's signature _____ Date _____

Instructor's signature _____ Date _____

PSY PROCEDURE 22-2 | **Using Sterile Transfer Forceps**

Name: _____ Date: _____ Time: _____ Grade: _____

EQUIPMENT/SUPPLIES: Sterile transfer forceps in a container with sterilization solution, sterile field, sterile items to be transferred

STANDARDS: Given the needed equipment and a place to work the student will perform this skill with _____% accuracy in a total of _____ minutes. *(Your instructor will tell you what the percentage and time limits will be before you begin.)*

KEY: 4 = Satisfactory   0 = Unsatisfactory   NA = This step is not counted

PROCEDURE STEPS	SELF	PARTNER	INSTRUCTOR
1. Slowly lift the forceps straight up and out of the container without touching the inside above the level of the solution or outside of the container.	☐	☐	☐
2. Hold the forceps with the tips down at all times.	☐	☐	☐
3. Keep the forceps above waist level.	☐	☐	☐
4. With the forceps, pick up the articles to be transferred and drop them onto the sterile field, but do not let the forceps come into contact with the sterile field.	☐	☐	☐
5. Carefully place the forceps back into the sterilization solution.	☐	☐	☐

CALCULATION

Total Possible Points: _____

Total Points Earned: _____ Multiplied by 100 = _____ Divided by Total Possible Points = _____ %

PASS   **FAIL**   **COMMENTS:**

☐   ☐

Student's signature _____ Date _____

Partner's signature _____ Date _____

Instructor's signature _____ Date _____

PSY PROCEDURE 22-3 Adding Sterile Solution to a Sterile Field

Name: _____ Date: _____ Time: _____ Grade: _____

EQUIPMENT/SUPPLIES: Sterile setup, container of sterile solution, sterile bowl or cup

STANDARDS: Given the needed equipment and a place to work the student will perform this skill with _____%
accuracy in a total of _____ minutes. *(Your instructor will tell you what the percentage and time limits will be
before you begin.)*

KEY: 4 = Satisfactory   0 = Unsatisfactory   NA = This step is not counted

PROCEDURE STEPS	SELF	PARTNER	INSTRUCTOR
1. Identify the correct solution by carefully reading the label.	☐	☐	☐
2. Check the expiration date on the label.	☐	☐	☐
3. If adding medications into the solution, show medication label to the physician.	☐	☐	☐
4. Remove the cap or stopper; avoid contamination of the inside of the cap.	☐	☐	☐
5. If it is necessary to put the cap down, place on side table with opened end facing up.	☐	☐	☐
6. Retain bottle to track amount added to field.	☐	☐	☐
7. Grasp container with label against the palm of your hand.	☐	☐	☐
8. Pour a small amount of the solution into a separate container or waste receptacle.	☐	☐	☐
9. Slowly pour the desired amount of solution into the sterile container.	☐	☐	☐
10. Recheck the label for the contents and expiration date and replace the cap.	☐	☐	☐
11. Return the solution to its proper storage area or discard the container after rechecking the label again.	☐	☐	☐

CALCULATION

Total Possible Points: _____

Total Points Earned: _____ Multiplied by 100 = _____ Divided by Total Possible Points = _____ %

PASS   **FAIL**   **COMMENTS:**

☐   ☐

Student's signature _____ Date _____

Partner's signature _____ Date _____

Instructor's signature _____ Date _____

PSY PROCEDURE 22-4 Performing Skin Preparation and Hair Removal

Name: _____ Date: _____ Time: _____ Grade: _____

EQUIPMENT/SUPPLIES: Nonsterile gloves; shave cream, lotion, or soap; new disposable razor; gauze or cotton balls; warm water; antiseptic; sponge forceps

STANDARDS: Given the needed equipment and a place to work the student will perform this skill with _____%
accuracy in a total of _____ minutes. *(Your instructor will tell you what the percentage and time limits will be before you begin.)*

KEY: 4 = Satisfactory   0 = Unsatisfactory   NA = This step is not counted

PROCEDURE STEPS	SELF	PARTNER	INSTRUCTOR
1. Wash your hands.	☐	☐	☐
2. Assemble the equipment.	☐	☐	☐
3. Greet and identify the patient; explain the procedure and answer any questions.	☐	☐	☐
4. Put on gloves.	☐	☐	☐
5. Prepare the patient's skin.	☐	☐	☐
6. If the patient's skin is to be shaved, apply shaving cream or soapy lather.	☐	☐	☐
a. Pull the skin taut and shave in the direction of hair growth.			
b. Rinse and pat the shaved area thoroughly dry using a gauze square.			
7. If the patient's skin is not to be shaved, wash with soap and water; rinse well and pat the area thoroughly dry using a gauze square.	☐	☐	☐
8. Apply antiseptic solution to the operative area using sterile gauze sponges.	☐	☐	☐
a. Wipe skin in circular motions starting at the operative site and working outward.			
b. Discard each sponge after a complete sweep has been made.			
c. If circles are not appropriate, the sponge may be wiped straight outward from the operative site and discarded.			
d. Repeat the procedure until the entire area has been thoroughly cleaned.			
9. Instruct the patient not to touch or cover the prepared area.	☐	☐	☐
10. **AFF** Explain how to respond to a patient who is developmentally challenged.	☐	☐	☐

11. Remove your gloves and wash your hands.	☐	☐	☐
12. Inform the physician that the patient is ready for the surgical procedure.	☐	☐	☐
13. Drape the prepared area with a sterile drape if the physician will be delayed more than 10 or 15 minutes.	☐	☐	☐

CALCULATION

Total Possible Points: _____

Total Points Earned: _____ Multiplied by 100 = _____ Divided by Total Possible Points = _____ %

PASS   **FAIL**   **COMMENTS:**

☐   ☐

Student's signature _____ Date _____

Partner's signature _____ Date _____

Instructor's signature _____ Date _____

PSY PROCEDURE 22-5 | Applying Sterile Gloves

Name: _____ Date: _____ Time: _____ Grade: _____

EQUIPMENT/SUPPLIES: One package of sterile gloves in the appropriate size

STANDARDS: Given the needed equipment and a place to work the student will perform this skill with _____%
accuracy in a total of _____ minutes. *(Your instructor will tell you what the percentage and time limits will be
before you begin.)*

KEY: 4 = Satisfactory 0 = Unsatisfactory NA = This step is not counted

PROCEDURE STEPS	SELF	PARTNER	INSTRUCTOR
1. Remove rings and other jewelry.	☐	☐	☐
2. Wash your hands.	☐	☐	☐
3. Place prepackaged gloves on a clean, dry, flat surface with the cuffed end toward you. **a.** Pull the outer wrapping apart to expose the sterile inner wrap. **b.** With the cuffs toward you, fold back the inner wrap to expose the gloves.	☐	☐	☐
4. Grasping the edges of the outer paper, open the package out to its fullest.	☐	☐	☐
5. Use your nondominant hand to pick up the dominant hand glove. **a.** Grasp the folded edge of the cuff and lift it up and away from the paper. **b.** Curl your fingers and thumb together and insert them into the glove. **c.** Straighten your fingers and pull the glove on with your nondominant hand still grasping the cuff.	☐	☐	☐
6. Unfold the cuff by pinching the inside surface and pull it toward your wrist.	☐	☐	☐
7. Place the fingers of your gloved hand under the cuff of the remaining glove. **a.** Lift the glove up and away from the wrapper. **b.** Slide your ungloved hand carefully into the glove with your fingers and thumb curled together. **c.** Straighten your fingers and pull the glove up and over your wrist by carefully unfolding the cuff.	☐	☐	☐
8. Settle the gloves comfortably onto your fingers by lacing your fingers together.	☐	☐	☐
9. Remove contaminated sterile gloves and discard them appropriately. Wash your hands.	☐	☐	☐

CALCULATION

Total Possible Points: _____

Total Points Earned: _____ Multiplied by 100 = _____ Divided by Total Possible Points = _____ %

PASS   **FAIL**   **COMMENTS:**

☐   ☐

Student's signature _____ Date _____

Partner's signature _____ Date _____

Instructor's signature _____ Date _____

PSY PROCEDURE 22-6 | Applying a Sterile Dressing

Name: _____ Date: _____ Time: _____ Grade: _____

EQUIPMENT/SUPPLIES: Sterile gloves, sterile gauze dressings, scissors, bandage tape, any medication to be applied to the dressing if ordered by the physician

STANDARDS: Given the needed equipment and a place to work the student will perform this skill with _____% accuracy in a total of _____ minutes. *(Your instructor will tell you what the percentage and time limits will be before you begin.)*

KEY: 4 = Satisfactory   0 = Unsatisfactory   NA = This step is not counted

PROCEDURE STEPS	SELF	PARTNER	INSTRUCTOR
1. Wash your hands.	☐	☐	☐
2. Assemble the equipment and supplies.	☐	☐	☐
3. Greet and identify the patient.	☐	☐	☐
4. Ask about any tape allergies before deciding on what type of tape to use.	☐	☐	☐
5. Cut or tear lengths of tape to secure the dressing.	☐	☐	☐
6. Explain the procedure and instruct the patient to remain still; avoid coughing, sneezing, or talking until the procedure is complete.	☐	☐	☐
7. Open the dressing pack to create a sterile field, maintaining sterile asepsis. **a.** If sterile gloves are to be used, open and place near dressing pack. **b.** If using a sterile transfer forceps, place it near the other supplies.	☐	☐	☐
8. Apply topical medication to the sterile dressing that will cover the wound.	☐	☐	☐
9. Apply the number of dressings necessary to properly cover and protect the wound.	☐	☐	☐
10. Apply sufficient cut lengths of tape over the dressing to secure.	☐	☐	☐
11. Remove contaminated gloves and discard in the proper receptacle. Wash your hands.	☐	☐	☐
12. Provide patient education and supplies as appropriate.	☐	☐	☐
13. **AFF** Explain how to respond to a patient who is visually impaired.	☐	☐	☐
14. Clean and sanitize the room and equipment.	☐	☐	☐
15. Record the procedure.	☐	☐	☐

CALCULATION

Total Possible Points: _____

Total Points Earned: _____ Multiplied by 100 = _____ Divided by Total Possible Points = _____ %

PASS   **FAIL**   **COMMENTS:**

☐   ☐

Student's signature _____ Date _____

Partner's signature _____ Date _____

Instructor's signature _____ Date _____

PSY PROCEDURE 22-7 Changing an Existing Sterile Dressing

Name: _____ Date: _____ Time: _____ Grade: _____

EQUIPMENT/SUPPLIES: Sterile gloves, nonsterile gloves, sterile dressing, prepackaged skin antiseptic swabs (or sterile antiseptic solution poured into a sterile basin and sterile cotton balls or gauze), tape, approved biohazard containers

STANDARDS: Given the needed equipment and a place to work the student will perform this skill with _____% accuracy in a total of _____ minutes. *(Your instructor will tell you what the percentage and time limits will be before you begin.)*

KEY: 4 = Satisfactory   0 = Unsatisfactory   NA = This step is not counted

PROCEDURE STEPS	SELF	PARTNER	INSTRUCTOR
1. Wash your hands.	☐	☐	☐
2. Assemble the equipment and supplies.	☐	☐	☐
3. Greet and identify the patient; explain the procedure and answer any questions.	☐	☐	☐
4. Prepare a sterile field including opening sterile dressings.	☐	☐	☐
5. Open a sterile basin and use the inside of the wrapper as the sterile field. 　**a.** Flip the sterile gauze or cotton balls into the basin. 　**b.** Pour antiseptic solution appropriately into the basin. 　**c.** If using prepackaged antiseptic swabs, carefully open an adequate number. 　**d.** Set swabs aside without contaminating them.	☐	☐	☐
6. Instruct the patient not to talk, cough, sneeze, laugh, or move during the procedure.	☐	☐	☐
7. **AFF** Explain how to respond to a patient who has dementia.	☐	☐	☐
_____			
_____			
_____			
_____			
8. Wear clean gloves and carefully remove tape from the wound dressing by pulling it toward the wound. 　**a.** Remove the old dressing. 　**b.** Discard the soiled dressing into a biohazard container.	☐	☐	☐
9. Inspect wound for the degree of healing, amount and type of drainage, and appearance of wound edges.	☐	☐	☐
10. Observing medical asepsis, remove and discard your gloves.	☐	☐	☐

11. Using proper technique, apply sterile gloves.	☐	☐	☐
12. Clean the wound with the antiseptic solution ordered by the physician.	☐	☐	☐
13. Clean in a straight motion with the cotton or gauze or the prepackaged antiseptic swab. Discard the wipe (cotton ball, swab) after each use.	☐	☐	☐
14. Remove your gloves and wash your hands.	☐	☐	☐
15. Change the dressing using the procedure for sterile dressing application (Procedure 22-6) and using sterile gloves (Procedure 22-5) or sterile transfer forceps (Procedure 22-2).	☐	☐	☐
16. Record the procedure.	☐	☐	☐

CALCULATION

Total Possible Points: _____

Total Points Earned: _____ Multiplied by 100 = _____ Divided by Total Possible Points = _____ %

PASS   **FAIL**   **COMMENTS:**

☐   ☐

Student's signature _____ Date _____

Partner's signature _____ Date _____

Instructor's signature _____ Date _____

Name: _____ Date: _____ Time: _____ Grade: _____

EQUIPMENT/SUPPLIES: Sterile gloves, local anesthetic, antiseptic wipes, adhesive tape, specimen container with completed laboratory request; *On the field:* basin for solutions, gauze sponges and cotton balls, antiseptic solution, sterile drape, dissecting scissors, disposable scalpel, blade of physician's choice, mosquito forceps, tissue forceps, needle holder, suture and needle of physician's choice

STANDARDS: Given the needed equipment and a place to work the student will perform this skill with _____% accuracy in a total of _____ minutes. *(Your instructor will tell you what the percentage and time limits will be before you begin.)*

KEY: 4 = Satisfactory 0 = Unsatisfactory NA = This step is not counted

PROCEDURE STEPS	SELF	PARTNER	INSTRUCTOR
1. Wash your hands.	☐	☐	☐
2. Assemble the equipment appropriate for the procedure and according to physician preference.	☐	☐	☐
3. Greet and identify the patient; explain the procedure and answer any questions.	☐	☐	☐
4. Set up a sterile field on a surgical stand with additional equipment close at hand.	☐	☐	☐
5. Cover the field with a sterile drape until the physician arrives.	☐	☐	☐
6. Position the patient appropriately.	☐	☐	☐
7. Put on sterile gloves (Procedure 22-5) or use sterile transfer forceps (Procedure 22-2) and cleanse the patient's skin (Procedure 22-4).	☐	☐	☐
8. Be ready to assist during the procedure: adding supplies as needed, assisting the physician, and comforting the patient.	☐	☐	☐
9. Assist with collecting tissue specimen in an appropriate container.	☐	☐	☐
10. At the end of the procedure, wash your hands and dress the wound using sterile technique (Procedure 22-6).	☐	☐	☐
11. Thank the patient and give appropriate instructions.	☐	☐	☐
12. **AFF** Explain how to respond to a patient who is hearing impaired.	☐	☐	☐
13. Sanitize the examining room in preparation for the next patient.	☐	☐	☐
14. Discard all disposables in the appropriate biohazard containers.	☐	☐	☐
15. Record the procedure.	☐	☐	☐

CALCULATION

Total Possible Points: _____

Total Points Earned: _____ Multiplied by 100 = _____ Divided by Total Possible Points = _____ %

PASS   **FAIL**   **COMMENTS:**

☐   ☐

Student's signature _____ Date _____

Partner's signature _____ Date _____

Instructor's signature _____ Date _____

Name: _____ Date: _____ Time: _____ Grade: _____

EQUIPMENT/SUPPLIES: Sterile gloves, local anesthetic, antiseptic wipes, adhesive tape, sterile dressings, packing gauze, a culture tube if the wound may be cultured; *On the field:* basin for solutions, gauze sponges and cotton balls, antiseptic solution, sterile drape, syringes and needles for local anesthetic, commercial I&D sterile setup *or* scalpel, dissecting scissors, hemostats, tissue forceps, 4 × 4 gauze sponges, probe (optional)

STANDARDS: Given the needed equipment and a place to work the student will perform this skill with _____%
accuracy in a total of _____ minutes. *(Your instructor will tell you what the percentage and time limits will be before you begin.)*

KEY: 4 = Satisfactory   0 = Unsatisfactory   NA = This step is not counted

PROCEDURE STEPS	SELF	PARTNER	INSTRUCTOR
1. Wash your hands.	☐	☐	☐
2. Assemble the equipment appropriate for the procedure and according to physician preference.	☐	☐	☐
3. Greet and identify the patient. Explain the procedure and answer any questions.	☐	☐	☐
4. Set up a sterile field on a surgical stand with additional equipment close at hand	☐	☐	☐
5. Cover the field with a sterile drape until the physician arrives.	☐	☐	☐
6. Position the patient appropriately.	☐	☐	☐
7. Put on sterile gloves (Procedure 22-5) or use sterile transfer forceps (Procedure 22-2) and cleanse the patient's skin (Procedure 22-4).	☐	☐	☐
8. Be ready to assist during the procedure: adding supplies as needed, assisting the physician, comforting the patient.	☐	☐	☐
9. Assist with collecting culturette specimen for culture and sensitivity.	☐	☐	☐
10. At the end of procedure, remove gloves, wash your hands, and dress the wound using sterile technique (Procedure 22-6).	☐	☐	☐
11. Thank the patient and give appropriate instructions.	☐	☐	☐
12. Sanitize the examining room in preparation for the next patient.	☐	☐	☐
13. Discard all disposables in appropriate biohazard containers.	☐	☐	☐
14. Record the procedure.	☐	☐	☐

CALCULATION

Total Possible Points: _____

Total Points Earned: _____ Multiplied by 100 = _____ Divided by Total Possible Points = _____ %

PASS   **FAIL**   **COMMENTS:**

☐   ☐

Student's signature _____ Date _____

Partner's signature _____ Date _____

Instructor's signature _____ Date _____

PSY PROCEDURE 22-10   Removing Sutures

Name: _____ Date: _____ Time: _____ Grade: _____

EQUIPMENT/SUPPLIES: Skin antiseptic, sterile gloves, prepackaged suture removal kit *or* thumb forceps, suture scissors, gauze

STANDARDS: Given the needed equipment and a place to work the student will perform this skill with _____% accuracy in a total of _____ minutes. *(Your instructor will tell you what the percentage and time limits will be before you begin.)*

KEY: 4 = Satisfactory   0 = Unsatisfactory   NA = This step is not counted

PROCEDURE STEPS	SELF	PARTNER	INSTRUCTOR
1. Wash your hands and apply clean examination gloves.	☐	☐	☐
2. Assemble the equipment.	☐	☐	☐
3. Greet and identify the patient; explain the procedure and answer any questions.	☐	☐	☐
4. If dressings have not been removed previously, remove them from the wound area.	☐	☐	☐
a. Properly dispose of the soiled dressings in the biohazard trash container.			
b. Remove your gloves and wash your hands.			
5. Put on another pair of clean examination gloves and cleanse the wound with an antiseptic.	☐	☐	☐
6. Open suture removal packet using sterile asepsis.	☐	☐	☐
7. Put on sterile gloves.	☐	☐	☐
a. With the thumb forceps, grasp the end of the knot closest to the skin surface and lift it slightly and gently up from the skin.			
b. Cut the suture below the knot as close to the skin as possible.			
c. Use the thumb forceps to pull the suture out of the skin with a smooth motion.			
8. Place the suture on the gauze sponge; repeat the procedure for each suture to be removed.	☐	☐	☐
9. Clean the site with an antiseptic solution and cover it with a sterile dressing.	☐	☐	☐
10. Thank the patient.	☐	☐	☐
11. **AFF** Explain how to respond to a patient who is developmentally challenged.	☐	☐	☐

12. Properly dispose of the equipment and supplies.	☐	☐	☐
13. Clean the work area, remove your gloves, and wash your hands.	☐	☐	☐
14. Record the procedure, including the time, location of sutures, the number removed, and the condition of the wound.	☐	☐	☐

CALCULATION

Total Possible Points: _____

Total Points Earned: _____ Multiplied by 100 = _____ Divided by Total Possible Points = _____ %

PASS   **FAIL**   **COMMENTS:**

☐   ☐

Student's signature _____ Date _____

Partner's signature _____ Date _____

Instructor's signature _____ Date _____

PSY PROCEDURE 22-11 Removing Staples

Name: _____ Date: _____ Time: _____ Grade: _____

EQUIPMENT/SUPPLIES: Antiseptic solution or wipes, gauze squares, sponge forceps, prepackaged sterile staple removal instrument, examination gloves, sterile gloves

STANDARDS: Given the needed equipment and a place to work the student will perform this skill with _____% accuracy in a total of _____ minutes. *(Your instructor will tell you what the percentage and time limits will be before you begin.)*

KEY: 4 = Satisfactory   0 = Unsatisfactory   NA = This step is not counted

PROCEDURE STEPS	SELF	PARTNER	INSTRUCTOR
1. Wash your hands.	☐	☐	☐
2. Assemble the equipment.	☐	☐	☐
3. Greet and identify the patient; explain the procedure and answer any questions.	☐	☐	☐
4. If the dressing has not been removed, put on clean examination gloves and do so.	☐	☐	☐
5. Dispose of the dressing properly in a biohazard container.	☐	☐	☐
6. Clean the incision with antiseptic solution.	☐	☐	☐
7. Pat dry using dry sterile gauze sponges.	☐	☐	☐
8. Put on sterile gloves.	☐	☐	☐
9. Gently slide the end of the staple remover under each staple to be removed; press the handles together to lift the ends of the staple out of the skin and remove the staple.	☐	☐	☐
10. Place each staple on a gauze square as it is removed.	☐	☐	☐
11. When all staples are removed, clean the incision as instructed for all procedures.	☐	☐	☐
12. Pat dry and dress the site if ordered to do so by the physician.	☐	☐	☐
13. Thank the patient and properly care for, or dispose of, all equipment and supplies.	☐	☐	☐
14. **AFF** Explain how to respond to a patient who is visually impaired.	☐	☐	☐
15. Clean the work area, remove your gloves, and wash your hands.	☐	☐	☐
16. Record the procedure.	☐	☐	☐

CALCULATION

Total Possible Points: _____

Total Points Earned: _____ Multiplied by 100 = _____ Divided by Total Possible Points = _____ %

PASS   **FAIL**   **COMMENTS:**

☐   ☐

Student's signature _____ Date _____

Partner's signature _____ Date _____

Instructor's signature _____ Date _____

Pharmacology

Cognitive Domain

1. Spell and define key terms
2. Describe the relationship between anatomy and physiology of all body systems and medications used for treatment in each
3. Identify chemical, trade, and generic drug names
4. Discuss all levels of governmental legislation and regulation as they apply to medical assisting practice, including food and drug administration and drug enforcement agency regulations
5. Explain the various drug actions and interactions, including pharmacodynamics and pharmacokinetics
6. Identify the classifications of medications, including desired effects, side effects, and adverse reactions
7. Name the sources for locating information on pharmacology

Affective Domain

1. Apply critical thinking skills in performing patient assessment and care
2. Demonstrate sensitivity to patient rights

ABHES Competencies

1. Properly utilize *Physicians' Desk Reference,* drug handbook, and other drug references to identify a drug's classification, usual dosage, usual side effects, and contradictions
2. Identify and define common abbreviations that are accepted in prescription writing
3. Understand legal aspects of writing prescriptions, including federal and state laws

Name: _____   Date: _____   Grade: _____

COG MULTIPLE CHOICE

Circle the letter preceding the correct answer.

1. A physician needs to register with the U.S. Attorney General:

   a. every 3 years.

   b. every 2 years.

   c. every 4 years.

   d. only once; registration is for life.

   e. every year.

2. When a drug is contraindicated, it:

   a. is not properly eliminated.

   b. is distributed throughout the bloodstream.

   c. should not be used.

   d. is detected in urine excretion.

   e. should be retested for accuracy.

3. Emetics are used to:

   a. dilate bronchi.

   b. prevent symptoms of menopause.

   c. control diabetes.

   d. dissolve blood clots.

   e. promote vomiting.

4. Which substance is an example of a Schedule I controlled substance?

   a. Morphine

   b. Ritalin

   c. Amphetamines

   d. Opium

   e. Tylenol with codeine

5. Which drug below is an example of an antipyretic?

   a. Aspirin

   b. Dramamine

   c. Lanoxin

   d. Zantac

   e. Benylin

6. A symptom of an allergic reaction is:

   a. nausea.

   b. drowsiness.

   c. dryness of mouth.

   d. hives.

   e. fever.

7. Two drugs when taken together that can create synergism are:

   a. sedatives and barbiturates.

   b. antacids and antibiotics.

   c. diuretics and decongestants.

   d. antibiotics and antifungals.

   e. antihypertensives and expectorants.

8. The DEA is a branch of the:

   a. BNDD.

   b. DOJ.

   c. FDA.

   d. AMA.

   e. AHFS.

9. All drugs cause:

   a. cellular and physiological change.

   b. cellular and psychological change.

   c. physiological and psychological change.

   d. physiological changes.

   e. cellular, physiological, and psychological change.

10. Green leafy vegetables can sometimes interact with:

    a. coumadin.

    b. verapamil.

    c. ibuprofen.

    d. amoxicillin.

    e. phenobarbital.

11. Drugs with a potential for abuse and currently accepted for medicinal use are:

    a. Schedule I drugs.

    b. Schedule II drugs.

    c. Schedule III drugs.

    d. Schedule IV drugs.

    e. Schedules I and IV drugs.

12. A drug is given a brand name when it:

    a. is first developed in laboratories.

    b. is used in field testing and studies.

    c. is assigned a sponsor for the research.

    d. is approved by the FDA.

    e. is available for commercial use.

Scenario for questions 13 and 14: A teenaged patient has called in saying that the pharmacy will not refill her painkiller prescription. It has been just over a month since she last refilled her prescription.

13. What is the first step you should take?

    a. Check her records to see how many more refills she has left.

    b. Inform the physician about the situation for directions.

    c. Call the pharmacy to find out how many refills she has gotten.

    d. Write out another prescription and fax it to the pharmacy.

    e. Inform the patient that she has no more refills remaining.

14. The patient still has three remaining refills on her prescription. After you call the pharmacy, however, you are informed that the patient has been purchasing over-the-counter painkillers along with her prescription. There is suspicion that the patient might be selling her medication and taking over-the-counter drugs. What do you do?

    a. Call the patient and confront her about the purchases.

    b. Discuss the possibility of drug abuse with the physician.

    c. Call the police immediately and report the patient.

    d. Tell the pharmacy to give her the prescriptions anyway.

    e. Gather information and report your findings.

15. The study of how drugs act on the body, including cells, tissues, and organs, is:

    a. pharmacokinetics.

    b. pharmacodynamics.

    c. synergism.

    d. antagonism.

    e. potentiation.

16. What kind of drug is used to increase the size of arterial blood vessels?

   a. Anticonvulsants

   b. Emetics

   c. Cholinergics

   d. Antihypertensives

   e. Immunologic agents

17. Which of the following is a trait of a Schedule I drug?

   a. No accepted safety standards

   b. Cannot be prescribed by a physician

   c. Lowest potential for abuse

   d. May be filled up to five times in 6 months

   e. Requires a handwritten prescription

18. When you are administering a controlled substance in a medical office, you must include:

   a. a drug schedule.

   b. the time of administration.

   c. patient allergies.

   d. your name.

   e. location.

19. If a patient is receiving a medication that has a high incidence of allergic reactions, how long should the patient wait before leaving the office?

   a. No wait time necessary

   b. 5 to 10 minutes

   c. 10 to 20 minutes

   d. 30 minutes to an hour

   e. Overnight observation

20. The chemical name of a drug is the:

   a. last name a drug is given before it is put on the market.

   b. description of the chemical compounds found in the drug.

   c. name given to the drug during research and development.

   d. name given to the drug by the FDA and AMA.

   e. name of the chemical the drug supplements in the body.

COG MATCHING

Grade: _____

Match each key term with its definition.

Key Terms

21. _____ allergy

22. _____ anaphylaxis

23. _____ antagonism

24. _____ chemical name

25. _____ contraindication

26. _____ drug

27. _____ generic name

28. _____ interaction

Definitions

a. effects, positive and negative, of two or more drugs taken by a patient

b. situation or condition that prohibits the prescribing or administering of a drug or medication

c. any substance that may modify one or more of the functions of an organism

d. study of drugs and their origin, nature, properties, and effects upon living organisms

e. exact chemical descriptor of a drug

f. official name given to a drug whose patent has expired

29. _____ pharmacodynamics

30. _____ pharmacokinetics

31. _____ pharmacology

32. _____ potentiation

33. _____ synergism

34. _____ trade name

g. name given to a medication by the company that owns the patent

h. study of the effects and reactions of drugs within the body

i. study of the action of drugs within the body from administration to excretion

j. harmonious action of two agents, such as drugs or organs, producing an effect that neither could produce alone or that is greater than the total effects of each agent operating by itself

k. mutual opposition or contrary action with something else; opposite of synergism

l. describes the action of two drugs taken together in which the combined effects are greater than the sum of the independent effects

m. acquired abnormal response to a substance (allergen) that does not ordinarily cause a reaction

n. severe allergic reaction that may result in death

COG MATCHING

Grade: _____

Match each drug term with its description.

Drug Terms

35. _____ therapeutic classification

36. _____ idiosyncratic reaction

37. _____ indications

38. _____ teratogenic category

39. _____ hypersensitivity

40. _____ contraindications

41. _____ adverse reactions

Descriptions

a. relates the level of risk to fetal or maternal health (These rank from Category A through D, with increasing danger at each level. Category X indicates that the particular drug should never be given during pregnancy.)

b. refers to an excessive reaction to a particular drug; also known as a _drug allergy_ (The body must build this response; the first exposures may or may not indicate that a problem is developing.)

c. indicates conditions or instances for which the particular drug should not be used

d. states the purpose for the drug's use (e.g., cardiotonic, anti-infective, antiarrhythmic)

e. refers to an abnormal or unexpected reaction to a drug peculiar to the individual patient; not technically an allergy

f. gives diseases for which the particular drug would be prescribed

g. refers to undesirable side effects of a particular drug

COG IDENTIFICATION

Grade: _____

42. Identify whether the following descriptions describe the chemical, generic, or trade name of a drug by writing C (chemical), G (generic), or T (trade) on the line preceding the description.

a. _____ The name of a drug that begins with a lowercase letter

b. _____ The name assigned to a drug during research and development

c. _____ The name given to a drug when it is available for commercial use

d. _____ The first name given to any medication

e. _____ The name that is registered by the U.S. patent office

f. _____ The name that identifies the chemical components of the drug

43. Determine if the information below can be found in the *Physicians' Desk Reference (PDR)* or the *United States Pharmacopeia Dispensing Information (USPDI)*. Place a check mark in the appropriate box below.

	Physicians' Desk Reference	United States Pharmacopeia Dispensing Information
a. Drug sources		
b. Indications		
c. Dosages		
d. Pictures		
e. Chemistry		
f. Physical properties		
g. Side effects		
h. Tests for identity		
i. Storage		
j. Contraindications		

44. Indicate where the following elements of a prescription go in sequential order.

Patient's name and address   Line 1: _____

Date   Line 2. _____

Inscription   Line 3. _____

Superscription   Line 4. _____

Subscription   Line 5. _____

Physician's signature   Line 6. _____

Signature   Line 7. _____

Generic   Line 8. _____

Refills   Line 9. _____

45. Indicate each drug's controlled substance category by writing I, II, III, IV, or V on the line preceding the drug name.

a. _____ morphine

b. _____ Tylenol with codeine

c. _____ cocaine

d. _____ codeine in cough medications

e. _____ marijuana

f. _____ Valium

g. _____ LSD

h. _____ Ritalin

i. _____ Librium

COG COMPLETION   Grade: _____

46. Each of the following statements about inventory of controlled substances is incorrect or incomplete. Rewrite each statement to make it correct or complete.

a. List only category III controlled substances on the appropriate inventory form.

_____

b. When you receive controlled substances, make sure that only the physician signs the receipt.

_____

c. Keep all controlled substance inventory forms for 10 years.

_____

d. When a controlled substance leaves the medical office inventory, record the following information: drug name and patient.

_____

e. Notify the office manager immediately if these drugs are lost or stolen.

_____

f. Store controlled substances in the same cabinet as other medications and supplies.

_____

COG SHORT ANSWER
Grade: _____

47. What are pharmacodynamics and pharmacokinetics? Explain the relationship between these two processes.

_____

_____

_____

_____

48. What four processes are connected to pharmacokinetics?

_____

_____

_____

_____

49. Why is it important for patients to know about food–drug interactions?

_____

_____

_____

_____

50. Explain the difference between drug side effects and allergic reactions.

_____

_____

_____

_____

51. List three common and predictable drug side effects.

_____

_____

_____

52. Compare and contrast the different types of drug interactions, including synergism, antagonism, and potentiation.

_____

_____

_____

_____

53. Compare the effect or action of the following therapeutic classifications: stimulants, diuretics, emetics, and immunologic agents.

_____

_____

_____

_____

COG TRUE OR FALSE?   Grade: _____

Indicate whether the statements are true or false by placing the letter T (true) or F (false) in the blank preceding the statement.

54. _____ The DEA is concerned with controlled substances only.

55. _____ Drugs are derived from natural and synthetic sources.

56. _____ Children have a slower response to drug intakes.

57. _____ Allergic reactions are always immediate.

58. _____ Side effects from drugs are often life threatening.

59. _____ A drug is a chemical substance that affects body function or functions.

60. _____ A drug administered for a systemic effect is applied topically.

61. _____ Women may react differently to certain drugs than men.

62. _____ Medications should always be taken on a full stomach.

COG AFF **CASE STUDIES FOR CRITICAL THINKING**   Grade: _____

1. You are doing an inventory of the controlled substances in your office and notice that the office's supply of morphine is off count. You double-check all written records of medications given for administration and still cannot account for the missing morphine. After realizing this, you immediately tell the physician. The physician tells you not to worry about it. Three weeks later you notice that more morphine is missing. What do you do?

   _____

   _____

   _____

   _____

2. A patient just received a shot of penicillin. Before the shot was administered, you advised the patient that she needs to remain in the physician's office for 30 minutes before leaving. However, the patient just remembers that she must pick her mother up for an appointment that her mother needs to attend. The patient is adamant that she must leave right away so as not to be late. How would you respond to this patient?

   _____

   _____

   _____

   _____

3. You have an elderly patient who is taking Lasix for his high blood pressure. This patient has recently called in to the office complaining of muscle weakness. What classification is the drug Lasix? What is possibly causing the patients' muscle weakness? How would you respond to this patient?

   _____

   _____

   _____

   _____

4. You have a patient with hepatic disease. After she consults with the physician, she asks you some general questions to clarify how her body processes medication. Think about the pharmacokinetic effects of drugs on her body. What processes would you discuss with her about her condition and medications?

_____

_____

_____

_____

5. Your patient tells you that she feels like she is coming down with a cold and has had a sore throat since yesterday. She also tells you that her friend gave her some leftover antibiotics that she did not finish when she had strep throat last month. How would you respond to this patient? Is this important information for the physician to know? Why or why not?

_____

_____

_____

_____

6. Louise asks Mr. Fujiwara about his medical history and if he has any allergies to any medications. Mr. Fujiwara says that he has an allergy to aspirin. Louise marks Mr. Fujiwara's drug allergy prominently on the front of his medication record before giving the record to the physician. What else should the medical assistant do?

_____

_____

_____

_____

Preparing and Administering Medications

Cognitive Domain

1. Spell and define the key terms
2. Demonstrate knowledge of basic math computations
3. Apply mathemathical computations to solve equations
4. Identify measurement systems
5. Define basic units of measurement in metric, apothecary, and household systems
6. Convert among measurement systems
7. Identify both abbreviations and symbols used in calculating medication dosages
8. List the safety guidelines for medication administration
9. Explain the differences between various parenteral and nonparenteral routes of medication administration
10. Describe the parts of a syringe and needle and name those parts that must be kept sterile
11. List the various needle lengths, gauges, and preferred sites for each type of injection
12. Compare the types of injections and locate the sites where each may be administered safely
13. Describe principles of intravenous therapy

Psychomotor Domain

1. Administer oral medications (Procedure 24-1)
2. Prepare injections (Procedure 24-2)
3. Prepare proper dosages of medication for administration
4. Administer an intradermal injection (Procedure 24-3)
5. Administer a subcutaneous injection (Procedure 24-4)
6. Administer an intramuscular injection (Procedure 24-5)
7. Administer an intramuscular injection using the Z-track method (Procedure 24-6)
8. Administer parenteral medications (excluding IV)
9. Select proper sites for administering parenteral medication
10. Apply transdermal medications (Procedure 24-7)
11. Obtain and prepare an intravenous site (Procedure 24-8)
12. Practice standard precautions
13. Document accurately in the patient record

Affective Domain

1. Apply critical thinking skills in performing patient assessment and care
2. Verify ordered doses/dosages prior to administration
3. Show awareness of patients' concerns regarding their perceptions related to the procedure being performed
4. Demonstrate empathy in communicating with patients, family, and staff
5. Apply active listening skills
6. Use appropriate body language and other nonverbal skills in communicating with patients, family, and staff
7. Demonstrate awareness of territorial boundaries of the person with you are whom communicating
8. Demonstrate sensitivity appropriate to the message being delivered
9. Demonstrate recognition of the patient's level of understanding in communications
10. Recognize and protect personal boundaries in communicating with others
11. Demonstrate respect for individual diversity, incorporating awareness of one's own biases in areas including gender, race, religion, age, and economic status

ABHES Competencies

1. Demonstrate accurate occupational math and metric conversions for proper medication administration
2. Apply principles of aseptic techniques and infection control
3. Maintain medication and immunization records
4. Use standard precautions
5. Prepare and administer oral and parenteral medications as directed by physician
6. Document accurately
7. Dispose of biohazardous materials

Name: _____   Date: _____   Grade: _____

COG **MULTIPLE CHOICE**

Circle the letter preceding the correct answer.

1. When administering an unfamiliar drug, you should look up information on:

   a. alternate formulations.

   b. the chemical name.

   c. generic alternatives.

   d. how the medication is stored.

   e. the route of administration.

2. When preparing medications you should:

   a. use previous medications and dosages listed on the patient's chart as a safety check.

   b. use a resource like the Internet to cross reference generic and brand names for medications.

   c. work in a quiet, well-lighted area.

   d. crush tablets so patients can swallow them easily.

   e. recap used needles to protect against accidental jabs.

3. Patient safety is protected by ensuring:

   a. a nurse prepares the medication for you to administer.

   b. you are administering the right drug to the right patient.

   c. medications are delivered to the right room for administration by the nurse.

   d. you are using the right type of syringe.

   e. you write down and document medications before you give them.

4. When dispensing drugs, make sure you convert the dosage ordered to the:

   a. apothecary system.

   b. household system.

   c. imperial units.

   d. system and units noted on the medication label.

   e. metric units.

5. The basic unit of weight in the metric system is the:

   a. grain.

   b. gram.

   c. liter.

   d. newton.

   e. pound.

6. What number do you multiply the base metric unit if the prefix is "milli"?

   a. 1,000

   b. 1,000,000

   c. 0.000001

   d. 0.001

   e. 0.01

7. Which of these measurements equals 2 cc?

   a. 2 mg

   b. 20 mg

   c. 2 mL

   d. 30 gr

   e. 120 mg

8. Which of these measurements equals 45 mL?

   a. 0.75 fl oz

   b. 1.5 fl oz

   c. 3.0 fl oz

   d. 4.5 fl oz

   e. 20.5 fl oz

9. The physician orders chloroquine syrup 100 mg oral for a 20-kg child. The concentration of the syrup is 50 mg/mL. How much medication do you give the child?

   a. 0.5 mL

   b. 2 mL

   c. 10 mL

   d. 40 mL

   e. 250 mL

10. Which method is the most accurate means of calculating pediatric dosages?

    a. Body weight method

    b. The Clarke rule

    c. The Fried rule

    d. BSA method

    e. The Young rule

11. Medicine administered under the tongue follows the:

    a. buccal route.

    b. dental route.

    c. dermal route.

    d. oral route.

    e. sublingual route.

12. Which item below could be a multiple-dose dispenser?

    a. Ampule

    b. Cartridge

    c. Carpuject

    d. Tubex

    e. Vial

13. How large is a tuberculin syringe?

    a. 10 U

    b. 5 mL

    c. 3 mL

    d. 1 mL

    e. 0.1 mL

14. A possible site for an intradermal injection is the:

    a. antecubital fossa.

    b. anterior forearm.

    c. upper arm.

    d. deltoid.

    e. vastus lateralis.

Scenario for questions 15 and 16: You are directed to set up an IV line delivering RL 30 mL/hr TKO with a 10-gtt/mL system.

15. How many drips per minute should the IV deliver?

    a. 1 gtt/min

    b. 3 gtt/min

    c. 5 gtt/min

    d. 10 gtt/min

    e. 20 gtt/min

16. A good site for the angiocatheter would be the:

    a. antecubital fossa.

    b. anterior forearm.

    c. upper arm.

    d. deltoid.

    e. vastus lateralis.

17. A good place to administer a 0.25 mL IM injection on a child is the:

    a. antecubital fossa.

    b. anterior forearm.

    c. upper arm.

    d. deltoid.

    e. vastus lateralis.

18. The physician orders Demerol 150 mg IM for a patient. The vial label indicates a total of 20 mL of medication with 100 mg/ml. Find the dosage.

    a. 0.67 mL

    b. 1.5 mL

    c. 2.5 mL

    d. 7.5 mL

    e. 30 mL

19. A good site to inject a medication ordered SC would be the:

a. antecubital fossa.

b. anterior forearm.

c. upper arm.

d. deltoid.

e. vastus lateralis.

20. You are told to administer a medicine by the otic route. This medicine should be administered into:

a. the ears.

b. inhaler.

c. the eyes

d. the mouth.

e. the nose.

COG MATCHING   Grade: _____

Match each key term with its definition.

Key Terms

21. _____ ampule

22. _____ apothecary system of measurement

23. _____ buccal

24. _____ diluent

25. _____ gauge

26. _____ induration

27. _____ infiltration

28. _____ Mantoux

29. _____ metric system

30. _____ nebulizer

31. _____ ophthalmic

32. _____ otic

33. _____ parenteral

34. _____ sublingual

35. _____ topical

36. _____ vial

Definitions

a. leakage of intravenous fluids into surrounding tissues

b. administration of medication between the cheek and gum of the mouth

c. all systemic administration routes excluding the gastrointestinal tract

d. a system of measurement that uses grams, liters, and meters

e. diameter of a needle lumen

f. device for administering respiratory medications as a fine inhaled spray

g. a tuberculosis screening test

h. small glass container that must be broken at the neck so that the solution can be aspirated into the syringe

i. administration route to a local spot on the outside of the body

j. administration route to the eyes

k. a system of measures based on drops, minims, grains, drams, and ounces

l. administration route to or by way of the ears

m. hardened area at the injection site after an intradermal screening test for tuberculosis

n. administration beneath the tongue

o. glass or plastic container sealed at the top by a rubber stopper

p. specified liquid used to reconstitute powder medications for injection

COG MATCHING   Grade: _____

Match the injection route to the proper location for administration. There may be more than one location for each injection.

Injection Routes   **Locations**

37. _____ intradermal (ID)   **a.** abdomen

38. _____ adult intramuscular (IM)   **b.** anterior forearm

39. _____ juvenile (<2 years old) intramuscular (IM)   **c.** back

40. _____ Z-track intramuscular (IM)   **d.** deltoid

41. _____ subcutaneous (SC)   **e.** dorsalgluteal

                                                        f. rectus femoris

                                                        g. thigh

                                                        h. upper arm

                                                        i. vastus lateralis

                                                        j. ventrogluteal

COG IDENTIFICATION   Grade: _____

42. When preparing medications, the patient's safety relies on good communication between the physician and yourself. Identify the safety rules you should use to prevent communication errors by placing a check mark on the line under "Yes" if the statement is a safety rule and check "No" if the rule does not apply.

Rule	Yes	No
a. Confirm all medications verbally. Do not try to interpret the physician's handwriting.		
b. Use previous medications and dosages listed on the patient's chart as a safety check.		
c. Check with the physician if you have any doubt about a medication or an order.		

43. Once you have correctly interpreted the medication order from the physician, you must locate and identify the correct drugs to dispense or administer. Choose the rules that prevent errors with identifying the correct medications by placing a check mark on the line under "Yes" if the statement is a safety rule and check "No" if the rule does not apply.

Rule	Yes	No
a. Check the label when taking the medication from the shelf, when preparing it, and again when replacing it on the shelf or disposing of the empty container.		
b. Peel off the label from the medication and place it in the patient's record.		
c. Place the order and the medication side by side to compare for accuracy.		
d. Only fill prescriptions written using brand names.		
e. Read labels carefully. Do not scan labels or medication orders.		
f. Use a resource like the Internet to cross reference generic and brand names for medications.		
g. It is always safer to give a medication poured or drawn up by someone more experienced.		

44. Once you have correctly interpreted the medication order from the physician and identified the correct medication, you must safely dispense and/or administer the medication. Identify which rules prevent mistakes in dispensing and administering medications by placing a check mark on the line under "Yes" if the statement is a safety rule and check "No" if the rule does not apply.

Rule	Yes	No
a. Know the policies of your office regarding the administration of medications.		
b. Never question the physician's written orders.		
c. Prepare medications in the presence of the patient so you can discuss what you are doing and answer the patient's questions.		
d. Check the strength of the medication (e.g., 250 versus 500 mg) and the route of administration.		
e. If you are interrupted, return the medicine to its original container so you can correctly identify it when you come back and finish.		
f. Work in a quiet, well-lit area.		
g. Check the patient's medical record for allergies to the actual medication or its components before administering.		
h. Measure exactly. Always read a meniscus where it touches the glass.		
i. Shake liquid medications vigorously before measuring to ensure they are well mixed.		
j. Never give a medication poured or drawn up by someone else		
k. Stay with the patient while he or she takes oral medication. Watch for any reaction and record the patient's response.		

45. Indicate whether the following are parenteral or enteral by writing P (parenteral) or E (enteral) on the line preceding the route.

   a. _____ buccal

   b. _____ inhalation

   c. _____ intramuscular

   d. _____ intravenous

   e. _____ oral

   f. _____ rectal

   g. _____ subcutaneous

   h. _____ sublingual

   i. _____ transdermal

46. Identify the medical term for the route for administration by placing the term on the line next to the administration method.

   a. ear drops _____

   b. eye drops _____

   c. nitroglycerine patch _____

   d. lotion _____

   e. TB test _____

   f. nebulizer_____

   g. suppositories _____

   h. cough syrup _____

COG COMPLETION

Grade: _____

For each of the dosage calculations, show your work and circle your answer.

47. The physician orders enoxaparin 40 mg SC. The label on the package reads 150 mg/mL. Find the correct dosage for this patient.

   _____

   _____

   _____

   _____

48. You are directed to give a heroin addict 30 mg of methadone PO. The medication comes in tablets labeled 20 mg/tablet. How many tablets would you give the patient?

_____

_____

_____

_____

49. As ordered by the physician, your patient needs 300,000 units of penicillin G IM. The label on the medication vial reads "Penicillin G 1 million units/2 mL." How many mL would you need to give?

_____

_____

_____

_____

50. The physician has written an order for you to give 40 mg of prednisone PO now before the patient leaves the office. You have on hand two strengths of prednisone: 10 mg/tablet and 5 mg/tablet. Choose the appropriate strength and calculate the number of tablets you would give to the patient.

_____

_____

_____

_____

51. Your patient has been ordered by the physician to receive 40 mg of furosemide IM. The ampule states "Furosemide 20 mg/mL." How much medication should you draw up to administer?

_____

_____

_____

_____

52. The patient seen in your office today is ordered by the physician to receive 750 mg of Rocephin™ deep IM. The label on the vial states "Rocephin 1 gm/2 cc." How much would you give?

_____

_____

_____

_____

53. The physician has ordered your patient to take doxycycline 100 mg BID for 7 days. She would like the patient to have a dose before leaving the office. The medication label on the doxycycline in your office reads "Doxycycline 50 mg/capsule." How many would you give to the patient?

_____

_____

_____

_____

54. Your patient arrives at the office with nausea and vomiting. The physician orders you to give 12.5 mg of Phenergan™ IM. The vial states "Phenergan 25 mg/ mL." How much would you give to the patient?

_____

_____

_____

_____

55. An order has been written by the physician for you to administer 7 mg of warfarin PO to your patient. You have three bottles of warfarin available: 2 mg/tablet; 2.5 mg/tablet; and 5 mg/tablet. Which tablet strength would you choose and how many tablets would you give the patient to ensure 7 mg were taken?

_____

_____

_____

_____

COG SHORT ANSWER

Grade: _____

56. What are the primary differences between enteral, parenteral, and topical medications?

_____

_____

_____

_____

57. List the four parts of a syringe that must be kept sterile.

_____

_____

_____

_____

58. What size needle (gauge and length) would you use for the following administration routes?

Route	Gauge	Length
a. IM		
b. SC		
c. ID		

COG TRUE OR FALSE?

Grade: _____

Indicate whether the statements are true or false by placing the letter T (true) or F (false) on the line preceding the statement.

59. _____ It is normal for frightened patients to have trouble breathing after taking a medication.

60. _____ A sip of water will help a patient take nitroglycerine sublingually.

61. _____ During SC and IM injections, a small amount of blood appears in the syringe when there is good penetration.

62. _____ Redness, swelling, pain, and discomfort are normal complications of IV therapy.

63. _____ Check the medication's expiration date, and use outdated medications first.

64. _____ Be alert for color changes, precipitation, odor, or any indication that the medication's properties have changed and discard appropriately.

65. _____ Keep narcotics on your person so others do not have access to them.

66. _____ Do not leave the medication cabinet unlocked when it is not in use.

67. _____ Never give keys for the medication cabinet to an unauthorized person.

Grade: _____

1. The parent of an 18 month old insists that you give the IM immunization in the child's "hip." How would you respond to the parent's request?

_____

_____

_____

_____

2. The patient you are monitoring is receiving intravenous fluids for rehydration. Unfortunately, the insertion site in the left anterior forearm has developed complications and must be removed. How would you respond to the patient who does not understand why the IV must be removed?

_____

_____

_____

_____

3. One of the physicians in your medical office would like to change office policy so that no abbreviations are used in the patients' medical charts for fear of potentially harmful errors. The office is divided on the issue. What is your opinion and why?

_____

_____

_____

_____

4. You are directed to give a Z-track IM injection to a patient. The patient's spouse observes you deliberately draw a bubble into the syringe and panics because you are about to inject air into the patient. How do you address the spouse's concerns?

_____

_____

_____

_____

PSY PROCEDURE 24-1 | Administer Oral Medications

Name: _____ Date: _____ Time: _____ Grade: _____

EQUIPMENT/SUPPLIES: Physician's order, oral medication, disposable calibrated cup, glass of water, patient's medical record

STANDARDS: Given the needed equipment and a place to work the student will perform this skill with _____% accuracy in a total of _____ minutes. *(Your instructor will tell you what the percentage and time limits will be before you begin.)*

KEY: 4 = Satisfactory   0 = Unsatisfactory   NA = This step is not counted

PROCEDURE STEPS	SELF	PARTNER	INSTRUCTOR
1. Wash your hands.	☐	☐	☐

2. Review the physician's medication order and select the correct oral medication.
  a. Compare the label with the physician's instructions.
  b. Note the expiration date.
  c. Check the label three times: when taking it from the shelf, while pouring, and when returning to the shelf.
	☐	☐	☐

3. Calculate the correct dosage to be given if necessary.	☐	☐	☐
4. If using a multidose container, remove cap from container. For single-dose medications, obtain the correct amount of medication.	☐	☐	☐

5. Remove the correct dose of medication.
  a. For solid medications:
    (1) Pour the capsule/tablet into the bottle cap,
    (2) Transfer the medication to a disposable cup.
  b. For liquid medications:
    (1) Open the bottle lid: place it on a flat surface with open end up.
    (2) Palm the label to prevent liquids from dripping onto the label.
    (3) With opposite hand, place the thumbnail at the correct calibration.
    (4) Pour the medication until the proper amount is in the cup.
	☐	☐	☐

6. Greet and identify the patient. Explain the procedure.	☐	☐	☐
7. Ask the patient about medication allergies that might not be noted on the chart.	☐	☐	☐
8. Give the patient a glass of water, unless contraindicated. Hand the patient the disposable cup containing the medication or pour the tablets or capsules into the patient's hand.	☐	☐	☐

9. Remain with the patient to be sure that all of the medication is swallowed.
    a. Observe any unusual reactions and report them to the physician.
    b. Record in the medical record.
	☐	☐	☐

10. Thank the patient and give any appropriate instructions.	☐	☐	☐
11. **AFF** Explain how to respond to a patient who is hearing impaired.	☐	☐	☐
12. Wash your hands.	☐	☐	☐
13. Record the procedure in the patient's medical record. Note the date, time, name of medication, dose administered, route of administration, and your name.	☐	☐	☐

CALCULATION

Total Possible Points: _____

Total Points Earned: _____ Multiplied by 100 = _____ Divided by Total Possible Points = _____ %

PASS   **FAIL**   **COMMENTS:**

☐   ☐

Student's signature _____ Date _____

Partner's signature _____ Date _____

Instructor's signature _____ Date _____

PSY PROCEDURE 24-2 Prepare Injections

Name: _____ Date: _____ Time: _____ Grade: _____

EQUIPMENT/SUPPLIES: Physician's order, medication for injection in ampule or vial, antiseptic wipes, gloves, appropriate-size needle and syringe, small gauze pad, biohazard sharps container, patient's medical record

STANDARDS: Given the needed equipment and a place to work the student will perform this skill with _____% accuracy in a total of _____ minutes. *(Your instructor will tell you what the percentage and time limits will be before you begin.)*

KEY: 4 = Satisfactory   0 = Unsatisfactory   NA = This step is not counted

PROCEDURE STEPS	SELF	PARTNER	INSTRUCTOR
1. Wash your hands.	☐	☐	☐
2. Review the physician's medication order and select the correct medication.	☐	☐	☐
a. Compare the label with the physician's instructions. Note the expiration date.			
b. Check the label three times: when taking it from the shelf, while drawing it up into the syringe, and when returning to the shelf.			
3. Calculate the correct dosage to be given, if necessary.	☐	☐	☐
4. Choose the needle and syringe according to the route of administration, type of medication, and size of the patient.	☐	☐	☐
5. Open the needle and syringe package. Assemble if necessary. Secure the needle to the syringe.	☐	☐	☐
6. Withdraw the correct amount of medication:			
a. From an ampule:	☐	☐	☐
(1) Tap the stem of the ampule lightly.			
(2) Place a piece of gauze around the ampule neck.			
(3) Grasp the gauze and ampule firmly. Snap the stem off the ampule.			
(4) Dispose of the ampule top in a biohazard sharps container.			
(5) Insert the needle lumen below the level of the medication.			
(6) Withdraw the medication.			
(7) Dispose of the ampule in a biohazard sharps container.			
(8) Remove any air bubbles in the syringe.			
(9) Draw back on the plunger to add a small amount of air; then gently push the plunger forward to eject the air out of the syringe.			

b. From a vial:	☐	☐	☐
(1) Using the antiseptic wipe, cleanse the rubber stopper of the vial.			
(2) Pull air into the syringe with the amount equivalent to the amount of medication to be removed from the vial.			
(3) Insert the needle into the vial top. Inject the air from the syringe.			
(4) With the needle inside the vial, invert the vial.			
(5) Hold the syringe at eye level.			
(6) Aspirate the desired amount of medication into the syringe.			
(7) Displace any air bubbles in the syringe by gently tapping the barrel.			
(8) Remove the air by pushing the plunger slowly and forcing the air into the vial.			
7. Carefully recap the needle using one-hand technique.	☐	☐	☐

CALCULATION

Total Possible Points: _____

Total Points Earned: _____ Multiplied by 100 = _____ Divided by Total Possible Points = _____ %

PASS   **FAIL**   **COMMENTS:**

  ☐   ☐

Student's signature _____ Date _____

Partner's signature _____ Date _____

Instructor's signature _____ Date _____

PSY PROCEDURE 24-3 **Administer an Intradermal Injection**

Name: _____ Date: _____ Time: _____ Grade: _____

EQUIPMENT/SUPPLIES: Physician's order, medication for injection in ampule or vial, antiseptic wipes, gloves, appropriate-size needle and syringe, small gauze pad, biohazard sharps container, patient's medical record

STANDARDS: Given the needed equipment and a place to work the student will perform this skill with _____% accuracy in a total of _____ minutes. *(Your instructor will tell you what the percentage and time limits will be before you begin.)*

KEY: 4 = Satisfactory   0 = Unsatisfactory   NA = This step is not counted

PROCEDURE STEPS	SELF	PARTNER	INSTRUCTOR
1. Wash your hands.	☐	☐	☐
a. Review the physician's medication order and select the correct medication.			
b. Compare the label with the physician's instructions. Note the expiration date.			
c. Check the label three times: when taking it from the shelf, while drawing it up into the syringe, and when returning it to the shelf.			
2. Prepare the injection according to the steps in Procedure 24-2.	☐	☐	☐
3. Greet and identify the patient. Explain the procedure.	☐	☐	☐
4. Ask patient about medication allergies.	☐	☐	☐
5. Select the appropriate site for the injection.	☐	☐	☐
6. Prepare the site by cleansing with an antiseptic wipe.	☐	☐	☐
7. Put on gloves. Remove the needle guard.	☐	☐	☐
8. Using your nondominant hand, pull the patient's skin taut.	☐	☐	☐
9. With the bevel of the needle facing upward, insert needle at a 10- to 15-degree angle into the upper layer of the skin.	☐	☐	☐
a. When the bevel of the needle is under the skin, stop inserting the needle.			
b. The needle will be slightly visible below the surface of the skin.			
c. It is not necessary to aspirate when performing an intradermal injection.			
10. Inject the medication slowly by depressing the plunger.	☐	☐	☐
a. A wheal will form as the medication enters the dermal layer of the skin.			
b. Hold the syringe steady for proper administration.			
11. Remove the needle from the skin at the same angle at which it was inserted.	☐	☐	☐
a. Do not use an antiseptic wipe or gauze pad over the site.			
b. Do not press or massage the site. Do not apply an adhesive bandage.			

12. Do not recap the needle.	☐	☐	☐
13. Dispose of the needle and syringe in an approved biohazard sharps container.	☐	☐	☐
14. **AFF** Explain how to respond to a patient with dementia.	☐	☐	☐
15. Remove your gloves, and wash your hands.	☐	☐	☐
16. Depending upon the type of skin test administered, the length of time required for the body tissues to react, and the policies of the medical office, perform one of the following: **a.** Read the test results. Inspect and palpate the site for the presence and amount of induration. **b.** Tell the patient when to return (date and time) to the office to have the results read. **c.** Instruct the patient to read the results at home. **d.** Make sure the patient understands the instructions.	☐	☐	☐
17. Document the procedure, the site, and the results. If instructions were given to the patient, document these also.	☐	☐	☐

CALCULATION

Total Possible Points: _____

Total Points Earned: _____ Multiplied by 100 = _____ Divided by Total Possible Points = _____ %

PASS   **FAIL**   **COMMENTS:**

  ☐   ☐

Student's signature _____ Date _____

Partner's signature _____ Date _____

Instructor's signature _____ Date _____

PSY PROCEDURE 24-4 **Administer a Subcutaneous Injection**

Name: _____ Date: _____ Time: _____ Grade: _____

EQUIPMENT/SUPPLIES: Physician's order, medication for injection in ampule or vial, antiseptic wipes, gloves, appropriate-size needle and syringe, small gauze pad, biohazard sharps container, patient's medical record

STANDARDS: Given the needed equipment and a place to work the student will perform this skill with _____% accuracy in a total of _____ minutes. *(Your instructor will tell you what the percentage and time limits will be before you begin.)*

KEY: 4 = Satisfactory   0 = Unsatisfactory   NA = This step is not counted

PROCEDURE STEPS	SELF	PARTNER	INSTRUCTOR
1. Wash your hands.	☐	☐	☐
a. Review the physician's medication order and select the correct medication.			
b. Compare the label with the physician's instructions. Note the expiration date.			
c. Check the label three times: when taking it from the shelf, while drawing it up into the syringe, and when returning it to the shelf.			
2. Prepare the injection according to the steps in Procedure 24-2.	☐	☐	☐
3. Greet and identify the patient. Explain the procedure.	☐	☐	☐
4. Ask the patient about medication allergies.	☐	☐	☐
5. Select the appropriate site for the injection.	☐	☐	☐
6. Prepare the site by cleansing with an antiseptic.	☐	☐	☐
7. Put on gloves.	☐	☐	☐
8. Using your nondominant hand, hold the skin surrounding the injection site.	☐	☐	☐
9. With a firm motion, insert the needle into the tissue at a 45-degree angle to the skin surface.	☐	☐	☐
10. Hold the barrel between the thumb and the index finger of your dominant hand.	☐	☐	☐
11. Insert the needle completely to the hub.	☐	☐	☐
12. Remove your nondominant hand from the skin.	☐	☐	☐
13. Holding the syringe steady, pull back on the syringe gently. If blood appears in the hub or the syringe, do not inject the medication; remove the needle and prepare a new injection.	☐	☐	☐
14. Inject the medication slowly by depressing the plunger.	☐	☐	☐
15. Place a gauze pad over the injection site and remove the needle.	☐	☐	☐
a. Gently massage the injection site with the gauze pad.			
b. Do not recap the used needle; place it in the biohazard sharps container.			
c. Apply an adhesive bandage if needed.			

16. Remove your gloves and wash your hands.	☐	☐	☐
17. **AFF** Explain how to respond to a patient who is deaf.	☐	☐	☐

18. An injection given for allergy desensitization requires:
 	
  a. Keeping the patient in the office for at least 30 minutes for observation.
 	
  b. Notifying the doctor of any reaction. (Be alert, anaphylaxis is possible.)
	☐	☐	☐

19. Document the procedure, the site, and the results. If instructions were given to the patient, document these also.	☐	☐	☐

CALCULATION

Total Possible Points: _____

Total Points Earned: _____ Multiplied by 100 = _____ Divided by Total Possible Points = _____ %

PASS   **FAIL**   **COMMENTS:**

☐   ☐

Student's signature _____ Date _____

Partner's signature _____ Date _____

Instructor's signature _____ Date _____

PSY PROCEDURE 24-5 **Administer an Intramuscular Injection**

Name: _____ Date: _____ Time: _____ Grade: _____

EQUIPMENT/SUPPLIES: Physician's order, medication for injection in ampule or vial, antiseptic wipes, gloves, appropriate-size needle and syringe, small gauze pad, biohazard sharps container, patient's medical record

STANDARDS: Given the needed equipment and a place to work the student will perform this skill with _____% accuracy in a total of _____ minutes. *(Your instructor will tell you what the percentage and time limits will be before you begin.)*

KEY: 4 = Satisfactory   0 = Unsatisfactory   NA = This step is not counted

PROCEDURE STEPS	SELF	PARTNER	INSTRUCTOR
1. Wash your hands.	☐	☐	☐
a. Review the physician's order and select the correct medication.			
b. Compare the label with the physician's instructions. Note the expiration date.			
c. Check the label three times: when taking it from the shelf, while drawing it up into the syringe, and when returning to the shelf.			
2. Prepare the injection according to the steps in Procedure 24-2.	☐	☐	☐
3. Greet and identify the patient. Explain the procedure.	☐	☐	☐
4. Ask the patient about medication allergies.	☐	☐	☐
5. Select the appropriate site for the injection.	☐	☐	☐
6. Prepare the site by cleansing with an antiseptic wipe.	☐	☐	☐
7. Put on gloves.	☐	☐	☐
8. Using your nondominant hand, hold the skin surrounding the injection site.	☐	☐	☐
9. While holding the syringe like a dart, use a quick, firm motion to insert the needle at a 90-degree angle to the skin surface. Hold the barrel between the thumb and the index finger of the dominant hand and insert the needle completely to the hub.	☐	☐	☐
10. Holding the syringe steady, pull back on the syringe gently. If blood appears in the hub or the syringe, do not inject the medication; remove the needle and prepare a new injection.	☐	☐	☐
11. Inject the medication slowly by depressing the plunger.	☐	☐	☐
12. Place a gauze pad over the injection site and remove the needle.	☐	☐	☐
a. Gently massage the injection site with the gauze pad.			
b. Do not recap the used needle. Place in biohazard sharps container.			
c. Apply an adhesive bandage if needed.			

13. [AFF] Explain how to respond to a patient who is visually impaired.	☐	☐	☐
14. Remove your gloves, and wash your hands.	☐	☐	☐
15. Notify the doctor of any reaction. (Be alert, anaphylaxis is possible.)	☐	☐	☐
16. Document the procedure, the site, and the results. If instructions were given to the patient, document these also.	☐	☐	☐

CALCULATION

Total Possible Points: _____

Total Points Earned: _____ Multiplied by 100 = _____ Divided by Total Possible Points = _____ %

PASS   **FAIL**   **COMMENTS:**

☐   ☐

Student's signature _____ Date _____

Partner's signature _____ Date _____

Instructor's signature _____ Date _____

Name: _____ Date: _____ Time: _____ Grade: _____

EQUIPMENT/SUPPLIES: Physician's order, medication for injection in ampule or vial, antiseptic wipes, gloves, appropriate-size needle and syringe, small gauze pad, biohazard sharps container, patient's medical record

STANDARDS: Given the needed equipment and a place to work the student will perform this skill with _____% accuracy in a total of _____ minutes. *(Your instructor will tell you what the percentage and time limits will be before you begin.)*

KEY: 4 = Satisfactory 0 = Unsatisfactory NA = This step is not counted

PROCEDURE STEPS	SELF	PARTNER	INSTRUCTOR
1. Follow steps 1 through 7 as described in Procedure 24-5.	☐	☐	☐
2. Pull the top layer of skin to the side and hold it with your nondominant hand throughout the injection.	☐	☐	☐
3. While holding the syringe like a dart, use a quick, firm motion to insert the needle at a 90-degree angle to the skin surface. a. Hold the barrel between the thumb and index finger of the dominant hand. b. Insert the needle completely to the hub.	☐	☐	☐
4. Aspirate by withdrawing the plunger slightly. a. If no blood appears, push the plunger in slowly and steadily. b. Count to 10 before withdrawing the needle.	☐	☐	☐
5. Place a gauze pad over the injection site and remove the needle. a. Gently massage the injection site with the gauze pad. b. Do not recap the used needle. Place in the biohazard sharps container. c. Apply an adhesive bandage if needed.	☐	☐	☐
6. Remove your gloves, and wash your hands.	☐	☐	☐
7. Notify the doctor of any reaction. (Be alert, anaphylaxis is possible.)	☐	☐	☐
8. Document the procedure, the site, and the results. If instructions were given to the patient, document these also.	☐	☐	☐

CALCULATION

Total Possible Points: _____

Total Points Earned: _____ Multiplied by 100 = _____ Divided by Total Possible Points = _____ %

PASS **FAIL**   **COMMENTS:**

☐   ☐

Student's signature _____ Date _____

Partner's signature _____ Date _____

Instructor's signature _____ Date _____

PSY PROCEDURE 24-7 Apply Transdermal Medications

Name: _____ Date: _____ Time: _____ Grade: _____

EQUIPMENT/SUPPLIES: Physician's order, medication, gloves, patient's medical record

STANDARDS: Given the needed equipment and a place to work the student will perform this skill with _____%
accuracy in a total of _____ minutes. *(Your instructor will tell you what the percentage and time limits will be
before you begin.)*

KEY: 4 = Satisfactory   0 = Unsatisfactory   NA = This step is not counted

PROCEDURE STEPS	SELF	PARTNER	INSTRUCTOR
1. Wash your hands.	☐	☐	☐
2. Review the physician's medication order and select the correct medication.	☐	☐	☐
a. Compare the label with the physician's instructions. Note the expiration date.			
b. Check the label three times: when taking it from the shelf, before taking it into the patient exam room, and before applying it to the patient's skin.			
3. Greet and identify the patient. Explain the procedure.	☐	☐	☐
4. Ask the patient about medication allergies that might not be noted on the medical record.	☐	☐	☐
5. Select the appropriate site and perform any necessary skin preparation. The sites are usually the upper arm, the chest or back surface, or behind the ear.	☐	☐	☐
a. Ensure that the skin is clean, dry, and free from any irritation.			
b. Do not shave areas with excessive hair; trim the hair closely with scissors.			
6. If there is a transdermal patch already in place, remove it carefully while wearing gloves. Discard the patch in the trash container. Inspect the site for irritation.	☐	☐	☐
7. Open the medication package by pulling the two sides apart. Do not touch the area of medication.	☐	☐	☐
8. Apply the medicated patch to the patient's skin, following the manufacturer's directions.	☐	☐	☐
a. Press the adhesive edges down firmly all around, starting at the center and pressing outward.			
b. If the edges do not stick, fasten with tape.			

9. **AFF** Explain how to respond to a patient who is uncomfortable exposing skin on areas such as the chest or arms due to cultural or religious beliefs.	☐	☐	☐

10. Wash your hands.	☐	☐	☐
11. Document the procedure and the site of the new patch in the medical record.	☐	☐	☐

CALCULATION

Total Possible Points: _____

Total Points Earned: _____ Multiplied by 100 = _____ Divided by Total Possible Points = _____ %

PASS   **FAIL**   **COMMENTS:**

☐   ☐

Student's signature _____ Date _____

Partner's signature _____ Date _____

Instructor's signature _____ Date _____

PSY PROCEDURE 24-8   Obtain and Prepare an Intravenous Site

Name: _____ Date: _____ Time: _____ Grade: _____

EQUIPMENT/SUPPLIES: Physician's order including the type of fluid to be used and the rate, intravenous solution, infusion administration set, IV pole, blank labels, appropriate size intravenous catheter, antiseptic wipes, tourniquet, small gauze pad, biohazard sharps container, clean examination gloves, bandage tape, adhesive bandage, patient's medical record, intravenous catheter (angiocath)

STANDARDS: Given the needed equipment and a place to work the student will perform this skill with _____% accuracy in a total of _____ minutes. *(Your instructor will tell you what the percentage and time limits will be before you begin.)*

KEY: 4 = Satisfactory   0 = Unsatisfactory   NA = This step is not counted

PROCEDURE STEPS	SELF	PARTNER	INSTRUCTOR
1. Wash your hands.	☐	☐	☐
2. Review the physician's order and select the correct IV catheter, solution, and administration set.	☐	☐	☐
a. Compare the label on the infusate solution and administration set with the physician's order.			
b. Note the expiration dates on the infusion solution and the administration set.			
3. Prepare the infusion solution by attaching a label to the solution indicating the date, time and name of the patient who will be receiving the IV.	☐	☐	☐
a. Hang the solution on an IV pole.			
b. Remove the administration set from the package and close the roller clamp.			
4. Remove the end of the administration set by removing the cover on the spike (located above the drip chamber).	☐	☐	☐
a. Remove the cover from the solution infusion port (located on the bottom of the bag).			
b. Insert the spike end of the administration set into the IV fluid.			
5. Fill the drip chamber on the administration set by squeezing the drip chamber until about half full.	☐	☐	☐
6. Open the roller clamp and allow fluid to flow from the drip chamber through the length of the tubing, displacing any air. Do not remove the cover protecting the end of the tubing.	☐	☐	☐
a. Close the roller clamp when the fluid has filled the tubing and no air is noted.			
b. Drape the filled tubing over the IV pole and proceed to perform a venipuncture.			
7. Greet and identify the patient. Explain the procedure.	☐	☐	☐

8. Ask the patient about medication allergies that might not be noted on the medical record.	☐	☐	☐
9. Prepare the IV start equipment by tearing or cutting two to three strips of tape that will be used to secure the IV catheter after insertion; also, inspect each arm for the best available vein.	☐	☐	☐

10. Wearing gloves, apply the tourniquet 1 to 2 inches above the intended venipuncture site.
  a. The tourniquet should be snug, but not too tight.
  b. Ask the patient to open and close the fist of the selected arm to distend the veins.
	☐	☐	☐

11. Secure the tourniquet by using the half-bow technique.	☐	☐	☐
12. Make sure the ends of the tourniquet extend upward to avoid contaminating the venipuncture site.	☐	☐	☐
13. Select a vein by palpating with your gloved index finger to trace the path of the vein and judge its depth.	☐	☐	☐
14. Release the tourniquet after palpating the vein if it has been left on for more than 1 minute.	☐	☐	☐
15. Prepare the site by cleansing with an antiseptic wipe using a circular motion.	☐	☐	☐
16. Place the end of the administration set tubing on the examination table for easy access after the venipuncture.	☐	☐	☐
17. Anchor the vein to be punctured by placing the thumb of your non-dominant hand below the intended site and holding the skin taut.	☐	☐	☐

18. Remove the needle cover from the IV catheter.
  a. While holding the catheter by the flash chamber, not the hub of the needle, use the dominant hand to insert the needle and catheter unit directly into the top of the vein, with the bevel of the needle up at a 15- to 20-degree angle for superficial veins.
  b. Observe for a blood flashback into the flash chamber.
	☐	☐	☐

19. When the blood flashback is observed, lower the angle of the needle until it is flush with the skin and slowly advance the needle and catheter unit about 14 inches.	☐	☐	☐

20. Once the needle and catheter unit has been inserted slightly into the lumen of the vein hold the flash chamber of the needle steady with the nondominant hand.
  a. Slide the catheter (using the catheter hub) off the needle and into the vein with the dominant hand.
  b. Advance the catheter into the vein up to the hub.
	☐	☐	☐

21. With the needle partly occluding the catheter, release the tourniquet.	☐	☐	☐

22. Remove the needle and discard into a biohazard sharps container.
  a. Connect the end of the administration tubing to the end of the IV catheter that has been inserted into the vein.
  b. Open the roller clamp and adjust the flow according the physician's order.
	☐	☐	☐

23. Secure the hub of the IV catheter with tape.	☐	☐	☐
a. Place one small strip, sticky side up, under the catheter.			
b. Cross one end over the hub and adhere onto the skin on the opposite side of the catheter.			
c. Cross the other end of the tape in the same fashion and adhere to the skin on the opposite side of the hub.			
d. A transparent membrane adhesive dressing can then be applied over the entire hub and insertion site.			
24. Make a small loop with the administration set tubing near the IV insertion site and secure with tape.	☐	☐	☐
25. **AFF** Explain how to respond to a patient who is from an older generation than you are.	☐	☐	☐
26. Remove your gloves, wash your hands, and document the procedure in the medical record indicating the size of the IV catheter inserted, the location, the type of infusion, and the rate.	☐	☐	☐

CALCULATION

Total Possible Points: _____

Total Points Earned: _____ Multiplied by 100 = _____ Divided by Total Possible Points = _____ %

PASS   **FAIL**   **COMMENTS:**

  ☐   ☐

Student's signature _____ Date _____

Partner's signature _____ Date _____

Instructor's signature _____ Date _____

Diagnostic Imaging

Cognitive Domain

1. Spell and define the key terms
2. Explain the theory and function of x-rays and x-ray machines
3. State the principles of radiology
4. Describe routine and contrast media, fluoroscopy, computed tomography, sonography, magnetic resonance imaging, nuclear medicine, and mammographic examinations
5. Explain the role of the medical assistant in radiologic procedures
6. Describe body planes, directional terms, quadrants, and cavities
7. Describe implications for treatment related to pathology
8. Identify critical information required for scheduling patient admissions and/or procedures

Psychomotor Domain

1. Assist with x-ray procedures (Procedure 25-1)
2. Instruct patients according to their needs to promote health maintenance and disease prevention
3. Prepare a patient for procedures and/or treatments
4. Document patient education
5. Schedule patient admissions and/or procedures
6. Perform within scope of practice

7. Apply local, state, and federal health care legislation and regulation appropriate to the medical assisting practice setting

Affective Domain

1. Apply critical thinking skills in performing patient assessment and care
2. Use language/verbal skills that enable a patient's understanding
3. Demonstrate respect for diversity in approaching patients and families
4. Explain the rationale for performance of a procedure to the patient
5. Demonstrate empathy in communicating with patients, family, and staff
6. Apply active listening skills
7. Use appropriate body language and other nonverbal skills in communicating with patients, family, and staff
8. Demonstrate awareness of the territorial boundaries of the person with whom you are communicating
9. Demonstrate sensitivity appropriate to the message being delivered
10. Demonstrate recognition of the patient's level of understanding communications
11. Recognize and protect personal boundaries in communicating with others
12. Demonstrate respect for individual diversity, incorporating awareness of one's own biases in areas including gender, race, religion, age, and economic status

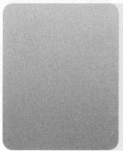

ABHES Competencies

1. Assist the physician with the regimen of diagnostic and treatment modalities as they relate to each body system
2. Comply with federal, state, and local health laws and regulations
3. Communicate on the recipient's level of comprehension
4. Serve as a liaison between the physician and others
5. Show empathy and impartiality when dealing with patients

Name: _____   Date: _____   Grade: _____

COG MULTIPLE CHOICE

Circle the letter preceding the correct answer.

1. Which term below means lying face downward?

    a. Supine

    b. Prone

    c. Decubitus

    d. Recumbent

    e. Relaxed

2. Which of the following is a form of nuclear medicine?

    a. Radiopaque

    b. Barium

    c. Iodine

    d. Radionuclides

    e. Radiolucent

3. Noises heard during an x-ray exposure may come from:

    a. the x-ray tube.

    b. x-rays.

    c. the positioning aid.

    d. high voltage.

    e. the sheet of film.

4. Which of the following is an example of radiopaque tissue?

    a. Lungs

    b. Bone

    c. Muscle

    d. Fat

    e. Veins

5. A minimum of two x-rays should be taken at:

    a. 180° of each other.

    b. 30° of each other.

    c. 70° of each other.

    d. 90° of each other.

    e. 50° of each other.

6. A type of radiography that creates cross-sectional images of the body is:

    a. fluoroscopy.

    b. echogram.

    c. computerized tomography.

    d. ultrasound.

    e. mammography.

7. Which of the following form of radiography does not use x-rays?

    a. MRI

    b. Nuclear medicine

    c. Fluoroscopy

    d. Teleradiology

    e. Tomography

8. Which procedure creates an image that depends on the chemical makeup of the body?

    a. Tomography

    b. Fluoroscopy

    c. MRI

    d. Mammography

    e. Nuclear medicine

9. Sonograms create images using:

    a. radioactive material.

    b. contrast media.

    c. magnetic resonance.

    d. chemotherapy.

    e. sound waves.

10. X-rays can be harmful to infants and young children because:

    a. their immune systems are not fully developed.

    b. their cells divide at a rapid pace.

    c. they have less muscle mass than adults.

    d. they have a smaller body mass.

    e. they have less body fat than adults.

11. Which of the following procedures may be done in a confined space?

    a. MRI

    b. Nuclear medicine

    c. Fluoroscopy

    d. Teleradiology

    e. Tomography

12. A physician who specializes in interpreting the images on the processed film is a(n):

    a. pulmonologist.

    b. internist.

    c. immunologist.

    d. ophthalmologist.

    e. radiologist.

Scenario for questions 13 and 14: A patient has come in for an x-ray. The physician wants you to get a clear image of the patient's liver.

13. What is another possible way to view the patient's liver without injections?

    a. Mammography

    b. Sonography

    c. Fluoroscopy

    d. Teleradiology

    e. Tomography

14. Which position would allow the best images of the liver?

    a. Supine

    b. Decubitus

    c. Posterior

    d. Left anterior oblique

    e. Right anterior oblique

15. Who owns the x-ray film after it has been developed?

    a. The patient

    b. The physician who ordered the x-rays

    c. The physician who will use the x-rays

    d. The lab that developed the film

    e. The site where the film was taken and developed.

16. You should wear a dosimeter to:

    a. lower the level of radiation.

    b. protect against radiation effects.

    c. monitor personal radiation exposure.

    d. enhance radiography images.

    e. collect data on different procedures.

17. Why do some tests require patients to be NPO before an administration of barium PO?

    a. Gastric juices may interfere with the readings.

    b. A full stomach may distort or alter an image.

    c. Patients are not allowed to relieve themselves.

    d. Undigested food might counteract contrast media.

    e. Instruments might become soiled during the procedure.

18. Images that partially block x-rays are called:

    a. radiographs.

    b. radiolucent.

    c. radiopaque.

    d. radionuclides.

    e. radiograms.

19. Why is radiology used as a form of cancer treatment?

    a. X-rays show the exact location of cancer.

    b. Radioactive cells produce more white blood cells.

    c. Radiation can destroy or weaken cancer cells.

    d. Radiation makes cancerous tumors benign.

    e. Chemotherapy is not as effective as radiation.

20. When explaining procedures to patients:

    a. let the physician go into detail.

    b. answer all the questions they ask.

    c. do not worry them with potential risk.

    d. soothe their fears without telling them anything.

    e. allow only the nurse to explain the procedure.

COG MATCHING

Grade: _____

Match each key term with its definition.

Key Terms

21. _____ cassette

22. _____ contrast medium

23. _____ film

24. _____ fluoroscopy

25. _____ magnetic resonance imaging

26. _____ nuclear medicine

27. _____ radiograph

28. _____ radiography

29. _____ radiologist

30. _____ radiology

31. _____ radiolucent

32. _____ radionuclide

33. _____ radiopaque

34. _____ teleradiology

35. _____ tomography

36. _____ ultrasound

37. _____ x-rays

Definitions

a. invisible electromagnetic radiation waves used in diagnosis and treatment of various disorders

b. a lightproof holder in which film is exposed

c. imaging technique that uses a strong magnetic field

d. a radioactive material with a short life that is used in small amounts in nuclear medicine studies

e. physician who interprets images to provide diagnostic information

f. imaging technique that uses sound waves to diagnose or monitor various body structures

g. not permeable to passage of x-rays

h. processed film that contains a visible image

i. a substance ingested or injected into the body to facilitate imaging of internal structures

j. the use of computed imaging and information systems to transmit diagnostic images to distant locations

k. a procedure in which the x-ray tube and film move in relation to each other during exposure, blurring out all structures except those in the focal plane

l. a raw material on which x-rays are projected through the body; prior to processing, this does not contain a visible image

m. permitting the passage of x-rays

n. a special x-ray technique for examining a body part by immediate projection onto a fluorescent screen

o. the branch of medicine involving diagnostic and therapeutic applications of x-rays

p. a branch of medicine that uses radioactive isotopes to diagnose and treat disease

q. the art and science of producing diagnostic images with x-rays

COG MATCHING   Grade: _____

Match the different types of radiography techniques with their individual characteristics.

Techniques

38. _____ Fluoroscopy

39. _____ Tomography

40. _____ Mammography

41. _____ Ultrasound

42. _____ Magnetic resonance imaging

43. _____ Radiation therapy

Characteristics

a. the image depends on the chemical makeup of the body, commonly used in prenatal testing

b. can create three-dimensional images, so that organs can be viewed from all angles

c. the area of the body exposed must be defined exactly so that each treatment is identical

d. used as an aid to other types of treatment, such as reducing fractures and implanting devices such as pacemakers

e. a vital adjunct to biopsy

f. designed to concentrate on specific areas of the body

COG SHORT ANSWER   Grade: _____

44. List the four processes by which radiographic film is produced.

_____

_____

_____

_____

45. List five radiation safety procedures for patients.

_____

_____

_____

_____

46. Fill in the full names for the abbreviations below.

    a. PET _____

    b. SPECT _____

    c. ALARA _____

47. Name two contrast mediums.

_____

_____

_____

_____

48. What are the three ways contrast media may be introduced into the body?

_____

_____

_____

_____

49. Name four types of interventional radiological procedures.

_____

_____

_____

_____

50. List five side effects of radiation therapy.

_____

_____

_____

_____

51. What is the difference between radiolucent and radiopaque tissues? How do these tissues appear differently on a radiograph? Give an example of each.

_____

_____

_____

_____

52. Why do x-ray examinations require a minimum of two exposures?

_____

_____

_____

_____

53. Why is it imperative to have an esophagogastroduodenoscopy done before other barium studies?

_____

_____

_____

_____

54. Compare and contrast fluoroscopy with tomography. How do these procedures use movement?

_____

_____

_____

_____

55. You have a patient who will have a radiographic exam using contrast media next week. You find out this patient has an allergy to shellfish. What should you do?

_____

_____

_____

COG **TRUE OR FALSE?**   Grade: _____

Indicate whether the statements are true or false by placing the letter T (true) or F (false) on the line preceding the statement.

56. _____ A patient may hear noises during an x-ray procedure.

57. _____ A mammogram is a minimally invasive procedure.

58. _____ You need to be proficient in the operation of your facility's equipment.

59. _____ The best way to explain procedures to a patient is with lots of detail.

COG **AFF** **CASE STUDIES FOR CRITICAL THINKING**   Grade: _____

1. Mrs. Kay has had several radiographic and contrast media studies over the past 5 years. She is now moving to another state and wants to know how to get copies of the films and reports to her new physician. What will you tell her about transferring these records?

   _____

   _____

   _____

   _____

2. You have a patient with a fear of enclosed spaces who is not able to have an open MRI at your outpatient radiographic center. How would you console this patient and explain x-ray procedures?

   _____

   _____

   _____

   _____

3. You have a patient coming in for radiation therapy who has been experiencing side effects such as weight loss, loss of appetite, and hair loss. She has concerns about the radiation therapy that she has been receiving and feels that it may be too much for her body. What would you say to her to help her better understand the situation?

_____

_____

_____

_____

4. You have a patient who has had radiographs taken with a referring physician. This patient has already spoken to his referral physician about the finding in his x-rays and would now like to consult with his primary care physician. However, the referring physician has not yet sent a summary of findings. Your patient is very anxious. What should you say?

_____

_____

_____

_____

PSY PROCEDURE 25-1   Assist with X-Ray Procedures

Name: _____ Date: _____ Time: _____ Grade: _____

EQUIPMENT/SUPPLIES: Patient gown and drape

STANDARDS: Given the needed equipment and a place to work the student will perform this skill with _____%
accuracy in a total of _____ minutes. *(Your instructor will tell you what the percentage
and time limits will be before you begin.)*

KEY: 4 = Satisfactory   0 = Unsatisfactory   NA = This step is not counted

PROCEDURE STEPS	SELF	PARTNER	INSTRUCTOR
1. Wash your hands.	☐	☐	☐
2. Greet the patient by name, introduce yourself, and escort him or her to the room where the x-ray equipment is maintained.	☐	☐	☐
3. Ask female patients about the possibility of pregnancy. If the patient is unsure or indicates pregnancy in any trimester, consult with the physician before proceeding with the x-ray procedure.	☐	☐	☐
4. **AFF** Explain how to respond to a patient who speaks English as a second language.	☐	☐	☐
5. After explaining what clothing should be removed, if any, give the patient a gown and privacy.	☐	☐	☐
6. Notify the x-ray technician or physician that the patient is ready for the x-ray procedure. Stay behind the lead-lined wall during the x-ray procedure to avoid exposure to x-rays during the procedure.	☐	☐	☐
7. After the x-ray, ask the patient to remain in the room until the film has been developed and checked for accuracy and readability.	☐	☐	☐
8. Once you have determined that the exposed film is adequate for the physician to view for diagnosis, have the patient get dressed and escort him or her to the front desk.	☐	☐	☐
9. Document the procedure in the medical record.	☐	☐	☐

CALCULATION

Total Possible Points: _____

Total Points Earned: _____ Multiplied by 100 = _____ Divided by Total Possible Points = _____ %

PASS   **FAIL**   **COMMENTS:**

☐   ☐

Student's signature _____ Date _____

Partner's signature _____ Date _____

Instructor's signature _____ Date _____

26 Medical Office Emergencies

Cognitive Domain

1. Spell and define key terms
2. State principles and steps of professional/provider cardiopulmonary resuscitation
3. Describe basic principles of first aid
4. Identify the five types of shock and the management of each
5. Describe how burns are classified and managed
6. Explain the management of allergic reactions
7. Describe the management of poisoning and the role of the poison control center
8. List the three types of hyperthermic emergencies and the treatment for each type
9. Discuss the treatment of hypothermia
10. Describe the role of the medical assistant in managing psychiatric emergencies

Psychomotor Domain

1. Administer oxygen (Procedure 26-1)
2. Perform cardiopulmonary resuscitation (Procedure 26-2)
3. Use an automatic external defibrillator (Procedure 26-3)
4. Manage a foreign body airway obstruction (Procedure 26-4)
5. Control bleeding (Procedure 26-5)
6. Respond to medical emergencies other than bleeding, cardiac/respiratory arrest, or foreign body airway obstruction (Procedure 26-6)

7. Perform first aid procedures
8. Practice standard precautions
9. Document accurately in the patient record
10. Perform within scope of practice
11. Select appropriate barrier/personal protective equipment for potentially infectious situations

Affective Domain

1. Apply critical thinking skills in performing patient assessment and care
2. Show awareness of patients' concerns regarding their perceptions related to the procedure being performed
3. Demonstrate empathy in communicating with patients, family, and staff
4. Apply active listening skills
5. Use appropriate body language and other nonverbal skills in communicating with patients, family, and staff
6. Demonstrate awareness of territorial boundaries of the person with whom you are communicating
7. Demonstrate sensitivity appropriate to the message being delivered
8. Demonstrate recognition of the patient's level of understanding in communications
9. Recognize and protect personal boundaries in communicating with others
10. Demonstrate respect for individual diversity, incorporating awareness of one's own biases in areas including gender, race, religion, age, and economic status

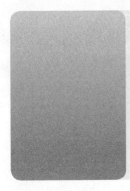

ABHES Competencies

1. Document accurately
2. Recognize and respond to verbal and nonverbal communication
3. Adapt to individualized needs
4. Apply principles of aseptic techniques and infection control
5. Recognize emergencies and treatments and minor office surgical procedures
6. Use standard precautions
7. Perform first aid and CPR
8. Demonstrate professionalism by exhibiting a positive attitude and sense of responsibility

Name: _____ Date: _____ Grade: _____

COG MULTIPLE CHOICE

Circle the letter preceding the correct answer.

1. During a primary assessment, you should check:

a. AVPU.

b. pupils.

c. responsiveness.

d. vital signs.

e. patient identification.

2. What signs and symptoms are consistent with heat stroke?

a. Cyanotic skin

b. Pale wet skin

c. Ecchymosis

d. Dry, flushed skin

e. Waxy, gray skin

3. Superficial burns are categorized as:

a. first degree.

b. second degree.

c. third degree.

d. partial thickness.

e. full thickness.

4. Which is an example of a closed wound?

a. Abrasion

b. Avulsion

c. Contusion

d. Laceration

e. Ecchymosis

5. What is the BSA of the anterior portion of an adult's trunk?

a. 1%

b. 9%

c. 13.5%

d. 18%

e. 36%

6. A patient with pneumonia is at risk for:

a. hypothermia.

b. hypovolemic shock.

c. septic shock.

d. seizures.

e. hyperthermia.

7. The first step to take when discovering an unresponsive patient is to:

a. begin CPR.

b. check circulation.

c. establish an airway.

d. go find help.

e. identify the patient.

8. During a physical examination of an emergency patient's abdomen, check for:

a. cerebral fluid.

b. distal pulses.

c. paradoxical movement.

d. tenderness, rigidity, and distension.

e. lethargy and slow movements.

9. A potential complication from a splint could be:

a. compartment syndrome.

b. dislocation.

c. hematoma.

d. injury from sharp bone fragments.

e. tissue ischemia and infarction.

10. Circulation after splinting can be tested using:

a. blood pressure.

b. brachial pulse.

c. carotid pulse.

d. distal pulse.

e. femoral pulse.

Scenario for questions 11 and 12: A patient complains about tightness in the chest, a feeling of warmth, and itching. After a minute the patient's breathing is labored.

11. You are most likely watching the early warning signs of:

    a. an allergic reaction.

    b. cardiogenic shock.

    c. a myocardial infarction.

    d. poisoning.

    e. ecchymosis.

12. What action is contraindicated should this patient go into shock?

    a. Cardiac monitoring

    b. Epinephrine (1:1,000)

    c. Establishing an IV line

    d. Intubation

    e. Providing high-flow oxygen

13. If a patient is having a seizure, you should:

    a. force something into the patient's mouth to protect the tongue.

    b. maintain spine immobilization.

    c. protect the patient from injury.

    d. restrain the patient.

    e. assist patient to supine position.

14. What is the difference between an emotional crisis and a psychiatric emergency?

    a. A psychiatric emergency results from substance abuse.

    b. A patient in a psychiatric emergency poses a physical threat to himself or others.

    c. An emotional crisis is a case of bipolar disorder.

    d. A psychiatric emergency involves a patient diagnosed with a psychiatric disorder.

    e. An emotional crisis does not include delusions.

15. A patient suffering hypothermia should be given:

    a. alcohol to promote circulation.

    b. hot chocolate to provide sugar.

    c. IV fluids for rehydration.

    d. warm coffee to raise his or her level of consciousness.

    e. dry heat to warm the surface.

16. What agency should be contacted first when a patient is exposed to a toxic substance?

    a. AMAA

    b. EMS

    c. MSDS

    d. Centers for Disease Control

    e. Poison Control Center

17. Which form of shock is an acute allergic reaction?

    a. Neurogenic shock

    b. Anaphylactic shock

    c. Cardiogenic shock

    d. Septic shock

    e. Hypovolemic shock

18. What does the "V" in AVPU stand for?

    a. Vocalization

    b. Vital signs

    c. Viscosity

    d. Voice recognition

    e. Verbal response

19. To manage open soft tissue injuries, you should:

    a. leave them open to the air.

    b. wrap loosely in bandages.

    c. immediately stitch closed.

    d. elevate the wound.

    e. apply direct pressure.

20. Which of the following items should be included in an emergency kit?

    a. Alcohol wipes

    b. Syringe

    c. Penicillin

    d. Oscilloscope

    e. Sample containers

COG MATCHING

Grade: _____

Match each key term with its definition.

Key Terms

21. _____ allergen

22. _____ anaphylactic shock

23. _____ cardiogenic shock

24. _____ contusion

25. _____ ecchymosis

26. _____ full-thickness burn

27. _____ heat cramps

28. _____ heat stroke

29. _____ hematoma

30. _____ hyperthermia

31. _____ hypothermia

32. _____ hypovolemic shock

33. _____ infarction

34. _____ ischemia

35. _____ melena

36. _____ neurogenic shock

37. _____ partial-thickness burn

38. _____ seizure

39. _____ septic shock

40. _____ shock

41. _____ splint

42. _____ superficial burn

Definitions

a. an abnormal discharge of electrical activity in the brain, resulting in erratic muscle movements, strange sensations, or a complete loss of consciousness

b. black, tarry stools caused by digested blood from the gastrointestinal tract

c. severe allergic reaction within minutes to hours after exposure to a foreign substance

d. an emergency where the body cannot compensate for elevated temperatures

e. a bruise or collection of blood under the skin or in damaged tissue

f. a burn limited to the epidermis

g. any device used to immobilize a sprain, strain, fracture, or dislocated limb

h. shock that results from dysfunction of the nervous system following a spinal cord injury

i. muscle cramping that follows a period of physical exertion and profuse sweating in a hot environment

j. a penetrating burn that has destroyed all skin layers

k. a characteristic black and blue mark from blood accumulation

l. below-normal body temperature

m. the general condition of excessive body heat

n. a blood clot that forms at an injury site

o. a burn that involves epidermis and varying levels of the dermis

p. a decrease in oxygen to tissue

q. a substance that causes manifestations of an allergy

r. shock that results from general infection in the bloodstream

s. shock caused by loss of blood or other body fluids

t. death of tissue due to lack of oxygen

u. condition resulting from the lack of oxygen to individual cells of the body

v. type of shock in which the left ventricle fails to pump enough blood for the body to function

COG IDENTIFICATION

Grade: _____

43. As a medical assistant, you may be called on to assist during an emergency. Review the list of tasks below and determine which tasks you may be responsible for as a medical assistant. Place a check mark in the "Yes" column for those duties you might assist with as a medical assistant and place a check mark in the "No" column for those tasks that not be the responsibility of the medical assistant.

Task	Yes	No
a. Obtain important patient information.		
b. Perform CPR.		
c. Set and splint bone fractures.		
d. Remove foreign body airway obstructions.		
e. Remain calm and react competently and professionally during a psychiatric crisis.		
f. Coordinate multiple ongoing events while rendering patient care in a cardiac emergency.		
g. Negotiate with or attempt to calm a violent patient during a psychiatric crisis.		
h. Know what emergency system is used in the community.		
i. Provide immediate care to the patient while the physician is notified.		
j. Perform rapid sequence intubation (RSI) on a patient who is suffering respiratory failure.		
k. Administer first aid.		
l. Document all actions taken.		
m. Complete routine scheduled tasks.		
n. Assist EMS personnel as necessary.		
o. Examine the patient for EMS personnel.		
p. Direct care of the patient for EMS personnel.		
q. Remove any obstacles that prevent speedy evacuation of the patient by stretcher.		
r. Direct family members to the reception area or a private room.		

44. Identify the type of shock described in the following scenarios.

   a. A very ill patient has been complaining of increasing pain in the pelvis and legs. Blood is present in the urine. The patient's temperature was elevated but is dropping.

   _____

   b. An elderly patient falls on her back while attempting to get out of bed. Her heart rate becomes rapid and thready, and her blood pressure drops quickly.

   _____

   c. A patient presents with fluid in the lungs, difficulty breathing, and chest pain.

   _____

d. A patient presents with labored breathing, grunting, wheezing, and swelling followed by fainting.

_____

e. A child is brought in for diarrhea. She has poor skin turgor and capillary refill. Her mental status appears to be deteriorating.

_____

45. Put a check mark on the line next to the correct signs and symptoms of shock.

a. _____low blood pressure

b. _____high blood pressure

c. _____calm or lethargic

d. _____restlessness or signs of fear

e. _____thirst

f. _____polyuria

g. _____hunger

h. _____nausea

i. _____hot, sweaty skin

j. _____cool, clammy skin

k. _____pale skin with cyanosis (bluish color) at the lips and earlobes

l. _____flushed skin

m. _____rapid and weak pulse

n. _____bounding pulse

46. Classify the type, severity, and coverage of the burns in each of these scenarios.

a. A contractor installing medical equipment accidentally touches exposed wires. He has burns on his right arm, but no sensation of pain.

• Type:

_____

• Severity:

_____

• Coverage:

_____

b. A child spills bleach on one leg. The leg is blistering and causing severe pain.

• Type:

_____

• Severity:

_____

• Coverage:

_____

c. A man watches a welder install handrails on your office's handicapped ramp. Now his face is red and painful, and his eyes have a painful itching sensation.

• Type:

_____

• Severity:

_____

• Coverage:

_____

d. A patient spills hot coffee while driving to your office, painfully blistering his genital area.

• Type:

_____

• Severity:

_____

• Coverage:

_____

47. Identify the hyperthermic and hypothermic emergencies from the list below and match them with the proper treatment. Place the number preceding the correct treatment on the line next to the heat or cold emergency.

a. _____ heat cramps

1. Remove wet clothing.
Cover the patient.
Give warm fluids by mouth if patient is alert and oriented.

b. _____ frostbite

2. Move the patient to a cool area.
Remove clothing that may be keeping in the heat.
Place cool, wet cloths or a wet sheet on the scalp, neck, axilla, and groin.
Administer oxygen as directed by the physician and apply a cardiac monitor.
Notify the EMS for transportation to the hospital as directed by the physician.

c. _____ heat stroke

3. Immerse the affected tissue in lukewarm water (41°C, 105°F) until the area becomes pliable and the color and sensation return.
Do not apply dry heat.
Do not massage the area; massage may cause further tissue damage.
Avoid breaking any blisters that may form.
Notify the EMS for transportation to a hospital.

d. _____ hypothermia

4. Move the patient to a cool area.
Give fluids (commercial electrolyte solution) by mouth if uncomplicated.
Give IV fluids if patient presents with nausea.

48. What are your responsibilities for managing an allergic reaction? Circle the letter preceding all tasks that apply.

  a. Leave the patient to bring the emergency kit or cart, oxygen, and to get a physician to evaluate the patient.

  b. Assist the patient to a supine position.

  c. Scrub patient's skin to remove allergens and urticaria.

  d. Assess the patient's respiratory and circulatory status by obtaining the blood pressure, pulse, and respiratory rates.

  e. Observe skin color and warmth.

  f. If the patient complains of being cold or is shivering, cover with a blanket.

  g. Intubate the patient.

  h. Upon the direction of the physician, start an intravenous line and administer oxygen.

  i. Administer medications as ordered by the physician.

  j. Document vital signs and any medications and treatments given, noting the time each set of vital signs is taken or medications are administered.

  k. Communicate relevant information to the EMS personnel, including copies of the progress notes or medication record as needed.

COG SHORT ANSWER   Grade: _____

49. List nine interventions or steps to manage burns.

_____

_____

_____

_____

50. A sullen and moody patient suddenly becomes threatening. Name three things the medical assistant should do.

_____

_____

_____

_____

51. What six pieces of information should be included in your office's emergency plan?

_____

_____

_____

_____

52. What are the elements of the AVPU scale for assessing a patient's level of consciousness?

A	
V	
P	
U	

53. List the first three steps you should use to control bleeding from an open wound.

_____

_____

_____

_____

54. You enter an exam room and unexpectedly find someone sprawled on the floor. What four things do you check on your primary assessment?

_____

_____

_____

_____

55. At what point do you assess the general appearance of the patient?

_____

_____

_____

56. A patient is found unconscious. You do not suspect trauma. In what order would you perform the physical examination?

_____

_____

_____

_____

57. An examination of the eyes can be done according to the acronym "PEARL," meaning _Pupils Equal And Reactive to Light_. What does this examination reveal?

_____

_____

_____

_____

58. A 55-year-old male begins complaining about nausea. He is clearly anxious or agitated. What could this be an early symptom of?

_____

_____

_____

_____

COG TRUE OR FALSE?   Grade: _____

Indicate whether the statements are true or false by placing the letter T (true) or F (false) on the line preceding the statement.

59. _____ During a primary assessment, you find a patient has inadequate respirations. You should proceed to the secondary assessment and physical examination to find out why.

60. _____ An impaled object should not be removed but requires careful immobilization of the patient and the injured area of the body.

61. _____ An allergic reaction will be evident immediately after exposure to an allergen.

62. _____ Closed wounds are not life threatening.

COG AFF **CASE STUDIES FOR CRITICAL THINKING**   Grade: _____

1. A male older adult falls in an exam room. He is conscious, but agitated and anxious. You are the first to discover him struggling on the floor. What is the only duty you will perform until others arrive, and why?

_____

_____

_____

_____

2. A patient in your office is in respiratory arrest. The physician is attending this patient. You have collected notes on the patient's vitals and SAMPLE history (signs and symptoms, allergies, medications, past pertinent history, last oral intake, and the events that led to the problem). A family member of the patient is present and is growing upset and intrusive. The EMTs arrive on the scene. What is your immediate responsibility? Explain.

_____

_____

_____

_____

3. A teenage patient is given an instant coldpack for an injury to the mouth. A few minutes later you discover the teenager misunderstood, and drank the contents of the cold pack. What information do you need to collect to prepare for a call to the poison control center?

_____

_____

_____

_____

4. Dante commutes to your office by public transportation. On a particularly cold day, Dante arrives late with cool, pale skin. He is lethargic and confused, with slow and shallow respirations and a slow and faint pulse. Describe what actions are appropriate.

_____

_____

_____

_____

5. You have just had a patient suffer anaphylactic shock and respiratory arrest due to an unsuspected penicillin allergy. EMS has transported the patient to a local hospital. The following week, the patient calls to ask what she can do to prevent this from happening in the future. What would you tell this patient? Are there any future precautions this patient should take? If so, what?

_____

_____

_____

_____

6. You have a 35-year-old patient who has religious reservations about some medical procedures. Normally, you and the physician carefully explain procedures to this patient so she has the opportunity to make informed consent decisions. Now she is lying unconscious in front of you with a medical emergency. How do you handle informed consent with an unconscious patient?

_____

_____

_____

_____

7. You have an elderly patient with a "do not resuscitate" order, because he does not want to receive CPR in the event of a heart attack. During treatment for another condition, he collapses in apparent anaphylactic shock. Do you provide emergency medical assistance?

_____

_____

_____

_____

PSY PROCEDURE 26-1 Administer Oxygen

Name: _____   Date: _____   Time: _____   Grade: _____

EQUIPMENT/SUPPLIES: Oxygen tank with a regulator and flow meter, an oxygen delivery system (nasal cannula or mask)

STANDARDS: Given the needed equipment and a place to work the student will perform this skill with _____% accuracy in a total of _____ minutes. *(Your instructor will tell you what the percentage and time limits will be before you begin.)*

KEY: 4 = Satisfactory   0 = Unsatisfactory   NA = This step is not counted

PROCEDURE STEPS	SELF	PARTNER	INSTRUCTOR
1. Wash your hands.	☐	☐	☐
2. Check the physician order.	☐	☐	☐
3. Obtain the oxygen tank and nasal cannula or mask.	☐	☐	☐
4. Greet and identify the patient.	☐	☐	☐
5. **AFF** Explain how to respond to a patient who has dementia.	☐	☐	☐
6. Connect the distal end of the nasal cannula or mask tubing to the adapter on the oxygen tank regulator, which is attached to the oxygen tank.	☐	☐	☐
7. Place the oxygen delivery device into the patient's nares (nasal cannula) or over the patient's nose and mouth (mask).	☐	☐	☐
8. Turn the regulator dial to the liters per minute ordered by the physician.	☐	☐	☐
9. Record the procedure in the patient's medical record.	☐	☐	☐

CALCULATION

Total Possible Points: _____

Total Points Earned: _____ Multiplied by 100 = _____ Divided by Total Possible Points = _____ %

PASS   **FAIL**   **COMMENTS:**

☐   ☐

Student's signature _____ Date _____

Partner's signature _____ Date _____

Instructor's signature _____ Date _____

PSY PROCEDURE 26-2 | **Perform Cardiopulmonary Resuscitation (Adult)**

Name: _____ Date: _____ Time: _____ Grade: _____

EQUIPMENT/SUPPLIES: CPR mannequin, mouth-to-mouth barrier device, gloves

STANDARDS: Given the needed equipment and a place to work the student will perform this skill with _____% accuracy in a total of _____ minutes. *(Your instructor will tell you what the percentage and time limits will be before you begin.)*

NOTE: All health care professionals should receive training for proficiency in CPR in an approved program. This skill sheet is not intended to substitute for proficiency training with a mannequin and structured protocol.

KEY: 4 = Satisfactory   0 = Unsatisfactory   NA = This step is not counted

PROCEDURE STEPS	SELF	PARTNER	INSTRUCTOR
1. Determine unresponsiveness by shaking the patient and shouting "Are you okay?"	☐	☐	☐
2. Instruct another staff member to get the physician, emergency cart/supplies, and AED.	☐	☐	☐
3. Put on clean exam gloves.	☐	☐	☐
4. If the patient does not respond, assess for cardiac function by feeling for a pulse using the carotid artery at the side of the patient's neck.	☐	☐	☐
5. If no pulse is present, follow the protocol for chest compressions according to the standards for training provided by an approved basic life support provider.	☐	☐	☐
6. After 30 compressions, check for airway patency and respiratory effort using the head-tilt, chin-lift maneuver with the patient in the supine position.	☐	☐	☐
7. After opening the airway, begin rescue breathing by placing a mask over the patient's mouth and nose and giving two slow breaths, causing the chest to rise without overfilling the lungs.	☐	☐	☐
8. Continue chest compressions and rescue breathing at a ratio of 30:1 until relieved by another health care provider or EMS arrives.	☐	☐	☐
9. Utilize the recovery position if the patient regains consciousness or a pulse and adequate breathing.	☐	☐	☐
10. Document the procedure and copy any records necessary for transport with EMS.	☐	☐	☐

CALCULATION

Total Possible Points: _____

Total Points Earned: _____ Multiplied by 100 = _____ Divided by Total Possible Points = _____ %

PASS	FAIL	COMMENTS:
☐	☐	

Student's signature _____ Date _____

Partner's signature _____ Date _____

Instructor's signature _____ Date _____

PSY PROCEDURE 26-3 | **Use an Automatic External Defibrillator (Adult)**

Name: _____ Date: _____ Time: _____ Grade: _____

EQUIPMENT/SUPPLIES: Practice mannequin, training automatic external defibrillator with chest pads and connection cables, scissors, gauze, gloves

STANDARDS: Given the needed equipment and a place to work the student will perform this skill with _____% accuracy in a total of _____ minutes. *(Your instructor will tell you what the percentage and time limits will be before you begin.)*

NOTE: All health care professionals should receive training for proficiency in CPR and using an AED in an approved program. This skill sheet is not intended to substitute for proficiency training with a mannequin and structured protocol.

KEY: 4 = Satisfactory   0 = Unsatisfactory   NA = This step is not counted

PROCEDURE STEPS	SELF	PARTNER	INSTRUCTOR
1. Determine unresponsiveness by shaking the patient and shouting "Are you okay?"	☐	☐	☐
2. Instruct another staff member to get the physician, emergency cart/supplies, and AED.	☐	☐	☐
3. While the other staff member continues CPR, remove the patient's shirt and prepare the chest for the AED electrodes: **a.** If there are medication patches on the chest where the electrodes will be placed, remove them and wipe away any excess medication with a towel. **b.** If there is excess hair on the chest that will prevent the AED electrodes from sticking, apply one set of electrodes and quickly remove, pulling any hair from the chest. **c.** If the chest is wet, dry with a towel or other cloth before applying the electrodes.	☐	☐	☐
4. After removing the paper on the back of the AED electrodes, apply the electrodes to the chest area, one to the upper right chest area and the other on the lower left chest area.	☐	☐	☐
5. Explain what should be done in the event the patient has an implantable device in the area where the chest electrodes should be applied.	☐	☐	☐
6. With the electrodes securely on the chest, connect the wire from the electrodes to the AED unit and turn the AED on.	☐	☐	☐
7. Advise everyone to not touch the patient while the AED is analyzing the heart rhythm.	☐	☐	☐
8. If no shock is advised by the AED, resume CPR.	☐	☐	☐
9. If a shock is advised by the AED, make sure no one is touching the patient before pressing the appropriate button on the AED.	☐	☐	☐

10. After a shock is delivered by the AED, resume CPR until the AED advises you that the heart rhythm is being analyzed again.	☐	☐	☐
11. Do not touch the patient while the heart rhythm is being reanalyzed at any point during the procedure.	☐	☐	☐
12. Continue to follow the instructions given by the AED and the physician until EMS has been notified and has arrived.	☐	☐	☐
13. Document the procedure and copy any records necessary for transport with EMS.	☐	☐	☐

CALCULATION

Total Possible Points: _____

Total Points Earned: _____ Multiplied by 100 = _____ Divided by Total Possible Points = _____ %

PASS   **FAIL**   **COMMENTS:**

☐   ☐

Student's signature _____ Date _____

Partner's signature _____ Date _____

Instructor's signature _____ Date _____

PSY PROCEDURE 26-4   Manage a Foreign Body Airway Obstruction (Adult)

Name: _____   Date: _____   Time: _____   Grade: _____

EQUIPMENT/SUPPLIES: Practice mannequin, mouth-to-mouth barrier device, gloves

STANDARDS: Given the needed equipment and a place to work the student will perform this skill with
_____% accuracy in a total of _____ minutes. *(Your instructor will tell you what the percentage and time limits will be before you begin.)*

NOTE: All health care professionals should receive training for proficiency in managing a foreign body airway obstruction in an approved program. This skill sheet is not intended to substitute for proficiency training with a mannequin and structured protocol.

KEY: 4 = Satisfactory   0 = Unsatisfactory   NA = This step is not counted

PROCEDURE STEPS	SELF	PARTNER	INSTRUCTOR
1. If the patient is conscious and appears to be choking, ask the patient, "Are you choking?"	☐	☐	☐
2. Do not perform abdominal thrusts if the patient can speak or cough because these are signs that the obstruction is not complete.	☐	☐	☐
3. If the patient cannot speak or cough but has indicated the he or she is choking, move behind the patient, wrapping your arms around his or her abdomen.	☐	☐	☐
4. Place the fist of your dominant hand with the thumb against the patient's abdomen, between the navel and xiphoid process.	☐	☐	☐
5. Put your other hand against your dominant hand and give quick, upward thrusts, forceful enough to dislodge the obstruction in the airway.	☐	☐	☐
6. If the patient is obese or pregnant, place your hands against the middle of the sternum, above the xiphoid process and proceed with quick thrusts inward.	☐	☐	☐
7. Continue with the abdominal thrusts until the object is expelled and the patient can breathe or the patient becomes unconscious.	☐	☐	☐
8. If the patient becomes unconscious or is found unconscious, open the airway and give two rescue breaths.	☐	☐	☐
9. If rescue breaths are obstructed, reposition the head, and try again.	☐	☐	☐
10. If rescue breaths continue to be obstructed after repositioning, begin abdominal thrusts by placing your palm against the patient's abdomen with your fingers facing his or her head (you may need to straddle the patient's hips). The palm of the hand should be located between the navel and the xiphoid process.	☐	☐	☐
11. Lace the fingers of the other hand into the fingers of the hand on the abdomen and give five abdominal thrusts.	☐	☐	☐

12. After five abdominal thrusts, open the patient's mouth using a tongue-jaw lift maneuver and do a finger-sweep of the mouth, removing any objects that may have been dislodged.	☐	☐	☐
13. If an item has been dislodged and can be removed easily, remove the object and attempt rescue breaths. Continue rescue breaths and chest compressions as necessary and appropriate.	☐	☐	☐
14. If the item has not been dislodged, attempt rescue breaths. If rescue breaths are successful, continue rescue breathing and chest compressions as necessary and appropriate.	☐	☐	☐
15. If the item has not been dislodged and rescue breaths are not successful, continue with abdominal thrusts.	☐	☐	☐
16. Repeat the pattern of abdominal thrusts, finger-sweep, and rescue breaths and follow the physician's orders until EMS is notified and arrives.	☐	☐	☐
17. Document the procedure and copy any records necessary for transport with EMS.	☐	☐	☐

CALCULATION

Total Possible Points: _____

Total Points Earned: _____ Multiplied by 100 = _____ Divided by Total Possible Points = _____ %

PASS   **FAIL**   **COMMENTS:**

☐   ☐

Student's signature _____ Date _____

Partner's signature _____ Date _____

Instructor's signature _____ Date _____

PSY PROCEDURE 26-5 | Control Bleeding

Name: _____ Date: _____ Time: _____ Grade: _____

EQUIPMENT/SUPPLIES: Gloves, sterile gauze pads

STANDARDS: Given the needed equipment and a place to work the student will perform this skill with _____% accuracy in a total of _____ minutes. *(Your instructor will tell you what the percentage and time limits will be before you begin.)*

KEY: 4 = Satisfactory 0 = Unsatisfactory NA = This step is not counted

PROCEDURE STEPS	SELF	PARTNER	INSTRUCTOR
1. Identify the patient and assess the extent of the bleeding and type of accident.	☐	☐	☐
2. Take the patient to an examination room and notify the physician if appropriate.	☐	☐	☐
3. Give the patient some gauze pads and have him or her apply pressure to the area while you put on a pair of clean examination gloves and open additional sterile gauze pads.	☐	☐	☐
4. Observe the patient for signs of dizziness or lightheadedness. Have the patient lie down.	☐	☐	☐
5. Using several sterile gauze pads, apply direct pressure to the wound.	☐	☐	☐
6. Maintain pressure until the bleeding stops.	☐	☐	☐
7. If the bleeding continues or seeps through the gauze, apply additional gauze on top of the saturated gauze while continuing to apply direct pressure.	☐	☐	☐
8. If directed by the physician to do so, apply pressure to the artery delivering blood to this area while continuing to apply direct pressure to the wound to control bleeding.	☐	☐	☐
9. Once the bleeding is controlled, prepare to assist the physician with a minor office surgical procedure to close the wound.	☐	☐	☐
10. Continue to monitor the patient for signs of shock and be prepared to treat the patient appropriately.	☐	☐	☐
11. Document the treatment in the patient's medical record.	☐	☐	☐

CALCULATION

Total Possible Points: _____

Total Points Earned: _____ Multiplied by 100 = _____ Divided by Total Possible Points = _____ %

PASS   **FAIL**   **COMMENTS:**

☐   ☐

Student's signature _____ Date _____

Partner's signature _____ Date _____

Instructor's signature _____ Date _____

PSY PROCEDURE 26-6 **Respond to Medical Emergencies Other than Bleeding, Cardiac/Respiratory Arrest, or Foreign Body Airway Obstruction**

Name: _____ Date: _____ Time: _____ Grade: _____

EQUIPMENT/SUPPLIES: A medical emergency kit that contains a minimum of personal protective equipment including gloves, low-dose aspirin tablets, 2 × 2 and 4 × 4 sterile gauze pads, vinegar or acetic acid solution, blood pressure cuff and stethoscope, sterile water or saline for irrigation, ice bags, and towel or rolled gauze bandage material

STANDARDS: Given the needed equipment and a place to work the student will perform this skill with _____% accuracy in a total of _____ minutes. *(Your instructor will tell you what the percentage and time limits will be before you begin.)*

KEY: 4 = Satisfactory   0 = Unsatisfactory   NA = This step is not counted

PROCEDURE STEPS	SELF	PARTNER	INSTRUCTOR
1. Identify the patient and assess the type of emergency involved.	☐	☐	☐
2. Escort the patient to an examination room.	☐	☐	☐
3. Have another staff member get the physician, medical emergency cart/supplies, and AED.	☐	☐	☐
4. Apply clean examination gloves and other PPE as appropriate.	☐	☐	☐
5. Assist the patient to the exam table and have him or her lie down.	☐	☐	☐
6. Treat the patient according to the physician's instructions and the most current guidelines for first aid procedures for the following:			
a. Chest pain	☐	☐	☐
b. Snakebite	☐	☐	☐
c. Jellyfish sting	☐	☐	☐
d. Dental injuries	☐	☐	☐
(1) Chipped tooth	☐	☐	☐
(2) Cracked or broken tooth	☐	☐	☐
(3) Tooth removed	☐	☐	☐
(4) Broken jaw	☐	☐	☐
7. If the patient develops cardiac or respiratory arrest, follow the procedure for CPR according to the most recent standards and guidelines.	☐	☐	☐
8. Document the treatment in the patient's medical record.	☐	☐	☐

CALCULATION

Total Possible Points: _____

Total Points Earned: _____ Multiplied by 100 = _____ Divided by Total Possible Points = _____ %

PASS   **FAIL**   **COMMENTS:**

☐   ☐

Student's signature _____ Date _____

Partner's signature _____ Date _____

Instructor's signature _____ Date _____

Clinical Duties Related to Medical Specialties

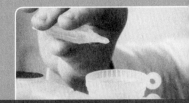

Dermatology

Learning Outcomes

Cognitive Domain

1. Spell and define key terms
2. Describe common skin disorders
3. Describe implications for treatment related to pathology
4. Explain common diagnostic procedures
5. Prepare the patient for examination of the integument
6. Assist the physician with examination of the integument
7. Explain the difference between bandages and dressings and give the purpose of each
8. Identify the guidelines for applying bandages

Psychomotor Domain

1. Apply a warm or cold compress (Procedure 27-1)
2. Assist physician with patient care
3. Practice standard precautions
4. Document patient care
5. Document patient education
6. Assist with therapeutic soaks (Procedure 27-2)
7. Apply a tubular gauze bandage (Procedure 27-3)
8. Practice within standard of care for a medical assistant

Affective Domain

1. Apply critical thinking skills in performing patient assessment and care
2. Use language/verbal skills that enable patients' understanding
3. Demonstrate empathy in communicating with patients, family, and staff

4. Use appropriate body language and other nonverbal skills in communicating with patients, family, and staff
5. Demonstrate awareness of the territorial boundaries of the person with whom you are communicating
6. Demonstrate sensitivity appropriate to the message being delivered
7. Demonstrate recognition of the patient's level of understanding in communications
8. Recognize and protect personal boundaries in communicating with others
9. Demonstrate respect for individual diversity, incorporating awareness of one's own biases in areas including gender, race, religion, age, and economic status
10. Apply active listening skills
11. Apply local, state, and federal health care legislation and regulation appropriate to the medical assisting practice setting

ABHES Competencies

1. Assist the physician with the regimen of diagnostic and treatment modalities as they relate to each body system
2. Comply with federal, state, and local health laws and regulations
3. Communicate on the recipient's level of comprehension
4. Serve as a liaison between the physician and others
5. Show empathy and impartiality when dealing with patients

Name: _____   Date: _____   Grade: _____

COG **MULTIPLE CHOICE**

Circle the letter preceding the correct answer.

1. Which of the following groups of people are most likely to develop impetigo?

   a. Older adults

   b. Women

   c. Young children

   d. Men

   e. Teenagers

2. What type of infection is herpes simplex?

   a. Bacterial

   b. Fungal

   c. Parasitic

   d. Viral

   e. Genetic

3. Public showers and swimming pools are common places to pick up fungal infections because:

   a. fungi thrive in moist conditions.

   b. areas that are highly populated increase the risk factor.

   c. sharing towels passes fungal infections from one person to another.

   d. fungi grow quickly on tile surfaces.

   e. antifungal medications do not work once they come into contact with water.

4. Which of these skin disorders may be caused by food allergies?

   a. Keloids

   b. Intertrigo

   c. Alopecia

   d. Eczema

   e. Seborrheic dermatitis

5. Which of the following statements is true about albinism?

   a. Respiratory problems are common among sufferers of albinism.

   b. Albinism is treated with benzoyl peroxide.

   c. Albinism usually occurs in exposed areas of the skin.

   d. People who suffer from albinism should have regular checkups.

   e. People who suffer from albinism should take particular care of their eyes in the sun.

6. Which statements are true about decubitus ulcers?

   a. They are frequently diagnosed in school-aged children.

   b. They are most common in aged, debilitated, and immobilized patients.

   c. They are highly contagious.

   d. They generally occur on the chin and forehead.

   e. They are effectively treated with antifungal creams.

7. When bandaging a patient, you should:

   a. fasten bandages only with safety pins.

   b. complete surgical asepsis before you begin.

   c. keep the area to be bandaged warm.

   d. leave fingers and toes exposed when possible.

   e. wrap the bandage as tightly as possible to prevent it from coming loose.

8. A person suffering from high stress levels is most likely to develop:

   a. urticaria.

   b. acne vulgaris.

   c. impetigo.

   d. leukoderma.

   e. herpes zoster.

9. How many people in the United States will typically develop malignant melanoma?

   a. 1 in 5

   b. 1 in 500

   c. 1 in 105

   d. 1 in 1,005

   e. 1 in 5,000

10. Which of the following conditions would be treated with topical antifungal cream?

    a. Folliculitis

    b. Vitiligo

    c. Tinea versicolor

    d. Urticaria

    e. Decubitus ulcers

11. What should patients do if they have an absence of melanin in their skin?

    a. Avoid coming into contact with other people.

    b. Protect their skin from the sun.

    c. Seek immediate medical assistance.

    d. Take supplementary vitamin pills.

    e. Stop sharing towels and bedding.

    Scenario for questions 12 and 13: A male patient comes into the physician's office to have a wart removed from his finger. While you are preparing him for the procedure, he tells you that he regularly gets verrucae on his feet.

12. How would you advise the patient to avoid further viral infections?

    a. Wash all bedding and clothing at high temperatures.

    b. Avoid sharing combs and toiletries with anyone.

    c. Avoid coming into direct contact with skin lesions.

    d. Wear comfortable footwear and avoid walking long distances.

    e. Frequently wash hands with antibacterial soap.

13. The patient should look for over-the-counter wart medication that contains:

    a. podophyllum resin.

    b. acyclovir.

    c. selenium sulfide.

    d. permethrin.

    e. prednisone.

14. Before you apply a bandage to an open wound, you should:

    a. moisten the bandage.

    b. keep the bandage at room temperature.

    c. apply pressure to the wound.

    d. apply a sterile dressing to the wound.

    e. check to see how the patient would like the bandage fastened.

15. How can you tell that a patient is suffering from stage I decubitus ulcers?

    a. The skin is blistered, peeling, or cracked.

    b. Red skin does not return to normal when massaged.

    c. The skin is scaly, dry, and flaky.

    d. The skin is extremely itchy.

    e. The patient is unable to feel pressure on the area.

16. When a physician performs a shave biopsy, he:

    a. cuts the lesion off just above the skin line.

    b. removes a small section from the center of the lesion.

    c. removes the entire lesion for evaluation.

    d. cuts the lesion off just below the skin line.

    e. removes a small section from the edge of the lesion.

17. Which of these is thought to be a cause of skin cancer in areas not exposed to the sun?

    a. Chemicals in toiletries

    b. Pet allergies

    c. Frequent irritation

    d. Second-hand smoke

    e. Excessive scratching

18. Treatment of impetigo involves:

    a. washing the area two to three times a day followed by application of topical antibiotics.

    b. cleaning with alcohol sponges twice a day.

    c. washing towels, washcloths, and bed linens daily.

    d. oral antibiotics for severe cases.

    e. the physician removing the infected area.

19. Which of the following statements is true about nevi?

    a. Nevi are usually malignant.

    b. Nevi are usually found on the back or legs.

    c. It is common for nevi to bleed occasionally.

    d. Nevi are congenital pigmented skin blemishes.

    e. Nevi are extremely rare in young patients.

20. Which part of the body is affected by tinea capitis?

    a. Hands

    b. Feet

    c. Hair follicles

    d. Groin

    e. Scalp

COG MATCHING

Grade: _____

Place the letter preceding the definition on the line next to the term.

Key Terms

21. _____ alopecia

22. _____ bulla

23. _____ carbuncle

24. _____ cellulitis

25. _____ dermatophytosis

26. _____ eczema

27. _____ erythema

28. _____ folliculitis

29. _____ furuncle

30. _____ herpes simplex

31. _____ herpes zoster

32. _____ impetigo

33. _____ macule

34. _____ neoplasm

35. _____ pediculosis

36. _____ pruritus

37. _____ psoriasis

38. _____ seborrhea

39. _____ urticaria

40. _____ verruca

41. _____ vesicle

42. _____ pustule

Definitions

a. a highly infectious skin infection causing erythema and progressing to honey-colored crusts

b. redness of the skin

c. an inflammation of hair follicles

d. a small, flat discoloration of the skin

e. an abnormal growth of new tissue; tumor

f. an infection of an interconnected group of hair follicles or several furuncles forming a mass

g. an inflammation or infection of the skin and deeper tissues that may result in tissue destruction if not treated properly

h. an infection caused by the herpes simplex virus

i. hives

j. an infection caused by reactivation of varicella zoster virus, which causes chicken pox

k. a wart

l. a large blister or vesicle

m. an infestation with parasitic lice

n. baldness

o. superficial dermatitis

p. itching

q. an overproduction of sebum by the sebaceous glands

r. an infection in a hair follicle or gland; characterized by pain, redness, and swelling with necrosis of tissue in the center

s. a skin lesion that appears as a small sac containing fluid; a blister

t. a fungal infection of the skin

u. a vesicle filled with pus

v. a chronic skin disorder that appears as red patches covered with thick, dry, silvery scales

COG MATCHING

Grade: _____

Place the letter of the description on the line preceding the skin disorder.

Disorders

43. _____ vitiligo

44. _____ decubitus ulcer

45. _____ corn

46. _____ acne vulgaris

47. _____ carbuncle

48. _____ squamous cell carcinoma

49. _____ seborrheic dermatitis

Descriptions

a. a skin disease characterized by pimples, comedones, and cysts

b. a pigmentation disorder thought to be an autoimmune disorder in patients with an inherited predisposition

c. an infection in an interconnected group of hair follicles

d. a skin inflammation caused by an overproduction of sebum that affects the scalp, eyelids, face, back, umbilicus, and body folds

e. a hard, raised thickening of the stratum corneum on the toes

f. an ulcerative lesion caused by impaired blood supply and insufficient oxygen to an area

g. a type of skin cancer that is a slow-growing, malignant tumor

COG MATCHING

Grade: _____

Place the letter of the description on the line preceding the type of bandage.

Bandages

50. _____ roller bandages

51. _____ elastic bandages

52. _____ tubular gauze bandages

Descriptions

a. These bandages can be given to the patient to take home to wash and reuse. You should be careful when applying them so as not to compromise circulation.

b. These bandages are made of soft, woven materials and are available in various lengths and widths. They can be either sterile or clean.

c. These bandages are very stretchy and are used to enclose fingers, toes, arms, legs, head, and trunk.

COG MATCHING Grade: _____

Although medical assistants do not prescribe treatments, match each of the following skin disorders with the most likely physician prescribed treatment. Place the letter of the possible treatment on the line next to the skin disorder.

Disorders

53. _____ decubitus ulcers

54. _____ casal cell carcinoma

55. _____ cellulitis

56. _____ folliculitis

57. _____ verruca

58. _____ urticaria

Treatments

a. saline soaks or compresses

b. antihistamines

c. antibiotic powder

d. surgical removal

e. keratolytic agents

f. antibiotics

COG IDENTIFICATION Grade: _____

59. Which of the following skin disorders cannot be treated? Circle the correct answer.

  a. Impetigo

  b. Folliculitis

  c. Albinism

  d. Malignant melanoma

  e. Decubitus ulcers

60. How would a physician be able to confirm a suspected case of malignant melanoma? Circle the correct answer.

  a. Wood light analysis

  b. inspection

  c. urine test

61. As a medical assistant, you'll be responsible for helping the physician perform physical examinations of the skin. Review the list of tasks below and determine which tasks you may be responsible for as a medical assistant. Place a check mark in the "Yes" column for duties that you might assist with and a check mark in the "No" column for tasks that would be completed by someone else.

Task	Yes	No
a. Assemble the equipment required by the physician.		
b. Perform a skin biopsy.		
c. Inject local anesthetic when needed.		
d. Direct specimens to the appropriate laboratories.		
e. Clean and disinfect the examination room.		
f. Diagnose and treat common skin inflammations.		
g. Reinforce the physician's instructions about caring for a skin condition at home.		

62. You are applying a bandage to a patient. Read the statements below and check the appropriate box to show whether the bandage has been applied correctly or incorrectly.

	Applied Correctly	Applied Incorrectly
a. You have fastened the bandage with adhesive tape.		
b. The area that you are about to bandage is clean and damp.		
c. You have dressed two burned fingers separately and then bandaged them together.		
d. The skin around the bandaged arm is pale and cool.		
e. You have bandaged a wounded foot by covering the toes to make it neater.		
f. You have bandaged an elbow with extra padding.		

63. Place a check mark in the appropriate box to show whether the person described is at a high risk or a low risk of developing impetigo.

	High Risk	Low Risk
a. A slightly overweight 34-year-old woman who showers twice a day		
b. A 55-year-old man who works at a hospital laundry room and does not wash his hands		
c. A 22-year-old woman with severe anorexia		
d. An 18-year-old drug addict who lives in an abandoned warehouse		
e. A 40-year-old mother of three who enjoys reading in the tub		

64. Read these descriptions of five of Dr. Marsh's patients then decide which of his patients is at the highest risk of developing malignant melanoma. Place a check mark on the line preceding the patient descriptions that are at the highest risk.

a. _____ Mrs. Pearson, 42-year-old mother of two. Light brown hair, brown eyes, enjoys reading and watching movies.

b. _____ Mr. Stevens, 50-year-old widower. Gray hair, brown eyes, enjoys walking and playing golf.

c. _____ Jessica Phillips, 24-year-old college student. Red hair, blue eyes, enjoys playing volleyball and surfing.

d. _____ Todd Andrews, 18-year-old student. Black hair, green eyes, enjoys running and swimming.

e. _____ Mr. Archer, 39-year-old father of three. Blond hair, blue eyes, lives in Minnesota and enjoys skiing.

COG SHORT ANSWER   Grade: _____

65. What are the symptoms of psoriasis?

_____

_____

_____

_____

66. A man brings his 85-year-old mother to the physician's office. He tells you that his mother lives in a local care home. When the physician examines the patient, you notice multiple decubitus ulcers on her body. Explain why this would be a particular cause of concern.

_____

_____

_____

_____

67. List the three types of skin biopsy performed by a physician.

_____

_____

_____

_____

68. List the three bacterial skin infections that develop in the hair follicles.

_____

_____

_____

_____

69. A patient has a band of lesions on his back made up of small red papules. What skin disorder does this person most likely have? Explain what causes the condition.

_____

_____

_____

_____

70. A father brings his 8-year-old son to the physician, who diagnoses the child with pediculosis. What advice could you give the father to ensure that no other members of the family become infected? List three things that the father could do to contain the problem.

_____

_____

_____

_____

71. What is the full version of the cancer prevention message "Slip! Slop! Slap! Wrap!"?

_____

_____

_____

_____

72. The physician suspects that a patient has ringworm. Explain what method the physician would most likely use to confirm the diagnosis?

_____

_____

_____

_____

COG TRUE OR FALSE?   Grade: _____

73. Indicate whether the statements are true or false by placing the letter T (true) or F (false) on the line preceding the statement.

a. _____ Before applying a bandage, you should perform surgical asepsis.

b. _____ Young women are more likely to develop keloids than young men.

c. _____ A wound culture is obtained by excising the wound.

d. _____ Erythema is best treated with antihistamines.

COG AFF CASE STUDIES FOR CRITICAL THINKING   Grade: _____

1. A patient has come into the physician's office for a skin biopsy on his thigh. After the physician has removed the tissue, she asks you to bandage the area. List three things you should do while you are bandaging the patient's thigh to ensure that it is both sterile and secure. Explain why they are important.

_____

_____

_____

_____

2. There are three patients waiting to be seen by a physician, and all of the appointments are slightly behind schedule. One of the patients is a young man who has clusters of wheals on his left arm. The second patient is a 7-year-old girl who has dry scaly crusts on her face and neck. The third patient is a 5-year-old boy with dried skin flakes and bald patches on his scalp. All three patients are itching, and the receptionist is concerned that they might be contagious. You have only one spare examination room. Which patient would you isolate in the examination room? Explain your answer.

_____

_____

_____

_____

3. Your patient is a 25-year-old female who has been to see the physician several times for severe sunburn. You know that her lifestyle can lead to long-term skin problems. Explain how you could educate her about staying safe in the sun. Include some of the early warning signs of skin cancer that she should keep an eye out for.

_____

_____

_____

_____

4. A mother brings her 8-year-old son to the physician's office, and the child is diagnosed with pediculosis. She insists that her child cannot possibly have lice because they live in a very clean home. The mother demands that the physician examine the child again. What do you say to the mother to calm her down? How do you reassure her?

_____

_____

_____

_____

5. A 14-year-old boy comes into the physician's office with severe acne vulgaris on his face and neck. He is embarrassed and depressed about his condition and is worried that it will never get better. He says that he has tried every over-the-counter medication and that this is his last hope. What would you say to this patient?

_____

_____

_____

_____

Name: _____ Date: _____ Time: _____ Grade: _____

EQUIPMENT/SUPPLIES: Warm compresses—appropriate solution (water with possible antiseptic if ordered), warmed to 110°F or recommended temperature; bath thermometer; absorbent material (cloths, gauze); waterproof barriers; hot water bottle (optional); clean or sterile basin; gloves. Cold compresses—appropriate solution; ice bag or cold pack; absorbent material (cloths, gauze); waterproof barriers; gloves

STANDARDS: Given the needed equipment and a place to work the student will perform this skill with _____% accuracy in a total of _____ minutes. *(Your instructor will tell you what the percentage and time limits will be before you begin.)*

KEY: 4 = Satisfactory   0 = Unsatisfactory   NA = This step is not counted

PROCEDURE STEPS	SELF	PARTNER	INSTRUCTOR
1. Wash your hands and put on gloves.	☐	☐	☐
2. Check the physician's order and assemble the equipment and supplies.	☐	☐	☐
3. Pour the appropriate solution into the basin. For hot compresses, check the temperature of the warmed solution.	☐	☐	☐
4. Greet and identify the patient. Explain the procedure.	☐	☐	☐
5. Ask patient to remove appropriate clothing.	☐	☐	☐
6. Gown and drape accordingly.	☐	☐	☐
7. **AFF** Explain how to respond to a patient who is hearing impaired.	☐	☐	☐
8. Protect the examination table with a waterproof barrier.	☐	☐	☐
9. Place absorbent material or gauze into the prepared solution. Wring out excess moisture.	☐	☐	☐
10. Place the compress on the patient's skin and ask about comfort of temperature.	☐	☐	☐
11. Observe the skin for changes in color.	☐	☐	☐
12. Arrange the wet compress over the area.	☐	☐	☐
13. Insulate the compress with plastic or another waterproof barrier.	☐	☐	☐
14. Check the compress frequently for moisture and temperature.	☐	☐	☐
a. Hot water bottles or ice packs may be used to maintain the temperature.			
b. Rewet absorbent material as needed.			

15. After the prescribed amount of time, usually 20–30 minutes, remove the compress.
   a. Discard disposable materials.
   b. Disinfect reusable equipment.
	☐	☐	☐

16. Remove your gloves and wash your hands.	☐	☐	☐

17. Document the procedure including:
   a. Length of treatment, type of solution, temperature of solution
   b. Skin color after treatment, assessment of the area, and patient's reactions
	☐	☐	☐

CALCULATION

Total Possible Points: _____

Total Points Earned: _____ Multiplied by 100 = _____ Divided by Total Possible Points = _____ %

PASS   **FAIL**   **COMMENTS:**

☐   ☐

Student's signature _____ Date _____

Partner's signature _____ Date _____

Instructor's signature _____ Date _____

PSY PROCEDURE 27-2 | **Assist with Therapeutic Soaks**

Name: _____ Date: _____ Time: _____ Grade: _____

EQUIPMENT/SUPPLIES: Clean or sterile basin or container to comfortably contain the body part to be soaked; solution and/or medication; dry towels; bath thermometer; gloves

STANDARDS: Given the needed equipment and a place to work the student will perform this skill with _____% accuracy in a total of _____ minutes. *(Your instructor will tell you what the percentage and time limits will be before you begin.)*

KEY: 4 = Satisfactory 0 = Unsatisfactory NA = This step is not counted

PROCEDURE STEPS	SELF	PARTNER	INSTRUCTOR
1. Wash your hands and apply your gloves.	☐	☐	☐
2. Assemble the equipment and supplies, including the appropriately sized basin or container. Pad surfaces of container for comfort.	☐	☐	☐
3. Fill the container with solution and check the temperature with a bath thermometer. The temperature should be below 110°F.	☐	☐	☐
4. Greet and identify the patient. Explain the procedure.	☐	☐	☐
5. **AFF** Explain how to respond to the patient who has dementia.	☐	☐	☐
6. Slowly lower the patient's extremity or body part into the container.	☐	☐	☐
7. Arrange the part comfortably and in easy alignment.	☐	☐	☐
8. Check for pressure areas and pad the edges as needed for comfort.	☐	☐	☐
9. Check the solution every 5–10 minutes for proper temperature.	☐	☐	☐
10. Soak for the prescribed amount of time, usually 15–20 minutes.	☐	☐	☐
11. Remove the body part from the solution and carefully dry the area with a towel.	☐	☐	☐
12. Properly care for the equipment and appropriately dispose of single-use supplies.	☐	☐	☐
13. Document the procedure including: a. Length of treatment, type of solution, temperature of solution b. Skin color after treatment, assessment of the area, and patient's reactions	☐	☐	☐

CALCULATION

Total Possible Points: _____

Total Points Earned: _____ Multiplied by 100 = _____ Divided by Total Possible Points = _____ %

PASS   **FAIL**   **COMMENTS:**

☐   ☐

Student's signature _____ Date _____

Partner's signature _____ Date _____

Instructor's signature _____ Date _____

PSY PROCEDURE 27-3 | **Apply a Tubular Gauze Bandage**

Name: _____ Date: _____ Time: _____ Grade: _____

EQUIPMENT/SUPPLIES: Tubular gauze, applicator, tape, scissors

STANDARDS: Given the needed equipment and a place to work the student will perform this skill with
_____% accuracy in a total of _____ minutes. *(Your instructor will tell you what the percentage and time limits will be before you begin.)*

KEY: 4 = Satisfactory   0 = Unsatisfactory   NA = This step is not counted

PROCEDURE STEPS	SELF	PARTNER	INSTRUCTOR
1. Wash your hands and assemble the equipment.	☐	☐	☐
2. Greet and identify the patient. Explain the procedure.	☐	☐	☐
3. **AFF** Explain how to respond to a patient who is visually impaired.	☐	☐	☐
4. Choose the appropriate-size tubular gauze applicator and gauze width.	☐	☐	☐
5. Select and cut or tear adhesive tape in lengths to secure the gauze ends.	☐	☐	☐
6. Place the gauze bandage on the applicator in the following manner: **a.** Be sure that the applicator is upright (open end up) and placed on a flat surface. **b.** Pull a sufficient length of gauze from the stock box, ready to cut. **c.** Open the end of the length of gauze and slide it over the upper end of the applicator. **d.** Push estimated amount of gauze needed for this procedure onto the applicator. **e.** Cut the gauze when the required amount of gauze has been transferred to the applicator.	☐	☐	☐
7. Place applicator over the distal end of the affected part. Hold it in place as you move to Step 7.	☐	☐	☐
8. Slide applicator containing the gauze up to the proximal end of the affected part.	☐	☐	☐
9. Pull the applicator 1–2 inches past the end of the affected part if the part is to be completely covered.	☐	☐	☐
10. Turn the applicator one full turn to anchor the bandage.	☐	☐	☐
11. Move the applicator toward the proximal part as before.	☐	☐	☐
12. Move the applicator forward about 1 inch beyond the original starting point.	☐	☐	☐
13. Repeat the procedure until the desired coverage is obtained.	☐	☐	☐

14. The final layer should end at the proximal part of the affected area. Remove the applicator.	☐	☐	☐
15. Secure the bandage in place with adhesive tape or cut the gauze into two tails and tie them at the base of the tear.	☐	☐	☐
16. Tie the two tails around the closest proximal joint.	☐	☐	☐
17. Use the adhesive tape sparingly to secure the end if not using a tie.	☐	☐	☐
18. Properly care for or dispose of equipment and supplies.	☐	☐	☐
19. Clean the work area. Wash your hands.	☐	☐	☐
20. Record the procedure.	☐	☐	☐

CALCULATION

Total Possible Points: _____

Total Points Earned: _____ Multiplied by 100 = _____ Divided by Total Possible Points = _____ %

PASS   **FAIL**   **COMMENTS:**

☐   ☐

Student's signature _____ Date _____

Partner's signature _____ Date _____

Instructor's signature _____ Date _____

28 Orthopedics

Cognitive Domain

1. Spell and define the key terms
2. List and describe disorders of the musculoskeletal system
3. Compare the different types of fractures
4. Identify and explain diagnostic procedures of the musculoskeletal system
5. Discuss the role of the medical assistant in caring for the patient with a musculoskeletal system disorder
6. Describe the various types of ambulatory aids
7. Identify common pathology related to each body system
8. Describe implications for treatment related to pathology

Psychomotor Domain

1. Apply an arm sling (Procedure 28-1)
2. Assist physician with patient care
3. Prepare a patient for procedures and/or treatments
4. Document patient care
5. Document patient education
6. Apply cold packs (Procedure 28-2)
7. Practice standard precautions
8. Use a hot water bottle or commercial hot pack (Procedure 28-3)
9. Measure a patient for axillary crutches (Procedure 28-4)
10. Instruct a patient in various crutch gaits (Procedure 28-5)
11. Practice within standard of care for a medical assistant

Affective Domain

1. Apply critical thinking skills in performing patient assessment and care
2. Use language/verbal skills that enable patients' understanding
3. Demonstrate empathy in communicating with patients, family, and staff
4. Use appropriate body language and other nonverbal skills in communicating with patients, family, and staff
5. Demonstrate awareness of the territorial boundaries of the person with whom you are communicating
6. Demonstrate sensitivity appropriate to the message being delivered
7. Demonstrate recognition of the patient's level of understanding in communications
8. Recognize and protect personal boundaries in communicating with others
9. Demonstrate respect for individual diversity, incorporating awareness of one's own biases in areas including gender, race, religion, age, and economic status
10. Apply active listening skills
11. Apply local, state, and federal health care legislation and regulation appropriate to the medical assisting practice setting

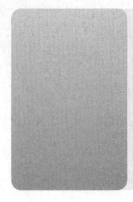

ABHES Competencies

1. Assist the physician with the regimen of diagnostic and treatment modalities as they relate to each body system
2. Comply with federal, state, and local health laws and regulations
3. Communicate on the recipient's level of comprehension
4. Serve as a liaison between the physician and others
5. Show empathy and impartiality when dealing with patients
6. Document accurately

Name: _____   Date: _____   Grade: _____

COG MULTIPLE CHOICE

Circle the letter preceding the correct answer.

1. The rebound phenomenon happens:

    a. when the body secretes callus, which fills in fractures and mends damaged bone.

    b. when the body experiences bulging discs or biomechanical stress as a result of poor posture.

    c. when the body overcompensates for a muscle sprain by increasing use of unaffected muscles.

    d. when the body responds to extremes of temperature for long periods of time by exerting an opposite effect.

    e. when the body releases fat droplets from the yellow marrow of the long bones.

2. In which crutch gait do both legs leave the floor together?

    a. One-arm gait

    b. Two-point gait

    c. Three-point gait

    d. Four-point gait

    e. Swing-through gait

3. A fracture that occurs in flat bones (like those of the skull) and results in a fragment being driven below the surface of the bone is called a(n):

    a. depressed fracture.

    b. impacted fracture.

    c. pathological fracture.

    d. compression fracture.

    e. spiral fracture.

4. A possible cause of gout is:

    a. a liver disorder.

    b. a degenerative strain.

    c. a diet high in purines.

    d. the wear and tear on weight-bearing joints.

    e. the release of fat droplets from the marrow of long bones.

Scenario for questions 5 and 6: The physician has determined that a male patient will need to wear a short arm cast on his left arm as part of the treatment for his fracture. The physician asks you to help her apply the cast to the patient. You assemble the items needed to apply the cast. As the physician prepares the limb for casting, you soak the casting material and press it until it is no longer dripping. Then, the physician wraps the affected limb with the material. After the cast has dried, the physician asks you to apply an arm sling to the patient's left arm.

5. How should the physician wrap the patient's affected arm with the soaked casting material?

    a. From the axilla to mid palm

    b. From mid palm to the axilla

    c. From the elbow to mid palm

    d. From mid palm to the elbow

    e. From the axilla to the elbow

6. Which of these steps will you follow when applying the arm sling?

    a. Cover the left arm with soft knitted tubular material.

    b. Position the hand of the left arm at a 90-degree angle.

    c. Instruct the patient in various gaits using auxiliary crutches.

    d. Check the patient's circulation by pinching each of his fingers.

    e. Insert the elbow of the right arm into the pouch end of the sling.

7. Rheumatoid arthritis is a(n):

    a. joint failure.

    b. bone fracture.

    c. skeletal tumor.

    d. autoimmune disease.

    e. spine disorder.

8. Tendonitis that is caused by calcium deposits is called:

   a. fibromyalgia.

   b. iontophoresis.

   c. hardened tendons.

   d. calcific tendonitis.

   e. depository tendonitis.

Scenario for questions 9 and 10: A 20-year-old female patient is visiting your office because of pain in her knee. During the patient interview, the patient tells you that she experiences pain when walking down stairs and getting out of bed. You learn that she is very active and is a member of her university's track and field team.

9. What musculoskeletal disorder does this patient have?

   a. Plantar fasciitis

   b. Lateral humeral epicondylitis

   c. Dupuytren contracture

   d. Chondromalacia patellae

   e. Ankylosing spondylitis

10. What surgical procedure may need to be performed to repair or remove damaged cartilage if the patient's case is severe?

   a. Arthrogram

   b. Arthroplasty

   c. Arthroscopy

   d. Phonophoresis

   e. Electromyography

11. You should *not* apply cold to:

   a. open wounds.

   b. the pregnant uterus.

   c. acute inflammation.

   d. the very young and older adults.

   e. a contusion.

12. Proper cane length calls for the cane to be level with the user's greater trochanter and for the user's elbow to be bent at a:

   a. 30-degree angle.

   b. 50-degree angle.

   c. 60-degree angle.

   d. 80-degree angle.

   e. 90-degree angle.

13. A subluxation is a(n):

   a. dislocation of a facet joint.

   b. partial dislocation of a joint.

   c. complete dislocation of a joint.

   d. dislocation that damages the tendons.

   e. injury to a joint capsule.

14. How is immobilization during closed reduction achieved?

   a. Casting

   b. Surgery

   c. Exercise

   d. Splinting

   e. Ultrasound

15. You and the physician must wear goggles during a cast removal to protect against:

   a. flying particles.

   b. dangerous waves.

   c. unsanitary material.

   d. bloodborne pathogens.

   e. disease and infection.

16. If a fat embolus becomes lodged in a patient's pulmonary or coronary vessels, the patient may experience:

   a. limited mobility.

   b. pain and swelling.

   c. a warm sensation.

   d. an infarction and death.

   e. swelling and numbness.

17. The most common site of bursitis is the:

   a. foot.

   b. wrist.

   c. elbow.

   d. shoulder.

   e. ankle.

18. Your patient has just received a fiberglass leg cast. Which of the following is a sign that proper circulation is present?

   a. Red, hot toes

   b. Swollen toes

   c. Clammy toes

   d. Cold, blue toes

   e. Warm, pink toes

19. Osteoporosis is a condition in which the bones lack:

   a. bursae.

   b. calcium.

   c. vitamin D.

   d. malignancies.

   e. marrow.

20. Your patient is recovering from a strain in his Achilles tendon. He is unable to use one leg, but he has coordination and upper body strength. Which of the following ambulatory assist devices should this patient use to gain mobility?

   a. Cast

   b. Cane

   c. Sling

   d. Walker

   e. Crutches

COG MATCHING

Grade: _____

Place the letter preceding the definition on the line next to the term.

Key Terms

21. _____ ankylosing spondylitis

22. _____ arthrogram

23. _____ arthroscopy

24. _____ arthroplasty

25. _____ bursae

26. _____ callus

27. _____ contracture

28. _____ contusion

29. _____ electromyography

30. _____ embolus

31. _____ goniometer

32. _____ iontophoresis

33. _____ kyphosis

34. _____ lordosis

Definitions

a. introduction of various chemical ions into the skin by means of electrical current

b. a deposit of new bone tissue that forms between the healing ends of broken bones

c. any artificial replacement for a missing body part, such as false teeth or an artificial limb

d. a mass of matter (thrombus, air, fat globule) freely floating in the circulatory system

e. small sacs filled with clear synovial fluid that surround some joints

f. a lateral curve of the spine, usually in the thoracic area, with a corresponding curve in the lumbar region, causing uneven shoulders and hips

g. an abnormal shortening of muscles around a joint caused by atrophy of the muscles and resulting in flexion and fixation

h. an abnormally deep ventral curve at the lumbar flexure of the spine; also known as swayback

i. ultrasound treatment used to force medications into tissues

j. surgical repair of a joint

k. an abnormally deep dorsal curvature of the thoracic spine; also known as humpback or hunchback

l. an examination of the inside of a joint through an arthroscope

m. x-ray of a joint

n. an instrument used to measure the angle of joints for range of motion

35. _____ Paget disease

36. _____ phonophoresis

37. _____ prosthesis

38. _____ reduction

39. _____ scoliosis

o. a collection of blood in tissues after an injury; a bruise

p. correcting a fracture by realigning the bones; may be closed (corrected by manipulation) or open (requires surgery)

q. a stiffening of the spine with inflammation

r. a recording of electrical nerve transmission in skeletal muscles

s. a degenerative bone disease usually in older persons with bone destruction and poor repair

---

COG MATCHING   Grade: _____

Place the letter preceding the condition on the line preceding the ambulatory assist device.

Devices

40. _____ crutches

41. _____ cane

42. _____ walker

Conditions

a. Patient A is a 53-year-old female who has recently undergone hip replacement surgery. She is able to walk and needs only slight assistance until she has fully healed from her surgery.

b. Patient B is a 17-year-old male with a sprained ankle. His condition is temporary, but he needs assistance walking with one affected leg.

c. Patient C is a 79-year-old female with osteoarthritis. She has trouble maintaining her balance when walking.

COG IDENTIFICATION   Grade: _____

43. Complete this chart to show the different types of fractures.

Type of Fracture	Description
Avulsion	Tearing away of bone fragments caused by sharp twisting force applied to ligaments or tendons attached to bone
Comminuted	**a.**
Compound or open	Broken end of bone punctures and protrudes through skin
b.	Damage to bone caused by strong force on both ends of the bone, such as through a fall
Depressed	Fracture of flat bones (typically the skull) which causes bone fragment to be driven below the surface of the bone
Greenstick	**c.**
Impacted	One bone segment driven into another
d.	Break is slanted across the axis of the bone

Pathological	Related to a disease such as osteoporosis, Paget disease, bone cysts, tumors, or cancers
Simple or closed	**e.**
Spiral	Appears as an S-shaped fracture on radiographs and occurs with torsion or twisting injuries
f.	A fracture at right angles to axis of bone that is usually caused by excessive bending force or direct pressure on bone

44. Complete this chart, which shows the variations of arthritis, the most commonly affected site, and the characteristics of the variation.

Disease	Affected Site	Characteristics
Osteoarthritis	Weight-bearing joints	**a.**
b.	Synovial membrane lining of the joint	Usually begins in non-weight-bearing joints, but can spread to many other joints; results in inflammation, pain, stiffness, and crippling deformities
Ankylosing spondylitis (or Marie-Strumpell disease)	**c.**	Rheumatoid arthritis of the spine; results in extreme forward flexion of the spine and tightness in the hip flexors
d.	Joint, usually the great toe	An overproduction of uric acid leads to a deposit of uric acid crystals in the joint; results in a painful, hot, inflamed joint; can become chronic

45. Review the list of tasks below and determine which tasks you may be responsible for as a medical assistant working in the clinical area. Place a check mark in the "Yes" column for those duties you may be responsible for doing and place a check mark in the "No" column for those tasks that you would not perform.

Task		Yes	No
a.	Instruct patients on how to use crutches, a cane, a walker, or a wheelchair.		
b.	Inform patients of the potential injury associated with heating pad use.		
c.	Perform arthroplasty to repair or remove cartilage damaged by chondromalacia patellae.		
d.	Assemble the supplies needed to cast a fractured bone.		
e.	Treat tendonitis with a transverse friction massage.		
f.	Help older adult patients avoid hip fractures by reviewing fall-prevention techniques.		
g.	Observe and report signs of a musculoskeletal disorder, such as skin color, temperature, tone, and tenderness.		
h.	Give patients specific and detailed instructions for applying heat or cold at home.		
i.	Identify the type of fracture and decide the method of treatment.		

46. Use the word bank to fill in the blanks in this paragraph about bone tumors.

The cause of malignant skeletal tumors is unknown but may be linked to rapid development of _____ during youth. An early sign of bone tumors is bone pain, which is most intense at night. Some bone tumors have the potential to spread to the skin and muscles. Bone tumors are identified by _____ after a bone scan reveals the need for further diagnosis. Treatments include surgery, amputation, and _____.

Word Bank:

biopsy   bone tissue   chemotherapy
CT scan   osteosarcomas

COG SHORT ANSWER   Grade: _____

47. Describe these three abnormal spine curvatures.

   a. Lordosis: _____

   b. Kyphosis: _____

   c. Scoliolis: _____

48. What is the difference between a sprain and a strain? How are they similar?

_____

_____

_____

_____

49. Name four common sites of dislocations.

_____

_____

_____

_____

50. Your patient is complaining of pain in his wrist. You learn that the pain began after he fell from a ladder and used his hand to break his fall. What would be signs that the patient has fractured his arm?

_____

_____

_____

_____

51. What is the difference between a spiral fracture and an avulsion fracture?

_____

_____

_____

_____

52. What test is performed that determines whether back pain results from a herniated intervertebral disc? How is the test done, and what is a positive indicator?

_____

_____

_____

_____

53. Both heat and cold treatments are used to relieve pain, but how do their uses differ?

_____

_____

_____

_____

54. List the five gaits utilized by patients who use crutches to assist them with walking.

_____

_____

_____

_____

55. The physician has just applied a plaster cast to a patient. What instructions and information should you give to the patient regarding her plaster cast?

_____

_____

_____

COG TRUE OR FALSE?

Grade: _____

Indicate whether the statements are true or false by placing the letter T (true) or F (false) on the line preceding the statement.

56. _____ Heat, such as heat from a heating pad or hot water bottle, should not be applied to the uterus of a pregnant woman.

57. _____ A greenstick fracture is a partial or incomplete fracture in which only one side of the bone is broken.

58. _____ The swing-through gait is the gait most commonly used to train patients to use crutches.

59. _____ Fibromyalgia is easy to diagnose because the symptoms are constant and centrally located in one joint socket.

COG **AFF** CASE STUDIES FOR CRITICAL THINKING

Grade: _____

1. Deirdre is a 52-year-old patient. She visits the office with a complaint of joint pain. After taking Deirdre's height and weight measurements, you notice that she is 1 1/2 inches shorter than she was just 2 years ago. After speaking with the patient, you learn that she does not exercise. The physician suspects Deirdre may have osteoporosis. What tests might the physician order to confirm his diagnosis? What preventative medicine information might be useful for Deirdre?

_____

_____

_____

_____

2. Maddy, a 9-year-old patient, needs to have her arm put into a cast after it is discovered that she has a greenstick fracture. The physician informs Maddy's mother that he will be using a fiberglass cast to immobilize Maddy's arm. Maddy's mother grows concerned after speaking with the physician. She has heard that fiberglass can be dangerous, and she wonders why the physician does not use a plaster like the cast she received when she was a child with a fractured arm. Explain to Maddy's mother the benefits of a fiberglass cast over a plaster cast, especially when the patient is a young, active child.

_____

_____

_____

_____

3. Your coworker Ben is moving some boxes from the reception area to a closet in the office. As you walk by, you observe him bending his back and lifting a box with extended arms. You know that this method of lifting could lead to serious back problems, so you decide to speak to Ben about avoiding back strain. What should you say to Ben? How would you respond if he laughs and tells you he is fine?

_____

_____

_____

_____

4. A 46-year-old patient has been advised by the physician to avoid using his strained knee. After you secure an ice pack to the patient's knee, you begin to instruct the patient in how to care for his knee at home. While you are speaking, the patient interrupts you saying that he has had this injury before and will "just throw a heating pad on there" like he has done in the past. How would you respond to the patient?

_____

_____

_____

_____

PSY PROCEDURE 28-1 **Apply an Arm Sling**

Name: _____ Date: _____ Time: _____ Grade: _____

EQUIPMENT/SUPPLIES: A canvas arm sling with adjustable straps.

STANDARDS: Given the needed equipment and a place to work the student will perform this skill with
_____% accuracy in a total of _____ minutes. *(Your instructor will tell you what the percentage and time limits will be before you begin.)*

KEY: 4 = Satisfactory 0 = Unsatisfactory NA = This step is not counted

PROCEDURE STEPS	SELF	PARTNER	INSTRUCTOR
1. Wash your hands.	☐	☐	☐
2. Assemble the equipment and supplies.	☐	☐	☐
3. Greet and identify the patient; explain the procedure.	☐	☐	☐
4. **AFF** Explain how to respond to a patient who does not speak English.	☐	☐	☐
5. Position the affected limb with the hand at slightly less than a 90° angle.	☐	☐	☐
6. Place the affected arm into the sling with the elbow snugly against the back of the sling, and the arm extended through the sling with the hand and/or fingers protruding out of the opposite end of the sling.	☐	☐	☐
7. Position the strap from the back of the sling around the patient's back, over the opposite shoulder.	☐	☐	☐
8. Secure the strap by inserting the end through the two metal rings on the top of the sling and further bringing the end of the strap back, looping it through the top metal ring only.	☐	☐	☐
9. Tighten the strap so that the patient's arm in the sling is slightly elevated. Make sure the strap coming around the patient's shoulder and neck is comfortable, padding if necessary to prevent friction and pressure areas.	☐	☐	☐
10. Check the patient's level of comfort and distal extremity circulation.	☐	☐	☐
11. Document the appliance in the patient's chart.	☐	☐	☐

CALCULATION

Total Possible Points: _____

Total Points Earned: _____ Multiplied by 100 = _____ Divided by Total Possible Points = _____ %

PASS   **FAIL**   **COMMENTS:**

☐   ☐

Student's signature _____ Date _____

Partner's signature _____ Date _____

Instructor's signature _____ Date _____

PSY PROCEDURE 28-2 | **Apply Cold Packs**

Name: _____ Date: _____ Time: _____ Grade: _____

EQUIPMENT/SUPPLIES: Ice bag and ice chips or small cubes, or disposable cold pack; small towel or cover for ice pack; gauze or tape.

STANDARDS: Given the needed equipment and a place to work the student will perform this skill with _____% accuracy in a total of _____ minutes. *(Your instructor will tell you what the percentage and time limits will be before you begin.)*

KEY: 4 = Satisfactory 0 = Unsatisfactory NA = This step is not counted

PROCEDURE STEPS	SELF	PARTNER	INSTRUCTOR
1. Wash your hands.	☐	☐	☐
2. Assemble the equipment and supplies, checking the ice bag, if used, for leaks. If using a commercial cold pack, read the manufacturer's directions.	☐	☐	☐

3. Fill a nondisposable ice bag about two-thirds full.
   a. Press it flat on a surface to express air from the bag.
   b. Seal the container.
	☐	☐	☐

4. If using a commercial chemical ice pack, activate it now.	☐	☐	☐
5. Cover the bag in a towel or other suitable cover.	☐	☐	☐
6. Greet and identify the patient. Explain the procedure.	☐	☐	☐
7. **AFF** Explain how to respond to a patient who has cultural or religious beliefs that prohibit disrobing.	☐	☐	☐
8. After assessing skin for color and warmth, place the covered ice pack on the area.	☐	☐	☐
9. Secure the ice pack with gauze or tape.	☐	☐	☐
10. Apply the treatment for the prescribed amount of time, but no longer than 30 minutes.	☐	☐	☐
11. During the treatment, assess the skin under the pack frequently for mottling, pallor, or redness.	☐	☐	☐
12. Properly care for or dispose of equipment and supplies. Wash your hands.	☐	☐	☐
13. Document the procedure, the site of the application, the results including the condition of the skin after the treatment, and the patient's reactions.	☐	☐	☐

CALCULATION

Total Possible Points: _____

Total Points Earned: _____ Multiplied by 100 = _____ Divided by Total Possible Points = _____ %

PASS   **FAIL**   **COMMENTS:**

☐   ☐

Student's signature _____ Date _____

Partner's signature _____ Date _____

Instructor's signature _____ Date _____

PSY PROCEDURE 28-3 | **Use a Hot Water Bottle or Commercial Hot Pack**

Name: _____ Date: _____ Time: _____ Grade: _____

EQUIPMENT/SUPPLIES: A hot water bottle or commercial hot pack, towel or other suitable covering for the hot pack

STANDARDS: Given the needed equipment and a place to work the student will perform this skill with _____% accuracy in a total of _____ minutes. *(Your instructor will tell you what the percentage and time limits will be before you begin.)*

KEY: 4 = Satisfactory   0 = Unsatisfactory   NA = This step is not counted

PROCEDURE STEPS	SELF	PARTNER	INSTRUCTOR
1. Wash your hands.	☐	☐	☐
2. Assemble equipment and supplies, checking the hot water bottle for leaks.	☐	☐	☐
3. Fill the hot water bottle about two-thirds full with warm (110°F) water.	☐	☐	☐
a. Place the bottle on a flat surface and the opening up; "burp" it by pressing out the air.			
b. If using a commercial hot pack, follow the manufacturer's directions for activating it.			
4. Wrap and secure the pack or bottle before placing it on the patient's skin.	☐	☐	☐
5. Greet and identify the patient. Explain the procedure.	☐	☐	☐
6. **AFF** Explain how to respond to a patient who is from a different generation (older) than you are.	☐	☐	☐
7. After assessing the color of the skin where the treatment is to be applied, place the covered hot pack on the area.	☐	☐	☐
8. Secure the hot pack with gauze or tape.	☐	☐	☐
9. Apply the treatment for the prescribed length of time, but no longer than 30 minutes.	☐	☐	☐
10. During treatment, assess the skin every 10 minutes for pallor (an indication of rebound), excessive redness (indicates temperature may be too high), and swelling (indicates possible tissue damage).	☐	☐	☐
11. Properly care for or dispose of equipment and supplies. Wash your hands.	☐	☐	☐
12. Document the procedure, the site of the application, the results including the condition of the skin after the treatment, and the patient's reactions.	☐	☐	☐

CALCULATION

Total Possible Points: _____

Total Points Earned: _____ Multiplied by 100 = _____ Divided by Total Possible Points = _____ %

PASS   **FAIL**   **COMMENTS:**

☐   ☐

Student's signature _____ Date _____

Partner's signature _____ Date _____

Instructor's signature _____ Date _____

PSY PROCEDURE 28-4 Measure a Patient for Axillary Crutches

Name: _____ Date: _____ Time: _____ Grade: _____

EQUIPMENT/SUPPLIES: Axillary crutches with tips, pads for the axilla, and hand rests, as needed

STANDARDS: Given the needed equipment and a place to work the student will perform this skill with _____% accuracy in a total of _____ minutes. *(Your instructor will tell you what the percentage and time limits will be before you begin.)*

KEY: 4 = Satisfactory   0 = Unsatisfactory   NA = This step is not counted

PROCEDURE STEPS	SELF	PARTNER	INSTRUCTOR
1. Wash your hands.	☐	☐	☐
2. Assemble the equipment including the correct-size crutches.	☐	☐	☐
3. Greet and identify the patient.	☐	☐	☐
4. Ensure that the patient is wearing low-heeled shoes with safety soles.	☐	☐	☐
5. Have the patient stand erect. Support the patient as needed.	☐	☐	☐
6. **AFF** Explain how to respond to a patient who is hearing impaired.	☐	☐	☐
7. While standing erect, have the patient hold the crutches in the tripod position.	☐	☐	☐
8. Adjust the central support in the base. a. Tighten the bolts for safety when the proper height is reached. b. Adjust the handgrips. Tighten bolts for safety. c. If needed, pad axillary bars and handgrips.	☐	☐	☐
9. Wash your hands and record the procedure.	☐	☐	☐

CALCULATION

Total Possible Points: _____

Total Points Earned: _____ Multiplied by 100 = _____ Divided by Total Possible Points = _____ %

PASS	**FAIL**	**COMMENTS:**
☐	☐	

Student's signature _____ Date _____

Partner's signature _____ Date _____

Instructor's signature _____ Date _____

PSY PROCEDURE 28-5 | **Instruct a Patient in Various Crutch Gaits**

Name: _____ Date: _____ Time: _____ Grade: _____

EQUIPMENT/SUPPLIES: Axillary crutches measured appropriately for a patient

STANDARDS: Given the needed equipment and a place to work the student will perform this skill with _____% accuracy in a total of _____ minutes. *(Your instructor will tell you what the percentage and time limits will be before you begin.)*

KEY: 4 = Satisfactory   0 = Unsatisfactory   NA = This step is not counted

PROCEDURE STEPS	SELF	PARTNER	INSTRUCTOR
1. Wash your hands.	☐	☐	☐
2. Have the patient stand up from a chair:	☐	☐	☐
a. The patient holds both crutches on the affected side.			
b. Then the patient slides to the edge of the chair.			
c. The patient pushes down on the chair arm on the unaffected side.			
d. Then the patient pushes to stand.			
3. With one crutch in each hand, rest on the crutches until balance is restored.	☐	☐	☐
4. Assist the patient to the tripod position.	☐	☐	☐
5. **AFF** Explain how to respond to a patient who is visually impaired.	☐	☐	☐
6. Depending upon the patient's weight-bearing ability, coordination, and general state of health, instruct the patient in one or more of the following gaits:			
a. *Three-point gait:*			
(1) Both crutches are moved forward with the unaffected leg bearing the weight.	☐	☐	☐
(2) With the weight supported by the crutches on the handgrips, the unaffected leg is brought past the level of the crutches.			
(3) The steps are repeated.			
b. *Two-point gait:*			
(1) The right crutch and left foot are moved forward.	☐	☐	☐
(2) As these points rest, the right foot and left crutch are moved forward.			
(3) The steps are repeated.			

   c. *Four-point gait:*

      (1) The right crutch moves forward. ☐ ☐ ☐

      (2) The left foot is moved to a position just ahead of the left crutch.

      (3) The left crutch is moved forward.

      (4) The right foot moves to a position just ahead of the right crutch.

      (5) The steps are repeated.

   d. *Swing-through gait:*

      (1) Both crutches are moved forward.

      (2) With the weight on the hands, the body swings through to a position ahead of the crutches with both legs leaving the floor together. ☐ ☐ ☐

      (3) The crutches are moved ahead.

      (4) The steps are repeated.

   e. *Swing-to gait:*

      (1) Both crutches are moved forward. ☐ ☐ ☐

      (2) With the weight on the hands, the body swings to the level of the crutches with both legs leaving the floor.

      (3) The crutches are moved ahead.

      (4) The steps are repeated.

7. Wash your hands and record the procedure	☐	☐	☐

CALCULATION

Total Possible Points: _____

Total Points Earned: _____ Multiplied by 100 = _____ Divided by Total Possible Points = _____ %

PASS   **FAIL**   **COMMENTS:**

  ☐   ☐

Student's signature _____ Date _____

Partner's signature _____ Date _____

Instructor's signature _____ Date _____

Cognitive Domain

1. Spell and define the key terms
2. List and define disorders associated with the eye and identify commonly performed diagnostic procedures
3. List and define disorders associated with the ear and identify commonly performed diagnostic procedures
4. List and define disorders associated with the nose and throat and identify commonly performed diagnostic procedures
5. Describe patient education procedures associated with the eye, ear, nose, and throat
6. Identify common pathology related to each body system
7. Describe implications for treatment related to pathology

Psychomotor Domain

1. Measure distance visual acuity with a Snellen chart (Procedure 29-1)
2. Assist physician with patient care
3. Prepare a patient for procedures and/or treatments
4. Document patient care
5. Perform patient screening using established protocols
6. Measure color perception with an Ishihara color plate book (Procedure 29-2)
7. Instill eye medication (Procedure 29-3)
8. Practice standard precautions
9. Irrigate the eye (Procedure 29-4)
10. Irrigate the ear (Procedure 29-5)
11. Administer an audiometric hearing test (Procedure 29-6)
12. Instill ear medication (Procedure 29-7)
13. Instill nasal medication (Procedure 29-8)
14. Practice within standard of care for a medical assistant

Affective Domain

1. Apply critical thinking skills in performing patient assessment and care
2. Use language/verbal skills that enable patients' understanding
3. Demonstrate empathy in communicating with patients, family, and staff
4. Use appropriate body language and other nonverbal skills in communicating with patients, family, and staff
5. Demonstrate awareness of the territorial boundaries of the person with whom you are communicating
6. Demonstrate sensitivity appropriate to the message being delivered
7. Demonstrate recognition of the patient's level of understanding in communications
8. Recognize and protect personal boundaries in communicating with others
9. Demonstrate respect for individual diversity, incorporating awareness of one's own biases in areas including gender, race, religion, age, and economic status
10. Apply active listening skills
11. Apply local, state, and federal health care legislation and regulation appropriate to the medical assisting practice setting

ABHES Competencies

1. Assist the physician with the regimen of diagnostic and treatment modalities as they relate to each body system
2. Comply with federal, state, and local health laws and regulations
3. Communicate on the recipient's level of comprehension
4. Serve as a liaison between the physician and others
5. Show empathy and impartiality when dealing with patients
6. Document accurately

Name: _____   Date: _____   Grade: _____

COG MULTIPLE CHOICE

Circle the letter preceding the correct answer.

1. The Ishihara method is used to test:

    a. hearing.

    b. color vision.

    c. cataract growth.

    d. corneal scarring.

    e. for multiple allergies.

2. A physician who specializes in disorders of the ears, nose, and throat is an:

    a. optician.

    b. ophthalmologist.

    c. optometrist.

    d. otolaryngologist.

    e. otitis externa.

3. A common cause of diminished hearing is:

    a. tinnitus.

    b. nasopharynx.

    c. cerumen.

    d. Ménière disease.

    e. strabismus.

4. Epistaxis is considered severe if bleeding continues how many minutes after treatment has begun?

    a. 5

    b. 10

    c. 15

    d. 20

    e. 30

5. Which of the following statements is true about preventive eye care?

    a. Patients should have regular checkups to maintain healthy eyes.

    b. Adults should wear UV protected sunglasses, but children are not as susceptible.

    c. Goggles do not need to be worn if you are wearing your regular glasses.

    d. Patients should thoroughly wash hands before rubbing their eyes.

    e. Contact lenses cause scarring, so glasses are safer to use.

6. It's important to treat sinusitis immediately because:

    a. it can lead to severe cases of upper respiratory infections.

    b. new allergies might develop while the nasal membrane is infected.

    c. mucus may infect areas of throat, nose, and ears if left unchecked.

    d. vision may be affected from pressure of sinus cavities on the eyes.

    e. complications in the ear and brain may occur, causing damage.

7. One symptom of laryngitis is:

    a. earache.

    b. muscle soreness.

    c. coughing.

    d. inflamed tonsils.

    e. excessive mucus.

8. An infection of any of the lacrimal glands of the eyelids is:

    a. hordeolum.

    b. cataract.

    c. glaucoma.

    d. conjunctivitis.

    e. astigmatism.

9. Which of the following could the physician treat with a warm compress?

   a. Nosebleed

   b. Ear infection

   c. Tonsillitis

   d. Astigmatism

   e. Tinnitus

10. The common term for *otitis externa* is:

    a. pink eye.

    b. nosebleed.

    c. Ménière disease.

    d. swimmer's ear.

    e. presbycusis.

Scenario for questions 11 and 12: A patient comes in for an annual exam, and the physician diagnoses her with presbycusis and presbyopia. She complains of an intermittent, high whistling in her right ear and cloudy vision in both eyes.

11. Reading the symptoms and diagnosis above, the patient is most likely:

    a. an infant or a toddler.

    b. a young child to early teen.

    c. an older teen to early 30s.

    d. middle aged.

    e. a senior citizen.

12. One possible cause of the cloudy vision is:

    a. presbyopia.

    b. glaucoma.

    c. Ménière disease.

    d. cataracts.

    e. sinusitis.

13. What is a safe way to remove cerumen?

    a. Gently inserting a tissue into the ear canal

    b. Using a cotton swab and digging out as much as possible

    c. Drops of hydrogen peroxide dropped into the ear

    d. Using an otoscope to melt the earwax

    e. Blowing your nose

14. It's important not to use nasal preparations more than four times a day because they:

    a. severely damage your nasal cavity.

    b. may become addictive.

    c. dry out sinuses and cause congestion.

    d. cause irritation to the throat.

    e. can lead to allergies.

15. Color blindness is a result of:

    a. people failing the Ishihara test.

    b. patients being unable to differentiate between colors.

    c. a deficiency in the number of rods in the eye.

    d. a deficiency in the number of cones in the eye.

    e. the size and shape of the eye.

16. What important advice can you give children when dealing with contagious diseases like pink eye?

    a. Keep your hands washed and clean.

    b. Do not play with children who are sick.

    c. If you sneeze, immediately cover your face with your hand.

    d. Do not go to school if you are sick.

    e. Try to keep from touching anything others have already touched.

17. To test for pharyngitis or tonsillitis, the physician would most likely order:

    a. a blood sample.

    b. a urine sample.

    c. a reflex test.

    d. a throat culture.

    e. radiology.

18. Which form of strabismus is known as *convergent eyes*, in which the eyes are crossed?

   a. Esotropic

   b. Exotropic

   c. Hypotropic

   d. Hypertropic

   e. Nonconcomitant

19. The purpose of a hearing aid is to:

   a. fully restore the ability to hear.

   b. assist patients with permanent nerve damage.

   c. amplify sound waves.

   d. differentiate between tones.

   e. permanently correct hearing disabilities.

20. A common treatment for allergic rhinitis is:

   a. sleep.

   b. antihistamine medication.

   c. surgery.

   d. antibiotics.

   e. ear irrigation.

COG MATCHING

Grade: _____

Place the letter preceding the definition on the line next to the term.

Key Terms	Definitions
21. _____ astigmatism	**a.** physician who specializes in treatment of diseases and disorders of the ears, nose, and throat
22. _____ cerumen	**b.** an extraneous noise heard in one or both ears, described as whirring, ringing, whistling, roaring, etc.; may be continuous or intermittent
23. _____ decibel	
24. _____ fluorescein angiography	**c.** specialist who can measure for errors of refraction and prescribe lenses but who cannot treat diseases of the eye or perform surgery
	d. an instrument used for visual examination of the ear canal and tympanic membrane
25. _____ hyperopia	**e.** an incision into the tympanic membrane to relieve pressure
26. _____ intraocular pressure	**f.** unit of intensity of sound
	g. an unfocused refraction of light rays on the retina
27. _____ myopia	**h.** a misalignment of eye movements usually caused by muscle incoordination
28. _____ myringotomy	**i.** loss of hearing associated with aging
29. _____ ophthalmologist	**j.** specialist who grinds lenses to correct errors of refraction according to prescriptions
30. _____ ophthalmoscope	**k.** yellowish or brownish waxlike secretion in the external ear canal; earwax
31. _____ optician	**l.** physician who specializes in treatment of disorders of the eyes
32. _____ optometrist	**m.** farsightedness
33. _____ otolaryngologist	**n.** pathological changes in the cell structure of the retina that impair or destroy its function, resulting in blindness
34. _____ otoscope	**o.** infection of any of the lacrimal glands of the eyelids
35. _____ presbycusis	**p.** intravenous injection of fluorescent dye; photographing blood vessels of the eye as dye moves through the vessels

36. _____ presbyopia

37. _____ refraction

38. _____ retinal degeneration

39. _____ tinnitus

40. _____ tonometry

41. _____ hordeolum

42. _____ strabismus

q. measurement of intraocular pressure using a tonometer

r. lighted instrument used to examine the inner surfaces of the eye

s. bending of light rays that enter the pupil to reflect exactly on the fovea centralis, the area of greatest visual acuity

t. pressure within the eyeball

u. vision change (farsightedness) associated with aging

v. nearsightedness

COG IDENTIFICATION

Grade: _____

43. Fill in the chart below with three types of vision testing charts, and when you should use each.

Type of Vision Testing Chart	When You Would Use It
a.	
b.	
c.	

44. Identify the seven causes of hearing loss.

a. _____

b. _____

c. _____

d. _____

e. _____

f. _____

g. _____

COG SHORT ANSWER

Grade: _____

45. List five preventive eye care tips that you may be asked to educate patients to follow.

a. _____

b. _____

c. _____

d. _____

e. _____

46. A patient complains of loss of vision and blurring, and cataracts are found in both eyes. How would surgery correct these symptoms?

_____

_____

_____

_____

47. What is the difference between an optometrist and an optician?

_____

_____

_____

_____

48. What is astigmatism?

_____

_____

_____

_____

49. An examination of a patient's eye reveals an irregular corneal surface. What is the method used to diagnose a corneal ulcer?

_____

_____

_____

_____

50. A patient comes in complaining of vertigo, nausea, and slight hearing loss. What might the patient be suffering from?

_____

_____

_____

51. Why is otitis media so common in infants and young children?

_____

_____

_____

_____

52. What is the difference between audiometry and tympanometry?

_____

_____

_____

_____

53. List the initial therapy for common epistaxis.

_____

_____

_____

_____

54. Why is it so important to treat upper respiratory infections?

_____

_____

_____

_____

55. When is the physician likely to suggest that a patient receive a tonsillectomy?

_____

_____

_____

_____

56. What is a way to isolate the protein causing allergic reactions in a patient directly?

_____

_____

_____

_____

57. Where do nasal polyps usually occur?

_____

_____

_____

_____

COG TRUE OR FALSE?

Grade: _____

Indicate whether the statements are true or false by placing the letter T (true) or F (false) on the line preceding the statement.

58. _____ Diagnosis of vision loss of any type is done by testing the hearing using an audiometer.

59. _____ Swimmer's ear goes away on its own and does not need to be treated.

60. _____ Allergic rhinitis is another name for hay fever.

61. _____ A patient with tonsillitis should be told to rest his voice and speak as little as possible.

COG AFF CASE STUDIES FOR CRITICAL THINKING

Grade: _____

1. A patient calls in to the physician's office saying that pink eye is going around her son's school. He has not been complaining of pain in either eye, but she has noticed that his eyes are red and that he has been sniffing and coughing lately. She wants to know if she should bring him in for a checkup. What should you tell her?

_____

_____

_____

_____

2. A patient is interested in getting LASIK surgery to correct her nearsightedness. She is 24 years old, and both of her parents have strong prescriptions for nearsightedness as well. She asks you what the surgery will be like, and if there is any chance that her eyes might revert back to their previous state. What is LASIK surgery and what are the advantages and disadvantages of this procedure? Are there any side effects?

_____

_____

_____

_____

3. A middle-aged patient comes in for a routine checkup, and mentions a slight loss of hearing since the last exam. What tests would most likely be ordered by the physician to check his hearing? Are there any preventative education tips that you can give him about hearing loss?

_____

_____

_____

_____

4. A swimmer comes into the office complaining of recurrent swimmer's ear. She says she has used cotton swabs in the past to clear her ear canals, and asks if there is any particular medication she can apply to help keep her ear canals clean. How would you respond to this patient?

_____

_____

_____

_____

5. A young man comes in for a routine checkup, and mentions that he will soon be learning to drive. However, the physician gives him the Ishihara test, and the teen fails to differentiate between colors. What information can you give him about color blindness, and what encouragement can you give him in regard to his upcoming driving test?

_____

_____

_____

_____

6. A young boy is brought in because he is complaining of headaches in school. The physician determines that the boy needs glasses and that the headaches are from eye strain. However, the boy states that he does not want glasses because he is afraid his classmates will make fun of him. What would you say to him?

_____

_____

_____

_____

PSY PROCEDURE 29-1   Measure Distance Visual Acuity with a Snellen Chart

Name: _____ Date: _____ Time: _____ Grade: _____

EQUIPMENT/SUPPLIES: Snellen eye chart, paper cup or eye paddle

STANDARDS: Given the needed equipment and a place to work the student will perform this skill with _____% accuracy in a total of _____ minutes. *(Your instructor will tell you what the percentage and time limits will be before you begin.)*

KEY: 4 = Satisfactory   0 = Unsatisfactory   NA = This step is not counted

PROCEDURE STEPS	SELF	PARTNER	INSTRUCTOR
1. Wash your hands.	☐	☐	☐
2. Prepare the examination area (well lit, distance marker 20 feet from the chart).	☐	☐	☐
3. Make sure the chart is at eye level.	☐	☐	☐
4. Greet and identify the patient. Explain the procedure.	☐	☐	☐
5. **AFF** Explain how to respond to a patient who is hearing impaired.	☐	☐	☐
6. Position the patient in a standing or sitting position at the 20-foot marker.	☐	☐	☐
7. If he or she is not wearing glasses, ask the patient about contact lenses. Mark results accordingly.	☐	☐	☐
8. Have patient cover the left eye with the eye paddle.	☐	☐	☐
9. Instruct the patient not to close the left eye, but to keep both eyes open during the test.	☐	☐	☐
10. Stand beside the chart and point to each row as the patient reads aloud. **a.** Point to the lines, starting with the 20/200 line. **b.** Record the smallest line that the patient can read with no errors.	☐	☐	☐
11. Repeat the procedure with the right eye covered and record.	☐	☐	☐
12. Wash your hands and document the procedure.	☐	☐	☐

CALCULATION

Total Possible Points: _____

Total Points Earned: _____ Multiplied by 100 = _____ Divided by Total Possible Points = _____ %

PASS   **FAIL**   **COMMENTS:**

☐   ☐

Student's signature _____ Date _____

Partner's signature _____ Date _____

Instructor's signature _____ Date _____

PSY PROCEDURE 29-2 | **Measuring Color Perception**

Name: _____ Date: _____ Time: _____ Grade: _____

EQUIPMENT/SUPPLIES: Ishihara color plates, gloves

STANDARDS: Given the needed equipment and a place to work the student will perform this skill with _____% accuracy in a total of _____ minutes. *(Your instructor will tell you what the percentage and time limits will be before you begin.)*

KEY: 4 = Satisfactory 0 = Unsatisfactory NA = This step is not counted

PROCEDURE STEPS	SELF	PARTNER	INSTRUCTOR
1. Wash your hands, put on gloves, and obtain the Ishihara color plate book.	☐	☐	☐
2. Prepare the examination area (adequate lighting).	☐	☐	☐
3. Greet and identify the patient. Explain the procedure.	☐	☐	☐
4. **AFF** Explain how to respond to a patient who is developmentally challenged.	☐	☐	☐
5. Hold the first bookplate about 30 inches from the patient.	☐	☐	☐
6. Ask if the patient can see the "number" within the series of dots.	☐	☐	☐
a. Record results of test by noting the number or figure the patient reports.			
b. If patient cannot distinguish a pattern, record plate number–x (e.g., 4–x).			
7. The patient should not take more than 3 seconds when reading the plates.			
a. The patient should not squint nor guess. These indicate that the patient is unsure.	☐	☐	☐
b. Record as plate number–x.			
8. Record the results for plates 1 through 10.			
a. Plate number 11 requires patient to trace a winding line between x's.			
b. Patients with a color deficit will not be able to trace the line.	☐	☐	☐
9. Store the book in a closed, protected area to protect the integrity of the colors.	☐	☐	☐
10. Remove your gloves and wash your hands.	☐	☐	☐

CALCULATION

Total Possible Points: _____

Total Points Earned: _____ Multiplied by 100 = _____ Divided by Total Possible Points = _____ %

PASS   **FAIL**   **COMMENTS:**

☐   ☐

Student's signature _____ Date _____

Partner's signature _____ Date _____

Instructor's signature _____ Date _____

PSY PROCEDURE 29-3 | **Instilling Eye Medication**

Name: _____ Date: _____ Time: _____ Grade: _____

EQUIPMENT/SUPPLIES: Physician's order and patient record, ophthalmic medications, 2 × 2 gauze pad, tissues, gloves

STANDARDS: Given the needed equipment and a place to work the student will perform this skill with _____% accuracy in a total of _____ minutes. *(Your instructor will tell you what the percentage and time limits will be before you begin.)*

KEY: 4 = Satisfactory   0 = Unsatisfactory   NA = This step is not counted

PROCEDURE STEPS	SELF	PARTNER	INSTRUCTOR
1. Wash your hands.	☐	☐	☐
2. Obtain the physician order, the correct medication, sterile gauze, and tissues.	☐	☐	☐
3. Greet and identify the patient. Explain the procedure.	☐	☐	☐
4. Ask the patient about any allergies not recorded in the chart.	☐	☐	☐
5. **AFF** Explain how to respond to a patient who does not speak English.	☐	☐	☐
6. Position the patient comfortably.	☐	☐	☐
7. Put on gloves. Ask the patient to look upward.	☐	☐	☐
8. Use gauze to gently pull lower lid down. Instill the medication.	☐	☐	☐

a. *Ointment:* Discard first bead of ointment without touching the end of the tube.
   (1) Place a thin line of ointment across inside of lower eyelid.
   (2) Move from the inner canthus outward.
   (3) Release ointment by twisting the tube slightly.
   (4) Do not touch the tube to the eye.
	☐	☐	☐

b. *Drops:* Hold dropper close to conjunctival sac, but do not touch the patient.
   (1) Release the proper number of drops into the sac.
   (2) Discard any medication left in the dropper.
	☐	☐	☐

9. Release the lower lid. Have patient gently close the eyelid and roll the eye.	☐	☐	☐
10. Wipe off any excess medication with tissue.	☐	☐	☐

11. Instruct patient to apply light pressure on the puncta lacrimale for several minutes.	☐	☐	☐
12. Properly care for or dispose of equipment and supplies. Clean the work area.	☐	☐	☐
13. Wash your hands.	☐	☐	☐
14. Record the procedure.	☐	☐	☐

CALCULATION

Total Possible Points: _____

Total Points Earned: _____ Multiplied by 100 = _____ Divided by Total Possible Points = _____ %

PASS   **FAIL**   **COMMENTS:**

☐   ☐

Student's signature _____ Date _____

Partner's signature _____ Date _____

Instructor's signature _____ Date _____

PSY PROCEDURE 29-4 | Irrigating the Eye

Name: _____ Date: _____ Time: _____ Grade: _____

EQUIPMENT/SUPPLIES: Physician's order and patient record, small basin, irrigating solution and medication if ordered, protective barrier or towels, emesis basin, sterile bulb syringe or 15 to 20 cc syringe, tissues, gloves

STANDARDS: Given the needed equipment and a place to work the student will perform this skill with _____% accuracy in a total of _____ minutes. *(Your instructor will tell you what the percentage and time limits will be before you begin.)*

KEY: 4 = Satisfactory   0 = Unsatisfactory   NA = This step is not counted

PROCEDURE STEPS	SELF	PARTNER	INSTRUCTOR
1. Wash your hands and put on your gloves.	☐	☐	☐

2. Assemble the equipment, supplies, and medication if ordered by the physician.
    a. Check solution label three times.
    b. Make sure that the label indicates for ophthalmic use.
	☐	☐	☐

3. Greet and identify the patient. Explain the procedure.	☐	☐	☐
4. **AFF** Explain how to respond to a patient who is hard of hearing.	☐	☐	☐
_____			

5. Position the patient comfortably.
    a. Sitting with head tilted with the affected eye lower.
    b. Lying with the affected eye downward.
	☐	☐	☐

6. Drape patient with the protective barrier or towel to avoid wetting the clothing.	☐	☐	☐

7. Place basin against upper cheek near eye with the towel under the basin.
    a. Wipe the eye from the inner canthus outward with gauze to remove debris.
    b. Separate the eyelids with your thumb and forefinger.
    c. Lightly support your hand, holding the syringe, on the bridge of the patient's nose.
	☐	☐	☐

8. Holding syringe 1 inch above the eye, gently irrigate from inner to outer canthus.
    a. Use gentle pressure and do not touch the eye.
    b. The physician will order the period of time or amount of solution required.
	☐	☐	☐

9. Use tissues to wipe any excess solution from the patient's face.	☐	☐	☐
10. Properly dispose of equipment or sanitize as recommended.	☐	☐	☐
11. Remove your gloves. Wash your hands.	☐	☐	☐
12. Record procedure, including amount, type, and strength of solution; which eye was irrigated; and any observations.	☐	☐	☐

CALCULATION

Total Possible Points: _____

Total Points Earned: _____ Multiplied by 100 = _____ Divided by Total Possible Points = _____ %

PASS   **FAIL**   **COMMENTS:**

☐   ☐

Student's signature _____ Date _____

Partner's signature _____ Date _____

Instructor's signature _____ Date _____

PSY PROCEDURE 29-5 | **Irrigating the Ear**

Name: _____ Date: _____ Time: _____ Grade: _____

EQUIPMENT/SUPPLIES: Physician's order and patient record, emesis basin or ear basin, waterproof barrier or towels, otoscope, irrigation solution, bowl for solution, gauze

STANDARDS: Given the needed equipment and a place to work the student will perform this skill with _____% accuracy in a total of _____ minutes. *(Your instructor will tell you what the percentage and time limits will be before you begin.)*

KEY: 4 = Satisfactory 0 = Unsatisfactory NA = This step is not counted

PROCEDURE STEPS	SELF	PARTNER	INSTRUCTOR
1. Wash your hands.	☐	☐	☐
2. Assemble the equipment and supplies.	☐	☐	☐
3. Greet and identify the patient. Explain the procedure.	☐	☐	☐
4. **AFF** Explain how to respond to a patient who has dementia.	☐	☐	☐
_____			
_____			
_____			
_____			
5. Position the patient comfortably in an erect position.	☐	☐	☐
6. View the affected ear with an otoscope to locate the foreign matter or cerumen. **a.** *Adults:* Gently pull up and back to straighten the auditory canal. **b.** *Children:* Gently pull slightly down and back to straighten the auditory canal.	☐	☐	☐
7. Drape the patient with a waterproof barrier or towel.	☐	☐	☐
8. Tilt the patient's head toward the affected side.	☐	☐	☐
9. Place the drainage basin under the affected ear.	☐	☐	☐
10. Fill the irrigating syringe or turn on the irrigating device	☐	☐	☐
11. Gently position the auricle as described above using your nondominant hand.	☐	☐	☐
12. With dominant hand, place the tip of the syringe into the auditory meatus.	☐	☐	☐
13. Direct the flow of the solution gently upward toward the roof of the canal.	☐	☐	☐
14. Irrigate for the prescribed period of time or until the desired results are obtained.	☐	☐	☐
15. Dry the patient's external ear with gauze.	☐	☐	☐

16. Inspect the ear with the otoscope to determine the results.	☐	☐	☐
17. Properly care for or dispose of equipment and supplies. Clean the work area.	☐	☐	☐
18. Wash your hands.	☐	☐	☐
19. Record the procedure in the patient's chart.	☐	☐	☐

CALCULATION

Total Possible Points: _____

Total Points Earned: _____ Multiplied by 100 = _____ Divided by Total Possible Points = _____ %

PASS   **FAIL**   **COMMENTS:**

☐   ☐

Student's signature _____ Date _____

Partner's signature _____ Date _____

Instructor's signature _____ Date _____

PSY PROCEDURE 29-6 Perform an Audiometric Hearing Test

Name: _____   Date: _____   Time: _____   Grade: _____

EQUIPMENT/SUPPLIES: Audiometer, otoscope

STANDARDS: Given the needed equipment and a place to work the student will perform this skill with _____% accuracy in a total of _____ minutes. *(Your instructor will tell you what the percentage and time limits will be before you begin.)*

KEY: 4 = Satisfactory   0 = Unsatisfactory   NA = This step is not counted

PROCEDURE STEPS	SELF	PARTNER	INSTRUCTOR
1. Wash your hands.	☐	☐	☐
2. Greet and identify patient. Explain the procedure.	☐	☐	☐
3. **AFF** Explain how to respond to a patient who is visually impaired.	☐	☐	☐
4. Take patient to a quiet area or room for testing.	☐	☐	☐
5. Visually inspect the ear canal and tympanic membrane before the examination.	☐	☐	☐
6. Choose the correct-size tip for the end of the audiometer.	☐	☐	☐
7. Attach a speculum to fit the patient's external auditory meatus.	☐	☐	☐

8. With the speculum in the ear canal, retract the pinna:
  a. *Adults:* Gently pull up and back to straighten the auditory canal.
  b. *Children:* Gently pull slightly down and back to straighten the auditory canal.
	☐
	☐
		☐
		☐
			☐
			☐

9. Follow audiometer instrument directions for use:
  a. Screen right ear.
  b. Screen left ear.
	☐
	☐
		☐
		☐
			☐
			☐

10. If the patient fails to respond at any frequency, re-screening is required.	☐	☐	☐
11. If the patient fails re-screening, notify the physician.	☐	☐	☐
12. Record the results in the medical record	☐	☐	☐

CALCULATION

Total Possible Points: _____

Total Points Earned: _____ Multiplied by 100 = _____ Divided by Total Possible Points = _____ %

PASS   **FAIL**   **COMMENTS:**

☐   ☐

Student's signature _____ Date _____

Partner's signature _____ Date _____

Instructor's signature _____ Date _____

PSY PROCEDURE 29-7 Instilling Ear Medication

Name: _____ Date: _____ Time: _____ Grade: _____

EQUIPMENT/SUPPLIES: Physician's order and patient record, otic medication with dropper, cotton balls

STANDARDS: Given the needed equipment and a place to work the student will perform this skill with _____% accuracy in a total of _____ minutes. *(Your instructor will tell you what the percentage and time limits will be before you begin.)*

KEY: 4 = Satisfactory   0 = Unsatisfactory   NA = This step is not counted

PROCEDURE STEPS	SELF	PARTNER	INSTRUCTOR
1. Wash your hands.	☐	☐	☐
2. Assemble the equipment, supplies, and medication if ordered by the physician.	☐	☐	☐
a. Check solution label three times.	☐	☐	☐
b. Make sure that the label indicates for otic use.			
3. Greet and identify the patient. Explain the procedure.	☐	☐	☐
4. Ask patient about any allergies not documented.	☐	☐	☐
5. **AFF** Explain how to respond to a patient who does not speak English.	☐	☐	☐
_____			
_____			
_____			
_____			
6. Have the patient seated with the affected ear tilted upward.	☐	☐	☐
7. Draw up the ordered amount of medication.			
a. *Adults:* Pull the auricle slightly up and back to straighten the S-shaped canal.	☐	☐	☐
b. *Children:* Pull the auricle slightly down and back to straighten the S-shaped canal.	☐	☐	☐
8. Insert the tip of dropper without touching the patient's skin.			
a. Let the medication flow along the side of the canal.	☐	☐	☐
b. Have patient sit or lie with affected ear upward for about 5 minutes.	☐	☐	☐
9. To keep medication in the canal, gently insert a moist cotton ball into the external auditory meatus.	☐	☐	☐
10. Properly care for or dispose of equipment and supplies. Clean the work area.	☐	☐	☐
11. Wash your hands.	☐	☐	☐
12. Record the procedure in the patient record.	☐	☐	☐

CALCULATION

Total Possible Points: _____

Total Points Earned: _____ Multiplied by 100 = _____ Divided by Total Possible Points = _____ %

PASS	FAIL	COMMENTS:
☐	☐	

Student's signature _____ Date _____

Partner's signature _____ Date _____

Instructor's signature _____ Date _____

PSY PROCEDURE 29-8 **Instilling Nasal Medication**

Name: _____ Date: _____ Time: _____ Grade: _____

EQUIPMENT/SUPPLIES: Physician's order and patient record; nasal medication, drops, or spray; tissues; gloves

STANDARDS: Given the needed equipment and a place to work the student will perform this skill with _____% accuracy in a total of _____ minutes. *(Your instructor will tell you what the percentage and time limits will be before you begin.)*

KEY: 4 = Satisfactory 0 = Unsatisfactory NA = This step is not counted

PROCEDURE STEPS	SELF	PARTNER	INSTRUCTOR
1. Wash your hands and put on gloves.	☐	☐	☐
2. Assemble the equipment and supplies. Check the medication label three times.	☐	☐	☐
3. Greet and identify the patient. Explain the procedure.	☐	☐	☐
4. Ask patient about any allergies not documented.	☐	☐	☐
5. **AFF** Explain how to respond to a patient who has dementia.	☐	☐	☐
_____			
6. Position the patient in a comfortable recumbent position.			
a. Extend patient's head beyond edge of examination table.	☐	☐	☐
b. Or place a pillow under the patient's shoulders.	☐	☐	☐
c. Support the patient's neck to avoid strain as the head is tilted back.	☐	☐	☐
7. Administering nasal medication:			
a. Nasal drops	☐	☐	☐
(1) Hold the dropper upright just above each nostril.			
(2) Drop the medication one drop at a time without touching the nares.			
(3) Keep the patient in a recumbent position for 5 minutes.	☐	☐	☐
b. Nasal spray			
(1) Place tip of the bottle at the naris opening without touching the patient.			
(2) Spray as the patient takes a deep breath.			

8. Wipe any excess medication from the patient's skin with tissues.	☐	☐	☐
9. Properly care for or dispose of equipment and supplies. Clean the work area.	☐	☐	☐
10. Remove your gloves and wash your hands.	☐	☐	☐
11. Record the procedure in the patient's chart.	☐	☐	☐

CALCULATION

Total Possible Points: _____

Total Points Earned: _____ Multiplied by 100 = _____ Divided by Total Possible Points = _____ %

PASS   **FAIL**   **COMMENTS:**

☐   ☐

Student's signature _____ Date _____

Partner's signature _____ Date _____

Instructor's signature _____ Date _____

Pulmonary Medicine

Cognitive Domain

1. Spell and define the key terms
2. Identify the primary defense mechanisms of the respiratory system
3. Identify common pathology related to each body system
4. Explain various diagnostic procedures of the respiratory system
5. Describe implications for treatment related to pathology
6. Describe the physician's examination of the respiratory system
7. Discuss the role of the medical assistant with regard to various diagnostic and therapeutic procedures

Psychomotor Domain

1. Instruct a patient in the use of the peak flowmeter (Procedure 30-1)
2. Assist physician with patient care
3. Prepare a patient for procedures and/or treatments
4. Practice standard precautions
5. Perform patient screening using established protocols
6. Document patient care
7. Document patient education
8. Administer a nebulized breathing treatment (Procedure 30-2)
9. Perform a pulmonary function test (Procedure 30-3)
10. Practice within the standard of care for a medical assistant

Affective Domain

1. Apply critical thinking skills in performing patient assessment and care
2. Use language/verbal skills that enable patients' understanding
3. Demonstrate empathy in communicating with patients, family, and staff
4. Use appropriate body language and other nonverbal skills in communicating with patients, family, and staff
5. Demonstrate awareness of the territorial boundaries of the person with whom you are communicating
6. Demonstrate sensitivity appropriate to the message being delivered
7. Demonstrate recognition of the patient's level of understanding in communications
8. Recognize and protect personal boundaries in communicating with others
9. Demonstrate respect for individual diversity, incorporating awareness of one's own biases in areas including gender, race, religion, age, and economic status
10. Apply active listening skills
11. Apply local, state, and federal health care legislation and regulation appropriate to the medical assisting practice setting

ABHES Competencies

1. Assist the physician with the regimen of diagnostic and treatment modalities as they relate to each body system
2. Comply with federal, state, and local health laws and regulations
3. Communicate on the recipient's level of comprehension
4. Serve as a liaison between the physician and others
5. Show empathy and impartiality when dealing with patients
6. Document accurately

Name: _____   Date: _____   Grade: _____

COG MULTIPLE CHOICE

Circle the letter preceding the correct answer.

1. A pulmonary function test measures:

   a. arterial blood gases.

   b. oxygen saturation.

   c. sputum cells.

   d. tidal volume.

   e. fluid in lungs.

2. A patient in need of an artificial airway will likely undergo:

   a. laryngectomy.

   b. tracheostomy.

   c. chemotherapy.

   d. bronchoscopy.

   e. pneumonectomy.

3. Which procedure necessitates a stethoscope?

   a. Percussion

   b. Palpation

   c. Inspection

   d. Radiation

   e. Auscultation

4. Which of the following would be a normal pulse oximetry reading for someone with no lung disease?

   a. 96%

   b. 94%

   c. 92%

   d. 90%

   e. 88%

5. One lower respiratory disorder is:

   a. laryngitis.

   b. bronchitis.

   c. sinusitis.

   d. pharyngitis.

   e. tonsillitis.

6. Which of the following is anesthetized by cigarette smoke?

   a. Alveoli

   b. Bronchioles

   c. Mucus

   d. Cilia

   e. Trachea

7. The most prominent symptom of bronchitis is:

   a. severe wheezing.

   b. repeated sneezing.

   c. productive cough.

   d. shortness of breath.

   e. coughing blood.

8. Viral pneumonia differs from bacterial pneumonia in that:

   a. it can be treated by antibiotics.

   b. it might result in hospitalization.

   c. it affects gas exchange in the lungs.

   d. it may lead to a fever and cough.

   e. it spreads throughout the lungs.

9. People with asthma have difficulty breathing because their:

   a. airways are narrow.

   b. cilia are inoperative.

   c. alveoli are collapsed.

   d. bronchioles are too wide.

   e. lungs are underdeveloped.

10. A productive cough refers to a cough that produces:

   a. blood.

   b. nasal mucus.

   c. sputum.

   d. oxygen.

   e. antibodies.

11. A type of medication that opens the bronchioles and controls bronchospasms is a(n):

    a. corticosteroid.

    b. bronchodilator.

    c. antibiotic.

    d. antihistamine.

    e. decongestant.

12. The public health department should be alerted about a diagnosis of:

    a. tuberculosis.

    b. pneumonia.

    c. bronchitis.

    d. asthma.

    e. COPD.

13. Which of the following is true of emphysema?

    a. It is not associated with bronchitis.

    b. It causes inflammation of the nasal passages.

    c. It can be cured with steroids.

    d. It is usually reversible.

    e. It usually takes many years to develop.

14. The purpose of a nebulizer is to:

    a. turn a vaporous medicine into a liquid.

    b. administer an asthma treatment.

    c. turn a liquid medicine into a vapor.

    d. cure COPD.

    e. pump oxygen.

15. Of the following diseases affecting the respiratory system, which, in most cases, is linked to cigarette smoking?

    a. Liver cancer.

    b. Cystic fibrosis

    c. Laryngitis

    d. Lung cancer

    e. Allergic rhinitis

16. In the case of a patient receiving oxygen treatment, a cannula:

    a. stores the oxygen.

    b. separates oxygen from the air in a room.

    c. delivers oxygen to the airways.

    d. ensures proper flow of oxygen.

    e. prevents accidents caused by oxygen's flammability.

17. COPD patients may take medications that are also prescribed for patients with:

    a. Influenza

    b. Pneumonia

    c. Meningitis

    d. Lung cancer

    e. Asthma

18. One acute disease of the lower respiratory tract is:

    a. asthma.

    b. pneumonia.

    c. emphysema.

    d. sinusitis.

    e. COPD.

19. The best way to thin mucus in the airways is:

    a. oxygen therapy.

    b. steroid medication.

    c. to increase oral fluid intake.

    d. to consume a balanced diet.

    e. frequent exercise.

20. A physician may perform an arterial blood gas test to:

    a. determine how much gas is in a patient's lungs.

    b. determine whether a patient has a normal respiratory rate.

    c. determine when a patient will be ready for respiratory surgery.

    d. determine whether a patient will be receptive to oxygen therapy.

    e. determine whether the patient's lungs are adequately exchanging gases.

COG MATCHING

Grade: _____

Place the letter preceding the definition on the line next to the term.

Key Terms

21. _____ atelectasis

22. _____ chronic obstructive pulmonary disease (COPD)

23. _____ dyspnea

24. _____ forced expiratory volume (FEV)

25. _____ hemoptysis

26. _____ laryngectomy

27. _____ palliative

28. _____ status asthmaticus

29. _____ thoracentesis

30. _____ tidal volume

31. _____ tracheostomy

Definitions

a. coughing up blood from the respiratory tract

b. easing symptoms without curing

c. a permanent surgical stoma in the neck with an indwelling tube

d. a surgical puncture into the pleural cavity for aspiration of serous fluid or for injection of medication

e. a progressive, irreversible condition with diminished respiratory capacity

f. the volume of air forced out of the lungs

g. difficulty breathing

h. the amount of air inhaled and exhaled during normal respiration

i. an asthma attack that is not responsive to treatment

j. collapsed lung fields; incomplete expansion of the lungs, either partial or complete

k. the surgical removal of the larynx

COG IDENTIFICATION

Grade: _____

32. Place a check mark on the line to indicate if each symptom is a possible symptom of laryngeal cancer.

a. _____ hoarseness lasting longer than three weeks

b. _____ pain in the throat when drinking hot liquids

c. _____ wheezing

d. _____ a feeling of a lump in the throat

e. _____ chest pain

f. _____ burning in the throat when drinking citrus juice

g. _____ dyspnea

h. _____ night sweats

i. _____ general malaise

33. Which of the following is/are an element/elements of the traditional examination of the chest? Circle the letter preceding all that apply.

    a. Palpation

    b. Auscultation

    c. Sputum culture

    d. Chest radiography

    e. Inspection

34. Which of the following pulmonary diagnostic methods is considered invasive? Place a check mark on the line next to the appropriate diagnostic methods.

    a. _____ Percussion

    b. _____ Bronchoscopy

    c. _____ Auscultation

    d. _____ Sputum culture

    e. _____ Posteroanterior x-ray

COG SHORT ANSWER

Grade: _____

35. What is the most common cause of chronic obstructive pulmonary disease?

    _____

    _____

    _____

    _____

36. Why is the term *chronic obstructive pulmonary disease* used to characterize a patient suffering from emphysema and chronic bronchitis?

    _____

    _____

    _____

    _____

37. What are two of the most common causes of upper respiratory problems?

_____

_____

_____

_____

38. In the case of a pneumonia patient, what prevents effective gas exchange?

_____

_____

_____

_____

39. What is usually the etiology of chronic bronchitis?

_____

_____

_____

_____

40. What is a symptomatic difference between viral and bacterial pneumonia?

_____

_____

_____

_____

41. What is the role of the medical assistant in the collection and analysis of a sputum specimen?

_____

_____

_____

42. What is the purpose of a peak flow meter?

_____

_____

_____

_____

43. Under what circumstance would a physician perform a laryngectomy?

_____

_____

_____

_____

44. Describe the difference between palliative care and a cure.

_____

_____

_____

_____

45. What measures ought to be taken in the case of an asthmatic patient who does not respond to medication?

_____

_____

_____

_____

46. If a patient is prescribed two bronchodilator inhalers, what is the most likely explanation? Why would two be prescribed?

_____

_____

_____

47. Describe the typical prognosis of a lung cancer patient.

_____

_____

_____

_____

COG **TRUE OR FALSE?**   Grade: _____

Indicate whether the statements are true or false by placing the letter T (true) or F (false) on the line preceding the statement.

48. _____ An asthma patient will, upon contracting the disease, suffer from it for her entire life.

49. _____ Emphysema entails chronic inflammation of the airways.

50. _____ A patient who tests positive for tuberculosis is contagious.

51. _____ Lung cancer, one of the most common causes of death in men and women, is believed to result usually from cigarette smoking.

COG **AFF** **CASE STUDIES FOR CRITICAL THINKING**   Grade: _____

1. Your patient comes to the office with shortness of breath. The physician asks you to perform an arterial blood gas and send it to the laboratory stat. How would you respond to the physician?

_____

_____

_____

_____

2. A patient with a severe lung disease explains that she has been smoking for decades. You explain that she ought to quit, but she contends that it does not matter. She says she has already damaged her lungs enough that continuing to smoke will do no further harm. How do you respond to this patient?

_____

_____

_____

3. A patient receiving oxygen therapy calls to complain that his machine is not working. He does not know what to do. What suggestions do you have for the patient? What will you do to assist him?

_____

_____

_____

_____

4. Your patient has just been diagnosed with tuberculosis. Explain to him ways in which he should act to protect others while he undergoes treatment.

_____

_____

_____

_____

5. A healthy patient worries that his exposure to secondhand smoke of his coworkers might cause his health to deteriorate. You are aware of research suggesting that this is so; however, much of the research is controversial. How would you advise the patient?

_____

_____

_____

_____

6. A patient has just been diagnosed with lung cancer that the physician described as "not terribly aggressive and potentially curable." The patient asks you if this means that he will be okay. How do you respond?

_____

_____

_____

_____

PSY PROCEDURE 30-1 Instruct a Patient on Using the Peak Flow Meter

Name: _____ Date: _____ Time: _____ Grade: _____

EQUIPMENT/SUPPLIES: Peak flow meter, recording documentation form

STANDARDS: Given the needed equipment and a place to work the student will perform this skill with _____% accuracy in a total of _____ minutes. *(Your instructor will tell you what the percentage and time limits will be before you begin.)*

KEY: 4 = Satisfactory   0 = Unsatisfactory   NA = This step is not counted

PROCEDURE STEPS	SELF	PARTNER	INSTRUCTOR
1. Wash your hands.	☐	☐	☐
2. Assemble the peak flow meter, disposable mouthpiece, and patient documentation form.	☐	☐	☐
3. Greet and identify the patient and explain the procedure.	☐	☐	☐
4. Holding the peak flow meter upright, explain how to read and reset the gauge after each reading.	☐	☐	☐
5. **AFF** Explain how to respond to a patient who is visually impaired.	☐	☐	☐
6. Instruct the patient to place the peak flow meter mouthpiece into the mouth, forming a tight seal with the lips. After taking a deep breath, the patient should blow hard into the mouthpiece without blocking the back of the flow meter.	☐	☐	☐
7. Note the number on the flow meter denoting the level at which the sliding gauge stopped after the hard blowing into the mouthpiece. Reset the gauge to zero.	☐	☐	☐
8. Instruct the patient to perform this procedure a total of three times consecutively, in both the morning and at night, and to record the highest reading on the form.	☐	☐	☐
9. Explain to the patient the procedure for cleaning the mouthpiece of the flow meter by washing with soapy water and rinsing without immersing the flow meter in water.	☐	☐	☐
10. Document the procedure.	☐	☐	☐

CALCULATION

Total Possible Points: _____

Total Points Earned: _____ Multiplied by 100 = _____ Divided by Total Possible Points = _____ %

PASS   **FAIL**   **COMMENTS:**

☐   ☐

Student's signature _____ Date _____

Partner's signature _____ Date _____

Instructor's signature _____ Date _____

Name: _____ Date: _____ Time: _____ Grade: _____

EQUIPMENT/SUPPLIES: Physician's order and patient's medical record, inhalation medication, nebulizer disposable setup, nebulizer machine

STANDARDS: Given the needed equipment and a place to work the student will perform this skill with _____% accuracy in a total of _____ minutes. *(Your instructor will tell you what the percentage and time limits will be before you begin.)*

KEY: 4 = Satisfactory   0 = Unsatisfactory   NA = This step is not counted

PROCEDURE STEPS	SELF	PARTNER	INSTRUCTOR
1. Wash your hands.	☐	☐	☐
2. Assemble the equipment and medication, checking the medication label three times as indicated when administering any medications.	☐	☐	☐
3. Greet and identify the patient and explain the procedure.	☐	☐	☐
4. **AFF** Explain how you would respond to a patient who is deaf.	☐	☐	☐
5. Remove the nebulizer treatment cup from the setup and add the medication ordered by the physician.	☐	☐	☐
6. Place the top on the cup securely, attach the "T" piece to the top of the cup, and position the mouthpiece firmly on one end of the "T" piece.	☐	☐	☐
7. Attach one end of the tubing securely to the connector on the cup and the other end to the connector on the nebulizer machine.	☐	☐	☐
8. Ask the patient to place the mouthpiece into the mouth and make a seal with the lips, without biting the mouthpiece. Instruct the patient to breathe normally during the treatment, occasionally taking a deep breath.	☐	☐	☐
9. Turn the machine on using the on/off switch. The medication in the reservoir cup will become a fine mist that is inhaled by the patient breathing through the mouthpiece.	☐	☐	☐
10. Before, during, and after the breathing treatment, take and record the patient's pulse.	☐	☐	☐
11. When the treatment is over and the medication is gone from the cup, turn the machine off and have the patient remove the mouthpiece.	☐	☐	☐
12. Disconnect the disposable treatment setup and dispose of all parts into a biohazard container. Properly put away the machine.	☐	☐	☐
13. Wash your hands and document the procedure, including the patient's pulse before, during, and after the treatment.	☐	☐	☐

CALCULATION

Total Possible Points: _____

Total Points Earned: _____ Multiplied by 100 = _____ Divided by Total Possible Points = _____ %

PASS   **FAIL**   **COMMENTS:**

☐   ☐

Student's signature _____ Date _____

Partner's signature _____ Date _____

Instructor's signature _____ Date _____

PSY PROCEDURE 30-3   Perform a Pulmonary Function Test

Name: _____   Date: _____   Time: _____   Grade: _____

EQUIPMENT/SUPPLIES: Physician's order and patient's medical record, spirometer and appropriate cables, calibration syringe and log book, disposable mouthpiece, printer, nose clip

STANDARDS: Given the needed equipment and a place to work the student will perform this skill with _____% accuracy in a total of _____ minutes. *(Your instructor will tell you what the percentage and time limits will be before you begin.)*

KEY: 4 = Satisfactory   0 = Unsatisfactory   NA = This step is not counted

PROCEDURE STEPS	SELF	PARTNER	INSTRUCTOR
1. Wash your hands.	☐	☐	☐
2. Assemble the equipment, greet and identify the patient, and explain the procedure.	☐	☐	☐
3. **AFF** Explain how to respond to a patient who has dementia.	☐	☐	☐
4. Turn the PFT machine on, and if the spirometer has not been calibrated according to the office policy, calibrate the machine using the calibration syringe according to the manufacturer's instructions, and record the calibration in the appropriate logbook.	☐	☐	☐
5. With the machine on and calibrated, attach the appropriate cable, tubing, and mouthpiece for the type of machine being used.	☐	☐	☐
6. Using the keyboard on the machine, input patient data into the machine including the patient's name or identification number, age, weight, height, sex, race, and smoking history.	☐	☐	☐
7. Ask the patient to remove any restrictive clothing, such as a necktie, and instruct the patient in applying the nose clip.	☐	☐	☐
8. Ask the patient to stand, breathe in deeply, and blow into the mouthpiece as hard as possible. He or she should continue to blow into the mouthpiece until the machine indicates that it is appropriate to stop blowing. A chair should be available in case the patient becomes dizzy or lightheaded.	☐	☐	☐
9. Continue the procedure until three adequate readings or maneuvers are performed.	☐	☐	☐

10. Before, during, and after the breathing treatment, take and record the patient's pulse.	☐	☐	☐
11. After printing the results, properly care for the equipment and dispose of the mouthpiece into the biohazard container. Wash your hands.	☐	☐	☐
12. Document the procedure and place the printed results in the patient's medical record.	☐	☐	☐

CALCULATION

Total Possible Points: _____

Total Points Earned: _____ Multiplied by 100 = _____ Divided by Total Possible Points = _____ %

PASS   **FAIL**   **COMMENTS:**

☐   ☐

Student's signature _____ Date _____

Partner's signature _____ Date _____

Instructor's signature _____ Date _____

Cognitive Domain

1. Spell and define key terms
2. List and describe common cardiovascular disorders
3. Identify and explain common cardiovascular procedures and tests
4. Describe the roles and responsibilities of the medical assistant during cardiovascular examinations and procedures
5. Discuss the information recorded on a basic 12-lead electrocardiogram
6. Explain the purpose of a Holter monitor
7. Identify common pathologies related to each body system
8. Describe implications for treatment related to pathology

Psychomotor Domain

1. Perform electrocardiography (Procedure 31-1)
2. Apply a Holter monitor for a 24-hour test (Procedure 31-2)
3. Assist physician with patient care
4. Prepare a patient for procedures and/or treatments
5. Practice standard precautions
6. Document patient care
7. Document patient education
8. Practice within the standard of care for a medical assistant

Affective Domain

1. Apply critical thinking skills in performing patient assessment and care
2. Use language/verbal skills that enable patients' understanding
3. Demonstrate empathy in communicating with patients, family, and staff
4. Use appropriate body language and other nonverbal skills in communicating with patients, family, and staff
5. Demonstrate awareness of the territorial boundaries of the person with whom you are communicating
6. Demonstrate sensitivity appropriate to the message being delivered
7. Demonstrate recognition of the patient's level of understanding in communications
8. Recognize and protect personal boundaries in communicating with others
9. Demonstrate respect for individual diversity, incorporating awareness of one's own biases in areas including gender, race, religion, age, and economic status
10. Apply active listening skills
11. Apply local, state, and federal health care legislation and regulation appropriate to the medical assisting practice setting

ABHES Competencies

1. Assist the physician with the regimen of diagnostic and treatment modalities as they relate to each body system
2. Perform electrocardiograms
3. Comply with federal, state, and local health laws and regulations
4. Communicate on the recipient's level of comprehension
5. Serve as a liaison between the physician and others
6. Show empathy and impartiality when dealing with patients
7. Document accurately

Name: _____   Date: _____   Grade: _____

COG **MULTIPLE CHOICE**

Circle the letter preceding the correct answer.

1. Chronic cases of myocarditis may lead to heart failure with:

   a. endocarditis.

   b. cardiomegaly.

   c. asthma.

   d. bronchitis.

   e. congestive heart failure.

2. To identify the causative agent, proper diagnosis of endocarditis requires a(n):

   a. chest radiograph.

   b. blood culture.

   c. electrocardiogram.

   d. x-ray.

   e. stool sample.

3. Arrhythmia may occur if the sinoatrial node initiates electrical impulses:

   a. too quietly or too loudly.

   b. too roughly or too smoothly.

   c. too fast or too slowly.

   d. always.

   e. 60 to 100 times a minute.

4. When a patient's heart conduction system cannot maintain normal sinus rhythm without assistance, an electrical source can be implanted to assist or replace the sinoatrial node. This device is called a(n):

   a. pacemaker.

   b. artifact.

   c. Holter monitor.

   d. aneurysm.

   e. lead.

5. Which condition may result from rheumatic heart disease?

   a. Valvular disease

   b. Cardiac arrhythmia

   c. Angina pectoris

   d. Mitral valve stenosis

   e. Endocarditis

6. One symptom of coronary artery disease is:

   a. bleeding around the heart.

   b. chronic head cold.

   c. swollen tongue.

   d. pressure or fullness in the chest.

   e. leg pain.

7. Patients who are considered hypertensive have a resting systolic blood pressure above _____ and a diastolic pressure above _____.

   a. 120 mm Hg; 70 mm Hg

   b. 130 mm Hg; 80 mm Hg

   c. 140 mm Hg; 90 mm Hg

   d. 150 mm Hg; 100 mm Hg

   e. 160 mm Hg; 110 mm Hg

8. Who is predisposed to varicose veins?

   a. People who use their brains more than their bodies

   b. People who run or jog excessively

   c. People who sit or stand for long periods of time without moving

   d. People who are obese over many years

   e. People who play a musical instrument

9. Another term for *thrombi* is:

   a. heart attack.

   b. blood clots.

   c. fever.

   d. racing heart.

   e. stroke.

10. Patients may refer to *anticoagulant medications* as:

    a. antipyretics.

    b. thrombolytics.

    c. sugar pills.

    d. thickening agents.

    e. blood thinners.

11. A common cause of cerebrovascular accident is:

    a. damage to the blood vessels in the heart.

    b. blockage of the cerebral artery by a thrombus.

    c. weakness or paralysis.

    d. pulmonary embolism.

    e. pleuritic chest pain.

12. Another term for *transient ischemic attack* is:

    a. peripheral vascular occlusion.

    b. mini-stroke.

    c. heart attack.

    d. brain damage.

    e. slurred speech.

13. Deficiencies in hemoglobin or in the numbers of red blood cells result in:

    a. tachycardia.

    b. thrombus.

    c. stroke.

    d. anemia.

    e. aneurysm.

14. During the physician's examination, what is used to evaluate the efficiency of the circulatory pathways and peripheral pulses?

    a. Palpation

    b. Blood pressure

    c. Weight

    d. Height

    e. Sign of fever

15. Electrocardiograms are not used to detect:

    a. ischemia.

    b. delays in impulse conduction.

    c. hypertrophy of the cardiac chambers.

    d. arrhythmias.

    e. heart murmurs.

16. How many leads does the standard ECG have?

    a. 2

    b. 10

    c. 12

    d. 18

    e. 20

17. A patient must keep a daily diary of activities when:

    a. wearing a Holter monitor.

    b. preparing for a cardiac examination.

    c. having an ECG.

    d. taking anticoagulants.

    e. completing a cardiac stress test.

18. Many patients with CHF have an enlarged:

    a. chest.

    b. throat.

    c. lung.

    d. heart.

    e. brain.

19. A person who can read and perform ECGs is called a(n):

    a. medical assistant.

    b. phlebotomist.

    c. ultrasonographer.

    d. sound technician.

    e. neurologist.

20. If atherosclerotic plaques are found during a catheterization, which procedure may be performed?

    a. Bypass graft

    b. Angioplasty

    c. Echocardiogram

    d. ECG

    e. Ultrasonograph

Grade: _____

Place the letter preceding the definition on the line next to the term.

Key Terms

21. _____ aneurysm

22. _____ angina pectoris

23. _____ artifact

24. _____ atherosclerosis

25. _____ bradycardia

26. _____ cardiomegaly

27. _____ cardiomyopathy

28. _____ cerebrovascular accident (CVA)

29. _____ congestive heart failure

30. _____ electrocardiography

31. _____ coronary artery bypass graft

32. _____ endocarditis

33. _____ leads

34. _____ myocardial infarction (MI)

35. _____ myocarditis

36. _____ palpitations

37. _____ percutaneous transluminal coronary angioplasty (PTCA)

38. _____ pericarditis

39. _____ tachycardia

40. _____ transient ischemic attack (TIA)

Definitions

a. a heart rate of less than 60 beats per minute

b. any disease affecting the myocardium

c. a surgical procedure that increases the blood flow to the heart by bypassing the occluded or blocked vessel with a graft

d. any activity recorded in an electrocardiogram caused by extraneous activity such as patient movement, loose lead, or electrical interference

e. a procedure that improves blood flow through a coronary artery by pressing the plaque against the wall of an artery with a balloon on a catheter, allowing for more blood flow

f. an inflammation of the inner lining of the heart

g. a death of cardiac muscle due to lack of blood flow to the muscle; also known as heart attack

h. a local dilation in a blood vessel wall

i. a heart rate of more than 100 beats per minute

j. an acute episode of cerebrovascular insuffiency, usually a result of narrowing of an artery by atherosclerotic plaques, emboli, or vasospasm; usually passes quickly, but should be considered a warning for predisposition to cerebrovascular accidents

k. electrodes or electrical connections attached to the body to record electrical impulses in the body, especially the heart or brain

l. paroxysmal chest pain usually caused by a decrease in blood flow to the heart muscle due to coronary occlusion

m. ischemia of the brain due to an occlusion of the blood vessels supplying blood to the brain, resulting in varying degrees of debilitation

n. a buildup of fatty plaque on the interior lining of arteries

o. the feeling of an increased heart rate or pounding heart that may be felt during an emotional response or a cardiac disorder

p. a condition in which the heart cannot pump effectively

q. an inflammation of the sac that covers the heart

r. a procedure that produces a record of the electrical activity of the heart

s. an enlarged heart muscle

t. an inflammation of the myocardial layer of the heart

COG **MATCHING**

Grade: _____

Place the letter preceding the description on the line preceding the cardiac condition.

Conditions	Descriptions
41. _____ congestive heart failure	**a.** occurs when some of the electrical signals originate in the ventricles rather than in the SA node
42. _____ myocardial infarction	**b.** a shock administered to restore normal cardiac electrical activity
43. _____ ventricular tachycardia	**c.** symptoms may be similar to those felt during angina pectoris
44. _____ ventricular fibrillation	**d.** may occur if the SA node initiates electrical impulses too fast or too slowly
45. _____ arrhythmia	**e.** failure of the left ventricle leads to pulmonary congestion

COG **MATCHING**

Grade: _____

Place the letter preceding the description on the line preceding the cardiac procedure.

Procedures	Descriptions
46. _____ electrocardiogram	**a.** provides valuable information about the anatomical location and gross structures of the heart, great vessels, and lungs
47. _____ chest radiography	**b.** uses sounds waves generated by a small device called a transducer
48. _____ cardiac stress test	**c.** a graphic record of the electrical current as it progresses through the heart
49. _____ echocardiography	**d.** common invasive procedure used to help diagnose or treat conditions affecting coronary arterial circulation
50. _____ cardiac catheterization	**e.** measures the response of the cardiac muscle to increased demands for oxygen

COG IDENTIFICATION

Grade: _____

51. Cardiac inflammation, or carditis, is a disorder of the heart that is usually the result of infection. In the chart below are descriptions of the three types of carditis. Read the descriptions and fill in the missing boxes with the correct type of carditis.

Disorder	Causes	Signs and Symptoms	Treatment
a. _____	a pathogen, neoplasm, or autoimmune disorder, such as lupus erythematosus or rheumatoid arthritis	sharp pain in the same locations as myocardial infarction	relieving the symptoms and, if possible, correcting the underlying cause, including administering an antibiotic for bacterial infection
b. _____	radiation, chemicals, and bacterial, viral, or parasitic infection	early signs: fever, fatigue, and mild chest pain chronic: cardiomegaly, arrhythmias, valvulitis	supportive care and medication as ordered by the physician to kill the responsible pathogen
c. _____	infection or inflammation of the inner lining of the heart, the endocardium	reflux, or backflow, of the valves or blood	directed at eliminating the infecting organism

Identify and circle the letter preceding the best answer.

52. Valvular disease is:

a. inflammatory lesions of the connective tissues, particularly in the heart joints, and subcutaneous tissues.

b. an acquired or congenital abnormality of any of the four cardiac valves.

c. a collection of fatty plaques made of calcium and cholesterol inside the walls of blood vessels.

d. a disordered blood flow within the valvular walls of the heart.

53. Atherosclerosis can sometimes result in:

a. rheumatic heart disease.

b. valvular disease.

c. coronary artery disease.

d. congestive heart failure.

54. Cerebrovascular accident (CVA) is sometimes called:

a. heart attack.

b. paralysis.

c. blood clot.

d. stroke.

55. Which of the following is a question you should ask the patient before a cardiovascular examination?

a. Are you currently pregnant?

b. How long have you had the pain/discomfort?

c. How often do you exercise?

d. What do you like to do in your free time?

56. A Holter monitor is used for:

    a. the diagnosis of intermittent cardiac arrhythmias and dysfunctions.

    b. obtaining a good-quality ECG without avoidable artifacts.

    c. obtaining basic information about the anatomical location and gross structures of the heart, great vessels, and lungs.

    d. measuring the response of the cardiac muscle to increased demands for oxygen.

57. Read the risk factors for developing thrombi below and indicate whether the risk factor is primary (P), or inherited, versus secondary (S), or acquired.

    a. _____hemolytic anemia

    b. _____long term immobility

    c. _____chronic pulmonary disease

    d. _____thrombophlebitis

    e. _____sickle cell disease

    f. _____varicosities

    g. _____defibrillation after cardiac arrest

58. Identify whether each description describes lead I, lead II, or lead III:

    a. _____ measures the difference in electrical potential between the right arm (RA) and the left leg (LL).

    b. _____ measures the difference in electrical potential between the right arm (RA) and the left arm (LA).

    c. _____ measures the difference in electrical potential between the left arm (LA) and the left leg (LL).

COG SHORT ANSWER

Grade: _____

59. List five symptoms of the various heart disorders.

_____

_____

_____

_____

60. List the four causes of congestive heart failure.

_____

_____

_____

_____

61. Explain how a pacemaker helps the heart maintain normal sinus rhythm.

_____

_____

_____

_____

62. List six potential causes of anemia.

_____

_____

_____

_____

63. Explain angiography, one of the procedures used to diagnose atherosclerosis.

_____

_____

_____

_____

64. Explain why a physician often requires several blood pressure readings before making the diagnosis of hypertension.

_____

_____

_____

_____

65. List the six elements that are taken into consideration during the ECG.

_____

_____

_____

66. Explain the role of the medical assistant during an ECG.

_____

_____

_____

_____

COG **TRUE OR FALSE?**   Grade: _____

Indicate whether the statements are true or false by placing the letter T (true) or F (false) on the line preceding the statement.

67. _____ Congestive heart failure (CHF) is a condition in which the heart cannot pump effectively.

68. _____ Ventricular fibrillation is a medical emergency that occurs when the heart is contracting rather than quivering in an organized fashion.

69. _____ Diagnosis of atherosclerosis is often made by electrocardiography.

70. _____ Patients who have cerebrovascular accidents usually have varying degrees of weakness or paralysis of one side of the body.

COG **AFF** **CASE STUDIES FOR CRITICAL THINKING**   Grade: _____

1. You are interviewing a patient prior to a physical examination of the cardiovascular system. This is his first time in a medical office after many years' absence, and he is considerably anxious. What do you say to him to calm him down? How would you explain the procedure?

_____

_____

_____

_____

2. A patient comes into the office complaining of chest pain, nausea, and vomiting. Will he likely be admitted to the hospital right away? Why or why not?

_____

_____

_____

_____

3. A patient is given an artificial pacemaker. She would like to know how the device works and what changes she can expect from it. What do you tell her?

_____

_____

_____

_____

4. Why is it important that a patient continue taking her prescribed antihypertensive medication, even if her blood pressure has reached a manageable level?

_____

_____

_____

_____

5. Many cardiac conditions are preventable with proper diet and exercise. It's important to stress prevention over cure, because in most instances, there is no quick "cure." How will you send this message to patients? What kinds of tools will you use?

_____

_____

_____

_____

PSY PROCEDURE 31-1 Perform a 12-Lead Electrocardiogram

Name: _____ Date: _____ Time: _____ Grade: _____

EQUIPMENT/SUPPLIES: Physician order, ECG machine with cable and lead wires, ECG paper, disposable electrodes that contain coupling gel, patient gown and drape, skin preparation materials including a razor and antiseptic wipes

STANDARDS: Given the needed equipment and a place to work the student will perform this skill with
_____% accuracy in a total of _____ minutes. *(Your instructor will tell you what the percentage and time limits will be before you begin.)*

KEY: 4 = Satisfactory   0 = Unsatisfactory   NA = This step is not counted

PROCEDURE STEPS	SELF	PARTNER	INSTRUCTOR
1. Wash your hands.	☐	☐	☐
2. Assemble the equipment.	☐	☐	☐
3. Greet and identify the patient. Explain the procedure.	☐	☐	☐
4. Turn the ECG machine on and enter appropriate data into it. Include the patient's name and/or identification number, age, sex, height, weight, blood pressure, and medications.	☐	☐	☐
5. Instruct the patient to disrobe above the waist.	☐	☐	☐
a. Provide a gown for privacy.	☐	☐	☐
b. Female patients should also be instructed to remove any nylons or tights.	☐	☐	☐
6. Position patient comfortably in a supine position.	☐	☐	☐
a. Provide pillows as needed for comfort.	☐	☐	☐
b. Drape the patient for warmth and privacy.	☐	☐	☐
7. Prepare the skin as needed.			
a. Wipe away skin oil and lotions with the antiseptic wipes.	☐	☐	☐
b. Shave hair that will interfere with good contact between skin and electrodes.	☐	☐	☐
8. Apply the electrodes:			
a. Arms and legs: snugly against the fleshy, muscular parts of upper arms and lower legs according to the manufacturer's directions.	☐	☐	☐
b. Chest: V_1 through V_6.	☐	☐	☐
9. Connect the lead wires securely according to the color codes.	☐	☐	☐
a. Untangle the wires before applying them to prevent electrical artifacts.	☐	☐	☐
b. Each lead must lie unencumbered along the contours of the patient's body to decrease the incidence of artifacts.	☐	☐	☐
c. Double-check the placement.			

10. Determine the sensitivity and paper speed settings on the ECG machine.	☐	☐	☐
11. Depress the automatic button on the ECG machine to obtain the 12-lead ECG.	☐	☐	☐
12. When the tracing is printed, check the ECG for artifacts and standardization mark.	☐	☐	☐
13. If the tracing is adequate, turn off the machine.	☐	☐	☐
a. Remove the electrodes from the patient's skin.	☐	☐	☐
b. Assist the patient to a sitting position and help him or her with dressing if needed.	☐	☐	☐
14. **AFF** Explain how to respond to a patient who has dementia.	☐	☐	☐
15. For a single-channel machine, roll the ECG strip.	☐	☐	☐
a. Do not secure the roll with clips.	☐	☐	☐
b. This ECG will need to be mounted on an 8 × 11-inch paper or form.	☐	☐	☐
16. Record the procedure in the patient's medical record.	☐	☐	☐
17. Place the ECG tracing and the patient's medical record on the physician's desk or give it directly to the physician as instructed.	☐	☐	☐

CALCULATION

Total Possible Points: _____

Total Points Earned: _____ Multiplied by 100 = _____ Divided by Total Possible Points = _____ %

PASS   **FAIL**   **COMMENTS:**

☐   ☐

Student's signature _____ Date _____

Partner's signature _____ Date _____

Instructor's signature _____ Date _____

PSY PROCEDURE 31-2 | **Apply a Holter Monitor for a 24-Hour Test**

Name: _____ Date: _____ Time: _____ Grade: _____

EQUIPMENT/SUPPLIES: Physician's order, Holter monitor with appropriate lead wires, fresh batteries, carrying case with strap, disposable electrodes that contain coupling gel, adhesive tape, patient gown and drape, skin preparation materials including a razor and antiseptic wipes, patient diary

STANDARDS: Given the needed equipment and a place to work the student will perform this skill with _____% accuracy in a total of _____ minutes. *(Your instructor will tell you what the percentage and time limits will be before you begin.)*

KEY: 4 = Satisfactory   0 = Unsatisfactory   NA = This step is not counted

PROCEDURE STEPS	SELF	PARTNER	INSTRUCTOR
1. Wash your hands.	☐	☐	☐
2. Assemble the equipment.	☐	☐	☐
3. Greet and identify the patient.	☐	☐	☐
4. Explain the procedure and importance of carrying out all normal activities.	☐	☐	☐
5. Explain the reason for the incident diary, emphasizing the need for the patient to carry it at all times during the test.	☐	☐	☐
6. Ask the patient to remove all clothing from the waist up; gown and drape appropriately for privacy.	☐	☐	☐
7. Prepare the patient's skin for electrode attachment.	☐	☐	☐
a. Provide privacy and have the patient in a sitting position.	☐	☐	☐
b. Shave the skin if necessary and cleanse with antiseptic wipes.	☐	☐	☐
8. Apply the Holter electrodes at the specified sites:	☐	☐	☐
a. The right manubrium border.	☐	☐	☐
b. The left manubrium border.	☐	☐	☐
c. The right sternal border at the fifth rib level.	☐	☐	☐
d. The fifth rib at the anterior axillary line.	☐	☐	☐
e. The right lower rib cage over the cartilage as a ground lead.	☐	☐	☐
9. To do this, expose the adhesive backing of the electrodes and follow the manufacturer's instructions to attach each firmly. Check the security of the attachments.	☐	☐	☐
10. Position electrode connectors downward toward the patient's feet.	☐	☐	☐
11. Attach the lead wires and secure with adhesive tape.	☐	☐	☐
12. Connect the cable and run a baseline ECG by hooking the Holter monitor to the ECG machine with the cable hookup.	☐	☐	☐
13. Assist the patient to carefully redress with the cable extending through the garment opening. *Note:* Instruct the patient that clothing that buttons down the front is more convenient.	☐	☐	☐

14. Plug the cable into the recorder and mark the diary.	☐	☐	☐
a. If needed, explain the purpose of the diary to the patient again.	☐	☐	☐
b. Give instructions for a return appointment to evaluate the recording and the diary.	☐	☐	☐
15. Record the procedure in the patient's medical record.	☐	☐	☐

CALCULATION

Total Possible Points: _____

Total Points Earned: _____ Multiplied by 100 = _____ Divided by Total Possible Points = _____ %

PASS   **FAIL**   **COMMENTS:**

☐   ☐

Student's signature _____ Date _____

Partner's signature _____ Date _____

Instructor's signature _____ Date _____

Gastroenterology

Cognitive Domain

1. Spell and define key terms
2. List and describe common disorders of the alimentary canal and accessory organs
3. Identify and explain the purpose of common procedures and tests associated with the gastrointestinal system
4. Describe the roles and responsibilities of the medical assistant in diagnosing and treating disorders of the gastrointestinal system
5. Identify common pathologies related to each body system
6. Describe implications for treatment related to pathology

Psychomotor Domain

1. Assisting with colon procedures (Procedure 32-1)
2. Assist physician with patient care
3. Prepare a patient for procedures and/or treatments
4. Practice standard precautions
5. Document patient care
6. Document patient education
7. Practice within the standard of care for a medical assistant

Affective Domain

1. Apply critical thinking skills in performing patient assessment and care
2. Use language/verbal skills that enable patients' understanding
3. Demonstrate empathy in communicating with patients, family, and staff
4. Use appropriate body language and other nonverbal skills in communicating with patients, family, and staff
5. Demonstrate awareness of the territorial boundaries of the person with whom you are communicating
6. Demonstrate sensitivity appropriate to the message being delivered
7. Demonstrate recognition of the patient's level of understanding in communications
8. Recognize and protect personal boundaries in communicating with others
9. Demonstrate respect for individual diversity, incorporating awareness of one's own biases in areas including gender, race, religion, age, and economic status
10. Apply active listening skills
11. Apply local, state, and federal health care legislation and regulation appropriate to the medical assisting practice setting

ABHES Competencies

1. Assist the physician with the regimen of diagnostic and treatment modalities as they relate to each body system
2. Prepare patient for examinations and treatments
3. Recognize and understand various treatment protocols
4. Comply with federal, state, and local health laws and regulations
5. Communicate on the recipient's level of comprehension
6. Serve as a liaison between the physician and others
7. Show empathy and impartiality when dealing with patients
8. Document accurately

Name: _____ Date: _____ Grade: _____

COG MULTIPLE CHOICE

Circle the letter preceding the correct answer.

1. Which of the following can trigger an outbreak of the herpes simplex virus?

   a. Food allergy

   b. Illness

   c. Lack of sleep

   d. Medication

   e. Poor diet

2. What commonly causes leukoplakia to develop?

   a. Hereditary genes

   b. Excessive alcohol intake

   c. Lack of exercise

   d. Tobacco irritation

   e. Obesity

3. Why should a patient complaining of heartburn be assessed immediately?

   a. The symptoms of gastroesophageal reflux disease may be similar to the chest pain of a patient with cardiac problems.

   b. A patient with heartburn is more likely to develop a serious heart condition.

   c. Heartburn is a symptom of a weak lower esophageal sphincter.

   d. It is important to assess any gastrointestinal disorder immediately because they are usually serious.

   e. Heartburn may be symptomatic of Barrett esophagus, which requires immediate surgery.

4. Abnormal contact between the upper teeth and lower teeth is:

   a. malocclusion.

   b. dental caries.

   c. stomatitis.

   d. candidiasis.

   e. gingivitis.

5. If a patient is suffering from peptic ulcers, the symptoms will be most severe when the patient:

   a. is hungry.

   b. has a bowel movement.

   c. lies on his back.

   d. chews his food.

   e. is digesting a meal.

6. Gastroenteritis could become life threatening if a patient:

   a. is pregnant.

   b. suffers from diabetes mellitus.

   c. needs a heart operation.

   d. consumes excess alcohol.

   e. does not receive treatment immediately.

7. The study of morbid obesity is called:

   a. orthodontistry.

   b. gerontology.

   c. bariatrics.

   d. gastroenterology.

   e. pediatrics.

8. What is the minimum body mass index that a patient must have to be considered for gastric bypass surgery?

   a. 25

   b. 30

   c. 35

   d. 40

   e. 45

9. Crohn disease becomes life threatening when:

   a. the bowel walls become inflamed and the lymph nodes enlarge.

   b. the fluid from the intestinal contents cannot be absorbed.

   c. edema of the bowel wall takes place.

   d. scarring narrows the colon and obstructs the bowel.

   e. patients have periods of constipation, anorexia, and fever.

10. How does irritable bowel syndrome differ from Crohn disease?

    a. It does not involve weight loss.

    b. It is easily treatable.

    c. It is thought to be genetic.

    d. It requires a colectomy.

    e. It causes scarring.

    Scenario for questions 11 and 12: A patient is diagnosed with diverticulitis.

11. Which of the following treatments would the physician most likely recommend?

    a. Antibiotics

    b. Bed rest

    c. Antifungal agent

    d. Bland food

    e. Drinking less water

12. What advice might the physician have you give to the patient to help maintain good bowel habits in future?

    a. Never eat spicy foods.

    b. Get some form of daily exercise.

    c. Try to force a bowel movement at least once a day.

    d. Use laxatives when suffering from constipation.

    e. Cut out food products that contain wheat.

13. How can a patient decrease his or her risk of developing a hernia?

    a. Avoid lifting heavy objects.

    b. Switch from processed to organic foods.

    c. Maintain good bowel habits.

    d. Have regular medical checkups.

    e. Walk at least a mile every day.

14. What is the most effective treatment for appendicitis?

    a. Antibiotics

    b. Ileostomy

    c. Appendectomy

    d. Cryosurgery

    e. Radiation

15. Which of these factors increases the production of intestinal gas?

    a. Excess water

    b. Spicy or fatty foods

    c. Peristalsis

    d. Fast metabolism

    e. Lack of exercise

16. The most likely method of contracting hepatitis B is:

    a. contaminated food.

    b. poor hygiene.

    c. contaminated blood.

    d. stagnant water.

    e. weak immune system.

17. For which of the following procedures would the patient usually be put under anesthesia?

    a. Anoscopy

    b. Sigmoidoscopy

    c. Nuclear imaging

    d. Ultrasonography

    e. Endoscopic retrograde cholangiopancreatography

18. What is the caustic chemical secreted by the lining of the stomach that may cause erosion if too much of it is secreted?

    a. Pepsin

    b. Hydrochloric acid

c. Insulin

d. Oral mucosa

e. Melena

19. How does lithotripsy break down gallstones to make them easy to pass?

a. Lasers

b. Sound waves

c. Acidic liquid

d. Heat

e. Air pressure

20. Which piece of advice could best be given to a patient with a malabsorption syndrome by the physician?

a. Drink more water.

b. Eat less processed food.

c. Take vitamin supplements.

d. Cut out spicy foods.

e. Exercise more often.

21. Which of these groups of people are at the highest risk of developing esophageal cancer?

a. Teenagers

b. Pregnant women

c. Young children

d. Elderly women

e. Elderly men

22. A male patient comes to the physician's office complaining of an acute pain in his upper abdomen and back. He also suffers from indigestion and nausea, particularly when he tries to eat foods that have a high fat content. Which of the following gastrointestinal disorders does the patient probably have?

a. Cholelithiasis

b. Peptic ulcers

c. Gastritis

d. Leukoplakia

e. Caries

COG MATCHING

Grade: _____

Place the letter preceding the definition on the line next to the term.

Key Terms

23. _____ anorexia

24. _____ ascites

25. _____ dysphagia

26. _____ guaiac

27. _____ hematemesis

28. _____ heptomegaly

29. _____ hepatotoxin

30. _____ insufflator

31. _____ leukoplakia

32. _____ malocclusion

Definitions

a. an enlarged liver

b. a substance used in a laboratory test for occult blood in the stool

c. a device for blowing air, gas, or powder into a body cavity

d. the sum of chemical processes that result in growth, energy production, elimination of waste, and body functions performed as digested nutrients are distributed

e. black, tarry stools caused by digested blood from the gastrointestinal tract

f. the contraction and relaxation of involuntary muscles of the alimentary canal, producing wavelike movements of products through the digestive system

g. difficulty speaking

h. loss of appetite

i. a substance that can damage the liver

j. an accumulation of serous fluid in the peritoneal cavity

k. the use of chemical agents to treat esophageal varices to produce fibrosis and hardening of the tissue

33. _____ melena

34. _____ metabolism

35. _____ obturator

36. _____ peristalsis

37. _____ sclerotherapy

38. _____ stomatitis

39. _____ turgor

l. an inflammation of the mucous membranes of the mouth

m. an abnormal contact between the teeth in the upper and lower jaw

n. the normal tension in a cell or the skin

o. vomiting blood or bloody vomitus

p. the smooth, rounded, removable inner portion of a hollow tube, such as an ano-scope, that allows for easier insertion

q. white, thickened patches on the oral mucosa or tongue that are often precancerous

COG MATCHING

Grade: _____

Place the letter preceding the description on the line next to the name of the gastrointestinal disorder.

Disorders

40. _____ esophageal varices

41. _____ cholecystitis

42. _____ peptic ulcers

43. _____ stomatitis

44. _____ gastroesophageal reflux disease (GERD)

45. _____ diverticulosis

46. _____ hiatal hernia

Descriptions

a. a chronic disorder characterized by discomfort in the chest due to the backflow of gastric contents into the esophagus

b. a condition that occurs when part of the stomach protrudes up through the diaphragm

c. varicose veins of the esophagus resulting from pressure within the esophageal veins

d. an acute or chronic inflammation of the gall bladder

e. erosions or sores in the GI tract left by sloughed tissue

f. a disorder that usually occurs in the sigmoid colon, attributed to a diet deficient in roughage

g. an inflammation of the oral mucosa, caused by a virus, bacteria, or fungus

COG MATCHING

Grade: _____

Place the letter preceding the description on the line next to the examination method.

Examination Methods

47. _____ endoscopic studies

48. _____ nuclear imaging

49. _____ ultrasonography

Descriptions

a. instilling barium into the GI tract orally or rectally to outline the organs and identify abnormalities

b. injecting radionuclides into the body and taking images using a nuclear scanning device to detect abnormalities

c. using high-frequency sound waves to diagnose disorders of internal structures

50. _____ radiology studies

51. _____ sigmoidoscopy

52. _____ endoscopic retrograde cholangiopancreatography (ERCP)

53. _____ anoscopy

d. passing soft, flexible tubes into the stomach, small intestine, or colon for direct visualization of the organs

e. a method of injecting dye into the ducts of the gallbladder and pancreas; used to visualize the esophagus, stomach, proximal duodenum, and pancreas with a flexible endoscope

f. the insertion of a metal or plastic anoscope into the rectal canal to inspect the anus and rectum and swab for cultures

g. a visual examination of the sigmoid colon

IDENTIFICATION

Grade: _____

54. A patient comes into the office with abdominal pain and indigestion. The physician diagnoses the patient with a hiatal hernia. Which of the following diet modifications and treatments would the physician most likely suggest to the patient? Circle the correct answers. There may be more than one.

a. Eat small, frequent meals.

b. Exercise vigorously three times a week.

c. Elevate the head of the bed when sleeping.

d. Do not eat for 2 hours before bedtime.

e. Drink less water.

f. Lose weight.

55. As a medical assistant, you may be called on to assist with colon procedures in the medical office. Place a check mark on the line next to the task(s) that the medical assistant would be responsible for performing in the medical office.

a. _____ Instruct the patient in the procedure of stool sample collection.

b. _____ Help to educate the patient about diet and the prevention of gastric disorders.

c. _____ Prescribe pain medication and antibiotics.

d. _____ Schedule radiographic and ultrasound procedures in an outpatient facility.

e. _____ Test the stool specimen when it is returned to the office.

f. _____ Compile detailed dietary regimens for obese patients.

g. _____ Assist the physician in performing colon examinations.

h. _____ Diagnose minor gastrointestinal disorders.

56. Which of the following factors increase a person's risk of developing pancreatic cancer? Circle all that apply.

   a. being female

   b. drinking alcohol

   c. smoking

   d. being of African American descent

   e. being male

   f. being of Caucasian descent

   g. eating high-fat foods

   h. a history of working with industrial chemicals

57. Some gastrointestinal disorders require specialist knowledge and equipment outside of the physician's office. In the table below, place a check mark in the appropriate box to indicate whether a procedure could be carried out in the physician's office or would likely require an outpatient facility.

Procedure	Physician's Office	Outpatient Facility
a. Ultrasonography		
b. Anoscopy		
c. Endoscopic retrograde cholangiopancreatography		
d. Nuclear imaging		
e. Sigmoidoscopy examination		

COG SHORT ANSWER   Grade: _____

58. Identify the part of the digestive system where the following gastrointestinal disorders occur.

   a. Appendicitis _____

   b. Hepatitis _____

   c. Cholelithiasis _____

   d. Crohn disease _____

   e. Peptic ulcers _____

   f. Ulcerative colitis _____

   g. Diverticulosis _____

59. List three symptoms that could indicate a patient is suffering from gastric cancer.

_____

_____

_____

_____

60. A 40-year-old woman comes to the physician's office complaining of severe stomach cramps and vomiting. To help the physician assess her condition and make a diagnosis, the medical assistant should obtain some personal information. List four things that the physician will ask the patient before continuing with the exam.

_____

_____

_____

_____

61. A 25-year-old woman comes to the physician's office complaining of fatigue and joint pain. She looks jaundiced, and when the physician asks her for her medical history, she says that she recently returned from a 3-month trip to Ghana. Which two tests will the physician most likely recommend?

_____

_____

_____

62. As a medical assistant, part of your job may be to educate patients about the care of teeth and gums. List three things that you could tell a patient to do that might help to prevent dental caries.

_____

_____

_____

63. Which is the more widely accepted instrument to use during an endoscopic study: a rigid sigmoidoscope or a flexible fiberoptic sigmoidoscope? Explain your answer.

_____

_____

_____

_____

COG **TRUE OR FALSE?** Grade: _____

Indicate whether the statements are true or false by placing the letter T (true) or F (false) on the line preceding the statement.

64. _____ Oral cancers are more common among people who smoke.

65. _____ Cancer of the esophagus is common and can easily be treated.

66. _____ A sign that a patient has a problem with malabsorption of fats includes stools that are loose.

67. _____ Irritable bowel syndrome usually results in chronic weight loss.

COG **AFF** **CASE STUDIES FOR CRITICAL THINKING** Grade: _____

1. A 55-year-old woman comes to the physician's office and asks about gastric bypass surgery. She says that she has tried every diet available and is unable to lose weight. She suffers from shortness of breath and an inability to walk for long distances. You take the woman's vital signs and measure her height and weight. She appears to be in good health, but is at least 60 pounds over the ideal weight for her height. The physician later confirms these facts. Is the patient likely to be a candidate for gastric bypass surgery? Explain your answer.

_____

_____

_____

_____

2. The physician tells a patient that he would like to schedule an endoscopic retrograde cholangiopancreatography in a local outpatient facility. After the physician leaves the room, you notice that the patient looks confused and worried. How would you explain the procedure to the patient to reassure him?

_____

_____

_____

_____

3. Mr. Thompson, a 50-year-old patient, is scheduled to have an endoscopic examination on Wednesday morning. You have given him all the necessary information to prepare for the examination, including taking a laxative the night before and eating only a light meal on Tuesday evening, with no breakfast Wednesday morning. Mr. Thompson calls you an hour before his appointment to tell you that he forgot to take the laxative the previous evening and has eaten breakfast. Explain what you would do.

_____

_____

_____

_____

4. A 15-year-old female patient comes into the physician's office with severe abdominal pains. She is extremely underweight for her height, and you suspect she might be anorexic. When the physician leaves the room, she confesses that she has been using laxatives every day to keep her weight down. Explain what you would do next.

_____

_____

_____

_____

5. A 50-year-old male patient has been diagnosed with pancreatic cancer. The patient is clearly devastated and tells you he has heard that people who develop pancreatic cancer have little chance of survival. What do you say to the patient?

_____

_____

_____

_____

PSY PROCEDURE 32-1 Assisting with Colon Procedures

Name: _____ Date: _____ Time: _____ Grade: _____

EQUIPMENT/SUPPLIES: Appropriate instrument (flexible or rigid sigmoidoscope, anoscope, or proctoscope); water-soluble lubricant; patient gown and drape; cotton swabs; suction (if not part of the scope); biopsy forceps; specimen container with preservative; completed laboratory requisition form; personal wipes or tissues; equipment for assessing vital signs; examination gloves

STANDARDS: Given the needed equipment and a place to work the student will perform this skill with
_____% accuracy in a total of _____ minutes. *(Your instructor will tell you what the percentage and time limits will be before you begin.)*

KEY: 4 = Satisfactory   0 = Unsatisfactory   NA = This step is not counted

PROCEDURE STEPS	SELF	PARTNER	INSTRUCTOR
1. Wash your hands.	☐	☐	☐
2. Assemble the equipment and supplies.	☐	☐	☐
a. Place the name of the patient on label on outside of specimen container.	☐	☐	☐
b. Complete the laboratory requisition.			
3. Check the illumination of the light source if a flexible sigmoidoscope. Turn off the power after checking for working order.	☐	☐	☐
4. Greet and identify the patient and explain the procedure.	☐	☐	☐
a. Inform patient that a sensation of pressure may be felt.	☐	☐	☐
b. Tell the patient that the pressure is from the instrument.	☐	☐	☐
c. Gas pressure may be felt when air is insufflated during the sigmoidoscopy.	☐	☐	☐
5. Instruct the patient to empty his or her urinary bladder.	☐	☐	☐
6. Assess the vital signs and record in the medical record.	☐	☐	☐
7. Have the patient undress from the waist down and gown and drape appropriately.	☐	☐	☐
8. Assist the patient onto the examination table.	☐	☐	☐
a. If the instrument is an anoscope or a fiberoptic device, the Sims position or a side-lying position is most comfortable.	☐	☐	☐
b. If a rigid instrument is used, position patient when doctor is ready: knee-chest position or on a proctological table.	☐	☐	☐
c. Drape the patient.	☐	☐	☐
9. Assist the physician with lubricant, instruments, power, swabs, suction, etc.	☐	☐	☐
10. Monitor the patient's response and offer reassurance.	☐	☐	☐
a. Instruct the patient to breathe slowly through pursed lips.	☐	☐	☐
b. Encourage relaxing as much as possible.	☐	☐	☐

11. When the physician is finished:	☐	☐	☐
a. Assist the patient into a comfortable position and allow a rest period.	☐	☐	☐
b. Offer personal cleaning wipes or tissues.	☐	☐	☐
c. Take the patient's vital signs before allowing him or her to stand.	☐	☐	☐
d. Assist the patient from the table and with dressing as needed.	☐	☐	☐
e. Give the patient any instructions regarding postprocedure care.			
12. Clean the room and route the specimen to the laboratory with the requisition.	☐	☐	☐
13. Disinfect or dispose of the supplies and equipment as appropriate.	☐	☐	☐
14. Wash your hands.	☐	☐	☐
15. Document the procedure.	☐	☐	☐

CALCULATION

Total Possible Points: _____

Total Points Earned: _____ Multiplied by 100 = _____ Divided by Total Possible Points = _____ %

PASS   **FAIL**   **COMMENTS:**

  ☐   ☐

Student's signature _____ Date _____

Partner's signature _____ Date _____

Instructor's signature _____ Date _____

Cognitive Domain

1. Spell and define key terms
2. Identify common diseases of the nervous system
3. Describe the physical and emotional effects of degenerative nervous system disorders
4. List potential complications of a spinal cord injury
5. Name and describe the common procedures for diagnosing nervous system disorders
6. Identify common pathologies related to each body system
7. Describe implications for treatment related to pathology

Psychomotor Domain

1. Assist with a lumbar puncture (Procedure 33-1)
2. Assist physician with patient care
3. Prepare a patient for procedures and/or treatments
4. Practice standard precautions
5. Document patient care
6. Document patient education
7. Practice within the standard of care for a medical assistant

Affective Domain

1. Apply critical thinking skills in performing patient assessment and care
2. Use language/verbal skills that enable patients' understanding
3. Demonstrate empathy in communicating with patients, family, and staff

4. Use appropriate body language and other nonverbal skills in communicating with patients, family, and staff
5. Demonstrate awareness of the territorial boundaries of the person with whom you are communicating
6. Demonstrate sensitivity appropriate to the message being delivered
7. Demonstrate recognition of the patient's level of understanding in communications
8. Recognize and protect personal boundaries in communicating with others
9. Demonstrate respect for individual diversity, incorporating awareness of one's own biases in areas including gender, race, religion, age, and economic status
10. Apply active listening skills
11. Apply local, state, and federal health care legislation and regulation appropriate to the medical assisting practice setting

ABHES Competencies

1. Assist the physician with the regimen of diagnostic and treatment modalities as they relate to each body system
2. Comply with federal, state, and local health laws and regulations
3. Communicate on the recipient's level of comprehension
4. Serve as a liaison between the physician and others
5. Show empathy and impartiality when dealing with patients
6. Document accurately

Name: _____   Date: _____   Grade: _____

COG MULTIPLE CHOICE

Circle the letter preceding the correct answer.

1. Initial symptoms of tetanus include:

   a. muscle spasms and stiff neck.

   b. paralysis and stiff neck.

   c. drooling and thick saliva.

   d. seizures and dysphagia.

   e. muscle spasms and clenched teeth.

2. What is another name for grand mal seizures?

   a. Absence seizures

   b. Tonic-clonic seizures

   c. Partial seizures

   d. Nervous seizures

   e. Flashing seizures

3. Febrile seizures occur in:

   a. teenagers.

   b. middle-aged men.

   c. young children.

   d. older adult women.

   e. people of all ages.

4. There may be no signs of external deformity with:

   a. meningocele.

   b. myelomeningocele.

   c. spina bifida occulta.

   d. amyotrophic lateral sclerosis.

   e. poliomyelitis.

5. To diagnose meningitis, the physician may order a(n):

   a. urine sample.

   b. x-ray.

   c. MRI.

   d. throat culture.

   e. complete blood count.

6. Hydrophobia often occurs after the onset of:

   a. rabies.

   b. tetanus.

   c. encephalitis.

   d. cerebral palsy.

   e. meningitis.

7. A herpes zoster breakout typically develops on:

   a. the legs and arms.

   b. the genitals and mouth.

   c. the stomach and chest.

   d. the face, back, and chest.

   e. the face and neck.

8. A disease closely related to poliomyelitis is:

   a. encephalitis.

   b. meningitis.

   c. Parkinson disease.

   d. PPMA syndrome.

   e. chicken pox.

9. Treatment for brain tumors may include:

   a. physical therapy and drug therapy.

   b. surgery and radiation therapy.

   c. surgery only.

   d. radiation therapy only.

   e. physical therapy and occupational therapy.

10. CSF removed and sent to the laboratory for a suspected diagnosis of meningitis may be tested for:

    a. red blood cell and white blood cell count.

    b. cholesterol and white blood cell count.

    c. red blood cells and viruses

    d. glucose and bacteria.

    e. glucose and fatty acids.

11. You should encourage slow, deep breathing for:

   a. electrical tests.

   b. a lumbar puncture.

   c. radiological tests.

   d. physical tests.

   e. the Romberg test.

12. Contrast medium helps distinguish between the soft tissues of the nervous system and:

   a. bones.

   b. tendons.

   c. tumors.

   d. muscles.

   e. arteries.

13. When assisting with a Queckenstedt test, you will be directed to:

   a. assist the patient into a side-curled position.

   b. support a forward-bending sitting position.

   c. maintain sterility of instruments.

   d. press against the patient's jugular vein.

   e. encourage the patient in slow, deep breathing.

14. AFP is generally performed:

   a. during the second trimester of pregnancy.

   b. during the first trimester of pregnancy.

   c. during the third trimester of pregnancy.

   d. before a woman gets pregnant.

   e. after the baby is born.

15. Which of the following is true of Lou Gehrig disease?

   a. It is officially known as multiple sclerosis.

   b. It is highly contagious.

   c. It is caused by a spinal cord injury.

   d. It is found most often in children.

   e. It is a terminal disease.

16. During the second phase of a grand mal seizure, the patient experiences:

   a. a tingling in extremities.

   b. a sensitivity to light.

   c. a complete loss of consciousness.

   d. an increased awareness of smell.

   e. a sense of drowsiness.

17. Which of the following is a cause of febrile seizures?

   a. Spinal cord damage

   b. Elevated body temperature

   c. Hypothermia

   d. Reye syndrome

   e. Neural tube defects

18. Paraplegia is:

   a. paralysis of all limbs.

   b. paralysis of the high thoracic vertebrae.

   c. paralysis on one side of the body, opposite the side of spinal cord involvement.

   d. paralysis of any part of the body above the point of spinal cord involvement.

   e. paralysis of any part of the body below the point of spinal cord involvement.

19. Which of the following is an infectious disorder of the nervous system?

   a. Tumors

   b. ALS

   c. Multiple sclerosis

   d. Encephalitis

   e. Febrile seizures

20. Parkinson disease is a:

   a. convulsive disorder.

   b. degenerative disorder.

   c. developmental disorder.

   d. neoplastic disorder.

   e. traumatic disorder.

COG MATCHING

Grade: _____

Place the letter preceding the definition on the line next to the term.

Key Terms

21. _____ cephalalgia

22. _____ concussion

23. _____ contusion

24. _____ convulsion

25. _____ dysphagia

26. _____ dysphasia

27. _____ electroencephalo-
gram (EEG)

28. _____ herpes zoster

29. _____ meningocele

30. _____ migraine

31. _____ myelogram

32. _____ myelomeningocele

33. _____ Queckenstedt test

34. _____ Romberg test

35. _____ seizure

36. _____ spina bifida occulta

Definitions

a. tracing of the electrical activity of the brain

b. a headache

c. meninges protruding through the spinal column

d. the protrusion of the spinal cord through the spinal defect

e. an invasive radiological test in which dye is injected into the spinal fluid

f. a test to determine presence of obstruction in the CSF flow performed during a lumbar puncture

g. an injury to the brain due to trauma

h. difficulty speaking

i. sudden, involuntary muscle contraction of a voluntary muscle group

j. an infection caused by reactivation of varicella zoster virus, which causes chicken pox

k. a collection of blood tissues after an injury; a bruise

l. a type of severe headache, usually unilateral; may appear in clusters

m. a congenital defect in the spinal column caused by lack of union of the vertebrae

n. an abnormal discharge of electrical activity in the brain, resulting in involuntary contractions of voluntary muscles

o. a test for the inability to maintain body balance when eyes are closed and feet are together; indication of spinal cord disease

p. inability to swallow or difficulty in swallowing

COG MATCHING

Grade: _____

Place the letter preceding the examination method on the line next to the cranial nerve.

Cranial Nerves

37. _____ Olfactory (I)

38. _____ Trochlear (IV)

39. _____ Facial (VII)

40. _____ Glossopharyngeal (IX)

41. _____ Vagus (X)

Examination Methods

a. Ask patient to raise eyebrows, smile, show teeth, puff out cheeks.

b. Test for downward, inward eye movement.

c. Test each nostril for smell reception, interpretation.

d. Ask patient to say "ah," yawn to observe upward movement of palate; elicit gag response, note ability to swallow.

e. Ask patient to swallow and speak; note hoarseness.

COG MATCHING

Grade: _____

Place the letter preceding the response on the line next to the reflex. Responses may be used more than once.

Reflexes

42. _____ Brachioradialis

43. _____ Biceps

44. _____ Triceps

45. _____ Patellar

46. _____ Achilles

47. _____ Corneal

Responses

a. Closure of eyelid

b. Extension of elbow

c. Flexion of elbow

d. Plantarflexion of foot

e. Extension of leg

cog IDENTIFICATION

Grade: _____

Indicate whether the following disorders are infectious (I), degenerative (DG), convulsive (C), developmental (DV), traumatic (T), neoplastic (N), or a type of headache (H) by placing the identifying letter(s) on the line preceding the disorder.

48. _____ Amyotrophic lateral sclerosis

49. _____ Focal or Jacksonian

50. _____ Hydrocephalus

51. _____ Meningitis

52. _____ Neural tube defects

53. _____ Poliomyelitis

54. _____ Brain astrocytoma

55. _____ Herpes zoster

56. _____ Cerebral palsy

57. _____ Tetanus

58. _____ Febrile seizures

59. _____ Multiple sclerosis

60. _____ Spinal cord injury

61. Identify whether the disorders listed below affect children, women, men, or older adults. Place a check mark on the line under the appropriate groups.

Disorder	Children	Women	Men	Older Adults
a. Parkinson disease				
b. Amyotrophic lateral sclerosis				
c. Multiple sclerosis				
d. Reye syndrome				
e. Febrile seizures				

62. Indicate whether the following symptoms occur at the onset of a migraine or after the migraine begins. Place a check mark on the line under the word "onset" or "after."

Symptoms	Onset	After Migraine Begins
a. experience of flashing lights		
b. photophobia		
c. nausea		
d. experience of wavy lines		
e. diplopia		

COG **SHORT ANSWER**　　　　　　　　　　　　　　　　　　　　　　　Grade: _____

63. Explain the difference between dysphagia and dysphasia.

_____

_____

_____

_____

64. Name three viral infections that lead to encephalitis.

_____

_____

_____

_____

65. What kind of outbreak might be caused by a varicella infection? What generally triggers this outbreak?

_____

_____

_____

_____

66. Which age group is most susceptible to traumatic brain injuries? Why? Which age group is most susceptible to spinal cord injuries? Why?

_____

_____

_____

_____

67. Name seven common diagnostic tests for the nervous system.

_____

_____

_____

_____

68. Explain the difference between the Romberg test and the Queckenstedt test and how or if you would assist the physician in each procedure.

_____

_____

_____

_____

69. List three responsibilities that you may have when working with patients with neurological disorders.

_____

_____

_____

_____

70. Below are some of the steps involved in assisting the physician with a lumbar puncture. Explain the reasons for performing each task listed.

a. Check that the consent form is signed and in the chart. Warn the patient not to move during the procedure. Tell the patient that the area will be numb but pressure may still be felt after the local anesthetic is administered.

_____

_____

_____

_____

b. Throughout the procedure, observe the patient closely for signs such as dyspnea or cyanosis. Monitor the pulse at intervals and record the vital signs after the procedure. Note the patient's mental alertness and any leakage at the site, nausea, or vomiting. Assess lower limb mobility. Assist the physician as necessary.

_____

_____

_____

_____

c. If the Queckenstedt test is to be performed, you may be required to press against the patient's jugular veins in the neck (right, left, or both) while the physician monitors the pressure of CSF.

_____

_____

_____

_____

COG TRUE OR FALSE?   Grade: _____

Indicate whether the statements are true or false by placing the letter T (true) or F (false) on the line preceding the statement.

71. _____ Ice and alcohol and sponge baths are preferable to cool compresses in returning a child's body temperature to normal.

72. _____ If a patient is bitten by an animal, a copy of the animal's rabies tag and certificate should be placed in the patient's chart.

73. _____ Multiple sclerosis is a contagious disease.

74. _____ A lumbar puncture is more commonly performed in outpatient clinics than in the medical office.

75. _____ Herpes zoster may develop in patients who had a previous varicella infection.

COG AFF **CASE STUDIES FOR CRITICAL THINKING**   Grade: _____

1. A patient comes in for treatment because of a severe dog bite. The patient has already cleaned the wound himself and the physician attends to the wound immediately. Your patient then receives antibiotic and vaccine therapy. What is the next course of action and what may you be responsible for?

   _____

   _____

   _____

   _____

2. A patient in your clinic has been treated for epilepsy and is now seizure free. This patient has decided that she is going to stop her medication regimen. She has also expressed her excitement about being able to drive again soon. How might you advise this patient before she makes her decisions?

   _____

   _____

   _____

   _____

3. There is a patient who has recently started coming to your clinic for treatment for herpes zoster. She doesn't understand why she has shingles. She is a single mom who has been supporting her children and taking care of one child with severe Down syndrome. What would you explain as the likely cause for the herpes zoster outbreak? What kind of advice might you offer this patient toward improving her health?

   _____

   _____

   _____

   _____

4. A 40-year-old patient has been suffering from severe migraines for the last year. He is concerned about his condition because he is a truck driver. He is worried that it is just a matter time before a migraine sets in while he is driving. Taking rests while he is on the road is a near impossibility. He is usually very tired, and he drinks a lot of coffee to keep himself awake on his long rides. How might you advise and educate this patient?

_____

_____

_____

_____

5. A patient comes in to the office and complains of headaches, blurred vision, and memory loss. What would your immediate concern be? What type of tests may need to be performed to learn more about this patient's symptoms?

_____

_____

_____

_____

PSY PROCEDURE 33-1 | Assist with a Lumbar Puncture

Name: _____ Date: _____ Time: _____ Grade: _____

EQUIPMENT/SUPPLIES: Sterile gloves, examination gloves, 3- to 5-inch lumbar needle with a stylet (physician will specify gauge and length), sterile gauze sponges, specimen containers, local anesthetic and syringe, needle, adhesive bandages, fenestrated drape, sterile drape, antiseptic, skin preparation supplies (razor), biohazard sharps container, biohazard waste container

STANDARDS: Given the needed equipment and a place to work the student will perform this skill with _____% accuracy in a total of _____ minutes. *(Your instructor will tell you what the percentage and time limits will be before you begin.)*

KEY: 4 = Satisfactory   0 = Unsatisfactory   NA = This step is not counted

PROCEDURE STEPS	SELF	PARTNER	INSTRUCTOR
1. Wash your hands.	☐	☐	☐
2. Assemble the equipment, identify the patient, and explain the procedure.	☐	☐	☐
3. Check that the consent form is signed and available in the chart.	☐	☐	☐
4. Explain the importance of not moving during the procedure and explain that the area will be numbed but pressure may still be felt.	☐	☐	☐
5. Have the patient void.	☐	☐	☐
6. Direct the patient to disrobe and put on a gown with the opening in the back.	☐	☐	☐
7. Prepare the skin unless this is to be done as part of the sterile preparation.	☐	☐	☐
8. Assist as needed with administration of the anesthetic.	☐	☐	☐
9. Assist the patient into the appropriate position.	☐	☐	☐
a. For the side-lying position:	☐	☐	☐
(1) Stand in front of the patient and help by holding the patient's knees and top shoulder.			
(2) Ask the patient to move, so the back is close to the edge of the table.			
b. For the forward-leaning, supported position:			
(1) Stand in front of the patient and rest your hands on the patient's shoulders.			
(2) Ask the patient to breathe slowly and deeply.			
10. Throughout the procedure, observe the patient closely for signs such as dyspnea or cyanosis.	☐	☐	☐
a. Monitor the pulse at intervals and record the vital signs after the procedure.			
b. Assess lower limb mobility.			

11. When the physician has the needle securely in place, if specimens are to be taken:
 	
    a. Put on gloves to receive the potentially hazardous body fluid.
 	
    b. Label the tubes in sequence as you receive them.
 	
    c. Label with the patient's identification and place them in biohazard bags.
	☐	☐	☐

12. If the Queckenstedt test is to be performed, you may be required to press against the patient's jugular veins in the neck, either right, left, or both, while the physician monitors the CSF pressure.	☐	☐	☐

13. At the completion of the procedure:
 	
    a. Cover the site with an adhesive bandage and assist the patient to a flat position.
 	
    b. The physician will determine when the patient is ready to leave.
	☐	☐	☐

14. Route the specimens as required.	☐	☐	☐
15. Clean the examination room and care for or dispose of the equipment as needed.	☐	☐	☐
16. Wash your hands.	☐	☐	☐
17. Chart all observations and record the procedure.			

CALCULATION

Total Possible Points: _____

Total Points Earned: _____ Multiplied by 100 = _____ Divided by Total Possible Points = _____ %

PASS   **FAIL**   **COMMENTS:**

  ☐   ☐

Student's signature _____ Date _____

Partner's signature _____ Date _____

Instructor's signature _____ Date _____

Cognitive Domain

1. Spell and define the key terms
2. List and describe the disorders of the urinary system and the male reproductive system
3. Describe and explain the purpose of various diagnostic procedures associated with the urinary system
4. Discuss the role of the medical assistant in diagnosing and treating disorders of the urinary system and the male reproductive system
5. Identify common pathologies related to each body system
6. Describe implications for treatment related to pathology

Psychomotor Domain

1. Perform a female urinary catheterization (Procedure 34-1)
2. Perform a male urinary catheterization (Procedure 34-2)
3. Instruct a male patient on the testicular self-examination (Procedure 34-3)
4. Assist physician with patient care
5. Prepare a patient for procedures and/or treatments
6. Practice standard precautions
7. Document patient care
8. Document patient education
9. Practice within the standard of care for a medical assistant

Affective Domain

1. Apply critical thinking skills in performing patient assessment and care
2. Use language/verbal skills that enable patients' understanding
3. Demonstrate empathy in communicating with patients, family, and staff
4. Use appropriate body language and other nonverbal skills in communicating with patients, family, and staff
5. Demonstrate awareness of the territorial boundaries of the person with whom you are communicating
6. Demonstrate sensitivity appropriate to the message being delivered
7. Demonstrate recognition of the patient's level of understanding in communications
8. Recognize and protect personal boundaries in communicating with others
9. Demonstrate respect for individual diversity, incorporating awareness of one's own biases in areas including gender, race, religion, age, and economic status
10. Apply active listening skills
11. Apply local, state, and federal health care legislation and regulation appropriate to the medical assisting practice setting

ABHES Competencies

1. Assist the physician with the regimen of diagnostic and treatment modalities as they relate to each body system
2. Comply with federal, state, and local health laws and regulations
3. Communicate on the recipient's level of comprehension
4. Serve as a liaison between the physician and others
5. Show empathy and impartiality when dealing with patients
6. Document accurately

Name: _____   Date: _____   Grade: _____

COG MULTIPLE CHOICE

Circle the letter preceding the correct answer.

1. Cystoscopy is:

   a. an inflammation of the urinary bladder.

   b. the direct visualization of the bladder and urethra.

   c. a procedure used to help patients pass calculi.

   d. the treatment used for men with an inguinal hernia.

   e. the use of a small camera inserted into the rectum.

2. Which of the following might contribute to psychogenic impotence?

   a. Disease in any other body system

   b. Injury to pelvic organs

   c. Medication

   d. Exhaustion

   e. Cardiovascular problems

3. Before scheduling a patient for an IVP or a retrograde pyelogram, you must check for a(n):

   a. protein allergy.

   b. lubricant allergy.

   c. iodine allergy.

   d. rubber allergy.

   e. latex allergy.

4. A procedure that cleanses the blood of waste products and excess fluid is:

   a. oliguria.

   b. lithotripsy.

   c. proteinuria.

   d. cystoscopy.

   e. dialysis.

5. Young girls are prone to urethritis because they:

   a. forget to practice good hand-washing technique.

   b. have a short urethra.

   c. don't take enough baths.

   d. urinate too frequently.

   e. wipe from front to back.

6. Which of the following instructions would be helpful for a patient trying to pass a stone?

   a. Eat a large amount of fiber.

   b. Get plenty of bed rest and relaxation.

   c. Drink lots of water.

   d. Go to the hospital when the stone passes.

   e. Do not consume anything until the stone has passed.

7. Orchiopexy is surgery to correct:

   a. undescended testes.

   b. enlarged prostate.

   c. inguinal hernia.

   d. impotence.

   e. hydrocele.

8. One common urinary disorder in females is:

   a. benign prostatic hyperplasia.

   b. nocturia.

   c. hydrocele.

   d. cryptorchidism.

   e. urinary tract infection.

Scenario for questions 9 and 10: An elderly patient comes in for a routine checkup, and the physician discovers his prostate gland is very enlarged.

9. What is a blood test you can run to look for prostate cancer?

   a. PSA test

   b. Proteinuria

   c. Snellen test

   d. Digital rectal exam

   e. Dialysis

10. A urinary condition that might indicate an enlarged prostate gland is:

    a. proteinuria.

    b. oliguria.

    c. nocturia.

    d. hematuria.

    e. pyuria.

11. Seventy-five percent of men with prostate cancer are over age:

    a. 15 years.

    b. 30 years.

    c. 34 years.

    d. 50 years.

    e. 75 years.

12. What kind of juice is recommended to patients to acidify urine?

    a. Tomato juice

    b. Orange juice

    c. Grape juice

    d. Cranberry juice

    e. Grapefruit juice

13. A patient should be given a catheter when:

    a. the patient suffers from nocturia.

    b. the patient has a urinary tract infection.

    c. the patient's urine has high PSA levels.

    d. the patient has calculi.

    e. the patient has dysuria.

14. Which of the following instruments is used to view the bladder and urethra?

    a. Catheter

    b. Cystoscope

    c. Dialysis machine

    d. Ultrasound

    e. Pyelogram

15. Which of the following patients is most likely to develop a urinary tract infection?

    a. A young boy who frequently urinates

    b. A teenaged girl who takes bubble baths

    c. An elderly woman who only wears loose-fitting dresses

    d. An adult woman who showers immediately after sexual intercourse

    e. A middle-aged man who does not wash his hands very often

16. Which of the following is the initial step in catheterization of a patient?

    a. Wash your hands.

    b. Open the catheterization kit.

    c. Put on sterile gloves.

    d. Use antiseptic swabs to clean area.

    e. Assist patient to assume position.

17. What is a symptom of hydronephrosis?

    a. Proteinuria

    b. Chills

    c. Swollen prostate

    d. Back pain

    e. High PSA levels

18. Which of the following is true for catheterizing both men and women?

    a. Tray may be placed on patient's lap for easy access to tools.

    b. Patient's position is on his or her back, legs apart.

    c. Catheter is inserted 5 inches.

    d. Nondominant hand is contaminated.

    e. Coudé catheter may be used.

19. Which of the following is a cause of organic impotence?

   a. Exhaustion

   b. Anxiety

   c. Depression

   d. Stress

   e. Endocrine imbalance

20. Ultrasonography can be used to treat which of the following?

   a. Renal failure

   b. Hydronephrosis

   c. Calculi

   d. Urinary tract infection

   e. Inguinal hernia

COG MATCHING   Grade: _____

Place the letter preceding the definition on the line next to the term.

Key Terms

21. _____ anuria

22. _____ blood urea nitrogen

23. _____ catheterization

24. _____ cystoscopy

25. _____ dialysis

26. _____ dysuria

27. _____ enuresis

28. _____ hematuria

29. _____ impotence

30. _____ incontinence

31. _____ intravenous pyelogram (IVP)

32. _____ lithotripsy

33. _____ nephrostomy

34. _____ nocturia

35. _____ oliguria

36. _____ prostate-specific antigen

37. _____ proteinuria

Definitions

a. an inability to achieve or maintain an erection

b. painful or difficult urination

c. crushing a stone with sound waves

d. the removal of waste in blood not filtered by kidneys by passing fluid through a semipermeable barrier that allows normal electrolytes to remain, either with a machine with circulatory access or by passing a balanced fluid through the peritoneal cavity

e. excessive urination at night

f. a blood test to determine the amount of nitrogen in blood or urea, a waste product normally excreted in urine

g. of psychological origin

h. a normal protein produced by the prostate that usually elevates in the presence of prostate cancer

i. the density of a liquid, such as urine, compared with water

j. radiography using contrast medium to evaluate kidney function

k. direct visualization of the urinary bladder through a cystoscope inserted through the urethra

l. an examination of the physical, chemical, and microscopic properties of urine

m. failure of kidneys to produce urine

n. blood in the urine

o. the presence of large quantities of protein in the urine; usually a sign of renal dysfunction

p. scant urine production

q. the urge to urinate occurring more often than is required for normal bladder elimination

r. a surgical opening to the outside of the body from the ureter to facilitate drainage of urine from an obstructed kidney

38. _____ psychogenic

39. _____ pyuria

40. _____ retrograde pyelogram

41. _____ specific gravity

42. _____ ureterostomy

43. _____ urinalysis

44. _____ urinary frequency

s. pus in the urine

t. bed wetting

u. the placement of a catheter in the kidney pelvis to drain urine from an obstructed kidney

v. the inability to control elimination of urine, feces, or both

w. a procedure for introducing a flexible tube into the body

x. an x-ray of the urinary tract using contrast medium injected through the bladder and ureters; useful in diagnosing obstructions

COG **SHORT ANSWER**   Grade: _____

45. What is the difference between hemodialysis and peritoneal dialysis?

_____

_____

_____

_____

46. What are calculi?

_____

_____

_____

_____

47. List five microorganisms that may cause epididymitis.

a. _____

b. _____

c. _____

d. _____

e. _____

48. What are the symptoms of a possible tumor in the urinary system?

_____

_____

_____

_____

49. Are stones more likely to form when urine is alkaline or acidic?

_____

_____

_____

_____

50. Why is a woman more likely to have cystitis than a man?

_____

_____

_____

_____

51. Why are infections in the male urinary tract likely to spread to the reproductive system?

_____

_____

_____

_____

52. What are the three characteristics of the prostate that the physician is checking when performing a digital rectal examination?

_____

_____

_____

53. An older adult male patient with prostatic hypertrophy must be given a catheter in order to obtain a urine sample. What is the best type of catheter to use, and why?

_____

_____

_____

_____

54. List three suggestions to help patients avoid urinary tract infections.

_____

_____

_____

_____

55. What is the difference between an intravenous pyelogram and a retrograde pyelogram? What might the medical assistant be responsible for with regards to the physician order for an intravenous pyelogram and retrograde pyelogram?

_____

_____

_____

_____

COG TRUE OR FALSE?   Grade: _____

Indicate whether the statements are true or false by placing the letter T (true) or F (false) on the line preceding the statement.

56. _____ Orchiopexy refers to either one or both undescended testes.

57. _____ A nephrologist is a physician who specializes in the physical characteristics of the urinary system.

58. _____ No other form of birth control is needed after a man receives a vasectomy.

59. _____ Your office is obligated to notify a patient if a procedure or medication is still in clinical trials, but likely to be approved.

COG **AFF** **CASE STUDIES FOR CRITICAL THINKING**   Grade: _____

1. A middle-aged patient in good shape comes in complaining of some pain in his groin. The physician suspects he might have an inguinal hernia. What is the procedure to diagnosis this, and how is it corrected?

_____

_____

_____

_____

2. An older adult patient has been diagnosed with renal failure and will need to undergo dialysis. However, he is not sure if hemodialysis or peritoneal dialysis would be better for his lifestyle. What information can you tell him about the two different processes, including the advantages and disadvantages of each?

_____

_____

_____

_____

3. The physician asks you to give information to one of the patients about passing small calculi. What would you tell the patient about calculi, and what suggestions would you give to help the patient pass the stones?

_____

_____

_____

_____

4. A man in his early 20s has come in for his physical, and the physician has instructed you to teach him about testicular disease. You will also need to teach him how to perform a self-examination. However, the man is shy and embarrassed about the procedure. What can you say to him to help him overcome his discomfort?

_____

_____

_____

5. An older adult woman has chronic renal failure, and the physician decides that she will need a catheter for peritoneal dialysis. The woman is upset that she needs this, because she believes that it will limit her movement and ability to participate in activities she likes. What can you tell her about catheters and how her lifestyle will change that might put her more at ease?

_____

_____

_____

_____

PSY PROCEDURE 34-1 Perform a Female Urinary Catheterization

Name: _____ Date: _____ Time: _____ Grade: _____

EQUIPMENT/SUPPLIES: Straight catheterization tray that includes a #14 or #16 French catheter, a sterile tray, sterile gloves, antiseptic, a specimen cup with a lid, lubricant, and a sterile drape; an examination light; an anatomically correct female torso model for performing the catheterization; a biohazard container

STANDARDS: Given the needed equipment and a place to work the student will perform this skill with _____% accuracy in a total of _____ minutes. *(Your instructor will tell you what the percentage and time limits will be before you begin.)*

KEY: 4 = Satisfactory   0 = Unsatisfactory   NA = this step is not counted

PROCEDURE STEPS	SELF	PARTNER	INSTRUCTOR
1. Wash your hands.	☐	☐	☐
2. Identify the patient.	☐	☐	☐
a. Explain the procedure and have the patient disrobe from the waist down.	☐	☐	☐
b. Provide adequate gowning and draping materials.			
3. Place the patient in the dorsal recumbent or lithotomy position.	☐	☐	☐
a. Drape carefully to prevent unnecessary exposure.	☐	☐	☐
b. Open the tray and place it between the patient's legs.	☐	☐	☐
c. Adjust examination light to allow adequate visualization of the perineum.	☐	☐	☐
4. Remove the sterile glove package and put on the sterile gloves.	☐	☐	☐
5. Remove sterile drape and place it under the patient's buttocks.	☐	☐	☐
6. Open the antiseptic swabs and place them upright inside the catheter tray.	☐	☐	☐
7. Open the lubricant and squeeze a generous amount onto the tip of the catheter.	☐	☐	☐
8. Remove the sterile urine specimen cup and lid and place them to the side of the tray.	☐	☐	☐
9. Using your nondominant hand, carefully expose the urinary meatus.	☐	☐	☐
10. Using your sterile dominant hand, use antiseptic swabs to cleanse the urinary meatus by starting at the top and moving the swab down each side of the urinary meatus and down the middle, using a new swab for each side and the middle. Do not contaminate the glove on this hand.	☐	☐	☐

11. Pick up the catheter with the sterile, dominant hand and:	☐	☐	☐
a. Carefully insert the lubricated tip into the urinary meatus approximately 3 inches.	☐	☐	☐
b. Leave the other end of the catheter in the tray.	☐	☐	☐
12. Once the urine begins to flow into the catheter tray, hold the catheter in position with your nondominant hand.	☐	☐	☐
13. Use your dominant hand to direct the flow of urine into the specimen cup.	☐	☐	☐
14. Remove catheter when urine flow slows or stops or 1,000 mL has been obtained.	☐	☐	☐
15. Wipe the perineum carefully with the drape that was placed under the buttocks.	☐	☐	☐
16. Dispose of urine appropriately and discard supplies in a biohazard container.	☐	☐	☐
a. Label the specimen container and complete the necessary laboratory requisition.	☐	☐	☐
b. Process the specimen according to the guidelines of the laboratory.	☐	☐	☐
17. Remove your gloves and wash your hands.	☐	☐	☐
18. Instruct patient to dress and give any follow-up information.	☐	☐	☐
19. Document the procedure in the patient's medical record.	☐	☐	☐

CALCULATION

Total Possible Points: _____

Total Points Earned: _____ Multiplied by 100 = _____ Divided by Total Possible Points = _____ %

PASS **FAIL** **COMMENTS:**

☐ ☐

Student's signature _____ Date _____

Partner's signature _____ Date _____

Instructor's signature _____ Date _____

PSY PROCEDURE 34-2 Perform a Male Urinary Catheterization

Name: _____ Date: _____ Time: _____ Grade: _____

EQUIPMENT/SUPPLIES: Straight catheterization tray that includes a #14 or #16 French catheter, a sterile tray, sterile gloves, antiseptic, a specimen cup with a lid, lubricant, and a sterile drape; an examination light; an anatomically correct male torso model for performing the catheterization; a biohazard container

STANDARDS: Given the needed equipment and a place to work the student will perform this skill with _____% accuracy in a total of _____ minutes. *(Your instructor will tell you what the percentage and time limits will be before you begin.)*

KEY: 4 = Satisfactory   0 = Unsatisfactory   NA = this step is not counted

PROCEDURE STEPS	SELF	PARTNER	INSTRUCTOR
1. Wash your hands.	☐	☐	☐
2. Identify the patient.	☐	☐	☐
a. Explain the procedure and have the patient disrobe from the waist down.			
b. Provide adequate gowning and draping materials.			
3. Place the patient in the supine position.	☐	☐	☐
a. Drape carefully to prevent unnecessary exposure.	☐	☐	☐
b. Open the tray and place it to the side or on the patient's thighs.	☐	☐	☐
c. Adjust examination light to allow adequate visualization of the perineum.	☐	☐	☐
4. Remove the sterile glove package and put on the sterile gloves.	☐	☐	☐
5. Carefully remove the sterile drape and place it under the glans penis.	☐	☐	☐
6. Open the antiseptic swabs and place them upright inside the catheter tray.	☐	☐	☐
7. Open lubricant and squeeze a generous amount onto the tip of the catheter.	☐	☐	☐
8. Remove sterile urine specimen cup and lid and place them to the side of the tray.	☐	☐	☐
9. Using your nondominant hand, pick up the penis to expose the urinary meatus.	☐	☐	☐
10. Using your sterile dominant hand, use antiseptic swabs to cleanse the urinary meatus by starting at the top and moving the swab around each side of the urinary meatus and down the middle, using a new swab for each side and the middle. Do not contaminate the glove on this hand.	☐	☐	☐

11. Using your sterile dominant hand, pick up the catheter.	☐	☐	☐
a. Carefully insert the lubricated tip into the meatus approximately 4 to 6 inches.	☐	☐	☐
b. The other end of the catheter should be left in the tray.	☐	☐	☐
12. Once the urine begins to flow into the catheter tray, hold the catheter in position.	☐	☐	☐
13. Use your dominant hand to direct the flow of urine into the specimen cup.	☐	☐	☐
14. Remove the catheter when urine flow slows or stops or 1,000 mL has been obtained.	☐	☐	☐
15. Wipe the glans penis carefully with the drape that was placed under the buttocks.	☐	☐	☐
16. Dispose of urine appropriately and discard supplies in a biohazard container.	☐	☐	☐
17. Label the specimen container and complete the necessary laboratory requisition.	☐	☐	☐
18. Process specimen according to the guidelines of the laboratory.	☐	☐	☐
19. Remove your gloves and wash your hands.	☐	☐	☐
20. Instruct patient to dress and give any follow-up information.	☐	☐	☐
21. Document the procedure in the patient's medical record.	☐	☐	☐

CALCULATION

Total Possible Points: _____

Total Points Earned: _____ Multiplied by 100 = _____ Divided by Total Possible Points = _____ %

PASS   **FAIL**   **COMMENTS:**

☐   ☐

Student's signature _____ Date _____

Partner's signature _____ Date _____

Instructor's signature _____ Date _____

PSY PROCEDURE 34-3 **Instruct a Male Patient on the Self-Testicular Examination**

Name: _____ Date: _____ Time: _____ Grade: _____

EQUIPMENT/SUPPLIES: A patient instruction sheet if available; a testicular examination model or pictures

STANDARDS: Given the needed equipment and a place to work the student will perform this skill with _____% accuracy in a total of _____ minutes. *(Your instructor will tell you what the percentage and time limits will be before you begin.)*

KEY: 4 = Satisfactory 0 = Unsatisfactory NA = This step is not counted

PROCEDURE STEPS	SELF	PARTNER	INSTRUCTOR
1. Wash your hands.	☐	☐	☐
2. Identify the patient and explain the procedure.	☐	☐	☐
3. Using the testicular model or pictures, explain the procedure.	☐	☐	☐
a. Tell the patient to examine each testicle by gently rolling between the fingers and the thumb with both hands.	☐	☐	☐
b. Check for lumps or thickenings.	☐	☐	☐
4. Explain that the epididymis is located on top of each testicle.	☐	☐	☐
a. Palpate to avoid incorrectly identifying it as an abnormal growth or lump.	☐	☐	☐
b. Instruct patient to report abnormal lumps or thickenings to the physician.	☐	☐	☐
5. Allow the patient to ask questions related to the testicular self-examination.	☐	☐	☐
6. Document the procedure in the patient's medical record.	☐	☐	☐

CALCULATION

Total Possible Points: _____

Total Points Earned: _____ Multiplied by 100 = _____ Divided by Total Possible Points = _____ %

PASS **FAIL** **COMMENTS:**

☐ ☐

Student's signature _____ Date _____

Partner's signature _____ Date _____

Instructor's signature _____ Date _____

Obstetrics and Gynecology

Cognitive Domain

1. Spell and define the key terms
2. List and describe common gynecologic and obstetric disorders
3. Identify your role in the care of gynecologic and obstetric patients
4. Describe the components of prenatal and postpartum patient care
5. Explain the diagnostic and therapeutic procedures associated with the female reproductive system
6. Identify the various methods of contraception
7. Describe menopause
8. Identify common pathologies related to each body system
9. Describe implications for treatment related to pathology

Psychomotor Domain

1. Instruct the patient on the breast self-examination (Procedure 35-1)
2. Assist with the pelvic examination and Pap smear (Procedure 35-2)
3. Assist with colposcopy and cervical biopsy (Procedure 35-3)
4. Assist physician with patient care
5. Prepare a patient for procedures and/or treatments
6. Practice standard precautions
7. Document patient care

8. Document patient education
9. Practice within the standard of care for a medical assistant

Affective Domain

1. Apply critical thinking skills in performing patient assessment and care
2. Use language/verbal skills that enable patients' understanding
3. Demonstrate empathy in communicating with patients, family, and staff
4. Use appropriate body language and other nonverbal skills in communicating with patients, family, and staff
5. Demonstrate awareness of the territorial boundaries of the person with whom you are communicating
6. Demonstrate sensitivity appropriate to the message being delivered
7. Demonstrate recognition of the patient's level of understanding in communications
8. Recognize and protect personal boundaries in communicating with others
9. Demonstrate respect for individual diversity, incorporating awareness of one's own biases in areas including gender, race, religion, age, and economic status
10. Apply active listening skills
11. Apply local, state, and federal health care legislation and regulation appropriate to the medical assisting practice setting

ABHES Competencies

1. Assist the physician with the regimen of diagnostic and treatment modalities as they relate to each body system
2. Comply with federal, state, and local health laws and regulations
3. Communicate on the recipient's level of comprehension
4. Serve as a liaison between the physician and others
5. Show empathy and impartiality when dealing with patients
6. Document accurately

Name: _____   Date: _____   Grade: _____

COG MULTIPLE CHOICE

Circle the letter preceding the correct answer.

1. Within 24 hours before a gynecological examination, a patient should avoid:

   a. showering.

   b. using vaginal medication.

   c. taking a home pregnancy test.

   d. performing a breast self-examination.

   e. taking a medication containing aspirin.

2. A cesarean section is used to:

   a. diagnose gynecological cancers.

   b. screen the fetus for defects in the neural tube.

   c. analyze fluid from the amniotic sac for nervous system disorders.

   d. deliver an infant when vaginal delivery is not possible or advisable.

   e. stabilize an infant that was delivered before the 37th week of pregnancy.

3. Morning sickness that has escalated to a serious condition is known as:

   a. eclampsia.

   b. proteinuria.

   c. abruptio placentae.

   d. hyperemesis gravidarum.

   e. endometriosis.

4. A pessary may be used to treat:

   a. leiomyomas.

   b. ovarian cysts.

   c. endometriosis.

   d. uterine prolapse.

   e. ectopic pregnancy.

5. The most common sexually transmitted disease in the United States is:

   a. syphilis.

   b. gonorrhea.

   c. chlamydia.

   d. herpes genitalis.

   e. AIDS.

6. Which of the following methods of contraception works hormonally and is worn on the skin for 3 out of 4 weeks to prevent ovulation?

   a. Pill

   b. Ring

   c. Patch

   d. Condom

   e. Spermicide

7. Which of the following is a presumptive sign of pregnancy?

   a. Goodell sign

   b. Fetal heart tone

   c. Nausea and vomiting

   d. HCG in urine and blood

   e. Visualization of the fetus

8. A contraction stress test (CST) should be performed in the:

   a. hospital.

   b. patient's home.

   c. obstetrician's office.

   d. gynecologist's office.

   e. laboratory.

9. A hysterosalpingography is used to determine:

   a. the location and severity of cervical lesions.

   b. whether the patient will abort or miscarry a fetus.

   c. the presence of abnormal cells associated with cervical cancer.

   d. the position of the uterus and the patency of the fallopian tubes.

   e. the size of the pelvic anatomy for a vaginal delivery.

Scenario for questions 10 and 11: Your patient is a pregnant 32-year-old woman in her 22nd week of gestation. She is complaining of edema, headaches, blurred vision, and vomiting. After laboratory results confirm proteinuria, the physician concludes that the patient has preeclampsia.

10. Which of the following would the physician advise the patient to increase in her diet?

    a. Protein

    b. Sodium

    c. Calcium

    d. Folic acid

    e. Iron

11. What more severe condition could result if her present condition does not improve?

    a. Epilepsy

    b. Eclampsia

    c. Posteclampsia

    d. Premature labor

    e. Hyperemesis gravidarum

12. An undiagnosed ectopic pregnancy could lead to:

    a. polymenorrhea.

    b. salpingo-oophorectomy.

    c. herniation of the ovaries.

    d. displacement of the uterus.

    e. rupture of the fallopian tube.

13. How should the lochia appear immediately and for up to 6 days after delivery?

    a. White

    b. Red

    c. Green

    d. Yellow

    e. Clear

14. The onset of eclampsia is marked by:

    a. seizures.

    b. vomiting.

    c. hypertension.

    d. premature labor.

    e. contractions.

15. A woman who is pregnant for the first time is:

    a. nulligravida.

    b. primigravida.

    c. nullipara.

    d. primipara.

    e. multipara.

16. If animal research indicates no fetal risk concerning the use of a medication, but no human studies have been completed, the medication can be found in which category of drugs?

    a. Category A

    b. Category B

    c. Category C

    d. Category D

    e. Category X

17. The onset of first menses is called:

    a. menarche.

    b. menses.

    c. menorrhagia.

    d. metrorrhagia.

    e. polymenorrhea.

18. Surgery to occlude the vagina is called:

    a. colporrhaphy.

    b. laparoscopy.

    c. ultrasound.

    d. pessary.

    e. colpocleisis.

19. The height of the fundus is determined each visit by:

    a. ultrasound.

    b. blood work.

    c. urinalysis.

    d. fetal heart monitor.

    e. palpation.

20. Elevated AFP levels in a pregnant woman may indicate:

a. fetal nervous system deformities.

b. preeclampsia.

c. hyperemesis gravidarum.

d. placenta previa.

e. uterine contractions.

COG MATCHING

Grade: _____

Place the letter preceding the definition on the line next to the term.

Key Terms

21. _____ abortion

22. _____ amenorrhea

23. _____ amniocentesis

24. _____ Braxton-Hicks

25. _____ Chadwick sign

26. _____ colpocleisis

27. _____ culdocentesis

28. _____ cystocele

29. _____ dysmenorrheal

30. _____ dyspareunia

31. _____ Goodell sign

32. _____ hirsutism

33. _____ human chorionic gonadotropin (HCG)

34. _____ hysterosalpingogram

35. _____ menorrhagia

36. _____ menarche

37. _____ metrorrhagia

38. _____ multipara

39. _____ nullipara

40. _____ pessary

Definitions

a. a woman who has never given birth to a viable fetus

b. softening of the cervix early in pregnancy

c. the presence of large amounts of protein in the urine; usually a sign of renal dysfunction

d. herniation of the rectum into the vaginal area

e. surgical puncture and aspiration of fluid from the vaginal cul-de-sac for diagnosis or therapy

f. when inserted into the vagina, device that supports the uterus

g. sign of early pregnancy in which the vaginal, cervical, and vulvar tissues develop a bluish violet color

h. herniation of the urinary bladder into the vagina

i. period of time (about 6 weeks) from childbirth until reproductive structures return to normal

j. hormone secreted by the placenta and found in the urine and blood of a pregnant female

k. irregular uterine bleeding

l. puncture of the amniotic sac to remove fluid for testing

m. termination of pregnancy or products of conception prior to fetal viability and/or 20 weeks' gestation

n. condition of not menstruating

o. painful coitus or sexual intercourse

p. a woman who has given birth to one viable infant

q. abnormally frequent menstrual periods

r. surgery to occlude the vagina

s. a woman who has given birth to more than one fetus

t. surgical excision of both the fallopian tube and the ovary

u. sporadic uterine contractions during pregnancy

v. painful menstruation

w. abnormal or excessive hair growth in women

41. _____ polymenorrhea

42. _____ primipara

43. _____ proteinuria

44. _____ puerperium

45. _____ rectocele

46. _____ salpingo-oophorectomy

x. radiograph of the uterus and fallopian tubes after injection with a contrast medium

y. onset of first menstruation

z. excessive bleeding during menstruation

COG MATCHING

Grade: _____

Place the letter preceding the description on the line next to the stage of lochia it describes.

STDs

47. _____ AIDS
48. _____ Syphilis
49. _____ Chlamydia
50. _____ Condylomata acuminata
51. _____ Gonorrhea
52. _____ Herpes genitalis

Microorganisms

a. Herpes simplex virus 2 (HSV2)

b. Human papilloma virus (HPV)

c. *Treponema pallidum*

d. *Chlamydia trachomatis*

e. Human immunodeficiency virus (HIV)

f. *Neisseria gonorrhoeae*

COG MATCHING

Grade: _____

Match each of the following stages of lochia with the correct description.

Lochia Stages

53. _____ Lochia rubra

54. _____ Lochia serosa

55. _____ Lochia alba

Descriptions

a. Thin, brownish discharge lasting about 3 to 4 days after the previous stage

b. Blood-tinged discharge within 6 days of delivery

c. White discharge that has no evidence of blood that can last up to week 6

COG IDENTIFICATION

56. Identify which of the following tasks may be the responsibility of the medical assistant in the care of the gynecological and obstetric patient by placing a check mark on the line preceding the task.

   a. _____ Give the patient instructions prior to her pelvic examination, such as refraining from douching, intercourse, and applying vaginal medication for 24 hours before her exam.

   b. _____ Warm the speculum prior to the pelvic exam.

   c. _____ Perform a breast examination.

   d. _____ Instruct the patient to change into an examining gown.

   e. _____ Inform patient of the effectiveness of different birth control methods.

   f. _____ Confirm whether a patient is gravid.

   g. _____ Decide whether a patient should go to the medical office, or go to the hospital after displaying signs and/or symptoms of labor.

   h. _____ Determine if the patient's medical history includes any over-the-counter medications known to be harmful to a developing fetus.

57. Identify the obstetric disorder associated with the following signs and symptoms by writing the name of the disorder on the line following the signs and symptoms.

   a. Nausea and vomiting (morning sickness) that has escalated to an unrelenting level, resulting in dehydration, electrolyte imbalance, and weight loss. _____

   b. The premature separation or detachment of the placenta from the uterus. _____

   c. Hypertension that is directly related to pregnancy and can be classified as either preeclampsia or eclampsia. _____

   d. The loss of pregnancy before the fetus is viable; preceded by vaginal bleeding, uterine cramps, and lower back pain. _____

   e. A fertilized ovum that has implanted somewhere other than the uterine cavity, such as the fallopian tubes, the abdomen, the ovaries, and the cervical os, causing breast enlargement or tenderness, nausea, pelvic pain, syncope, abdominal symptoms, painful sexual intercourse, and irregular menstrual bleeding. _____

58. During the first prenatal visit, you will be responsible for instructing the patient to contact the physician if she experiences certain alarming signs or symptoms. Below, eliminate the signs or symptoms that should not be included in the list by placing a check mark on the line next to the sign or symptom that should *not* be included.

   a. _____ Vaginal bleeding or spotting

   b. _____ Persistent vomiting

   c. _____ Weight gain

   d. _____ Increased appetite

   e. _____ Fever or chills

f. _____ Dysuria

g. _____ Frequent urination

h. _____ Unusual food cravings

i. _____ Abdominal or uterine cramping

j. _____ Leaking amniotic fluid

k. _____ Alteration in fetal movement

l. _____ Depressed mood

m. _____ Dizziness or blurred vision

59. Review the list of contraceptive methods. Then place a check mark on the line under the column to identify the type of contraceptive that describes the method.

Methods	Surgical	Hormonal	Barrier	Other
a. The pill				
b. Vasectomy				
c. Male condom				
d. Spermicide				
e. Injection				
f. The patch				
g. Emergency contraception				
h. Female condom				
i. The ring				
j. Diaphragm/spermicide				
k. Fertility awareness				
l. IUD				

COG SHORT ANSWER

Grade: _____

60. Some ovarian cysts are functional, whereas others are problematic. Give an example of each.

_____

_____

_____

_____

61. How is premenstrual dysphoric disorder (PMDD) diagnosed and treated?

_____

_____

_____

_____

62. What is the difference between HIV and AIDS?

_____

_____

_____

_____

63. A pregnant patient is listed as gr iv, pret 0, ab 2, p i. What does this listing describe?

_____

_____

_____

_____

64. What is a cesarean section, and list the reasons that this procedure would be necessary?

_____

_____

_____

_____

65. Which muscles are strengthened by Kegel exercises? How can these exercises benefit a patient?

_____

_____

_____

_____

66. A patient has just learned she is pregnant. What will you tell her to expect during her first prenatal visit? How often will you schedule the patient's subsequent prenatal visits?

_____

_____

_____

_____

67. After a patient's AFP (alpha-fetoprotein) levels were found to be abnormal, the physician has ordered an amniocentesis and a fetal ultrasonography. Describe the responsibilities of the medical assistant regarding these procedures performed in the medical office.

_____

_____

_____

_____

68. What signs differentiate true labor from false labor?

_____

_____

_____

_____

69. What should a patient nearing the age range of 45 to 50 years be told to expect during menopause?

_____

_____

_____

_____

Grade: _____

70. Complete this chart, which shows common gynecological disorders, their signs and symptoms, and possible treatments.

Disorder	Signs and Symptoms	Treatment
Dysfunctional uterine bleeding	**a.**	Hormone therapy, contraceptives, curettage, hysterectomy
Premenstrual syndrome	Severe physical, psychological, and behavioral signs and symptoms during the 7 to 10 days before menses	**b.**
Endometriosis	**c.**	Hormone and drug therapy, laparoscopic excision, hysterectomy, bilateral salpingo-oophorectomy
Uterine prolapse and displacement	Pelvic pressure, dyspareunia, urinary problems, constipation	**d.**
Leiomyomas	**e.**	Monitoring, myomectomy, hysterectomy
f.	Anovulation, irregular menses or amenorrhea, hirsutism	Hormone therapy, oral contraceptives
Infertility	Inability to conceive	**g.**

71. Complete this chart, which shows common diagnostic and therapeutic procedures and their purposes.

Procedure	Description	Purpose
Pelvic examination	**a.**	To identify or diagnose any abnormal conditions
Breast examination	Examination of the breast and surrounding tissue; performed with the hands	**b.**
Papanicolaou (Pap) test	**c.**	To detect signs of cervical cancer
Colposcopy	Visual examination of the vaginal and cervical surfaces using a stereoscopic microscope called a *colposcope*	**d.**
e.	Injection of a contrast medium into the uterus and fallopian tubes followed by a radiograph, using a hysterosalpingogram	To determine the configuration of the uterus and the patency of the fallopian tubes for patients with infertility
Dilation and curettage	**f.**	To remove uterine tissue for diagnostic testing, to remove endocrine tissue, to prevent or treat menorrhagia, or to remove retained products of conception after a spontaneous abortion or miscarriage

COG **TRUE OR FALSE?**

Grade: _____

Indicate whether the statements are true or false by placing the letter T (true) or F (false) on the line preceding the statement.

72. _____ A woman's first Pap test and pelvic examination should be performed about 3 years after her first sexual inter-course or by age 21 years, whichever comes first, as recommended by the American College of Obstetricians and Gynecologists (ACOG).

73. _____ A pelvic examination is performed for a pregnant patient during each prenatal visit to the obstetrician's office.

74. _____ The presence of Braxton-Hicks contractions is a conclusive sign of pregnancy and leads to a formal diagnosis of pregnancy.

75. _____ The date on which the patient last had sexual intercourse is used to calculate the expected date of delivery.

COG **AFF** **CASE STUDIES FOR CRITICAL THINKING**

Grade: _____

1. A patient at your medical office tested positive for a sexually transmitted disease (STD). What will be your responsibilities in connection with this diagnosis?

_____

_____

_____

_____

2. While working at a gynecological/obstetrics office, you receive a frantic phone call from a pregnant patient who is experiencing vaginal bleeding, uterine cramps, and lower back pain. You put the patient on hold in order to consult the physician, but you learn that the physician has just been called to the hospital for a delivery. How would you handle this call?

_____

_____

_____

_____

3. Your 34-year-old patient is concerned about gynecological cancers because there are cases of breast cancer and cervical cancer in her family history. What can you recommend the patient do to ensure early detection of any gynecological problems? Describe these procedures to her in a way that will ease her anxieties.

_____

_____

_____

_____

4. A 20-year-old female patient has made an appointment with the physician because she believes that she has PMDD, which she blames for her failing grades and damaged personal relationships. When you meet with the patient to assess her medical history, she asks you to write a note to her professors excusing her from any missed assignments. What should you do next?

_____

_____

_____

_____

PSY PROCEDURE 35-1   Instruct the Patient on the Breast Self-Examination

Name: _____ Date: _____ Time: _____ Grade: _____

EQUIPMENT/SUPPLIES: Patient education instruction sheet, if available; breast examination model, if available

STANDARDS: Given the needed equipment and a place to work the student will perform this skill with _____% accuracy in a total of _____ minutes. *(Your instructor will tell you what the percentage and time limits will be before you begin.)*

KEY: 4 = Satisfactory   0 = Unsatisfactory   NA = This step is not counted

PROCEDURE STEPS	SELF	PARTNER	INSTRUCTOR
1. Wash your hands.	☐	☐	☐
2. Explain the purpose and frequency of examining the breasts.	☐	☐	☐
3. Describe three positions necessary for the patient to examine the breasts: in front of a mirror, in the shower, and while lying down.	☐	☐	☐
4. In front of a mirror:			
a. Disrobe and inspect the breasts with her arms at sides and with arms raised above her head.	☐	☐	☐
b. Look for any changes in contour, swelling, dimpling of the skin, or changes in the nipple.	☐	☐	☐
5. In the shower:			
a. Feel each breast with hands over wet skin using the flat part of the first three fingers.	☐	☐	☐
b. Check for any lumps, hard knots, or thickenings.	☐	☐	☐
c. Use right hand to lightly press over all areas of left breast.	☐	☐	☐
d. Use left hand to examine right breast.	☐	☐	☐
6. Lying down:			
a. Place a pillow or folded towel under the right shoulder, and place the right hand behind head to examine the right breast.	☐	☐	☐
b. With left hand, use flat part of the fingers to palpate the breast tissue.	☐	☐	☐
c. Begin at the outermost top of the right breast.	☐	☐	☐
d. Work in a small circular motion around the breast in a clockwise rotation.	☐	☐	☐
7. Encourage patient to palpate the breast carefully moving her fingers inward toward the nipple and palpating every part of the breast including the nipple.	☐	☐	☐
8. Repeat the procedure for the left breast. Place a pillow or folded towel under the left shoulder with the left hand behind the head.	☐	☐	☐

9. Gently squeeze each nipple between the thumb and index finger.	☐	☐	☐
a. Report any clear or bloody discharge to the physician.	☐	☐	☐
b. Promptly report any abnormalities found in the breast self-examination to the physician.	☐	☐	☐
10. **AFF** Explain how to respond to a patient who is visually impaired.	☐	☐	☐
11. Document the patient education.	☐	☐	☐

CALCULATION

Total Possible Points: _____

Total Points Earned: _____ Multiplied by 100 = _____ Divided by Total Possible Points = _____ %

PASS   **FAIL**   **COMMENTS:**

☐   ☐

Student's signature _____ Date _____

Partner's signature _____ Date _____

Instructor's signature _____ Date _____

PSY PROCEDURE 35-2 | Assist with the Pelvic Examination and Pap Smear

Name: _____ Date: _____ Time: _____ Grade: _____

EQUIPMENT/SUPPLIES: Patient gown and drape, appropriate size vaginal speculum, cotton-tipped applicators, water-soluble lubricant, examination gloves, examination light, tissues *Materials for Pap smear:* Cervical spatula and/or brush, liquid cytology preparation, laboratory request form, identification labels *or* the materials required according to the laboratory, biohazard container

STANDARDS: Given the needed equipment and a place to work the student will perform this skill with _____% accuracy in a total of _____ minutes. *(Your instructor will tell you what the percentage and time limits will be before you begin.)*

KEY: 4 = Satisfactory   0 = Unsatisfactory   NA = This step is not counted

PROCEDURE STEPS	SELF	PARTNER	INSTRUCTOR
1. Wash your hands.	☐	☐	☐
2. Assemble the equipment and supplies.	☐	☐	☐
a. Warm vaginal speculum by running under warm water.	☐	☐	☐
b. Do not use lubricant on the vaginal speculum before insertion.	☐	☐	☐
3. Label each slide with date and type of specimen on the frosted end with a pencil.	☐	☐	☐
4. Greet and identify the patient. Explain the procedure.	☐	☐	☐
5. Ask the patient to empty her bladder and, if necessary, collect a urine specimen.	☐	☐	☐
6. Provide a gown and drape, and ask the patient to disrobe from the waist down.	☐	☐	☐
7. Position patient in the dorsal lithotomy position—buttocks at bottom edge of table.	☐	☐	☐
8. Adjust drape to cover patient's abdomen and knees but expose the genitalia.	☐	☐	☐
9. Adjust light over the genitalia for maximum visibility.	☐	☐	☐
10. Assist physician with the examination as needed.	☐	☐	☐
11. Put on examination gloves.	☐	☐	☐
a. Hold cytology liquid container for physician *or* insert brush as directed and mix with cytology liquid.	☐	☐	☐
b. Spray or cover each slide with fixative solution.	☐	☐	☐
12. Have a basin or other container ready to receive the now-contaminated speculum.	☐	☐	☐
13. Apply lubricant across the physician's two fingers.	☐	☐	☐
14. Encourage the patient to relax during the bimanual examination as needed.	☐	☐	☐

15. After the examination, assist the patient in sliding up to the top of the examination table and remove both feet at the same time from the stirrups.	☐	☐	☐
16. Offer the patient tissues to remove excess lubricant.	☐	☐	☐
a. Assist her to a sitting position if necessary.	☐	☐	☐
b. Watch for signs of vertigo.	☐	☐	☐
c. Ask the patient to get dressed and assist as needed.	☐	☐	☐
d. Provide for privacy as the patient dresses.	☐	☐	☐
17. Reinforce any physician instructions regarding follow-up appointments needed.	☐	☐	☐
a. Advise patient on the procedure for obtaining results from the Pap smear.	☐	☐	☐
18. **AFF** Explain how to respond to a patient who has dementia.	☐	☐	☐

_____

_____

_____

_____

_____

19. Properly care for or dispose of equipment and clean the examination room.	☐	☐	☐
20. Wash your hands.	☐	☐	☐
21. Document your responsibilities during the procedure.	☐	☐	☐

CALCULATION

Total Possible Points: _____

Total Points Earned: _____ Multiplied by 100 = _____ Divided by Total Possible Points = _____ %

PASS   **FAIL**   **COMMENTS:**

  ☐   ☐

Student's signature _____ Date _____

Partner's signature _____ Date _____

Instructor's signature _____ Date _____

PSY PROCEDURE 35-3 **Assist with Colposcopy and Cervical Biopsy**

Name: _____ Date: _____ Time: _____ Grade: _____

EQUIPMENT/SUPPLIES: Patient gown and drape, vaginal speculum, colposcope, specimen container with preservative (10% formalin), sterile gloves, appropriate size sterile cotton-tipped applicators, sterile normal saline solution, sterile 3% acetic acid, sterile povidone-iodine (Betadine), silver nitrate sticks or ferric subsulfate (Monsel's solution), sterile biopsy forceps or punch biopsy instrument, sterile uterine curet, sterile uterine dressing forceps, sterile 4 × 4 gauze pad, sterile towel, sterile endocervical curet, sterile uterine tenaculum, sanitary napkin, examination gloves, examination light, tissues, biohazard container

STANDARDS: Given the needed equipment and a place to work the student will perform this skill with _____% accuracy in a total of _____ minutes. *(Your instructor will tell you what the percentage and time limits will be before you begin.)*

KEY: 4 = Satisfactory 0 = Unsatisfactory NA = This step is not counted

PROCEDURE STEPS	SELF	PARTNER	INSTRUCTOR
1. Wash your hands.	☐	☐	☐
2. Verify that the patient has signed the consent form.	☐	☐	☐
3. Assemble the equipment and supplies.	☐	☐	☐
4. Check the light on the colposcope.	☐	☐	☐
5. Set up the sterile field without contaminating it.	☐	☐	☐
6. Pour sterile normal saline and acetic acid into their respective sterile containers.	☐	☐	☐
7. Cover the field with a sterile drape.	☐	☐	☐
8. Greet and identify the patient. Explain the procedure.	☐	☐	☐
9. When the physician is ready to proceed with the procedure:	☐	☐	☐
a. Assist the patient into the dorsal lithotomy position.	☐	☐	☐
b. Put on sterile gloves after positioning the patient if necessary.	☐	☐	☐
10. Hand the physician:			
a. The applicator immersed in normal saline.	☐	☐	☐
b. Followed by the applicator immersed in acetic acid.	☐	☐	☐
c. The applicator with the antiseptic solution (Betadine).	☐	☐	☐
11. If you did not apply sterile gloves to assist the physician:			
a. Apply clean examination gloves.	☐	☐	☐
b. Accept the biopsy specimen into a container of 10% formalin preservative.	☐	☐	☐
12. Provide the physician with Monsel's solution or silver nitrate sticks.	☐	☐	☐

13. When the physician is finished with the procedure:			
a. Assist the patient from the stirrups and into a sitting position.	☐	☐	☐
b. Explain to the patient that a small amount of bleeding may occur.	☐	☐	☐
c. Have a sanitary napkin available for the patient.	☐	☐	☐
d. Ask the patient to get dressed and assist as needed.	☐	☐	☐
e. Provide for privacy as the patient dresses.	☐	☐	☐
f. Reinforce any physician instructions regarding follow-up appointments.	☐	☐	☐
g. Advise the patient on how to obtain the biopsy results.	☐	☐	☐
14. **AFF** Explain how to respond to a patient who does not speak English or speaks English as a second language.	☐	☐	☐

_____

_____

_____

_____

15. Label the specimen container with the patient's name and date.	☐	☐	☐
a. Prepare the laboratory request.	☐	☐	☐
b. Transport the specimen and form to the laboratory.	☐	☐	☐
16. Properly care for, or dispose of, equipment and clean the examination room.	☐	☐	☐
17. Wash your hands.	☐	☐	☐
18. Document your responsibilities during the procedure.	☐	☐	☐

CALCULATION

Total Possible Points: _____

Total Points Earned: _____ Multiplied by 100 = _____ Divided by Total Possible Points = _____ %

PASS   **FAIL**   **COMMENTS:**

  ☐   ☐

Student's signature _____ Date _____

Partner's signature _____ Date _____

Instructor's signature _____ Date _____

Cognitive Domain

1. Spell and define key terms
2. Identify abnormal conditions of the thyroid, pancreas, adrenal, and pituitary glands
3. Describe the tests commonly used to diagnose disorders of these endocrine system glands
4. Explain your role in working with patients with endocrine system disorders
5. Identify common pathologies related to each body system
6. Describe implications for treatment related to pathology

Psychomotor Domain

1. Manage a patient with a diabetic emergency (Procedure 36-1)
2. Assist physician with patient care
3. Prepare a patient for procedures and/or treatments
4. Practice standard precautions
5. Document patient care
6. Document patient education
7. Practice within the standard of care for a medical assistant

Affective Domain

1. Apply critical thinking skills in performing patient assessment and care
2. Use language/verbal skills that enable patients' understanding
3. Demonstrate empathy in communicating with patients, family, and staff
4. Use appropriate body language and other nonverbal skills in communicating with patients, family, and staff
5. Demonstrate awareness of the territorial boundaries of the person with whom you are communicating
6. Demonstrate sensitivity appropriate to the message being delivered
7. Demonstrate recognition of the patient's level of understanding in communications
8. Recognize and protect personal boundaries in communicating with others
9. Demonstrate respect for individual diversity, incorporating awareness of one's own biases in areas including gender, race, religion, age, and economic status
10. Apply active listening skills
11. Apply local, state, and federal health care legislation and regulation appropriate to the medical assisting practice setting

ABHES Competencies

1. Assist the physician with the regimen of diagnostic and treatment modalities as they relate to each body system
2. Comply with federal, state, and local health laws and regulations
3. Communicate on the recipient's level of comprehension
4. Serve as a liaison between the physician and others
5. Show empathy and impartiality when dealing with patients
6. Document accurately

Name: _____   Date: _____   Grade: _____

COG MULTIPLE CHOICE

Circle the letter preceding the correct answer:

1. A patient with hypothyroidism must take hormone replacements:

   a. for as many years as he has had the disease.

   b. until the conclusion of puberty.

   c. for his entire life.

   d. until middle age.

   e. for 10 years.

2. Diabetics may need supplemental insulin to:

   a. test blood glucose levels.

   b. reverse vascular changes.

   c. reduce the presence of ketones.

   d. restore pancreatic function.

   e. control blood glucose levels.

3. One symptom of ketoacidosis is:

   a. shallow respirations.

   b. low blood glucose levels.

   c. overhydration.

   d. abdominal pain.

   e. pale, moist skin.

4. Diabetes mellitus affects metabolism of which type of molecule?

   a. Neurotransmitters

   b. Carbohydrates

   c. Hormones

   d. Vitamins

   e. Lipids

5. One symptom of type 1 diabetes mellitus is:

   a. polyuria.

   b. exophthalmia.

   c. anorexia.

   d. weight gain.

   e. a goiter.

6. Hyperpigmentation of the skin might be an indication of:

   a. Cushing syndrome.

   b. Hashimoto thyroiditis.

   c. Graves disease.

   d. Addison disease.

   e. diabetes insipidus.

7. To control gestational diabetes, a blood glucose specimen should be taken from a pregnant woman between:

   a. 28 and 32 weeks of gestation.

   b. 24 and 28 weeks of gestation.

   c. 20 and 24 weeks of gestation.

   d. 16 and 20 weeks of gestation.

   e. 12 and 16 weeks of gestation.

8. Cushing syndrome sufferers may experience accelerated:

   a. Addison disease.

   b. endocarditis.

   c. osteoporosis.

   d. arthritis.

   e. dementia.

9. Acromegaly results primarily in:

   a. an increase in bone width.

   b. muscular atrophy.

   c. an increase in bone length.

   d. muscular hypertrophy.

   e. an increase in bone density.

10. Growth can be stimulated for children with dwarfism by:

    a. repairs in the pituitary gland.

    b. administration of growth hormone.

    c. psychotherapy.

    d. increased physical activity.

    e. a high-protein diet.

11. Diabetes inspidus results from a deficiency of:

    a. adrenocorticotropic hormone.

    b. anterior pituitary hormones.

    c. human growth hormone.

    d. antidiuretic hormone.

    e. thyroid hormones.

12. Insulin shock is a result of:

    a. Cushing syndrome.

    b. Addison disease.

    c. Graves disease.

    d. hyperglycemia.

    e. hypoglycemia.

13. Diabetes mellitus patients need to care for their feet because:

    a. they regularly develop ingrown toenails.

    b. their peripheral circulation may be poor.

    c. they suffer severe joint pain.

    d. they have weak calves.

    e. foot pain occurs.

14. Exophthalmia is a protrusion of the:

    a. thyroid gland.

    b. pancreas.

    c. gall bladder.

    d. eyes.

    e. liver.

15. Patients taking corticosteroids may be at risk for:

    a. Cushing disease.

    b. Addison disease.

    c. type 2 diabetes mellitus.

    d. Graves disease.

    e. Hashimoto thyroiditis.

16. The A1C test determines how well blood glucose has been controlled during the previous:

    a. 2 to 3 hours.

    b. 2 to 3 days.

    c. 2 to 3 weeks.

    d. 2 to 3 months.

    e. 2 to 3 years.

17. Gigantism is a disorder of the:

    a. adrenal glands.

    b. pancreas.

    c. liver.

    d. thyroid.

    e. pituitary gland.

18. A thyroid scan relies on a radioactive isotope of what element?

    a. Iodine

    b. Barium

    c. Indium

    d. Bismuth

    e. Iridium

19. Addison disease is a disorder of the:

    a. pituitary gland.

    b. pancreas.

    c. thyroid.

    d. adrenal gland.

    e. salivary glands.

20. Both Graves disease and goiters are examples of:

    a. hypothyroidism.

    b. hypoglycemia.

    c. hyperthyroidism.

    d. hyperglycemia.

    e. hypertension.

COG MATCHING

Place the letter preceding the definition on the line next to the term.

Key Terms	Definitions
21. _____ acromegaly	**a.** an enlargement of the thyroid gland
22. _____ Addison disease	**b.** a substance that is produced by an endocrine gland and travels through the blood to a distant organ or gland where it acts to modify the structure or function of that gland or organ
23. _____ Cushing syndrome	**c.** an adrenal gland disorder that results in an increased production of ACTH from the pituitary glands
24. _____ diabetes insipidus	
25. _____ dwarfism	**d.** excess quantities of thyroid hormone in tissues
26. _____ endocrinologist	**e.** excessive proliferation of normal cells in the normal tissue arrangement of an organism
27. _____ exophthalmia	**f.** the end products of fat metabolism
28. _____ gigantism	**g.** itching
	h. pronounced hyperthyroidism with signs of enlarged thyroid and exophthalmos
29. _____ glycosuria	**i.** a type of diabetes in which patients do not require insulin to control blood sugar
30. _____ goiter	**j.** a deficiency in insulin production that leads to an inability to metabolize carbohydrates
31. _____ Graves disease	**k.** partial or complete failure of the adrenal cortex functions, causing general physical deterioration
32. _____ Hashimoto thyroiditis	
33. _____ hormones	**l.** the presence of glucose in the urine
34. _____ hyperglycemia	**m.** a disease of the immune system in which the tissue of the thyroid gland is replaced with fibrous tissue
35. _____ hyperplasia	**n.** excessive thirst
36. _____ hypoglycemia	**o.** abnormal underdevelopment of the body with extreme shortness but normal proportion; achondroplastic dwarfism is an inherited growth disorder characterized by shortened limbs and a large head but almost normal trunk proportions
37. _____ insulin-dependent diabetes mellitus	
	p. acidosis accompanied by an accumulation of ketones in the body
38. _____ ketoacidosis	**q.** excessive size and stature caused most frequently by hypersecretion of the human growth hormone
39. _____ ketones	**r.** deficiency of sugar in the blood
	s. an unusual protrusion of the eyeballs as a result of a thyroid disorder
40. _____ non–insulin-dependent diabetes mellitus	**t.** a disorder of metabolism characterized by polyuria and polydipsia; caused by a deficiency in ADH or an inability of the kidneys to respond to ADH
41. _____ polydipsia	**u.** excessive excretion and elimination of urine
42. _____ polyphagia	**v.** hyperfunction of the anterior pituitary gland near the end of puberty that results in increased bone width.

43. _____ polyuria

44. _____ pruritus

45. _____ radioimmunoassay

46. _____ thyrotoxicosis

w. the introduction of radioactive substances in the body to determine the concentration of a substance in the serum, usually the concentration of antigens, antibodies, or proteins

x. a doctor who diagnoses and treats disorders of the endocrine system and its hormone-secreting glands

y. abnormal hunger

z. an increase in blood sugar, as in diabetes mellitus

COG IDENTIFICATION   Grade: _____

47. Read the following list of symptoms. Are these symptoms representative of hyperglycemia or hypoglycemia? Place the prefix "hyper" on the line preceding the symptoms for hyperglycemia and "hypo" for hypoglycemia.

a. _____ Pale complexion

b. _____ Deep respirations

c. _____ Moist skin

d. _____ Shallow respirations

e. _____ Abdominal pain

f. _____ Rapid, bounding pulse

g. _____ Fruity breath

h. _____ Subnormal blood glucose levels

COG SHORT ANSWER   Grade: _____

48. When does ketoacidosis occur?

_____

_____

_____

_____

49. A patient is stunned to learn that she has been diagnosed with type 2 diabetes mellitus. She is 43 years old and in excellent health. As a personal trainer and nutritionist, she has always taken good care of her body. What potential cause of type 2 diabetes mellitus might she be overlooking?

_____

_____

_____

_____

50. A patient complains that, lately, his appetite has been ferocious, but he is actually losing weight. He does not understand why this is happening. What do you tell him?

_____

_____

_____

_____

51. Why is it difficult for many sufferers of endocrine disorders to comply with physicians' orders?

_____

_____

_____

_____

52. A patient who has been diagnosed with type 2 diabetes mellitus explains that a friend told him the disease is sometimes called _non-insulin-dependent diabetes mellitus._ He asks if this means that he will not need to take insulin. Is he correct? Why, or why not?

_____

_____

_____

_____

53. Who might be at risk for gestational diabetes mellitus?

_____

_____

_____

_____

54. What is the cause of hypoglycemia?

_____

_____

_____

_____

55. How is Addison disease treated?

_____

_____

_____

_____

56. A patient is diagnosed with dwarfism, and the patient's mother is extremely distressed, wondering if certain body parts will grow normally while others will not. She also wonders if her daughter could ever grow normally. What could you tell the mother?

_____

_____

_____

_____

57. What do the fasting glucose test and glucose tolerance test for diabetes mellitus have in common?

_____

_____

_____

58. What is the purpose of the A1C blood test?

_____

_____

_____

_____

59. Cushing syndrome and Addison disease are both disorders of which gland?

_____

_____

_____

_____

60. Why is it important that patients with diseases of the endocrine system wear a medical alert bracelet or necklace?

_____

_____

_____

_____

COG TRUE OR FALSE?   Grade: _____

Indicate whether the statements are true or false by placing the letter T (true) or F (false) on the line preceding the statement.

61. _____ Endocrine glands are unlike other glands in the body because they are ductless.

62. _____ Hashimoto thyroiditis is a disease of the endocrine system.

63. _____ Type 1 diabetes mellitus occurs only in children and young adults.

64. _____ Addison disease has no effect on the pituitary gland.

COG AFF **CASE STUDIES FOR CRITICAL THINKING**   Grade: _____

1. A patient is worried that a thyroid function test requires the use of radioactive material. Explain, to the best of your ability, how the test works and why there is no need to be concerned about radiation. If necessary, do additional research on thyroid function tests to prepare your answer.

_____

_____

_____

_____

2. After an examination, a pregnant patient asks why the physician performed a test on her blood glucose level. She says she does not have diabetes. Explain why the physician chose to do the test.

_____

_____

_____

_____

3. Young children are sometimes afflicted with diabetes mellitus. This can be difficult for both the child and the family. What is your perspective of the medical assistant's role in this situation?

_____

_____

_____

_____

4. A patient with hyperthyroidism says she would prefer not to be treated because she has few negative symptoms, and the increased metabolic rate helps keep her thin. How would you respond to this?

_____

_____

_____

_____

PSY PROCEDURE 36-1 Manage a Patient with a Diabetic Emergency

Name: _____ Date: _____ Time: _____ Grade: _____

EQUIPMENT/SUPPLIES: Gloves, blood glucose monitor and strips, fruit juice or oral glucose tablets

STANDARDS: Given the needed equipment and a place to work the student will perform this skill with _____% accuracy in a total of _____ minutes. *(Your instructor will tell you what the percentage and time limits will be before you begin.)*

KEY: 4 = Satisfactory   0 = Unsatisfactory   NA = This step is not counted

PROCEDURE STEPS	SELF	PARTNER	INSTRUCTOR
1. Wash your hands.	☐	☐	☐
2. Recognize the signs and symptoms of hyperglycemia and hypoglycemia.	☐	☐	☐
3. Identify the patient and escort him or her into the examination room.	☐	☐	☐
4. Determine if the patient has been previously diagnosed with diabetes mellitus.	☐	☐	☐
5. Ask the patient if he or she has eaten today or taken any medication.	☐	☐	☐
6. Notify the physician about the patient and perform a capillary stick for a blood glucose as directed.	☐	☐	☐
7. Notify the physician with the results of the blood glucose and treat the patient as ordered by the physician. **a.** Administer insulin subcutaneously to a patient with hyperglycemia. **b.** Administer a quick-acting sugar, such as an oral glucose tablet or fruit juice, for a patient with hypoglycemia.	☐	☐	☐
8. **AFF** Explain how to respond to a patient who is developmentally challenged.	☐	☐	☐
9. Be prepared to notify EMS as directed by the physician if the symptoms do not improve or worsen.	☐	☐	☐
10. Document any observations and treatments given.	☐	☐	☐

CALCULATION

Total Possible Points: _____

Total Points Earned: _____ Multiplied by 100 = _____ Divided by Total Possible Points = _____ %

PASS   **FAIL**   **COMMENTS:**

☐   ☐

Student's signature _____ Date _____

Partner's signature _____ Date _____

Instructor's signature _____ Date _____

37 Pediatrics

Learning Outcomes

Cognitive Domain

1. Spell and define key terms
2. List safety precautions for the pediatric office
3. Explain the difference between a well-child and a sick-child visit
4. List types and schedule of immunizations
5. Describe the types of feelings a child might have during an office visit
6. List and explain how to record the anthropometric measurements obtained in a pediatric visit
7. Identify two injection sites to use on an infant and two used on a child
8. Describe the role of the parent during the office visit
9. List the names, symptoms, and treatments for common pediatric illnesses
10. Identify common pathologies related to each body system
11. Describe implications for treatment related to pathology

Psychomotor Domain

1. Obtain an infant's length and weight (Procedure 37-1)
2. Obtain the head and chest circumference (Procedure 37-2)
3. Apply a urinary collection device (Procedure 37-3)
4. Assist physician with patient care
5. Prepare a patient for procedures and/or treatments

6. Practice standard precautions
7. Document patient care
8. Document patient education
9. Practice within the standard of care for a medical assistant

Affective Domain

1. Apply critical thinking skills in performing patient assessment and care
2. Use language/verbal skills that enable patients' understanding
3. Demonstrate empathy in communicating with patients, family, and staff
4. Use appropriate body language and other nonverbal skills in communicating with patients, family, and staff
5. Demonstrate awareness of the territorial boundaries of the person with whom you are communicating
6. Demonstrate sensitivity appropriate to the message being delivered
7. Demonstrate recognition of the patient's level of understanding in communications
8. Recognize and protect personal boundaries in communicating with others
9. Demonstrate respect for individual diversity, incorporating awareness of one's own biases in areas including gender, race, religion, age, and economic status
10. Apply active listening skills
11. Apply local, state, and federal health care legislation and regulation appropriate to the medical assisting practice setting

ABHES Competencies

1. Assist the physician with the regimen of diagnostic and treatment modalities as they relate to each body system
2. Comply with federal, state, and local health laws and regulations
3. Communicate on the recipient's level of comprehension
4. Serve as a liaison between the physician and others
5. Show empathy and impartiality when dealing with patients
6. Document accurately

Name: _____   Date: _____   Grade: _____

COG MULTIPLE CHOICE

Circle the letter preceding the correct answer.

1. The top priority in a pediatrics office is:

    a. organization.

    b. safety.

    c. efficiency.

    d. location.

    e. size.

2. In a pediatrician's waiting room, it's most important that the toys are:

    a. trendy.

    b. interesting to all age groups.

    c. large enough to share.

    d. washable.

    e. educational.

3. Which method of taking a temperature is most readily accepted by children of all ages?

    a. Tympanic

    b. Oral

    c. Rectal

    d. Axillary

    e. Touch

4. One symptom of meningitis is:

    a. dysuria.

    b. disorientation.

    c. coughing.

    d. stiff neck.

    e. chills.

5. Which of the following has been associated with Reye syndrome?

    a. Pyloric stenosis

    b. Aspirin

    c. Cerebral palsy

    d. Phenylalanine hydroxylase

    e. Otitis media

6. Which of the following is something that is routinely done at a child's wellness exam?

    a. Blood test

    b. Urine test

    c. Immunization

    d. Radiography

    e. Measurements

7. To minimize a child's anxiety during a visit, you should:

    a. avoid talking to the child.

    b. speak directly to the parent.

    c. be gentle but firm.

    d. ask the child to be quiet.

    e. spend as little time in the room as possible.

8. Which of the following statements is true?

    a. The reflexes present in a newborn disappear by age 3 months.

    b. A pediatrician is responsible for a child's physical and mental health.

    c. Disinfectants should be kept in patient rooms for easy access.

    d. Vaccination Information Statements may be provided upon request.

    e. The DDST measures all physical and mental aspects of a child.

9. One warning sign of child abuse is a child who:

    a. comes in with scraped knees.

    b. shrinks away as you approach.

    c. has a poor growth pattern.

    d. has a bloody nose.

    e. screams when you administer a shot.

10. What might make the examination more fun for a 4- or 5-year-old child?

    a. Allowing the child to crawl on the floor

    b. Answering all the questions he or she asks

    c. Showing the child medical pictures

    d. Letting the child listen to his or her heartbeat

    e. Asking the parent to assist with the exam

    Scenario for questions 11 and 12: A child comes in for a well-child visit and begins to panic when she hears she will need to get a vaccination.

11. What should you do?

    a. Let another assistant give her the shot.

    b. Ask the parent or caregiver to calm her down.

    c. Show her the needle ahead of time.

    d. Tell her gently that it won't hurt at all.

    e. Hide the needle until you give her the shot.

12. After you administer the medication, the girl becomes sullen and withdrawn. What is the best way to address this behavior?

    a. Leave and allow her mother to comfort her.

    b. Praise and comfort her before you leave.

    c. Ask her if the shot was really that bad.

    d. Promise it won't hurt so much next time.

    e. Laugh and say it was just a little shot.

13. Which of the following disorders has symptoms that may become obvious only with the passage of time?

    a. Meningitis

    b. Croup

    c. Epiglottitis

    d. Cerebral palsy

    e. Pyloric stenosis

14. Children are more likely to develop ear infections than adults because they have:

    a. an immature nervous system.

    b. short and straight Eustachian tubes.

    c. decreased resistance to diseases.

    d. more exposure to bacteria.

    e. poor handwashing skills.

15. Which infant reflex is a result of the cheek being stroked?

    a. Rooting

    b. Moro

    c. Stepping

    d. Fencing

    e. Babinski

16. Children have lower blood pressure than adults because:

    a. they cannot sit still for long periods of time.

    b. they require a smaller cuff for measurements.

    c. their hearts do not pump as quickly as adults' hearts.

    d. their vessels are softer and less resistant.

    e. you must use a standard sphygmomanometer.

17. At what age does a child's respiratory rate slow to that of an adult's?

    a. 0–1 year

    b. 1–5 years

    c. 5–10 years

    d. 10–15 years

    e. 15–20 years

18. Which of the following can help a physician test an infant for pyloric stenosis?

    a. Blood tests

    b. Urine tests

    c. Parental history

    d. Percentile comparisons

    e. Weight

19. Which of the following disorders cannot be cured at this time?

    a. Meningitis

    b. Impetigo

    c. Tetanus

    d. Syphilis

    e. Cerebral palsy

20. A sharp barking cough is a symptom of:

    a. meningitis.

    b. croup.

    c. tetanus.

    d. encephalitis.

    e. impetigo.

COG MATCHING
        Grade: _____

Place the letter preceding the definition on the line next to the term.

Key Terms

21. _____ aspiration

22. _____ autonomous

23. _____ congenital anomaly

24. _____ immunization

25. _____ neonatologist

26. _____ pediatrician

27. _____ pediatrics

28. _____ psychosocial

29. _____ restrain

30. _____ sick-child visit

31. _____ varicella zoster

32. _____ well-child visit

Definitions

a. to control or confine movement

b. a physician who specializes in the care and treatment of newborns

c. a viral infection manifested by the characteristic rash of successive crops of vesicles that scab before resolution; also called *chicken pox*

d. a physician who specializes in the care of infants, children, and adolescents

e. a visit to the medical office for the administration of immunizations and evaluation of growth and development

f. drawing in or out by suction, as in breathing objects into the respiratory tract or suctioning substances from a site

g. an abnormality, either structural or functional, present at birth

h. a pediatric visit for the treatment of illness or injury

i. a specialty of medicine that deals with the care of infants, children, and adolescents

j. existing or functioning independently

k. relating to mental and emotional aspects of social encounters

l. the act or process of rendering an individual immune to specific disease

COG MATCHING
        Grade: _____

Place the letter preceding the pulse rate range on the line preceding the appropriate age.

Ages

33. _____ newborn

34. _____ 3 months to 2 years

35. _____ 2 years to 10 years

36. _____ 10 years and older

Pulse Rate Ranges

a. 80–150/minute

b. 60–100/minute

c. 100–180/minute

d. 65–130/minute

COG IDENTIFICATION

Grade: _____

37. Review the pediatric immunization schedule in your textbook to answer the following questions:

   a. How many doses of the rotavirus vaccine are given? When?

   _____

   b. How many immunizations do children receive at 4 months? Which ones?

   _____

   c. When do children start receiving a yearly influenza vaccination?

   _____

   d. How many doses of the hepatitis B vaccine are administered?

   _____

38. What are five different ways to check a child's temperature?

   a. _____

   b. _____

   c. _____

   d. _____

   e. _____

39. What are the seven "rights" of drug administration?

   a. _____

   b. _____

   c. _____

   d. _____

   e. _____

   f. _____

   g. _____

40. Identify six symptoms of meningitis:

   _____

COG **SHORT ANSWER**   Grade: _____

41. What does the Federal Child Abuse Prevention and Treatment Act mandate?

_____

_____

_____

_____

42. What is the VIS? Why do you give the parent or caregiver of a child a copy?

_____

_____

_____

_____

43. Why do sick-child visits occur frequently during early childhood?

_____

_____

_____

_____

44. What is the difference between a well-child and a sick-child visit?

_____

_____

_____

_____

45. List five feelings a child might have during an office visit.

_____

_____

_____

_____

46. What role does a parent or caregiver play in the child's exam?

_____

_____

_____

_____

47. How is a child's medication dosage calculated?

_____

_____

_____

_____

48. Why is epiglottitis considered more serious than croup?

_____

_____

_____

_____

49. If a child has been reported as being easily distracted, forgetful, extremely talkative, impulsive, and showing a dislike for school activities, does the child have ADHD?

_____

_____

_____

_____

50. A worried mother calls in because her newborn baby is vomiting. She wants to know if she should bring her baby into the office for examination. What do you tell her?

_____

_____

_____

_____

COG COMPLETION   Grade: _____

51. Complete the chart below with information about childhood reflexes. Briefly describe each response and note the age it generally disappears.

Reflex	Response	Age When It Generally Disappears
a. Sucking, or rooting		
b. Moro, or startle		
c. Grasp		
d. Tonic neck, or fencing		
e. Placing, or stepping		
f. Babinski		

COG TRUE OR FALSE?   Grade: _____

Indicate whether the statements are true or false by placing the letter T (true) or F (false) on the line preceding the statement.

52. _____ Infant scales should always be placed on the floor next to the adult scale.

53. _____ It is a violation of HIPAA to have two separate waiting rooms for sick children and well children.

54. _____ There should be no toys in the waiting room because they may help spread germs.

55. _____ Children outgrow child-sized furniture too quickly, so it is not a worthwhile investment.

56. _____ Many childhood diseases are highly contagious and can be controlled by stringent handwashing measures.

57. _____ Immunization schedules change every 5 years.

58. _____ A child's heartbeat is much slower than an adult's heart rate.

59. _____ Asthma is a respiratory problem that usually develops after puberty.

60. _____ Minors do not need to be informed of what you're going to do.

COG **AFF** **CASE STUDIES FOR CRITICAL THINKING**   Grade: _____

1. A mother calls in, saying her 15-month-old daughter has been fussy and tugging at her ear. There is no fever, but the girl has been tired and had a cold a few days before. What do you tell her to do?

_____

_____

_____

_____

2. A young boy, accompanied by his mother, greets you in the examination room and starts asking all kinds of questions about things you do. He enjoys helping you test his reflexes and reading the vision chart, but he firmly refuses to cooperate when you try to give him a shot. What can you or his mother do to get him settled down enough to give him the shot?

_____

_____

_____

_____

3. A 16-year-old boy has been diagnosed as obese, and his parents have come in to find out what they can do to help their son achieve a healthy weight. The physician wants the boy to exercise at a local gym and to return in 6 months to check his progress. What education can you provide that will help the boy and his parents start a healthier lifestyle?

_____

_____

_____

_____

4. A young child has come in with a broken arm. During the examination, you notice the child also has several scrapes and bruises on his legs and feet as well. His mother says he got them from playing outdoors. Do you report this as child abuse to the physician? If not, what do you do?

_____

_____

_____

_____

5. Spanking children for misbehaving is sometimes considered child abuse. However, the parents who spank their children say that they were spanked when they were young, and they believe it is the best way to safely punish bad behavior. They also say that children who are not spanked become spoiled and difficult to control. What do you think? Is it your duty to report spanking as child abuse?

_____

_____

_____

_____

PSY PROCEDURE 37-1 Obtain an Infant's Length and Weight

Name: _____ Date: _____ Time: _____ Grade: _____

EQUIPMENT/SUPPLIES: Examining table with clean paper, tape measure, infant scale, protective paper for the scale, appropriate growth chart

STANDARDS: Given the needed equipment and a place to work the student will perform this skill with _____% accuracy in a total of _____ minutes. *(Your instructor will tell you what the percentage and time limits will be before you begin.)*

KEY: 4 = Satisfactory   0 = Unsatisfactory   NA = This step is not counted

PROCEDURE STEPS	SELF	PARTNER	INSTRUCTOR
1. Wash your hands.	☐	☐	☐
2. Explain the procedure to the parent.	☐	☐	☐
3. Ask parent to remove the infant's clothing except for the diaper.	☐	☐	☐
4. Place the child on a firm examination table covered with clean table paper.	☐	☐	☐
5. Fully extend the child's body by holding the head in the midline.	☐	☐	☐
6. Grasp the knees and press flat onto the table gently but firmly.	☐	☐	☐
7. Make a mark on table paper with pen at the top of the head and heel of the feet.	☐	☐	☐
8. Measure between marks in either inches or centimeters.	☐	☐	☐
9. Record the child's length on the growth chart and in the patient's chart.	☐	☐	☐
10. Either carry the infant or have the parent carry the infant to the scale.	☐	☐	☐
11. Place a protective paper on the scale and balance the scale.	☐	☐	☐
12. Remove the diaper just before laying the infant on the scale.	☐	☐	☐
13. Place the child gently on the scale. Keep one of your hands over or near the child on the scale at all times.	☐	☐	☐
14. Balance the scale quickly but carefully.	☐	☐	☐
15. Pick the infant up and instruct the parent to replace the diaper if removed.	☐	☐	☐
16. Record the infant's weight on the growth chart and in the patient chart.	☐	☐	☐
17. Wash your hands.	☐	☐	☐

CALCULATION

Total Possible Points: _____

Total Points Earned: _____ Multiplied by 100 = _____ Divided by Total Possible Points = _____ %

PASS   **FAIL**   **COMMENTS:**

☐   ☐

Student's signature _____ Date _____

Partner's signature _____ Date _____

Instructor's signature _____ Date _____

PSY PROCEDURE 37-2 Obtain the Head and Chest Circumference

Name: _____ Date: _____ Time: _____ Grade: _____

EQUIPMENT/SUPPLIES: Paper or cloth measuring tape, growth chart

STANDARDS: Given the needed equipment and a place to work the student will perform this skill with _____% accuracy in a total of _____ minutes. *(Your instructor will tell you what the percentage and time limits will be before you begin.)*

KEY: 4 = Satisfactory 0 = Unsatisfactory NA = This step is not counted

PROCEDURE STEPS	SELF	PARTNER	INSTRUCTOR
1. Wash your hands.	☐	☐	☐
2. Place the infant in the supine position on the examination table, or ask the parent to hold the infant.	☐	☐	☐
3. Measure around the head above the eyebrow and posteriorly at the largest part of the occiput.	☐	☐	☐
4. Record the child's head circumference on the growth chart.	☐	☐	☐
5. With the infant's clothing removed from the chest, measure around the chest at the nipple line, keeping the measuring tape at the same level anteriorly and posteriorly.	☐	☐	☐
6. Record the child's chest circumference on the growth chart.	☐	☐	☐
7. Wash your hands.	☐	☐	☐

CALCULATION

Total Possible Points: _____

Total Points Earned: _____ Multiplied by 100 = _____ Divided by Total Possible Points = _____ %

PASS **FAIL** **COMMENTS:**

☐ ☐

Student's signature _____ Date _____

Partner's signature _____ Date _____

Instructor's signature _____ Date _____

PSY PROCEDURE 37-3 | **Apply a Urinary Collection Device**

Name: _____ Date: _____ Time: _____ Grade: _____

EQUIPMENT/SUPPLIES: Gloves, personal antiseptic wipes, pediatric urine collection bag, completed laboratory request slip, biohazard transport container

STANDARDS: Given the needed equipment and a place to work the student will perform this skill with _____% accuracy in a total of _____ minutes. *(Your instructor will tell you what the percentage and time limits will be before you begin.)*

KEY: 4 = Satisfactory   0 = Unsatisfactory   NA = This step is not counted

PROCEDURE STEPS	SELF	PARTNER	INSTRUCTOR
1. Wash your hands.	☐	☐	☐
2. Assemble the equipment and supplies.	☐	☐	☐
3. Explain the procedure to the child's parents.	☐	☐	☐
4. Place the child in a supine position. Ask for help from the parents as needed.	☐	☐	☐
5. After putting on gloves, clean the genitalia with the antiseptic wipes:			
a. For females:			
(1) Cleanse front to back with separate wipes for each downward stroke on the outer labia.	☐	☐	☐
(2) The last clean wipe should be used between the inner labia.	☐	☐	☐
b. For males:			
(1) Retract the foreskin if the baby has not been circumcised.	☐	☐	☐
(2) Cleanse the meatus in an ever-widening circle.	☐	☐	☐
(3) Discard the wipe and repeat the procedure.	☐	☐	☐
(4) Return the foreskin to its proper position.	☐	☐	☐
5. Holding the collection device:			
a. Remove the upper portion of the paper backing and press it around the mons pubis.	☐	☐	☐
b. Remove the second section and press it against the perineum.	☐	☐	☐
c. Loosely attach the diaper.	☐	☐	☐
6. Give the baby fluids unless contraindicated, and check the diaper frequently.	☐	☐	☐
7. When the child has voided, remove the device, clean the skin of residual adhesive, and re-diaper.	☐	☐	☐
8. Prepare the specimen for transport to the laboratory.	☐	☐	☐
9. Remove your gloves and wash your hands.	☐	☐	☐
10. Record the procedure.	☐	☐	☐

CALCULATION

Total Possible Points: _____

Total Points Earned: _____ Multiplied by 100 = _____ Divided by Total Possible Points = _____ %

PASS   **FAIL**   **COMMENTS:**

☐   ☐

Student's signature _____ Date _____

Partner's signature _____ Date _____

Instructor's signature _____ Date _____

Geriatrics

Cognitive Domain

1. Spell and define key terms
2. Explain how aging affects thought processes
3. Describe methods to increase compliance with health maintenance programs among older adults
4. Discuss communication problems that may occur with older adults and list steps to maintain open communication
5. Recognize and describe the coping mechanisms used by older adults to deal with multiple losses
6. Name the risk factors and signs of older adult abuse
7. Explain the types of long-term care facilities available
8. Describe the effects of aging on the way the body processes medication
9. Discuss the responsibility of medical assistants with regard to teaching older adult patients
10. List and describe physical changes and diseases common to the aging process
11. Identify common pathologies related to each body system
12. Describe implications for treatment related to pathology

Psychomotor Domain

1. Assist physician with patient care
2. Prepare a patient for procedures and/or treatments

3. Practice standard precautions
4. Document patient care
5. Document patient education
6. Practice within the standard of care for a medical assistant

Affective Domain

1. Apply critical thinking skills in performing patient assessment and care
2. Use language/verbal skills that enable patients' understanding
3. Demonstrate empathy in communicating with patients, family, and staff
4. Use appropriate body language and other nonverbal skills in communicating with patients, family, and staff
5. Demonstrate awareness of the territorial boundaries of the person with whom you are communicating
6. Demonstrate sensitivity appropriate to the message being delivered
7. Demonstrate recognition of the patient's level of understanding in communications
8. Recognize and protect personal boundaries in communicating with others
9. Demonstrate respect for individual diversity, incorporating awareness of one's own biases in areas including gender, race, religion, age, and economic status
10. Apply active listening skills
11. Apply local, state, and federal health care legislation and regulation appropriate to the medical assisting practice setting

ABHES Competencies

1. Assist the physician with the regimen of diagnostic and treatment modalities as they relate to each body system
2. Comply with federal, state, and local health laws and regulations
3. Communicate on the recipient's level of comprehension
4. Serve as a liaison between the physician and others
5. Show empathy and impartiality when dealing with patients
6. Document accurately

Name: _____   Date: _____   Grade: _____

COG MULTIPLE CHOICE

Circle the letter preceding the correct answer.

1. Which of the following statements is true about older adult patients who require long-term medication?

   a. If older adult patients take their medication every day, they are unlikely to forget a dosage.

   b. Compliance over a long period of time can become problematic in older adult patients.

   c. With a chronic illness, an older adult patient can neglect to take his or her medication for a few weeks with no side effects.

   d. Patients who take their medications for a long period of time will eventually notice a significant improvement.

   e. Older adult patients will eventually become immune to long-term medication.

2. Which of these conditions can sometimes be improved by taking the herbal supplement gingko?

   a. Arthritis

   b. Parkinson disease

   c. Loss of appetite

   d. Poor concentration

   e. Alzheimer disease

3. The purpose of an advance directive is to:

   a. divide a person's possessions in the event of death.

   b. inform the physician of any allergies that an individual has to specific medications.

   c. outline a person's wishes about end-of-life care.

   d. transfer a patient's medical records between physicians' offices.

   e. order a physician not to resuscitate a patient under any circumstances.

4. Which of these is a task performed by a home health aide?

   a. Light housecleaning

   b. Refilling prescriptions

   c. Reorganizing bulky furniture

   d. Writing daily task lists and reminders

   e. Keeping the older adult occupied

5. Which of these is a good place to find information about respite care for older adult relatives?

   a. Local newspaper

   b. Television advertisement

   c. Community senior citizen program

   d. Local business directory

   e. Library bulletin board

6. What is an example of passive neglect of an older adult patient?

   a. Withholding medication from the patient

   b. Locking the patient in a room

   c. Overmedicating the patient to make him or her easier to care for

   d. Isolating the patient from friends and family

   e. Forgetting to give the patient regular baths

7. Which of the following statements is true about the aging process?

   a. Longevity is based entirely on environmental factors.

   b. People who have dangerous occupations will not live as long as people who do not.

   c. Longevity is hereditary, so it does not make a difference how you live your life.

   d. Longevity is largely hereditary, but environmental factors play a significant role.

   e. An obese, physically inactive smoker will have a shorter lifespan than a healthy nonsmoker.

8. What is the best way to deal with a patient who is hearing impaired?

   a. Raise your voice until the patient can hear you.

   b. Give written instructions whenever possible.

   c. Talk to the patient with your back to the light.

   d. Talk directly into the patient's ear.

   e. Find a coworker who is able to communicate using sign language.

Scenario for questions 9-11: A 55-year-old patient comes into the physician's office and tells you that he thinks he is suffering from Parkinson disease.

9. The physician would diagnose the patient by:

   a. taking a blood test.

   b. performing dexterity tasks.

   c. excluding other causes.

   d. performing an MRI scan.

   e. testing his reflexes.

10. How would you explain deep brain stimulation to the patient?

   a. It increases the levels of dopamine in the brain.

   b. It lowers a person's acetylcholine levels.

   c. It blocks the impulses that cause tremors.

   d. It controls a person's stress and anxiety levels.

   e. It acts as a muscle relaxant and prevents rigidity.

11. What would you tell the patient about Levodopa?

   a. It has no serious side effects.

   b. It remains effective for the entire length of the disease.

   c. It can cause headaches and migraines.

   d. It should not be taken with alcohol.

   e. It may aggravate stomach ulcers.

12. When older adult patients are beginning a new exercise regime, it is a good idea for them to:

   a. rest when they get tired.

   b. start with a brisk 30-minute jog.

   c. keep to the same weekly routine.

   d. exercise alone so they are not distracted.

   e. work through any initial pain or discomfort.

13. Which of the following statements is true about the nutritional requirements of older adult patients?

   a. Older adult patients need less food and water than younger patients because older adults are not as active.

   b. It is easier for older adult patients to maintain good nutrition because they have more time to prepare meals.

   c. Vitamin and mineral requirements are lower in older adult patients than in younger patients.

   d. Older adult patients should eat smaller, more frequent meals to aid digestion.

   e. Older adult patients can replace meals with liquid dietary supplements without damaging their health.

14. A caregiver can help increase safety in the home of an older adult patient by:

   a. installing handrails in the bathtub and near the commode.

   b. placing childproof locks on the kitchen cupboards.

   c. encouraging the patient to exercise regularly.

   d. covering highly polished floors with scatter rugs.

   e. keeping the patient's medicine in a locked bathroom cabinet.

15. What action should you take if you suspect older adult abuse?

   a. Try to separate the caregiver from the patient for the examination.

   b. Tell the caregiver you will be reporting him/her to the authorities.

   c. Question the patient about suspicious injuries until she tells you the truth.

   d. Call the police while the patient is in the examination room.

   e. Wait to inform the physician of your suspicions until you are sure they are correct.

16. What does the acronym HOH mean in a patient's chart?

   a. Has ordinary hearing

   b. Head of household

   c. Has own home

   d. Hard on health

   e. Hard of hearing

17. Another name for the herbal supplement gingko is:

   a. folic acid.

   b. kew tree.

   c. aloe vera.

   d. green tea.

   e. milk thistle.

18. What is the best advice to give a patient who is having difficulty swallowing medication?

    a. Grind the medication into powder.

    b. Ask the pharmacist for smaller pills.

    c. Put the medication on the back of the tongue, and drink water with a straw.

    d. Lie down and swallow the medication with a lot of water.

    e. Dissolve the medication in a hot drink.

19. A physician who specializes in disorders that affect the aging population is called a(n):

    a. gastroenterologist.

    b. gerontologist.

    c. oncologist.

    d. otorhinolaryngologist.

    e. rheumatologist.

20. An eye condition that causes increased intraocular pressure and intolerance to light is:

    a. cataracts.

    b. kyphosis.

    c. bradykinesia.

    d. osteoporosis.

    e. glaucoma.

COG **MATCHING**   Grade: _____

Place the letter preceding the definition on the line next to the term.

Key Terms

21. _____ activities of daily living (ADL)

22. _____ biotransform

23. _____ bradykinesia

24. _____ cataracts

25. _____ cerebrovascular accident (CVA)

26. _____ compliance

27. _____ degenerative joint disease (DJD)

28. _____ dementia

29. _____ dysphagia

30. _____ gerontologist

31. _____ glaucoma

32. _____ Kegel exercises

Definitions

a. a specialist who studies aging

b. general mental deterioration associated with old age

c. to convert the molecules of a substance from one form to another, as in medications within the body

d. a sensation of whirling of oneself or the environment, dizziness

e. abnormally slow voluntary movements

f. a sudden fall in blood pressure or cerebral hypoxia resulting in loss of consciousness

g. progressive organic mental deterioration with loss of intellectual function

h. a skin condition characterized by overgrowth and thickening

i. difficulty speaking

j. an abnormal porosity of the bone, most often found in the older adult, predisposing the affected bony tissue to fracture

k. an acute episode of cerebrovascular insufficiency, usually a result of narrowing of an artery by atherosclerotic plaques, emboli, or vasospasm; usually passes quickly but should be considered a warning for predisposition to cerebrovascular accidents

l. a progressive loss of transparency of the lens of the eye, resulting in opacity and loss of sight

m. describes the actions of two drugs taken together in which the combined effects are greater than the sum of the independent effects

33. _____ keratosis (senile)

34. _____ kyphosis (dowager's hump)

35. _____ lentigines

36. _____ osteoporosis

37. _____ potentiation

38. _____ presbycusis

39. _____ presbyopia

40. _____ senility

41. _____ syncope

42. _____ transient ischemic attack (TIA)

43. _____ vertigo

n. a vision change (farsightedness) associated with aging

o. isometric exercises in which the muscles of the pelvic floor are voluntarily contracted and relaxed while urinating

p. brown skin macules occurring after prolonged exposure to the sun; freckles

q. a loss of hearing associated with aging

r. an abnormally deep dorsal curvature of the thoracic spine; also known as humpback or hunchback

s. activities usually performed in the course of the day, i.e., bathing, dressing, feeding oneself

t. also known as _osteoarthritis_; arthritis characterized by degeneration of the bony structure of the joints, usually noninflammatory

u. willingness of a patient to follow a prescribed course of treatment

v. ischemia of the brain due to an occlusion of the blood vessels supplying the brain, resulting in varying degrees of debilitation

w. an abnormal increase in the fluid of the eye, usually as a result of obstructed outflow, resulting in degeneration of the intraocular components and blindness

COG MATCHING

Grade: _____

Place the letter preceding the description of the facility on the line preceding the type of facility.

Facilities

44. _____ Group homes or assisted living facilities

45. _____ Long-term care facilities

46. _____ Skilled-nursing facilities

Descriptions

a. Facilities for those who need help with most areas of personal care and moderate medical supervision

b. Facilities for those who are gravely or terminally ill and need constant supervision

c. Facilities for those who can tend to their own activities of daily living but need companionship and light supervision for safety

COG IDENTIFICATION

Grade: _____

47. Some older adult patients suffer from memory loss, which may make it difficult for them to remember to take their medications. As a medical assistant, it is important to give these patients tools to help them remember and maintain their medication regimens. Identify and list five ways you can help older adult patients remember their medication regimens.

_____

_____

_____

_____

48. Which of the following are common reasons for older adult patients not taking their medications correctly? Place a check mark on the line next to all that apply.

a. _____ Financial difficulties

b. _____ To attract attention

c. _____ Forgetfulness

d. _____ Tiring of the constraints of taking long-term medication

e. _____ Deliberate defiance

49. Mrs. Kim is 89 years old and suffers from memory lapses. It is apparent that she is both frustrated and lonely. Identify and list three ways that you can maintain good communication with her and help her express her feelings.

_____

_____

_____

_____

50. Mrs. Driscoll is 84 years old with poor eyesight who suffers from forgetfulness. She needs to take two different types of medication three times a day. Identify and list four ways that you could help ensure that Mrs. Driscoll adheres to her medication regimen.

_____

_____

_____

51. Patients who react negatively to moving to a long-term care facility can show signs of grief. Identify and list five symptoms that could indicate that a patient is suffering from a sense of loss.

_____

_____

_____

_____

52. Sometimes an older adult patient will turn to alcohol as a way of coping. The effects of drinking alcohol can often be mistaken for other ailments. Identify and list three conditions that exhibit symptoms similar to the influence of alcohol.

_____

_____

_____

_____

53. Suicide is a risk for older adult patients, especially those who have recently lost a spouse to death or divorce. Which of the following warning signs indicate that an older adult patient is contemplating suicide? Place a check mark on the line next to all that apply.

   a. _____ Giving away favored objects

   b. _____ Increased interest in family affairs

   c. _____ Secretive behavior

   d. _____ Increased anger, hostility, or isolation

   e. _____ Increased forgetfulness

   f. _____ Increased alcohol or drug use

   g. _____ Loss of interest in matters of health

54. Which of the following indicate that a patient is suffering from older adult abuse? Place a check mark on the line preceding all that apply.

   a. _____ Disturbed sleep patterns

   b. _____ Signs of restraint on the wrists or ankles

   c. _____ Large, deep pressure ulcers

   d. _____ Incontinence

   e. _____ Poor hygiene or poor nutrition

   f. _____ Untreated injury or condition

   g. _____ Dehydration not caused by disease

55. Which of the following are symptoms of Parkinson disease? Circle the letter preceding all that apply.

    a. Muscle rigidity

    b. Increased anger

    c. Involuntary tremors

    d. Difficulty walking

    e. Loss of memory

    f. Dysphagia and drooling

    g. Expressionless face and infrequent blinking

56. Identify and list three reasons why an older adult patient can have difficulty maintaining good nutrition.

    a. _____

    b. _____

    c. _____

COG SHORT ANSWER   Grade: _____

57. You ask Mr. Walton if he is taking his blood pressure medication and he tells you that he is taking it every day. Later, the physician tells you that Mr. Walton has been taking three pills a day instead of just one. How could this situation be avoided with other older adult patients?

_____

_____

_____

_____

58. Mrs. Dawson is a widow who lives in a long-term care facility. Her family is worried that she has recently become withdrawn and uncommunicative. Before her husband died, Mrs. Dawson led an active life and took a large role in running the household. What could you say to Mrs. Dawson's family to help her cope with the loss of her spouse and her independence?

_____

_____

_____

_____

59. Mr. Gonzalez is an 85-year-old patient who lives alone. He is still fairly active and is able to carry out most activities of daily living by himself. However, members of his family have expressed some concerns that he is lonely and that they are not able to visit him as often as they would like. What options could you discuss with the family?

_____

_____

_____

_____

COG COMPLETION

Grade: _____

60. Older adult patients whose health and economic situation are unstable may experience feelings of grief and loss. These feelings can be about both specific and nonspecific aspects of their lives. Fill in the chart below, listing five specific and nonspecific losses older adult patients may find difficult to cope with.

Specific Losses	Nonspecific Losses
a.	
b.	
c.	
d.	
e.	

61. The passage below describes how medications affect the body of an older adult. However, some of the important terms are missing. Read the passage and fill in the correct words from the list below.

The _____ system no longer moves medications along as efficiently because _____ has slowed. The _____ system does not absorb dissolved medication from the _____ or the _____ and deliver it to the target tissue as quickly. The _____ does not _____ medication as quickly, causing medications to remain in the body longer than desirable and possibly add to the cumulative effect. Finally, the _____ receive less blood, so less medication is filtered and removed from the body. These decreases in body system function can result in possible _____ of medications in the older adult.

circulatory system	*gastrointestinal system*	*intestines*	*biotransform*	*kidneys*
toxic effects		*liver*	*peristalsis*	*injection site*

62. Complete the following table by indicating whether the following suggestions are appropriate for a patient with Parkinson disease or for a patient with Alzheimer disease. Place a checkmark in the appropriate box.

Suggestion	Patient with Parkinson Disease	Patient with Alzheimer Disease
a. Speak calmly and without condescension.		
b. Do not argue with the patient.		
c. Tell the patient to take small bites and chew each mouthful carefully before swallowing.		
d. Encourage the patient to use no-spill cups, plates with high sides, and special utensils.		
e. Free the home from rugs and loose cords that may cause tripping.		
f. Speak in short, simple, direct sentences and explain one action at a time.		
g. Listen to the patient and stimulate his intelligence.		
h. Remind the patient who you are and what you must do.		

COG TRUE OR FALSE?

Grade: _____

Indicate whether the statements are true or false by placing the letter T (true) or F (false) on the line preceding the statement.

63. _____ Newspaper word puzzles are just a temporary distraction to help entertain older adults.

64. _____ Attempts to commit suicide by older adults are usually just a cry for help.

65. _____ If a patient has an advance directive on file somewhere other than the medical office, it should be noted in her medical record.

66. _____ Most older adult abuse is committed by workers in long-term care facilities.

COG AFF **CASE STUDIES FOR CRITICAL THINKING**   Grade: _____

1. Read the following case studies and think about what you know about the causes of older adult abuse. Circle the letter preceding the case study that describes the patient who falls in the highest risk category for abuse.

   a. Mr. Simpson is an 89-year-old widower who lives alone. He is still fairly active and is able to carry out most daily activities by himself. He has a daughter and a son, who take turns visiting him every week and doing his shopping and laundry for him. Mr. Simpson takes medication for high blood pressure and angina.

   b. Mrs. Lewis is an 83-year-old patient who lives in a long-term care facility. She suffers from mild senile dementia, which her family sometimes finds frustrating, but is learning to cope with. Mrs. Lewis has a home health aide and private nurse to help her carry out activities of daily living. She sleeps for most of the day.

   c. Mrs. Beddowes is a 90-year-old widow who lives with her son. She suffers from senile dementia, incontinence, and insomnia. Her family members cannot afford to place her in a long-term care facility, so they share the responsibility of taking care of her. However, most of the responsibility falls onto her son, who helps Mrs. Beddowes carry out most activities of daily living.

   d. Mr. Williams is an 81-year-old patient who lives in an assisted living facility. He was recently widowed and is having difficulty coming to terms with his wife's death. Mr. Williams used to be extremely active, but has recently become withdrawn and has started drinking heavily. He has two daughters who visit him regularly.

2. Your patient is a 90-year-old man with various age-associated health problems. He has been recently diagnosed with dementia, but during his recent visits to the physician's office you have smelled alcohol on his breath. How would you handle this situation? What would you do?

   _____

   _____

   _____

   _____

3. Your patient is an 82-year-old woman who suffers from mild hearing loss. She recently lost her husband and has been making frequent appointments at the physician's office for minor complaints. You suspect that the patient is lonely and is visiting the office for company and human interaction. Explain what you would do.

   _____

   _____

   _____

   _____

4. Your patient is an 80-year-old woman who has recently lost a noticeable amount of weight. She tells you that she has not been very hungry lately and has not felt like eating very much. The physician has asked you to write a list of nutritional guidelines for her to follow and explain why they are important. What would you put in the guidelines?

_____

_____

_____

_____

5. Your patient is a 91-year-old man with Alzheimer disease. After his appointment with the physician, you overhear his family trying to get him into the car. The patient has forgotten where he is and refuses to leave the physician's office. His daughter loses her temper and shouts at her father loudly until he complies. What would you do? Explain your actions.

_____

_____

_____

_____

6. You overhear a coworker asking a 77-year-old patient about her medical history. When the patient tells your coworker that she is taking gingko to improve her memory, your coworker tells her that she needs to know only about actual medications. What would you say to your coworker?

_____

_____

_____

_____

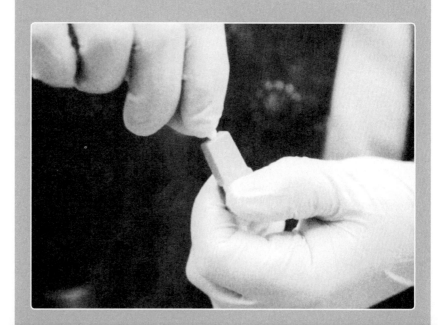

PART

IV

The Clinical Laboratory

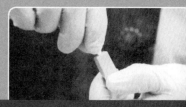

Learning Outcomes

Cognitive Domain

1. Spell and define key terms
2. Identify the kinds of laboratories where medical assistants work and the functions of each
3. Identify the types of departments found in most large laboratories and give their purposes
4. Identify the types of personnel in laboratories and describe their jobs
5. Describe the medical assistant's responsibility in the clinical laboratory
6. Define scope of practice for the medical assistant and comprehend the conditions for practice within the state that the medical assistant is employed
7. Identify body systems
8. Describe the panels defined by the American Medical Association for national standardization of nomenclature and testing and list the test results provided in each panel
9. Identify the equipment found in most small laboratories and give the purpose of each
10. Describe the parts of a microscope

Psychomotor Domain

1. Care for the microscope (Procedure 39-1)

Name: _____   Date: _____   Grade: _____

COG MULTIPLE CHOICE

Circle the letter preceding the correct answer.

1. Laboratory test results are evaluated to determine the relative health of body systems or organs by comparison with:

   a. panels.

   b. constituents.

   c. reference intervals.

   d. calibration ranges.

   e. quality control ranges.

2. A large facility in which thousands of tests of various types are performed each day is a:

   a. hospital laboratory.

   b. POL.

   c. waived-testing laboratory.

   d. clinical chemistry laboratory.

   e. referral laboratory.

3. Specimen processors send portions of specimens used for testing by preparing:

   a. antibodies.

   b. aliquots.

   c. diagnostic tests.

   d. kits.

   e. panels.

4. Medical assistants frequently work with referral laboratory customer service personnel to:

   a. answer questions and provide special handling for specimens from their patients.

   b. suggest medication replacements.

   c. establish reference intervals for their patient results.

   d. obtain orders for laboratory tests.

   e. explain to the patient the reasons for performing the test.

5. How must a centrifuge be set up in order to work properly?

   a. Tubes must be equidistant.

   b. All tubes must have the same substance.

   c. Only one tube may be spun at a time.

   d. The lid must be down at all times.

   e. Spin must alternate every 30 minutes.

6. A Pap test specimen would be sent to which department for analysis?

   a. Histology

   b. Cytology

   c. Immunohematology

   d. Microbiology

   e. Clinical chemistry

7. Hematology includes the study of:

   a. etiology, diagnosis, and treatment of blood diseases.

   b. analysis of body fluids.

   c. the study of hormones.

   d. the study of the immune system and antibodies.

   e. the study of drugs.

8. Hemophilia is a:

   a. common skin pathogen.

   b. test performed on a urine specimen.

   c. blood clotting disease.

   d. shortage of red blood cells.

   e. type of leukemia.

9. The two most common tests performed in the coagulation laboratory are:

   a. red blood cell and white blood cell counts.

   b. prothrombin time and partial thromboplastin time.

   c. hemoglobin and hematocrit.

   d. iron and total iron-binding capacity.

   e. vitamin B$_{12}$ and folate.

10. The lipid panel tests are performed in:

    a. toxicology.

    b. urinalysis.

    c. cytology.

    d. coagulation.

    e. chemistry.

11. Mycology is the study of:

    a. protozoa and worms.

    b. viruses.

    c. bacteria.

    d. tuberculosis.

    e. fungi and yeasts.

12. The laboratory instrument used to prepare serum for laboratory testing is the:

    a. centrifuge.

    b. incubater.

    c. chemistry analyzer.

    d. cell counter.

    e. microscope diaphragm.

13. The test panel defined by the American Medical Association (AMA) for national standardization of nomenclature and testing used to test cholesterol, triglycerides, HDL, and LDL is the:

    a. comprehensive metabolic panel.

    b. basic metabolic panel.

    c. electrolyte panel.

    d. hepatic panel.

    e. lipid panel.

14. Sjögren syndrome, diagnosed using the antithyoglobulin antibody test, the rheumatoid arthritis test, and the antinuclear antibody test, is a disease of which body system?

    a. Endocrine

    b. Muscular

    c. Sensory

    d. Nervous

    e. Lymphatic

15. Klinefelter syndrome, diagnosed using serum and urine gonadotropin measurements, semen analysis, and chromosome studies, is a disease of which body system?

    a. Endocrine

    b. Lymphatic

    c. Nervous

    d. Reproductive

    e. Urinary

16. Osteomalacia and rickets, diagnosed using the comprehensive metabolic panel, vitamin D level, and the erythrocyte sedimentation rate, are diseases of which body system?

    a. Muscular

    b. Skeletal

    c. Nervous

    d. Respiratory

    e. Endocrine

17. Meningitis, diagnosed using cerebrospinal fluid levels of WBCs, protein, glucose, and a cerebrospinal fluid culture, is a disease of which body system?

    a. Muscular

    b. Skeletal

    c. Nervous

    d. Respiratory

    e. Endocrine

18. A graduate of an associate (2-year) degree program (or equivalent) in medical laboratory science who is nationally certified and performs specimen testing is a:

   a. cytologist.

   b. phlebotomist.

   c. medical laboratory technician.

   d. medical laboratory technologist.

   e. laboratory assistant.

19. A technician trained to process and evaluate tissue samples, such as biopsy or surgical samples, is a:

   a. medical laboratory technician.

   b. histologist.

   c. cytologist.

   d. medical laboratory technologist.

   e. pathologist.

20. What information is required on a laboratory requisition form?

   a. Date and time the physician ordered the test(s)

   b. Temperature of the room at the time of specimen collection

   c. Credit card number

   d. Birth date and gender of patient

   e. Signature of patient

COG MATCHING

Grade: _____

Match each key term with the correct definition.

Key Terms

21. _____ aliquots

22. _____ analytes

23. _____ antibodies

24. _____ antigen

25. _____ anticoagulant

26. _____ autoimmunity

27. _____ biohazard

28. _____ centrifugation

29. _____ Centers for Medicare and Medicaid Services (CMS)

30. _____ coagulation

31. _____ coagulopathies

32. _____ cytogenetics

33. _____ cytology

Definitions

a. substance or constituent for which a laboratory conducts testing

b. anything that prevents or delays blood clotting

c. diseases associated with abnormal blood clotting functions

d. specimens requiring a legal chain of custody

e. testing based on the reactions of antibodies in the presence of antigens

f. proteins formed in the body in response to foreign substances

g. substance that, when introduced into the body, cause the development of immune responses

h. disorder of the immune system in which parts of the immune system fail to provide an adequate response

i. disorders of the immune system in which the immune system attacks its own host's body

j. disorders in which the immune system responds inappropriately to harmless compounds or responds too intensely

k. study of the microscopic structure of tissue; samples of tissue are prepared, stained, and evaluated under a microscope to determine whether disease is present

l. involves a wide variety of procedures used in donor selection, component preparation and use, and techniques used to detect antigen/antibody reactions which may adversely affect a patient receiving a transfusion

m. study of the microscopic structure of cells; individual cells in body fluids and other specimens are evaluated microscopically for the presence of disease such as cancer

34. ____ for cause

35. ____ hematology

36. ____ histology

37. ____ hypersensitivities

38. ____ immunodeficiency

39. ____ immunohematology

40. ____ immunology

41. ____ kit

42. ____ microbiology

n. genetic structure of the cells obtained from tissue, blood, or body fluids, such as amniotic fluid, are examined or tested for chromosome deficiencies related to genetic disease

o. the process of separating blood or other body fluid cells from liquid components

p. portions of the original specimen

q. substance that is a potential carrier of blood-borne pathogens

r. require the use of test panels created by the AMA

s. the study of blood and blood forming tissues

t. packaged set of supplies needed to perform a test

u. the study of the blood's ability to clot

v. the study of pathogen identification and antiobiotic susceptibilty determination

---

COG MATCHING

Grade: _____

Match each key term with the correct definition.

Key Terms

43. ____ oncology

44. ____ panels

45. ____ pathogen

46. ____ physician office laboratory (POL)

47. ____ plasma

48. ____ procedure manual

49. ____ product insert

50. ____ quality assurance (QA)

51. ____ quality control (QC)

52. ____ reference intervals

53. ____ referral laboratory

54. ____ serum

55. ____ specimens

56. ____ surgical pathology

Definitions

a. acceptable ranges for a healthy population

b. designed to ensure thorough patient care

c. procedures to monitor and evaluate testing procedures, supplies, and equipment to ensure accuracy in laboratory performance

d. standard groups of laboratory tests organized to effectively evaluate disease processes or organ systems

e. contains instructions and critical details for performing a test

f. a handbook that contains test methods and other information needed to perform testing, suggested by the United States Department of Health and Human Services (HHS) and the Centers for Disease Control and Prevention (CDC) as a valuable resource for CW sites

g. top layer of a whole blood specimen if the specimen was anticoagulated and not allowed to clot

h. the study and medical treatment of cancer

i. a limited testing laboratory in a medical office

j. a large facility in which thousands of tests of various types are performed each day

k. blood containing all its cellular and liquid components

l. disease-causing microorganism

m. the liquid portion of the blood after the blood has been allowed to clot

n. examination of the physical, chemical, and microscopic properties of urine

57. ____ toxicology

58. ____ unitized test device

59. ____ urinalysis

60. ____ whole blood

o. the pathologist in this department gives a diagnosis of the presence or absence of disease in tissue that is surgically removed from a patient

p. used for a single test and discarded after testing

q. small portions of anything used to evaluate the nature of the whole

r. branch of chemistry that studies the amounts and identification of chemicals foreign to the body

---

COG **MATCHING**   Grade: _____

Match the following panel(s) defined by AMA and mandated by CMS to the correct analytes. Place the letter preceding the panel name on the line next to the analyte that it includes. There may be more than one correct panel name for some analytes. You must list all the corresponding panels for a correct answer.

Analytes

61. _____ Glucose

62. _____ Sodium

63. _____ Albumin

64. _____ Cholesterol

65. _____ Potassium

66. _____ Total protein

67. _____ Triglycerides

68. _____ Chloride

69. _____ Alkaline phosphatase (ALP)

70. _____ HDL

71. _____ CO_2

72. _____ Alanine aminotransferase (ALT)

73. _____ LDL

74. _____ Creatinine

75. _____ Direct bilirubin

Panels

a. Comprehensive metabolic

b. Basic metabolic

c. Electrolyte

d. Hepatic function

e. Lipid

COG **IDENTIFICATION**   Grade: _____

Each of the medical assistants below needs a laboratory test completed for a patient. Review the task that must be performed and then decide which laboratory department should handle each task.

76. Ericka needs to send in blood for a complete blood count. _____

77. Kwon needs results of the chemical properties of a patient's urine. _____

78. Darren has to send a patient to the lab for glucose testing. _____

79. Don has a mole removed and sent to the lab for analysis. _____

80. Rochelle collects a clean catch urine for culture. _____

For each list of organs, name the corresponding body system.

81. Bone marrow, thymus gland, spleen, lymph nodes: _____

82. Heart, blood vessels: _____

83. Small and large intestines, rectum, anus: _____

84. Heart, arteries, capillaries, veins: _____

85. Mouth, esophagus, stomach, liver, gallbladder: _____

86. Skin, hair, nails, sweat glands: _____

87. Hypothalamus, pituitary, thyroid, parathyroids: _____

88. Smooth, cardiac, and skeletal muscles: _____

89. Sight, hearing, feeling, smell, taste, balance: _____

90. Bone, bone marrow, joints, teeth: _____

91. Ducts, lymph nodes: _____

92. Brain, spinal cord, nerves: _____

93. Kidneys, ureter, urethra: _____

94. Penis, testes, vagina, uterus, ovaries: _____

95. Nose, pharynx, larynx: _____

96. Pancreas, small intestine, large intestine: _____

97. Adrenals, pancreas, pineal body, ovaries, testes: _____

98. Ligaments, cartilage: _____

99. Bronchioles, lungs: _____

100. Palatine tonsil, thymus gland: _____

101. Trachea, bronchi, alveoli: _____

COG IDENTIFICATION

Grade: _____

102. For each disease or syndrome given, fill in the corresponding body system followed by laboratory tests used in diagnosing that disease or syndrome. Use Table 39-1, "Body Systems and Laboratory Testing," in the textbook for assistance.

Disease	Body System	Laboratory Tests
a. Gout		
b. Sarcoidosis		
c. Tonsillitis		
d. Myasthenia gravis		
e. Colorectal cancer		
f. Menopause		
g. Pancreatitis		
h. Myocardial infarction		
i. Sjögren syndrome		
j. Tuberculosis		

COG SHORT ANSWER

Grade: _____

103. What items are included in the patient database and why?

_____

_____

_____

_____

104. Why does the laboratory need the patient's birth date and gender?

_____

_____

_____

_____

105. How does the laboratory use the date and time of collection?

_____

_____

_____

_____

106. How does the laboratory use the physician's name and address?

_____

_____

_____

_____

107. What other specimen information may be required?

_____

_____

_____

_____

108. List six good laboratory practices for POLs performing POC testing.

_____

_____

_____

_____

COG FILL IN THE BLANK

Grade: _____

109. The physician you work for is beginning his practice and has asked you to purchase the laboratory equipment the office will need. List six pieces of equipment found in most POLs and their functions.

Equipment	Function
a.	
b.	
c.	
d.	
e.	
f.	

AFF CASE STUDIES FOR CRITICAL THINKING

Grade: _____

1. Jacob works for a large primary care practice and is the medical assistant assigned to the laboratory. When Jacob arrives in the laboratory, he finds 12 urine samples and requisitions waiting for testing. After quality control results for urine tests are acceptable, Jacob prepares to perform the urine tests. He reads each requisition to set up appropriate testing supplies. He notices that one urine specimen has no patient identification of any kind. How should Jacob handle this specimen?

_____

_____

_____

_____

2. Dr. Oyakawa calls to say he will be 30 minutes late. His medical assistant, Paula, brings Dr. Oyakawa's first patient to the laboratory with a test requisition. This is the patient's first visit with Dr. Oyakawa. Dr. Oyakawa has not called in a verbal order for this patient. Paula fills out the requisition in front of you and selects tests for you to perform. How do you respond to Paula?

_____

_____

_____

_____

3. This is your first day working in the laboratory at a university outpatient clinic. You are the only person working in the laboratory. You completed your orientation and training prior to today, but today is your first day being responsible for patient testing. Dr. Rayshawdhury brings a throat swab to the laboratory and requests a STAT streptococcus test. You know that the test is performed using a waived-testing kit. You open the test box expecting to use the package insert as a guide for performing the test, but the package insert is not there. You look for the Laboratory Manual and cannot locate one. How do you obtain directions for performing the test?

_____

_____

_____

_____

PSY PROCEDURE 39-1   Care for the Microscope

Name: _____ Date: _____ Time: _____ Grade: _____

EQUIPMENT/SUPPLIES: Lens paper, lens cleaner, gauze, mild soap solution, microscope, hand disinfectant, surface disinfectant

STANDARDS: Given the needed equipment and a place to work, the student will perform this skill with _____% accuracy in a total of _____ minutes. *(Your instructor will tell you what the percentage and time limits will be before you begin practicing.)*

KEY: 4 = Satisfactory   0 = Unsatisfactory   NA = This step is not counted

PROCEDURE STEPS	SELF	PARTNER	INSTRUCTOR
1. Wash your hands.	☐	☐	☐
2. Assemble the equipment.	☐	☐	☐
3. If you need to move the microscope, carry it in both hands, one holding the base and the other holding the arm.	☐	☐	☐
4. Clean the optical areas.	☐	☐	☐
a. Place a drop or two of lens cleaner on a piece of lens paper.			
b. Wipe each eyepiece thoroughly with the lens paper. Do not touch the optical areas with your fingers. Wipe each eyepiece with lens paper and lens cleaner.			
c. Wipe each objective lens, starting with the lowest power and continuing to the highest power (usually an oil immersion lens). If the lens paper appears to have dirt or oil on it, use a clean section of the lens paper or a new piece of lens paper with cleaner. Wipe each objective lens with lens paper and lens cleaner. Clean the oil objective last so you do not carry its oil to the other objective lenses.			
d. Using a new piece of dry lens paper, wipe each eyepiece and objective lens so that no cleaner remains.			
e. With a new piece of lens paper moistened with lens cleaner, clean the condenser and illuminator optics. Clean and dry the condenser and illuminator optics.			
5. Clean the areas other than the optics.	☐	☐	☐
a. Moisten gauze with mild soap solution or use an alcohol wipe and wipe all areas other than the optics, including the stage, base, and adjustment knobs.			
b. Moisten another gauze with water and rinse the washed areas.			
6. To store the cleaned microscope, ensure that the light source is turned off. Rotate the nosepiece so that the low-power objective is pointed down toward the stage. Cover the microscope with the plastic dust cover that came with it or a small trash bag.	☐	☐	☐
7. Document microscope cleaning on the microscope maintenance log sheet (sample instrument log sheet).	☐	☐	☐

CALCULATION

Total Possible Points: _____

Total Points Earned: _____ Multiplied by 100 = _____ Divided by Total Possible Points = _____ %

PASS   **FAIL**   **COMMENTS:**

☐   ☐

Student's signature _____ Date _____

Partner's signature _____ Date _____

Instructor's signature _____ Date _____

CLIA Compliance and Laboratory Safety

Cognitive Domain

1. Spell and define the key terms
2. Explain the significance of CLIA and describe how to maintain compliance in the physician office laboratory
3. Discuss the practices physician office laboratories must define to assure good performance of waived testing
4. Using CLIA guidelines, identify laboratory tests that are and are not within the scope of practice for a medical assistant
5. Identify disease processes that are indications for CLIA-waived tests
6. Identify the consequences of practicing outside CLIA guidelines
7. Identify the role of the Centers for Disease Control regulations in health care settings
8. Define critical values and document the proper notification to the health care professional
9. Identify results that require follow-up and document action in chart
10. Identify how to handle all test results whether inside or outside the reference interval and document on a flow sheet
11. Identify and use quality control methods
12. Define proficiency testing and describe why CLIA requires it to maintain laboratory quality
13. Identify the source of instrument maintenance and calibration instructions

14. Analyze charts, graphs, and/or tables in the interpretation of health care results
15. Define OSHA and state its purpose
16. Discuss the application of standard precautions with regards to: a) all body fluids, secretions, and excretions; b) blood; c) nonintact skin; and d) mucous membranes
17. Identify safety techniques that can be used to prevent accidents and maintain a safe work environment
18. List the types and uses of personal protective equipment
19. Identify safety signs, symbols, and labels
20. Describe the reasons to file an incident report
21. Describe the Needlestick Safety and Prevention Act and list its requirements

Psychomotor Domain

1. Practice standard precautions
2. Participate in training on standard precautions
3. Comply with safety signs, symbols, and labels
4. Evaluate the work environment to identify safe versus unsafe working conditions
5. Screen and follow up test results and document laboratory results appropriately (Procedure 40-1)
6. Use methods of quality control (Procedure 40-2)

7. Document accurately
8. Perform routine maintenance of clinical equipment (Procedure 40-3)
9. Perform patient screening using established protocols
10. Assist with patient care

ABHES Competencies

1. Define scope of practice for the medical assistant, and comprehend the conditions for practice within CLIA regulations
2. Document accurately
3. Understand the various medical terminology for each specialty
4. Comply with federal, state, and local health laws and regulations
5. Apply principles of aseptic techniques and infection control
6. Screen and follow up patient test results
7. Use standard precautions
8. Advise patients of office policies and procedures
9. Practice quality control
10. Dispose of biohazardous materials

Name: _____   Date: _____   Grade: _____

COG MULTIPLE CHOICE

1. What body regulates nonresearch laboratory testing in the United States?

   a. The Centers for Disease Control and Prevention

   b. The Centers for Medicare and Medicaid Services

   c. The Food and Drug Administration

   d. The Department of Labor

   e. Congress

2. A laboratory must have a written quality assurance policy that:

   a. is communicated to all staff.

   b. is stored neared the site of use.

   c. includes all HazCom requirements.

   d. includes all MSDSs supplied by the manufacturers.

   e. is updated once a week.

3. A pronounced and immediate change in test performance is known as a:

   a. control.

   b. trend.

   c. reagent.

   d. flow.

   e. shift.

4. What might the yellow quadrant of the National Fire Safety Association diamond indicate?

   a. Health hazard

   b. Fire hazard

   c. Reaction hazard

   d. Biological hazard

   e. Natural hazard

5. OSHA is a federal agency within the:

   a. Department of the Interior.

   b. Department of Health and Human Services.

   c. Department of Labor.

   d. Department of Commerce.

   e. Department of the Treasury.

6. All hazardous chemicals must be:

   a. placed on top shelves out of a patient's reach.

   b. placed near a sink in case a person's skin is exposed.

   c. labeled with a warning and statement of the hazard.

   d. used only by medical professionals while wearing heavy boots.

   e. stored away from sunlight.

7. The best source of normal values for the POL is:

   a. the *Physicians' Desk Reference.*

   b. the manufacturer's packaging insert.

   c. the ICD-9 CM.

   d. the Laboratory Procedure Manual.

   e. the CLIA certificate.

8. The presence of a panic value in test results indicates:

   a. an outbreak of a contagious virus.

   b. imminent death of the patient.

   c. general good health.

   d. a potentially life threatening situation.

   e. negligence on the part of the laboratory.

9. Who provides quality control instructions for a given test?

   a. FDA

   b. CLSI

   c. Laboratory director

   d. Manufacturer

   e. OSHA

10. What document describes the appropriate methods for performing every test offered by a laboratory?

    a. Quality assurance plan

    b. CLIA certificate

    c. Laboratory Procedure Manual

    d. Flow sheet

    e. Material safety data sheet

11. Which of the following does OSHA require the employer to make available to the medical assistant in the laboratory?

    a. Health insurance

    b. Hepatitis B vaccine

    c. Prescription refills

    d. Performance evaluations

    e. Measles vaccine

12. Hazardous waste materials include

    a. Supply packaging

    b. Laboratory reports

    c. Used needles and sharps

    d. Unopened supplies

    e. Documents in the patient's chart

13. Urine dipsticks and pregnancy tests are examples of

    a. Waived tests

    b. Moderately complex tests

    c. Provider performed microscopy

    d. High complexity tests

    e. Referral tests

14. What CLIA-waived test may be ordered on a patient presenting with a sore throat?

    a. Hematocrit

    b. Urine dipstick

    c. Glucose meter measurement

    d. Rapid strep test

    e. CBC

15. The laboratory receives a patient report from the referral laboratory. What is the next responsibility of the medical assistant?

    a. Place the results in the patient's chart.

    b. Place the results on the physician's desk.

    c. Screen and follow up the test results.

    d. Ask Medical Records to follow up.

    e. Phone the results to the patient.

16. The physician orders a urine dipstick test on a patient. What is required before reporting the test results to the physician?

    a. Acceptable quality control results

    b. The test to be duplicated

    c. A microscopic evaluation

    d. A signed release from the patient

    e. Review of the results with the patient

17. You bring your lunch to work and need to refrigerate it. You would:

    a. store it in the laboratory refrigerator. It is nearest to you while you work.

    b. store it in the refrigerator in the break room. That refrigerator does not have a biohazard label.

    c. store it in the refrigerator with drugs and vaccines.

    d. store it in a drawer in the laboratory.

    e. store it in an empty drawer in the procedure room.

18. How do you choose the shoes you wear in the laboratory?

    a. It is summer so you choose sandals.

    b. Your canvas sport shoes are so comfortable.

    c. You choose a completely closed shoe to protect from physical and chemical hazards.

    d. You choose a clog. You have heard they are really ergonomic.

    e. You do not wear scrubs in your office, so you wear a casual, open-toed shoe with your casual work outfit.

19. You are just getting over a cold and have a lingering cough. How do you protect your patients?

   a. Turn your head when you cough.

   b. Wear a mask.

   c. Call in sick.

   d. Cough into your arm.

   e. Open a lozenge and slip it in your mouth so you won't cough while collecting a patient's specimen.

20. You are cleaning the laboratory counters at the end of the day. What is the cleaning product of choice?

   a. Boiling water

   b. Dish soap and warm water.

   c. Ammonia

   d. Full strength bleach

   e. A 10% bleach solution

COG MATCHING

Grade: _____

Match each key term with its definition.

Key Terms

21. _____ aerosol

22. _____ calibration

23. _____ biohazardous waste

24. _____ blood-borne pathogens

25. _____ chemical hygiene plan (CHP)

26. _____ confirmatory test

27. _____ control

28. _____ critical values

29. _____ external control

30. _____ flow sheet

31. _____ internal control

32. _____ material safety data sheet (MSDS)

33. _____ precision

Definitions

a. an additional more specific test performed to rule out or confirm a preliminary test result to provide a final result

b. a device or solution used to monitor the test for accuracy and precision

c. life-threatening test results

d. a form used to collect important data regarding a patient's condition

e. similar results if asked to repeat the test

f. control built into the testing device

g. control that acts just like a patient specimen

h. particles suspended in gas or air

i. the manufacturer's instructions for storage, handling, and disposal of the chemical

j. pathogens when present in human blood cause disease

k. infectious waste or biomedical waste

l. a method provided by the manufacturer to standardize a test or laboratory instrument

m. a part of the HazCom standard that must address chemical hazards present in the medical office

cog MATCHING

Grade: _____

Match each key term with its definition.

Key Terms

34. _____ proficiency testing

35. _____ qualitative test

36. _____ quantitative test

37. _____ reagent

38. _____ reconstitution

39. _____ sensitivity

40. _____ shifts

41. _____ specificity

42. _____ standard precautions

43. _____ therapeutic range

44. _____ trends

45. _____ universal precautions

Definitions

a. testing programs provide unknown samples to test as if they were patient specimens

b. a substance that produces a reaction with a patient specimen so the analyte can be detected or measured

c. the test result range the physician wants for the patient

d. test has positive or negative results

e. tests are measured and reported in a number value

f. when QC results make an obvious change

g. when results increase or decrease over time

h. used in medical offices to reduce the risk for transmission of pathogens

i. human blood and most body fluids are handled as if they are infectious for HIV, hepatitis B virus, hepatitis C virus, and other blood-borne pathogens

j. adding water to bring a material back to its liquid state

k. the lowest concentration of an analyte that can reliably be detected or measured by a test system

l. the ability of a test to detect a particular substance or constituent without interferences or false reactions by other substances

cog IDENTIFICATION

Grade: _____

For each listed purpose, identify the organization, law, or standard initiating the purpose.

Organization, Law, or Standard	Purpose
46.	regulatory program that sets standards for the quality of laboratory testing
47.	regulates all laboratory testing performed on humans
48.	U.S. government's agency for protecting the health of all Americans and providing essential human services
49.	works to protect public health and safety
50.	responsible for protecting and promoting public health through the regulation and supervision of blood transfusions products
51.	works to support the health care industry by providing knowledge and resources for maintaining quality laboratory operations
52.	required by any group that performs even one test, including a waived test

53.	state agency requiring notification of the occurrence of a reportable disease
54.	establishes rules to ensure the safety, standards, and integrity of all testing performed on human specimens
55.	standards protect workers by eliminating or minimizing chemical, physical, and biological hazards and preventing accidents
56.	requires all medical employers to provide training for their employees in techniques that will protect them from occupational exposure to infectious agents, including blood-borne pathogens
57.	the right to know law
58.	a part of the HazCom standard that must address potential chemical exposure by the employee
59.	requires medical offices to keep an injury log to record the details of sharps injuries

COG IDENTIFICATION

Grade: _____

Identify laboratory tests that a medical assistant (MA) can perform and those that must be performed by a medical technologist/clinical laboratory scientist (MT/CLS).

60. _____ Urine dipstick

61. _____ Urine microscopic

62. _____ Hematocrit

63. _____ WBC differential

64. _____ Thyroid panel

65. _____ Specific gravity

66. _____ Glucose by glucose meter

67. _____ Pregnancy test by waived kit

68. _____ Rapid strep by waived kit

69. _____ Strep identification by microbiology culture

cog IDENTIFICATION   Grade: _____

Identify requirements to maintain CLIA compliance in the POL. Note required (R) or not applicable (NA).

70. _____ Test complexity

71. _____ CLIA certification

72. _____ Quality assurance plan

73. _____ Critical values

74. _____ Personnel training

75. _____ Personnel Competency Assessment

76. _____ Screen and follow up test results

77. _____ Maintain flow sheets

78. _____ Proficiency testing

79. _____ Patient test management

80. _____ Laboratory Procedure Manual

81. _____ Quality control

82. _____ Report communicable diseases

83. _____ Reagent management

84. _____ Instrument calibration and maintenance

85. _____ Documentation

COG IDENTIFICATION

Grade: _____

Identify the waived test used in the identification of the disease process. Answers may be used more than once.

86. Strep throat: _____

87. Pregnancy: _____

88. Mononucleosis: _____

89. Glycosuria: _____

90. Hypoglycemia: _____

91. Inflammation: _____

92. Anemia: _____

93. Proteinuria: _____

94. Bilirubinuria: _____

95. Hyperglycemia: _____

A. Erythrocyte sedimentation rate

B. Urine HCG test

C. Hematocrit

D. Mono test

E. Rapid Strep test

F. Urine dipstick

G. PT/INR meter

H. Glucose meter

COG AFF SHORT ANSWER

Grade: _____

96. Why did the Needlestick Safety and Prevention Act become law, and what are its requirements?

_____

_____

_____

_____

97. Define proficiency testing and describe why CLIA requires it to maintain laboratory quality?

_____

_____

_____

_____

98. Identify the source of instrument maintenance and calibration instructions.

_____

_____

_____

_____

99. Describe the difference between a flow sheet and a patient history.

_____

_____

_____

_____

100. In the context of laboratory medical testing, what is the purpose of a control?

_____

_____

_____

_____

101. Explain the difference between qualitative and quantitative tests.

_____

_____

_____

_____

102. How do you identify whether patient values are inside or outside the reference interval?

_____

_____

_____

_____

103. In reviewing patient results, how do you determine patient values requiring followup?

_____

_____

_____

_____

104. Give four reasons an incident report may be needed.

_____

_____

_____

_____

105. Using the hazardous materials rating system, give the type of hazard identified by the following colors.

a. Blue: _____

b. Red: _____

c. Yellow: _____

106. A bottle of sodium hydroxide, a common alkali, has the diamond-shaped symbol of the National Fire Protection Association printed on it. The number "3" is printed in the blue quadrant. What does this number indicate?

_____

_____

_____

_____

COG IDENTIFICATION

Grade: _____

Identify safety techniques that can be used to prevent accidents and maintain a safe work environment. Identify each action as S (safe) or NS (not safe).

107. _____ Eating, drinking, or smoking in the laboratory area.

108. _____ Touching your face, mouth, or eyes with your gloves or with items, such as a pen or pencil used in the laboratory.

109. _____ Wash your hands prior to inserting your contact lens in the laboratory.

110. _____ Label all specimen containers with biohazard labels.

111. _____ Store all chemicals according to the manufacturer's recommendations.

112. _____ Wash hands frequently for infection control.

113. _____ Wear gloves to protect from needlestick accidents.

114. _____ Wear gloves to protect yourself and the patient from biohazard contamination.

115. _____ Do not discuss a work injury or biohazard exposure to minimize concern.

COG IDENTIFICATION

Grade: _____

For each item of personal protective equipment listed, describe the type of protection provided.

116. Gloves: _____

_____

_____

117. Lab coats: _____

_____

_____

118. Masks: _____

_____

_____

119. Goggles and face shields: _____

_____

_____

120. Respirators: _____

_____

_____

COG **PSY** **AFF** **CASE STUDIES FOR CRITICAL THINKING**   Grade: _____

1. The Levey-Jennings QC Chart for a test commonly performed in your office appears to suggest that the test is producing progressively higher results. How would you go about researching this phenomenon? What information should you present to the physician?

_____

_____

_____

_____

2. A test is showing systematically low results; that is, in each case, the result is proportionately lower than expected. The results are precise, but inaccurate. What must you do to ensure proper results? Document this appropriately in the QC log and in the patient's chart.

_____

_____

_____

_____

3. You are performing a glucose test on your patient using a glucose meter. The patient's glucose result is below the level the meter can detect. The glucose meter can detect values as low as 40 mg/dl. What kind of value is this? What steps should you take with the test results? Using the space below, demonstrate recording this information in the patient's chart.

_____

_____

_____

_____

4. Patient Jacob Wisliki is on coumadin therapy following a stroke. Dr. Wilson requests that you maintain a flow sheet on this patient. Today is November 11, 2012. Mr. Wisliki's INR is 1.8. His current medication dose is 2 mg qd. Dr. Wilson orders weekly INR testing. Maintain Mr. Wisliki's flow chart using the information provided below.

- Mr. Wisliki's INR is below Dr. Wilson's target range today, so Dr. Wilson increases Mr. Wisliki's dose to 2.5 mg qd. You instruct Mr. Wisliki to return in a week as Dr. Wilson ordered.

- Mr. Wisliki returns. His INR today is 2.1. This is in Dr. Wilson's therapeutic range, but Dr. Wilson would like to see the value run higher. He increases Mr. Wisliki's dose to 3.5 mg qd. You instruct Mr. Wisliki to return in a week as Dr. Wilson ordered.

- Mr. Wisliki returns the following week. His INR today is 3.5. This value is higher than Dr. Wilson's therapeutic range, so he decreases Mr. Wisliki's dose to 3.0 mg qd. You instruct Mr. Wisliki to return in a week as Dr. Wilson ordered.

- Mr. Wisliki returns on schedule. His INR today is 3.1. Dr. Wilson is concerned that Mr. Wisliki's INR did not respond as usual to the decrease in the dose. He asks Mr. Wisliki about any changes in his diet. Mr. Wilson says that he has been eating more spinach lately because it is ripe in his garden. Dr. Wilson tells Mr. Wisliki that eating green leafy vegetables will cause the anticoagulant to not work as well in his body and can cause increased INR. He instructs Mr. Wisliki to avoid eating green leafy vegetables while on anticoagulant therapy. Dr. Wilson does not change Mr. Wisliki's dose as he expects the INR to go down when Mr. Wisliki stops eating as much green leafy vegetables. You instruct Mr. Wisliki to return in a week as Dr. Wilson ordered.

- Mr. Wisliki is back for his weekly INR check. Today his INR is 2.5. This is exactly where Dr. Wilson wants Mr. Wisliki's INR to be so he does not change his dose today. You instruct Mr. Wisliki to return in a week as Dr. Wilson ordered.

- Mr. Wisliki is back for his INR. Today his INR is 2.5. As Mr. Wisliki's INR is stable, Dr. Wilson does not change his dose. You instruct Mr. Wisliki to return in a week as Dr. Wilson ordered.

Anticoagulation Flowsheet

Patient's name: _Jacob Wisliki _____ Date of Birth: _03/20/1940 _____

Target International Normalized Ratio (INR): √ 2.0–3.0 ☐ 2.5–3.5 ☐ Other: _____

Date	Current Dose	INR	Complications	New Dose	Next INR	Initials
11/23/2011	2 mg qd	1.8				
	2.5 mg qd	2.1				
	3.5 mg qd	3.2				
	3.0 mg qd	3.1				
	3.0 mg qd	2.5				
	3.0 mg qd	2.5				

PSY PROCEDURE 40-1: Screen and Follow Up Test Results and Document Laboratory Results Appropriately

Name: _____ Date: _____ Time: _____ Grade: _____

EQUIPMENT/SUPPLIES: Patient laboratory results, critical values list for office, patient's chart, telephone (as needed)

STANDARDS: Given the needed equipment and a place to work, the student will perform this skill with _____% accuracy in a total of _____ minutes. *(Your instructor will tell you what the percentage and time limits will be before you begin practicing.)*

KEY: 4 = Satisfactory 0 = Unsatisfactory NA = This step is not counted

PROCEDURE STEPS	SELF	PARTNER	INSTRUCTOR
1. Review laboratory reports received from reference laboratory.	☐	☐	☐
2. Note which reports may be placed directly on the patient's chart and which require immediate notification due to critical results.	☐	☐	☐
3. Notify the physician of the result. Take any immediate instructions from the physician.	☐	☐	☐
4. Follow instructions and document notification and follow-up.	☐	☐	☐
5. Chart remaining reports appropriately.	☐	☐	☐

CALCULATION

Total Possible Points: _____

Total Points Earned: _____ Multiplied by 100 = _____ Divided by Total Possible Points = _____ %

PASS **FAIL** **COMMENTS:**

☐ ☐

Student's signature _____ Date _____

Partner's signature _____ Date _____

Instructor's signature _____ Date _____

PSY PROCEDURE 40-2 | **Quality Control Monitoring Using a QC Chart**

Name: _____ Date: _____ Time: _____ Grade: _____

EQUIPMENT/SUPPLIES: Instrument test results, quality control charts

STANDARDS: Given the needed equipment and a place to work, the student will perform this skill with _____% accuracy in a total of _____ minutes. *(Your instructor will tell you what the percentage and time limits will be before you begin practicing.)*

KEY: 4 = Satisfactory   0 = Unsatisfactory   NA = This step is not counted

PROCEDURE STEPS	SELF	PARTNER	INSTRUCTOR
1. Assemble the charts and data.	☐	☐	☐
2. On the QC chart, plot the control results obtained for the test run.	☐	☐	☐
3. Evaluate chart for acceptability of results.	☐	☐	☐
4. If results are within accepted limits, report patient results.	☐	☐	☐
5. If results are not within accepted limits, do not report patient results. Troubleshoot the test. Repeat testing on the patient and control specimens.	☐	☐	☐
6. If results are within accepted limits, report patient results. Document corrective action and acceptable control results.	☐	☐	☐
7. If results are not within accepted limits, notify the physician of test malfunction. Arrange to have patient specimen referred for testing or store the specimen appropriately until repairs can be made.	☐	☐	☐
8. Troubleshoot within manufacturer's guidelines for operator troubleshooting. Document in the maintenance log. If this is not successful, arrange repairs for the instrument. Document any manufacturer-supplied repairs in the maintenance log.	☐	☐	☐
9. Keep physician informed of testing status.	☐	☐	☐
10. Before returning the instrument to service, validate calibration and quality control. Document appropriately.	☐	☐	☐

CALCULATION

Total Possible Points: _____

Total Points Earned: _____ Multiplied by 100 = _____ Divided by Total Possible Points = _____ %

PASS   **FAIL**   **COMMENTS:**

☐   ☐

Student's signature _____ Date _____

Partner's signature _____ Date _____

Instructor's signature _____ Date _____

PSY PROCEDURE 40-3 Perform Routine Maintenance of Clinical Equipment

Name: _____ Date: _____ Time: _____ Grade: _____

EQUIPMENT/SUPPLIES: Laboratory instrument to be maintained, instrument manual from manufacturer, instrument maintenance log, maintenance supplies as indicated in the instrument manual, personal protective equipment, hand sanitizer, surface sanitizer, contaminated waste container

STANDARDS: Given the needed equipment and a place to work, the student will perform this skill with _____% accuracy in a total of _____ minutes. *(Your instructor will tell you what the percentage and time limits will be before you begin practicing.)*

KEY: 4 = Satisfactory   0 = Unsatisfactory   NA = This step is not counted

PROCEDURE STEPS	SELF	PARTNER	INSTRUCTOR
1. Wash your hands. Put on gloves.	☐	☐	☐
2. Read or review the maintenance section of the instrument manual.	☐	☐	☐
3. Follow the manufacturer's step-by-step instructions for maintaining the instrument.	☐	☐	☐
4. Turn on the instrument and ensure that it is calibrated.	☐	☐	☐
5. Perform the test on the quality control material. Record results. Determine whether QC is within control limits. If yes, proceed with patient testing. If no, take corrective action and recheck controls. Document corrective action. Proceed with patient testing when acceptable QC results are obtained.	☐	☐	☐
6. Document maintenance procedures performed in instrument maintenance log.	☐	☐	☐
7. Properly care for or dispose of equipment and supplies.	☐	☐	☐
8. Clean the work area. Remove personal protective equipment, and wash your hands.	☐	☐	☐

CALCULATION

Total Possible Points: _____

Total Points Earned: _____ Multiplied by 100 = _____ Divided by Total Possible Points = _____ %

PASS   FAIL   COMMENTS:

☐   ☐

Student's signature _____ Date _____

Partner's signature _____ Date _____

Instructor's signature _____ Date _____

41

Phlebotomy

Cognitive Domain

1. Spell and define the key terms
2. Describe the proper patient identification procedures
3. Identify equipment and supplies used to obtain a routine venous specimen and a routine capillary skin puncture
4. Describe proper use of specimen collection equipment
5. List the major anticoagulants, their color codes, and the suggested order in which they are filled from a venipuncture
6. Describe the location and selection of the blood collection sites for capillaries and veins
7. Describe specimen labeling and requisition completion
8. Differentiate between the feel of a vein, tendon, and artery
9. Describe the steps in preparation of the puncture site for venipuncture and skin puncture
10. Describe care for a puncture site after blood has been drawn
11. Describe safety and infection control procedures
12. Describe quality assessment issues in specimen collection procedures
13. List six areas to be avoided when performing venipuncture and the reasons for the restrictions
14. Summarize the problems that may be encountered in accessing a vein, includ-

ing the procedure to follow when a specimen is not obtained
15. List several effects of exercise, posture, and tourniquet application upon laboratory values

Psychomotor Domain

1. Demonstrate proper use of sharps disposal containers
2. Practice standard precautions
3. Participate in standard precautions training
4. Perform handwashing
5. Obtain a blood specimen by evacuated tube or winged infusion set (Procedure 41-1)
6. Obtain a blood specimen by capillary puncture (Procedure 41-2)
7. Use medical terminology, pronouncing medical terms correctly, to communicate information
8. Prepare a patient for procedures and/or treatments
9. Document patient care accurately in the patient record
10. Respond to issues of confidentiality
11. Perform within scope of practice
12. Perform patient screening using using established protocols

Affective Domain

1. Display sensitivity to patient rights and feelings in collecting specimens
2. Explain the rationale for performance of a procedure to the patient

3. Show awareness of patients' concerns regarding their perceptions related to the procedure being performed
4. Demonstrate sensitivity to patients' rights
5. Apply critical thinking skills in performing patient assessment and care
6. Use language/verbal skills that enable patients' understanding
7. Demonstrate respect for diversity in approaching patients and families
8. Demonstrate empathy in communicating with patients, family, and staff
9. Apply active listening skills
10. Demonstrate awareness of the territorial boundaries of the person with whom you are communicating
11. Demonstrate sensitivity appropriate to the message being delivered
12. Demonstrate recognition of the patient's level of understanding in communications
13. Demonstrate respect for individual diversity, incorporating awareness of one's own biases in areas including gender, race, religion, age, and economic status

ABHES Competencies

1. Define and use entire basic structure of medical words and be able to accurately identify in the correct context, i.e. root, prefix, suffix, combinations, spelling, and definitions

2. Build and dissect medical terms from roots/suffixes to understand the word element combinations that create medical terminology
3. Document accurately
4. Comply with federal, state, and local health laws and regulations
5. Identify and respond appropriately when working/caring for patients with special needs
6. Maintain inventory equipment and supplies
7. Communicate on the recipient's level of comprehension
8. Use pertinent medical terminology
9. Recognize and respond to verbal and nonverbal communication
10. Use standard precautions
11. Dispose of biohazardous materials
12. Collect, label, and process specimens
13. Perform venipuncture
14. Perform capillary puncture

Name: _____   Date: _____   Grade: _____

COG MULTIPLE CHOICE

Circle the letter preceding the correct answer.

1. When obtaining a blood specimen from a winged infusion set you need all of the following except:

   a. evacuated tubes.

   b. tourniquet.

   c. gauze pads.

   d. syringe.

   e. permanent marker.

2. A source of error in venipuncture is:

   a. puncturing the wrong area of an infant's heel.

   b. inserting needle bevel side down.

   c. prolonged tourniquet application.

   d. pulling back on syringe plunger too forcefully.

   e. all of the above

3. When your patient is feeling faint during venipuncture, you should do all of the following except:

   a. remove the tourniquet and withdraw the needle.

   b. divert attention from the procedure.

   c. have patient breathe deeply.

   d. loosen a tight collar or tie.

   e. apply a cold compress or washcloth.

4. To avoid hemoconcentration the phlebotomist should:

   a. ensure the tourniquet is not too tight.

   b. have patient make a fist.

   c. use occluded veins.

   d. draw blood from the heel.

   e. use a needle with a small diameter.

5. If you accidentally puncture an artery, you should:

   a. hold pressure over the site for a full 5 minutes.

   b. use a cold compress to reduce pain.

   c. perform a capillary puncture.

   d. use a multisample needle instead.

   e. use a flatter angle when inserting the needle.

6. What is the difference between NPO and fasting?

   a. Fasting is no food, and NPO is no water.

   b. Fasting and NPO are basically the same.

   c. Fasting allows the patient to drink water, whereas NPO does not.

   d. NPO requires that the patient drink water, whereas fasting does not.

   e. Fasting is for surgery, and NPO is for getting true test results.

7. Aseptic techniques to prevent infection of the venipuncture site include:

   a. using sterile gloves.

   b. wearing a lab coat.

   c. using a gel separator.

   d. not opening bandages ahead of time.

   e. not speaking while you draw blood.

8. When collecting a blood sample from the fingers, you should use:

   a. the thumb.

   b. the second finger.

   c. the fifth finger.

   d. all fingers.

   e. the third and fourth fingers.

9. You should not draw blood using a small gauge needle because:

   a. there is a greater likelihood of it breaking off in the vein.

   b. blood cells will rupture, causing hemolysis of the specimen.

   c. the luer adaptor will not fit venipuncture cuffs.

   d. the small needles are awkward to hold and manipulate.

   e. the small needles do not allow you to collect enough blood.

10. Which of the following may trigger hematoma formation?

    a. Pressure is applied after venipuncture.

    b. The needle is removed after the tourniquet is removed.

    c. The needle penetrates all the way through the vein.

    d. The needle is fully inserted into the vein.

    e. The patient has not properly followed preparation instructions.

11. If you are exposed to blood by needlestick, it is necessary to:

    a. wash the needle with hot soap and water.

    b. notify your supervisor.

    c. determine the type of needle involved in the injury.

    d. alert the patient.

    e. activate the safety device on the needle.

12. Gloves that are dusted with powder may:

    a. contaminate blood tests collected by capillary puncture.

    b. transfer disease from patient to patient.

    c. inhibit the growth of bacteria.

    d. cause an allergic reaction in the patient.

    e. hold up better than regular latex gloves.

13. The purpose of antiseptics is to:

    a. hold needles.

    b. clean biohazardous spills.

    c. inhibit the growth of bacteria.

    d. promote anticoagulation.

    e. prevent hematomas.

14. The most commonly used antiseptic for routine blood collection is:

    a. 70% isopropyl alcohol.

    b. povidone iodine.

    c. 0.5% chlorhexidine gluconate.

    d. benzalkonium chloride.

    e. sodium chloride.

15. The end of the needle that pierces the vein is cut into a slant called a:

    a. bevel.

    b. hub.

    c. gauge.

    d. shaft.

    e. adapter.

16. Gauze pads are used to:

    a. prevent hemolysis

    b. prevent blood clots at the venipuncture site.

    c. handle used needles.

    d. hold pressure on the venipuncture site following removal of the needle.

    e. reduce the spread of bloodborne pathogens.

17. Which tubes must be first in the order of the draw?

    a. Blood culture tubes

    b. Coagulation tubes

    c. Heparin tubes

    d. Serum separator tubes (SSTs)

    e. Plain tubes

18. Which of the following is true of ethylenediaminetetraacetic acid (EDTA) tubes?

    a. They cause the least interference in tests.

    b. They should be filled after hematology tubes.

    c. They are the same as PSTs.

    d. They minimize the chance of microbial contamination.

    e. They elevate sodium and potassium levels.

19. What safety features are available for the holder used with the evacuated tube system?

    a. Shields that cover the needle, or devices that retract the needle into the holder

    b. A self-locking cover for recapping the needle

    c. A gripper to clamp the holder to the Vacutainer tube, preventing slippage

    d. Orange color as a reminder to discard in biohazard container

    e. A beveled point on only one end

20. What example explains the best advantage of using the evacuated tube system?

a. Multiple tubes may be filled from a single venipuncture.

b. The tubes are color coded according to the tests to be done.

c. The vacuum draws the blood into the tubes.

d. It is a universal system, used in all phlebotomy laboratories around the country.

e. It is the least painful way to draw blood from a patient.

COG MATCHING

Grade: _____

Match each key term with the correct definition.

Key Terms

21. _____ anchor

22. _____ antecubital space

23. _____ anticoagulant

24. _____ antiseptic

25. _____ barrier precautions

26. _____ bevel

27. _____ blood cultures

28. _____ bore

29. _____ breathing the syringe

30. _____ butterfly

31. _____ cultured

32. _____ distal

33. _____ microcontainers

34. _____ edematous

35. _____ evacuated tube

36. _____ fasting

37. _____ flanges

38. _____ gauge

39. _____ gauze sponges

Definitions

a. physical products, equipment, or methods used specifically for the purpose of protecting the patient and the health care worker from exposure to potentially infectious material

b. blood collection tube additive used because it prevents clotting

c. forms a physical barrier between the cellular portion of a specimen and the serum or plasma portion after the specimen has been centrifuged

d. specimens drawn to culture the blood for pathogens

e. the end of the needle that pierces the vein that is cut on a slant

f. diameter of the needle

g. measure of the diameter of the needle

h. winged infusion set

i. extensions on the sides of the rim of the holder to aid in tube placement and removal

j. grown in the laboratory

k. solution used to inhibit the growth of bacteria

l. pads that come in multiple sizes depending upon their use in various clinical areas

m. pull back the plunger to about halfway up the barrel, and then push it back

n. the inside of the elbow

o. away from the origin

p. swollen area due to excess tissue fluid

q. the patient must eat nothing after midnight until the blood specimen is drawn, including chewing gum, breath mints, and coffee; the patient *can* have water

r. extend beyond the normal range of motion

s. hold a vein in place so that it does not roll

t. formation caused by blood leaking into the tissues during or after venipuncture

u. packed red blood cell volume

40. _____ gel separator

41. _____ hemachromatosis

42. _____ hematocrit

43. _____ hematoma

44. _____ hemoconcentration

45. _____ hemolysis

46. _____ hyperextend

v. a condition that causes an elevated hematocrit

w. disorder that increases the amount of iron in the blood to dangerous levels

x. small, nonsterile plastic tubes with color-coded stoppers that indicate the presence or absence of an additive; contains no vacuum to remove very small amounts of blood from the patient

y. tubes that fill with a predetermined volume of blood because of the vacuum inside the tube (the vacuum is premeasured by the manufacturer to draw the precise amount of blood into the tube; the tube fills until the vacuum is exhausted)

z. rupturing of red blood cells, causing release of intracellular contents into the plasma

COG MATCHING

Grade: _____

Match each key term with the correct definition.

Key Terms

47. _____ luer adapter

48. _____ lumen

49. _____ lymphedema

50. _____ multisample needle

51. _____ needle disposal unit

52. _____ NPO

53. _____ order of draw

54. _____ palpate

55. _____ peak level

56. _____ polycythemia vera

57. _____ probing

58. _____ prophylaxis

59. _____ requisition

60. _____ sharps container

61. _____ syncope

62. _____ syringe

Definitions

a. protective treatment for the prevention of disease once exposure has occurred

b. an order form for laboratory tests

c. system that facilitates collecting multiple tubes with a single venipuncture

d. tube filling sequence for both collection of evacuated tubes and filling evacuated tubes from a syringe

e. opening of a needle

f. needle holder

g. disease of having too many red blood cells; abnormally high hematocrit

h. puncture-resistant, leak-proof disposable container

i. sharps container

j. made of disposable plastic and vary in volume from 1 to 50 mL

k. veins that have been injured, lack resilience, and roll easily

l. lymphatic obstruction

m. using the tip of the index finger to evaluate veins by feeling to determine their suitability

n. the patient must have absolutely nothing by mouth after midnight until the procedure is done; in this case, the patient _cannot_ have water

o. fainting

p. digging with a needle

q. the highest serum level of a drug in a patient based on a dosing schedule, which is usually measured about 60 minutes after the end of the infusion

r. drug level drawn immediately prior to a dose

63. _____ taut

64. _____ therapeutic phlebotomy

65. _____ thrombosed

66. _____ trough level

s. phlebotomy done as part of the patient's treatment for certain blood disorders

t. so that there is no give or slack

COG SHORT ANSWER

Grade: _____

67. List four techniques for avoiding hemoconcentration.

    a. _____

    b. _____

    c. _____

    d. _____

68. List three problems using the correct order of draw enables you to avoid.

    _____

    _____

    _____

    _____

69. What is a warming device? What is its purpose in capillary puncture?

    _____

    _____

    _____

    _____

70. List six reasons not to choose a specific site for venipuncture.

    _____

    _____

    _____

71. What should you do if a hematoma begins to form during venipuncture?

_____

_____

_____

_____

72. List four sites to reject for capillary puncture.

_____

_____

_____

_____

73. Name eight sources of error in venipuncture procedure.

_____

_____

_____

_____

COG FILL IN THE BLANK

Grade: _____

74. Fill in the blanks on situations that may trigger hematoma formation.

a. The vein is _____ or too _____ for the needle.

b. The needle _____ all the way through the _____.

c. The needle is only _____ inserted into the vein.

d. _____ or _____ probing is used to find the vein.

e. The needle is _____ while the _____ is still on.

f. _____ is not adequately _____ after venipuncture.

COG MATCHING

Grade: _____

Match each tube with its description.

Tubes

75. _____ Heparin tubes

76. _____ Tubes for coagulation testing

77. _____ EDTA tubes

78. _____ Tubes for blood cultures

79. _____ PST tubes

80. _____ Serum separator gel tubes

81. _____ Plain (nonadditive) tubes

Descriptions

a. Drawn first to minimize chance of microbial contamination

b. Prevents contamination by additives in other tubes

c. Must be the first additive tube in the order because all other additive tubes affect coagulation tests

d. Come after coagulation tests because silica particles activate clotting and affect coagulation tests; carryover of silica into subsequent tubes can be overridden by the anticoagulant in them

e. Affects coagulation tests and interferes in collection of serum specimens; causes the least interference in tests other than coagulation tests

f. Causes more carryover problems than any other additive; elevates sodium and potassium levels; chelates and decreases calcium and iron levels; elevates prothrombin time and partial thromboplastin time results

g. Causes the least interference in tests other than coagulation tests and contains a gel separator to separate plasma from the blood cells in the specimen

COG TRUE OR FALSE?

Grade: _____

Indicate whether the statements are true or false by placing the letter T (true) or F (false) on the line preceding the statement.

82. _____ Winged sets cause increased numbers of needlesticks to phlebotomists.

83. _____ For finger puncture sites, it is best to have the hand below the heart.

84. _____ Never believe patients when they say they faint during venipuncture.

85. _____ Warmers decrease blood flow before the skin is punctured.

86. _____ Excessive massaging of the puncture site is a source of error in skin puncture.

COG SHORT ANSWER

87. The properly labeled sample is essential so that the results of the test match the patient. List the four key elements in labeling.

_____

_____

_____

_____

88. List the use of each item of equipment used to obtain a routine venous specimen and a routine capillary skin puncture.

a. Evacuated collection tubes:

_____

_____

_____

_____

b. Multisample needles:

_____

_____

_____

_____

c. Winged infusion sets:

_____

_____

_____

_____

    d. Holders/adapters:

_____

_____

_____

_____

    e. Tourniquets:

_____

_____

_____

_____

    f. Alcohol wipes:

_____

_____

_____

_____

    g. Gauze sponges:

_____

_____

_____

_____

    h. Bandages:

_____

_____

_____

_____

i. Needle disposal units (sharps containers):

_____

_____

_____

_____

j. Gloves:

_____

_____

_____

_____

k. Syringes:

_____

_____

_____

_____

l. Puncture devices:

_____

_____

_____

_____

m. Microhematocrit tubes:

_____

_____

_____

_____

n. Microcollection containers:

_____

_____

_____

_____

o. Filter paper test requisitions:

_____

_____

_____

_____

p. Warming devices:

_____

_____

_____

_____

89. What are the two parts of patient identification in the medical office?

_____

_____

_____

_____

90. Supply the color code for each type of blood collection tube.

a. Blood cultures _____

b. Coagulation tests _____

c. Serum separator tubes _____

d. Ethylenediaminetetraacetic acid _____

e. Plain (nonadditive) tubes _____

f. Plasma tubes and plasma separator tubes _____

91. List the 7 items required for completing test requisitions.

_____

_____

_____

_____

COG IDENTIFICATION

Grade: _____

92. Fill in artery (A), tendon (T), or vein (V) by the feeling when palpating a vein.

a. _____ cordlike

b. _____ lacks resilience

c. _____ most elastic

d. _____ palpable

e. _____ pulsatile

f. _____ resilient

g. _____ trackable

COG PLACE IN ORDER

Grade: _____

93. Numbering from 1–25, place the steps for performing a venipuncture in the correct order.

_____ Properly care for or dispose of all equipment and supplies. Clean the work area. Remove personal protective equipment and wash your hands.

_____ Greet and identify the patient. Explain the procedure. Ask for and answer any questions.

_____ Tap the tubes that contain additives to ensure that the additive is dislodged from the stopper and wall of the tube. Insert the tube into the adaptor until the needle slightly enters the stopper. Do not push the top of the tube stopper beyond the indentation mark. If the tube retracts slightly, leave it in the retracted position.

_____ Check the requisition slip to determine the tests ordered and specimen requirements.

_____ If a fasting specimen is required, ask the patient the last time he or she ate or drank anything other than water.

_____ Select a vein by palpating. Use your gloved index finger to trace the path of the vein and judge its depth.

_____ Wash your hands.

_____ Apply the tourniquet around the patient's arm 3–4 inches above the elbow.

_____ Cleanse the venipuncture site with an alcohol pad, starting in the center of puncture site and working outward in a circular motion. Allow the site to dry or dry the site with sterile gauze. Do not touch the area after cleansing.

_____ With the bevel up, line up the needle with the vein approximately one quarter to half an inch below the site where the vein is to be entered. At a 15- to 30-degree angle, rapidly and smoothly insert the needle through the skin. Place two fingers on the flanges of the adapter and with the thumb push the tube onto the needle inside the adapter. Allow the tube to fill to capacity. Release the tourniquet and allow the patient to release the fist. When blood flow ceases, remove the tube from the adapter by gripping the tube with your nondominant hand and placing your thumb against the flange during removal. Twist and gently pull out the tube. Steady the needle in the vein. Avoid pulling up or pressing down on the needle while it is in the vein. Insert any other necessary tubes into adapter and allow each to fill to capacity.

_____ Assemble the equipment. Check the expiration date on the tubes.

_____ Record the procedure.

_____ Put on nonsterile latex or vinyl gloves. Use other personal protective equipment as defined by facility policy.

_____ Place a sterile gauze pad over the puncture site at the time of needle withdrawal. Do not apply any pressure to the site until the needle is completely removed. After the needle is removed, immediately activate the safety device and apply pressure or have the patient apply direct pressure for 3–5 minutes. Do not bend the arm at the elbow.

_____ Instruct the patient to sit with a well-supported arm.

_____ Label the tubes with patient information as defined in facility protocol.

_____ Release tourniquet after palpating the vein if it has been left on for more than 1 minute. Have patient release his or her fist.

_____ Test, transfer, or store the blood specimen according to the medical office policy.

_____ Remove the needle cover. Hold the needle assembly in your dominant hand, thumb on top of the adaptor and fingers under it. Grasp the patient's arm with the other hand, using your thumb to draw the skin taut over the site. This anchors the vein about 1–2 inches below the puncture site and helps keep it in place during needle insertion.

_____ If the vacuum tubes contain an anticoagulant, they must be mixed immediately by gently inverting the tube 8–10 times. Do not shake the tube.

_____ If blood being drawn for culture will be used in diagnosing a septic condition, make sure the specimen is sterile. To do this, apply alcohol to the area for 2 full minutes. Then apply a 2% iodine solution in ever widening circles. Never move the wipes back over areas that have been cleaned; use a new wipe for each sweep across the area.

_____ Thank the patient. Instruct the patient to leave the bandage in place at least 15 minutes and not to carry a heavy object (such as a purse) or lift heavy objects with that arm for 1 hour.

_____ Properly care for or dispose of all equipment and supplies. Clean the work area. Remove personal protective equipment and wash your hands.

_____ Reapply the tourniquet if it was removed after palpation. Ask patient to make a fist.

_____ Check the puncture site for bleeding. Apply a dressing, a clean 2 × 2 gauze pad folded in quarters, and hold in place by an adhesive bandage or 3-inch strip of tape.

_____ With the tourniquet released, remove the tube from the adapter before removing the needle from the arm.

94. Numbering from 1–16, place the steps for performing a capillary puncture in the correct order.

_____ Thank the patient. Instruct the patient to leave the bandage in place at least 15 minutes.

_____ Greet and identify the patient. Explain the procedure. Ask for and answer any questions.

_____ Check the requisition slip to determine the tests ordered and specimen requirements.

_____ Select the puncture site. Use the appropriate puncture device for the site selected.

_____ Obtain the first drop of blood. Wipe away the first drop of blood with dry gauze. Apply pressure toward the site but do not milk the site.

_____ Wash your hands.

_____ Grasp the finger firmly between your non-dominant index finger and thumb, or grasp the infant's heel firmly with your index finger wrapped around the foot and your thumb wrapped around the ankle. Cleanse the selected area with 70% isopropyl alcohol and allow to air dry.

_____ Record the procedure.

_____ Assemble the equipment.

_____ Hold the patient's finger or heel firmly and make a swift, firm puncture. Perform the puncture perpendicular to the whorls of the fingerprint or footprint. Dispose of the used puncture device in a sharps container.

_____ Test, transfer, or store the specimen according to the medical office policy.

_____ Put on gloves.

_____ Collect the specimen in the chosen container or slide. Touch only the tip of the collection device to the drop of blood. Blood flow is encouraged if the puncture site is held downward and gentle pressure is applied near the site. Cap micro collection tubes with the caps provided and mix the additives by gently tilting or inverting the tubes 8–10 times.

_____ Make sure the site chosen is warm and not cyanotic or edematous. Gently massage the finger from the base to the tip or massage the infant's heel.

_____ Properly care for or dispose of equipment and supplies. Clean the work area. Remove gloves and wash your hands.

_____ When collection is complete, apply clean gauze to the site with pressure. Hold pressure or have the patient hold pressure until bleeding stops. Label the containers with the proper information. Do not apply a dressing to a skin puncture of an infant under age 2 years. Never release a patient until the bleeding has stopped.

COG IDENTIFICATION

Grade: _____

Note if the following is acceptable (A) or unacceptable (U) treatment of the puncture site.

95. _____ If the venipuncture process is interrupted, leave the clean venipuncture site open to the air.

96. _____ Place pressure on the puncture site and remove needle.

97. _____ Do not have the patient fold the arm following venipuncture.

98. _____ Have the patient hold light pressure on the venipuncture site, if possible, while you secure the exposed needle.

99. _____ Dismiss the patient after holding light pressure on the venipuncture site.

100. _____ Avoid overly massaging the capillary puncture site.

101. _____ When finished, elevate the heel, place a clean gauze sponge on the puncture site and hold it in place until the bleeding has stopped.

102. _____ Gauze pads folded in fourths are used to hold pressure over the puncture site when secured by a bandage.

COG TRUE OR FALSE?

Grade: _____

Indicate whether the statements are true or false by placing the letter T (true) or F (false) on the line preceding the statement.

103. _____ After the needle is removed, activate the safety device as soon as possible.

104. _____ The phlebotomy station should be central to all of the clinical areas so that it is easily accessible by everyone.

105. _____ A safety device locks the armrest in place in front of the patient to prevent falling from the chair if fainting occurs.

106. _____ Needle holders do not include a safety device, so needle safety devices are required.

107. _____ The Needlestick Safety and Prevention Act requires each phlebotomist to be responsible for his or her own safety.

108. _____ Quick activation of the safety device relieves the phlebotomist of concern for caution.

109. _____ Holder safety features may include a shield that covers the needle or a device that retracts the needle into the holder after it is withdrawn from the vein.

110. _____ Regardless of safety features, immediately dispose of used needles, lancets, and other sharp objects in a puncture-resistant, leak-proof disposable container called a sharps container.

COG LIST

Grade: _____

111. List six actions that provide safety and infection control.

_____

_____

_____

_____

112. List nine factors that must be monitored to assure quality in phlebotomy.

_____

_____

_____

_____

113. Exercise causes changes in the blood levels of which four analytes?

_____

_____

_____

_____

COG FILL IN THE BLANK   Grade: _____

114. Postural changes (_____, _____, _____) are known
     to vary laboratory results of some analytes. The differences in these lab values have been attributed to shifts in
     _____ _____. Fluids tend to stay in the vascular compartment (bloodstream)
     when the patient is _____ or _____. This tends to _____ the
     blood. There is a _____ of fluids to the interstitial spaces upon standing or ambulation. The lab
     tests that are the most affected by this phenomenon are proteins (_____, _____,
     _____) and protein-bound substances, such as _____,
     _____, _____, and _____.

115. The maximum time limit for leaving the tourniquet in place is _____ minutes. Extending
     the time limit can alter test results by causing _____ and _____. The
     _____ of fluid in hemoconcentrated blood results in a(n) _____ of cellular
     components in that blood. This _____ elevation results in _____ labora-
     tory measurement of _____, _____, and some _____.
     _____ tourniquet placement may significantly increase total protein, aspartate aminotransferase
     (AST), total lipids, cholesterol, iron, and hematocrit.

116. The most common complication of venipuncture is _____ formation caused by blood leaking into
     the tissues during or after venipuncture.

117. Situations that may trigger hematoma formation include:

     a. The vein is _____ or too _____ for the needle.

     b. The needle _____ all the way through the _____.

     c. The needle is only _____ _____ into the vein.

     d. Excessive or _____ _____ is used to find the vein.

     e. The needle is removed while the _____ _____ _____
     _____.

     f. _____ is not adequately applied after venipuncture.

118. _____ veins (lack resilience) feel like rope or cord and _____ easily.

119. Accidental puncture of an _____ is recognized by the blood's bright red color and the
     _____ of the specimen into the tube.

120. Permanent _____ damage may result from _____ site selection, move-
     ment of the _____ during needle insertion, inserting the needle too _____ or
     _____, or excessive blind _____.

121. Make sure the needle fully _____ the _____ most wall of the vein. (Partial
     _____ allow blood to leak into the soft tissue surrounding the vein by way of the needle
     _____.)

122. If an insufficient amount or no blood is collected:

a. Change the _____ of the _____. Move it forward (it may not be in the _____). Or, move it backward (it may have _____ _____ _____).

b. Adjust the angle (the _____ may be against the vein _____).

c. Loosen the tourniquet; it may be _____ blood _____.

d. Try _____ tube. There may be no _____ in the _____ _____ _____.

e. _____ the vein. Veins sometimes _____ _____ from the _____ of the needle and puncture site.

f. The vein may have _____; _____ the tourniquet to increase _____ filling. If this is not successful, remove the _____, take care of the _____ site, and _____.

g. The _____ may have pulled _____ _____ _____ _____ when switching tubes. _____ equipment firmly and place _____ against patient's arm, using the _____ for leverage when withdrawing and inserting _____.

CASE STUDIES FOR CRITICAL THINKING   Grade: _____

1. You have a patient who says that he always becomes nervous at the sight of his own blood, but has never fainted before. You ask the patient to lie down during the procedure. Your patient is fine with the needle insertion, but as soon as he sees the sight of his own blood, he passes out. What should you do?

_____

_____

_____

_____

2. It is your first time performing a skin puncture on the heel of an infant, and as much as the father tries to comfort his baby, the baby won't stop crying or hold still. How would you handle this situation?

_____

_____

_____

_____

3. An older adult patient comes in for a venipuncture procedure. You insert the needle at a narrow angle because of the shallowness of her veins. However, her vein "rolls" during this procedure, and, after needle removal, she begins to develop a huge hematoma and becomes very anxious. How do you treat your patient's condition and console her?

_____

_____

_____

_____

4. Write a narrative note that describes the procedure in the exercise above. Include all necessary details, as this will be included in the patient's chart.

_____

_____

_____

_____

_____

5. You are reviewing test results received from the referral laboratory. You notice that the HIV results on your neighbor, Alice Sihotang, are positive. Your friend Kaylene Oyakawa meets you for lunch. She tells you that all of your neighbors are worried about about Alice because she looks so ill and has been losing weight. Kaylene says that she knows Alice is a patient at your medical office and asks you what is wrong with Alice. What do you say?

_____

_____

_____

_____

6. After drawing blood with a winged set, you inadvertently stick yourself with the needle. How would you handle this situation?

_____

_____

_____

_____

7. Your last patient of the day, a young child accompanied by her mother, accidentally knocks over your collection tubes that were within her reach as you were disposing of sharps. How would you handle this situation?

_____

_____

_____

_____

8. Jordan, your 5-year-old patient, is afraid to have a skin puncture. She is extremely agitated, and her mother is having a difficult time trying to get her to sit still. Gloria, the phlebotomist, decides to have the parent restrain the child by firmly holding the child's finger very still. Gloria notices that the screaming child's hands are cold and clammy. With gloves on, Gloria quickly performs the skin puncture, capturing every drop. Identify the mistakes Gloria made in preparing the patient and list possible effects.

_____

_____

_____

_____

9. You are preparing to draw blood from your patient. When you begin to palpate for a vein, the patient asks what the doctor has ordered and why he ordered those tests. What do you say?

_____

_____

_____

_____

10. Jenna, your 15-year-old patient, is waiting with her mother. She is extremely nervous. You are greeting the patient and reviewing the requisition. The doctor has ordered a serum pregnancy test on Jenna. Jenna's mother asks what test the doctor has requested. What is the cause of Jenna's anxiety and how do you handle the situation?

_____

_____

_____

11. Medical ethics limit your discussion with a patient regarding the physician's orders and why she ordered them. To stress the key role patients play in staying healthy, what can you say to the patient about his rights and responsibilities?

_____

_____

_____

_____

12. In reviewing the physician's orders on the requisition, you see that your patient needs to collect a urine specimen in addition to having blood drawn. You tell the patient you will need a urine specimen and that the containers are in the bathroom. Your patient stares at you and does not move toward the restroom. What is the reason and what action do you take?

_____

_____

_____

_____

13. Nick is preparing to draw blood from a 55-year-old, very obese female. In preparing to tie the tourniquet 3–4 inches above the elbow, he accidently brushes the patient's breast. How should Nick handle completing this phlebotomy? How should Nick plan to handle this type of situation in the future?

_____

_____

_____

_____

14. The medical office has closed and you are completing preparation of specimens for the reference laboratory pick-up. You find you have two requisitions without labeled specimens to accompany them. You have two unlabeled blood tubes. There is no way to identify the two specimens. What do you do?

_____

_____

_____

_____

PSY PROCEDURE 41-1   **Obtaining a Blood Specimen by Evacuated Tube or Winged Infusion Set**

Name: _____ Date: _____ Time: _____ Grade: _____

EQUIPMENT/SUPPLIES: Multisample needle and adaptor or winged infusion set, evacuated tubes, tourniquet, sterile gauze pads, bandages, sharps container, 70% alcohol pad, permanent marker or pen, appropriate personal protective equipment (e.g., gloves, impervious gown, face shield)

STANDARDS: Given the needed equipment and a place to work, the student will perform this skill with _____% accuracy in a total of _____ minutes. *(Your instructor will tell you what the percentage and time limits will be before you begin practicing.)*

KEY: 4 = Satisfactory   0 = Unsatisfactory   NA = This step is not counted

PROCEDURE STEPS	SELF	PARTNER	INSTRUCTOR
1. Check the requisition slip to determine the tests ordered and specimen requirements.	☐	☐	☐
2. Wash your hands.	☐	☐	☐
3. Assemble the equipment. Check the expiration date on the tubes.	☐	☐	☐
4. **AFF** Greet and identify the patient. Explain the procedure. Ask for and answer any questions.	☐	☐	☐
5. **AFF** Demonstrate recognition of the patient's level of understanding communications. Apply active listening skills. Modify communication to the patient's level of understanding, or obtain assistance with language differences.	☐	☐	☐
6. If a fasting specimen is required, ask the patient the last time he or she ate or drank anything other than water.	☐	☐	☐
7. Put on nonsterile latex or vinyl gloves. Use other personal protective equipment as defined by facility policy.	☐	☐	☐
8. For evacuated tube collection: Break the seal of the needle cover and thread the sleeved needle into the adaptor, using the needle cover as a wrench. For winged infusion set collection: Extend the tubing. Thread the sleeved needle into the adaptor. For both methods: Tap the tubes that contain additives to ensure that the additive is dislodged from the stopper and wall of the tube. Insert the tube into the adaptor until the needle slightly enters the stopper. Do not push the top of the tube stopper beyond the indentation mark. If the tube retracts slightly, leave it in the retracted position.	☐	☐	☐
9. Instruct the patient to sit with a well-supported arm.	☐	☐	☐

10. Apply the tourniquet around the patient's arm 3–4 inches above the elbow.
 	
   a. Apply the tourniquet snuggly, but not too tightly.
 	
   b. Secure the tourniquet by using the half-bow knot.
 	
   c. Make sure the tails of the tourniquet extend upward to avoid contaminating the venipuncture site.
 	
   d. Ask the patient to make a fist and hold it, but not to pump the fist.
	☐	☐	☐

11. Select a vein by palpating. Use your gloved index finger to trace the path of the vein and judge its depth.	☐	☐	☐
12. Release tourniquet after palpating the vein if it has been left on for more than one minute. Have patient release fist.	☐	☐	☐
13. Cleanse the venipuncture site with an alcohol pad, starting in the center of puncture site and working outward in a circular motion. Allow the site to dry or dry the site with sterile gauze. Do not touch the area after cleansing.	☐	☐	☐
14. If blood being drawn for culture will be used in diagnosing a septic condition, make sure the specimen is sterile. To do this, apply alcohol to the area for 2 full minutes. Then apply a 2% iodine solution in ever widening circles. Never move the wipes back over areas that have been cleaned; use a new wipe for each sweep across the area.	☐	☐	☐
15. Reapply the tourniquet if it was removed after palpation. Ask patient to make a fist.	☐	☐	☐
16. Remove the needle cover. Hold the needle assembly in your dominant hand, thumb on top of the adaptor and fingers under it. Grasp the patient's arm with the other hand, using your thumb to draw the skin taut over the site. This anchors the vein about 1–2 inches below the puncture site and helps keep it in place during needle insertion.	☐	☐	☐
17. With the bevel up, line up the needle with the vein approximately one quarter to half an inch below the site where the vein is to be entered. At a 15- to 30-degree angle, rapidly and smoothly insert the needle through the skin. Use a lesser angle for winged infusion set collections. Place two fingers on the flanges of the adapter and with the thumb push the tube onto the needle inside the adapter. Allow the tube to fill to capacity. Release the tourniquet and allow the patient to release the fist. When blood flow ceases, remove the tube from the adapter by gripping the tube with your non-dominant hand and placing your thumb against the flange during removal. Twist and gently pull out the tube. Steady the needle in the vein. Avoid pulling up or pressing down on the needle while it is in the vein. Insert any other necessary tubes into adapter and allow each to fill to capacity.	☐	☐	☐
18. With the tourniquet released, remove the tube from the adapter before removing the needle from the arm.	☐	☐	☐

19. Place a sterile gauze pad over the puncture site at the time of needle withdrawal. Do not apply any pressure to the site until the needle is completely removed. **a.** After the needle is removed, immediately activate the safety device and apply pressure or have the patient apply direct pressure for 3–5 minutes. Do not bend the arm at the elbow.	☐	☐	☐
20. After the needle is removed, immediately activate the safety device and apply pressure, or have the patient apply direct pressure for 3–5 minutes. Do not bend the arm at the elbow.	☐	☐	☐
21. If the vacuum tubes contain an anticoagulant, they must be mixed immediately by gently inverting the tube 8–10 times. Do not shake the tube.	☐	☐	☐
22. Label the tubes with patient information as defined in facility protocol.	☐	☐	☐
23. Check the puncture site for bleeding. Apply a dressing, a clean 2 × 2 gauze pad folded in quarters, and hold in place by an adhesive bandage or 3-inch strip of tape.	☐	☐	☐
24. **AFF** Thank the patient. Instruct the patient to leave the bandage in place at least 15 minutes and not to carry a heavy object (such as a purse) or lift heavy objects with that arm for 1 hour.	☐	☐	☐
25. Properly care for or dispose of all equipment and supplies. Clean the work area. Remove personal protective equipment and wash your hands.	☐	☐	☐
26. Test, transfer, or store the blood specimen according to the medical office policy.	☐	☐	☐
27. Record the procedure.	☐	☐	☐
28. **AFF** Explain how to respond to a patient who is deaf, hearing impaired, visually impaired, developmentally challenged, or speaks English as a second language (ESL) or who has dementia, cultural or religious concerns, or generational differences.	☐	☐	☐

CALCULATION

Total Possible Points: _____

Total Points Earned: _____ Multiplied by 100 = _____ Divided by Total Possible Points = _____ %

PASS   **FAIL**   **COMMENTS:**

☐   ☐

Student's signature _____ Date _____

Partner's signature _____ Date _____

Instructor's signature _____ Date _____

PSY PROCEDURE 41-2 Obtaining a Blood Specimen by Capillary Puncture

Name: _____ Date: _____ Time: _____ Grade: _____

EQUIPMENT/SUPPLIES: Skin puncture device, 70% alcohol pads, 2 × 2 gauze pads, microcollection tubes or containers, heel warming device if needed, small band aids, pen or permanent marker and personal protective equipment (e.g., gloves, impervious gown, face shield)

STANDARDS: Given the needed equipment and a place to work, the student will perform this skill with _____% accuracy in a total of _____ minutes. *(Your instructor will tell you what the percentage and time limits will be before you begin practicing.)*

KEY: 4 = Satisfactory   0 = Unsatisfactory   NA = This step is not counted

PROCEDURE STEPS	SELF	PARTNER	INSTRUCTOR
1. Check the requisition slip to determine the tests ordered and specimen requirements.	☐	☐	☐
2. Wash your hands.	☐	☐	☐
3. Assemble the equipment.	☐	☐	☐
4. **AFF** Greet and identify the patient. Explain the procedure. Ask for and answer any questions.	☐	☐	☐
5. **AFF** Evaluate your patient for his or her ability to understand your instructions. When indicated, whether the problem is deafness, hearing impairment, visual impairment, a developmental challenge, English as a second language (ESL), dementia, cultural or religious concerns, or generational differences, you are responsible for helping the patient understand the procedure before beginning the phlebotomy. This may include help from the person who brought the patient to the office or from a translator.	☐	☐	☐
6. Put on gloves.	☐	☐	☐
7. Select the puncture site (the lateral portion of the tip of the middle or ring finger of the non-dominant hand or lateral curved surface of the heel of an infant). The puncture should be made in the fleshy central portion of the second or third finger, slightly to the side of center, and perpendicular to the grooves of the fingerprint. Perform heel puncture only on the plantar surface of the heel, medial to an imaginary line extending from the middle of the great toe to the heel, and lateral to an imaginary line drawn from between the fourth and fifth toes to the heel. Use the appropriate puncture device for the site selected.	☐	☐	☐

8. Make sure the site chosen is warm and not cyanotic or edematous. Gently massage the finger from the base to the tip or massage the infant's heel.	☐	☐	☐
9. Grasp the finger firmly between your nondominant index finger and thumb, or grasp the infant's heel firmly with your index finger wrapped around the foot and your thumb wrapped around the ankle. Cleanse the selected area with 70% isopropyl alcohol and allow to air dry.	☐	☐	☐
10. Hold the patient's finger or heel firmly and make a swift, firm puncture. Perform the puncture perpendicular to the whorls of the fingerprint or footprint. Dispose of the used puncture device in a sharps container.	☐	☐	☐

11. Obtain the first drop of blood.
    a. Wipe away the first drop of blood with dry gauze.
    b. Apply pressure toward the site but do not milk the site.
	☐	☐	☐

12. Collect the specimen in the chosen container or slide. Touch only the tip of the collection device to the drop of blood. Blood flow is encouraged if the puncture site is held downward and gentle pressure is applied near the site. Cap micro-collection tubes with the caps provided and mix the additives by gently tilting or inverting the tubes 8–10 times.	☐	☐	☐
13. When collection is complete, apply clean gauze to the site with pressure. Hold pressure or have the patient hold pressure until bleeding stops. Label the containers with the proper information. Do not apply a dressing to a skin puncture of an infant under age 2 years. Never release a patient until the bleeding has stopped.	☐	☐	☐
14. **AFF** Thank the patient. Instruct the patient to leave the bandage in place at least 15 minutes.	☐	☐	☐
15. Properly care for or dispose of equipment and supplies. Clean the work area. Remove gloves and wash your hands.	☐	☐	☐
16. Test, transfer, or store the specimen according to the medical office policy.	☐	☐	☐
17. Record the procedure.	☐	☐	☐

CALCULATION

Total Possible Points: _____

Total Points Earned: _____ Multiplied by 100 = _____ Divided by Total Possible Points = _____ %

PASS   **FAIL**   **COMMENTS:**

  ☐   ☐

Student's signature _____ Date _____

Partner's signature _____ Date _____

Instructor's signature _____ Date _____

Cognitive Domain

1. Spell and define the key terms
2. List the parameters measured in the complete blood count and their normal ranges
3. State the conditions associated with selected abnormal complete blood count findings
4. Explain the functions of the three types of blood cells
5. Describe the purpose of testing for the erythrocyte sedimentation rate
6. List the leukocytes seen normally in the blood and their functions
7. Analyze a table in the interpretation of healthcare results
8. Distinguish between normal and abnormal test results
9. Explain the hemostatic mechanism of the body
10. List and describe the tests that measure the body's ability to form a fibrin clot
11. Explain how to determine the prothrombin time and partial thromboplastin time

Psychomotor Domain

1. Make a peripheral blood smear (Procedure 42-1)
2. Stain a peripheral blood smear (Procedure 42-2)
3. Perform a hemoglobin determination (Procedure 42-3)
4. Perform a microhematocrit determination (Procedure 42-4)
5. Determine a Westergren erythrocyte sedimentation rate (Procedure 42-5)
6. Obtain information on proper collection methods for hematology testing
7. Practice standard precautions
8. Use medical terminology, pronouncing medical terms correctly, to communicate information
9. Instruct patients according to their needs to promote disease prevention
10. Prepare a patient for procedures
11. Document patient care
12. Respond to issues of confidentiality
13. Perform within scope of practice
14. Practice within the standard of care for a medical assistant
15. Document accurately in the patient record
16. Perform quality control measures
17. Perform hematology testing
18. Screen test results

Affective Domain

1. Display sensitivity to patient rights and feelings in collecting specimens
2. Explain the rationale for performance of a procedure to the patient within parameters set by the physician
3. Show awareness of patients' concerns regarding their preceptions related to the procedure being performed

ABHES Competencies

1. Apply principles of aseptic techniques and infection control
2. Collect and process specimens
3. Perform selected CLIA-waived tests that assist with diagnosis and treatment
4. Dispose of biohazardous waste
5. Practice standard precautions
6. Perform hematology testing
7. Document appropriately
8. Use methods of quality control
9. Adhere to OSHA compliance rules and regulations

Name: _____   Date: _____   Grade: _____

COG MULTIPLE CHOICE

Circle the letter preceding the correct answer.

1. Hematopoiesis is:

   a. the ability of a person's blood to form a clot.

   b. creation of new blood cells.

   c. the proportion of red blood cells to plasma.

   d. a protein released by the kidneys to stimulate red blood cell creation.

   e. the shape of red blood cells.

2. Leukocytosis is most likely caused by:

   a. chemical toxicity.

   b. inflammation.

   c. nutritional deficiencies.

   d. infection.

   e. anticoagulant therapy.

3. What indicates a vitamin B_{12} deficiency?

   a. The presence of bands

   b. Neutrophils with more than five lobes in their nuclei

   c. High numbers of lymphocytes

   d. Erythrocytes that lack a nucleus

   e. Microcytosis or a mean cell volume (MCV) less than 80 fL

4. Which white blood cells produce antibodies?

   a. Neutrophils

   b. Lymphocytes

   c. Monocytes

   d. Eosinophils

   e. Basophils

5. Where in the body are red blood cells produced?

   a. Bone marrow

   b. Fatty tissue

   c. Liver

   d. Kidney

   e. Heart

6. Which food is a good natural source of folate?

   a. Chicken

   b. Leafy green vegetables

   c. Liver

   d. Oysters

   e. Root vegetables

7. A parasitic infection is indicated by increased numbers of which leukocytes?

   a. Neutrophils

   b. Lymphocytes

   c. Monocytes

   d. Eosinophils

   e. Basophils

8. Which condition could be caused by chemotherapy?

   a. Anemia

   b. Folate deficiency

   c. Leukocytosis

   d. Monocytosis

   e. Thrombocytopenia

9. One symptom of vitamin K deficiency is:

   a. left shift.

   b. macrocytosis.

   c. prolonged ESR.

   d. prolonged PT.

   e. thrombocytosis.

10. ESR tests should be read:

   a. after 1 minute.

   b. at 15 minutes.

   c. at 30 minutes.

   d. at 60 minutes.

   e. at any time; the exact time is not important.

11. Which of the following is true of thrombocytosis?

    a. It indicates bacterial infection.

    b. It indicates bleeding.

    c. It is benign.

    d. It results from nutritional deficiency.

    e. It is a warning sign of embolism.

12. Microcytosis indicates:

    a. B_{12} deficiency.

    b. the presence of gamma globins.

    c. liver disorders.

    d. iron deficiency.

    e. sickle cell anemia.

13. Patients with iron deficiencies should be encouraged to eat:

    a. dairy.

    b. fish.

    c. fruit.

    d. liver.

    e. tofu.

14. Erythropoiesis is driven by chemical signals from:

    a. the brain.

    b. the kidneys.

    c. the liver.

    d. the marrow.

    e. the spleen.

15. What is the most direct measurement of the blood's ability to deliver oxygen available in the CBC?

    a. RBC count

    b. Hemoglobin (Hgb) determination

    c. Hematocrit (Hct) determination

    d. Mean cell volume (MCV)

    e. Mean corpuscular hemoglobin (MCH)

16. A patient has a platelet count of 75,000/mm³. What visible symptom might appear on the patient?

    a. Circular rash

    b. Edema

    c. Bruising

    d. Sloughing of skin

    e. Hair loss

17. Increased numbers of which leukocyte correspond to allergies and asthma?

    a. Neutrophils

    b. Lymphocytes

    c. Monocytes

    d. Eosinophils

    e. Basophils

18. Which is a normal platelet count for women?

    a. 4,300 to 10,800/mm³

    b. 200,000 to 400,000/mm³

    c. 4.2 to 5.4 million/mm³

    d. 4.6 to 6.2 million/mm³

    e. 27 to 31 million/mm³

19. Which is the normal RBC count for women?

    a. 4,300 to 10,800/mm³

    b. 200,000 to 400,000/mm³

    c. 4.2 to 5.4 million/mm³

    d. 4.6 to 6.2 million/mm³

    e. 27 to 31 million/mm³

20. Which is the normal WBC count for men?

    a. 4,300 to 10,800/mm³

    b. 200,000 to 400,000/mm³

    c. 4.2 to 5.4 million/mm³

    d. 4.6 to 6.2 million/mm³

    e. 27 to 31 million/mm³

COG MATCHING

Match each key terms with the correct definition.

Key Terms

21. _____ adhesion

22. _____ band

23. _____ basophil

24. _____ coagulation

25. _____ complete blood count

26. _____ eosinophil

27. _____ erythrocytes

28. _____ erythrocyte indices

29. _____ erythrocyte sedimentation rate

30. _____ erythropoietin

31. _____ folate

32. _____ hematocrit

33. _____ hemoglobin

34. _____ leukocytes

35. _____ monocyte

36. _____ morphology

37. _____ neutrophil

38. _____ plasma

39. _____ platelets

40. _____ point-of-care testing (POC or POCT)

41. _____ sickle cell anemia

42. _____ spherocytosis

Definitions

a. tests performed for a patient outside of a central laboratory

b. red blood cells or RBCs

c. white blood cells or WBCs

d. platelets

e. yellow liquid part of the blood that is 90% water

f. the functioning unit of the red blood cell

g. influences RBC production when it is released from the kidneys

h. cell type that makes up only a small portion of the number of white blood cells but are important parts of the body's immune response

i. cells active at the end of allergic responses and of parasite elimination

j. third most abundant leukocyte that engulfs foreign material

k. cell that defends against foreign invaders by engulfing them

l. deficiency causes hypersegmented neutrophils

m. a younger, less mature version of the neutrophils

n. critical elements of clot formation

o. contains WBC count and differential, RBC count, hemoglobin (Hgb) determination, hematocrit (Hct) determination, mean cell volume (MCV), mean corpuscular hemoglobin (MCH), mean corpuscular hemoglobin concentration (MCHC), and platelet count

p. 100 WBCs are counted, tallied according to type, and reported as percentages

q. how cells appear under the microscope

r. the disease caused by a defect in the globin chains resulting in an abnormal hemoglobin

s. percentage of RBCs in whole blood

t. measurements indicating the size of the RBC and how much hemogobin the RBC holds

u. RBC's are small and round

v. the rate in millimeters per hour at which RBCs settle out in a tube

w. process which changes blood from a fluid to a solid

x. platelets stick across the injured surface

y. blood clotting inside a blood vessel

43. _____ thrombocytes

44. _____ thrombosis

45. _____ WBC differential

COG **FILL IN THE BLANK**

Grade: _____

List the parameters measured in the complete blood count and their normal ranges

Test	Reference Interval
46.	
47.	
48.	
49.	
50.	
51.	
52.	
53.	

COG **MATCHING**

Grade: _____

Match each condition with the correct abnormal finding.

Conditions

54. _____ Increased bleeding

55. _____ Infection

56. _____ Anemia

57. _____ Low iron level

58. _____ Dehydration

Abnormal Findings

a. hemoglobin of 10 g/dL

b. thrombocytopenia

c. hematocrit of 55%

d. leukocytosis

e. macrocytosis

f. red cell count of 3.9 million/mL

59. _____ Liver disorders

60. _____ Microcytic anemia

61. _____ Thalassemia

g. MCHC of 28 g/dL

h. MCH of 22 picograms/red cell

COG IDENTIFICATION

Grade: _____

Indicate whether following cell function is that of a red blood cell (RBC), a white blood cell (WBC), or a platelet (PLA).

62. _____ body's primary defense against bacteria found inside cells

63. _____ contribute to inflammatory reactions

64. _____ critical elements of clot formation

65. _____ defend against foreign invaders by engulfing them

66. _____ important parts of the body's immune response

67. _____ may indicate any of a variety of acute conditions that necessitate immediate attention

68. _____ plug can arrest bleeding

69. _____ process the antigens and through a series of cell transitions, produce the antibodies that can now fight that antigen in the body

70. _____ release carbon dioxide that was picked up from the tissues and then bind oxygen

71. _____ signal of a viral infection

72. _____ transport gases (mainly oxygen and carbon dioxide) between the lungs and the tissues

COG FILL IN THE BLANK

Grade: _____

73. Fill in the blanks in this description of the purpose of testing for the erythrocyte sedimentation rate.
The reference interval for men is _____, and for women, it is _____. Elevations in ESR values are _____ _____ for any disorder but indicate either _____ or any other condition that causes increased or altered _____ in the blood (e.g., rheumatoid arthritis). The more _____ the RBCs fall in the column, the greater the degree of inflammation. The ESR can be elevated with infection and _____.

FILL IN THE BLANK   Grade: _____

List the leukocytes seen normally in the blood and their functions.

White Blood Cell Type	Function
74.	
75.	
76.	
77.	
78.	

ANALYSIS

79. Analyze a graph in the interpretation of health care results.

You have centrifuged your capillary collection tubes to calculate the patient's hematocrit.

a. _____ Which tube is placed correctly on the measurement grid? (Place the letter identifying the correct tube in the space provided.)

b. How did you verify the correct placement of the tube on the grid?

_____

_____

_____

_____

c. Beacuse this graph is difficult to interpret, estimate the approximate hematocrit for this patient.

_____

_____

_____

_____

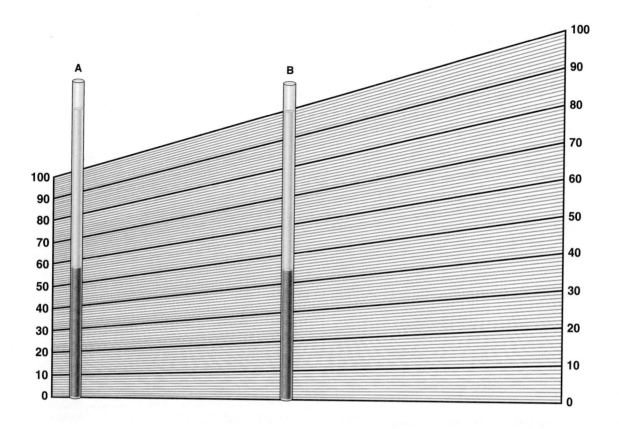

Indicate whether each laboratory result is normal (N) or abnormal (A).

80. _____ Platelet count = 150,000/mm^3

81. _____ Hemoglobin in a male = 16 g/dL

82. _____ Hematocrit in a male = 49%

83. _____ MCV = 75 fL

84. _____ MCH = 29 picograms

85. _____ MCHC = 35 g/dL

86. _____ RBC in a female = 3.71 x 10^{12}/L

87. _____ WBC = 5.9 x 10^9/L

88. _____ ESR = 5 mm/hr

List the four main steps of hemostasis.

89. _____

90. _____

91. _____

92. _____

COG IDENTIFICATION   Grade: _____

Indicate whether each statement is related to a prothrombin time (PT) or a partial thromboplastin time (PTT).

93. _____ normal range is 12 to 15 seconds

94. _____ prolonged in certain factor deficiencies, especially those that cause hemophilia

95. _____ normal range is 32 to 51 seconds

96. _____ prolonged by liver disease, vitamin K deficiency, and warfarin (Coumadin; oral anticoagulant) therapy

97. _____ primary monitor of Coumadin anticoagulant therapy

98. _____ reported along with its corresponding international normalized ratio (INR) to standardize results

99. _____ point-of-care instruments allow medical assistants to perform this test in the medical office

---

PSY AFF CASE STUDIES FOR CRITICAL THINKING   Grade: _____

1. Men over age 35 years and alcoholics frequently have difficulty absorbing vitamin B. What symptoms would you expect to see in an older male who drinks, and how could these be best addressed?

_____

_____

_____

_____

2. A trauma patient arrives in the hospital with extensive bleeding and internal injuries. The next day you are asked to run lab tests on this patient's bloodwork. How do you expect her results to differ from those of a healthy patient?

_____

_____

_____

3. Your patient presents with a persistent headache and nasal congestion. His WBC count is normal, but the eosinophil count is high. What is the probable cause of the patient's complaint?

_____

_____

_____

4. You are performing an erythrocyte sedimentation rate. After 60 minutes you look at the tube to report the test results. You cannot determine the separation between the cells and the plasma. The separation is not straight, and there are bubbles in the tube. What are the probable causes of your problem?

_____

_____

_____

5. You are preparing to collect a fingerstick specimen from your patient for a PT and INR test. The puncture wound continues to bleed heavily after the specimen is completed. How do you stop the bleeding and reassure the patient?

_____

_____

_____

6. Explain the rationale used when explaining a procedure to the patient within parameters set by the physician.

_____

_____

_____

_____

7. Your patient arrives for a fingerstick hematocrit test. She tells you she is worried because she continues to have anemia and treatment does not seem to be helping. How do you show awareness of the patient's feelings within the scope of practice of a medical assistant?

_____

_____

_____

_____

PSY PROCEDURE 42-1 | Making a Peripheral Blood Smear

Name: _____ Date: _____ Time: _____ Grade: _____

EQUIPMENT/SUPPLIES: Clean glass slides with frosted ends, pencil, well-mixed whole blood specimen, transfer pipette, hand disinfectant, surface disinfectant, gloves, biohazard container

STANDARDS Given the needed equipment and a place to work, the student will perform this skill with _____% accuracy in a total of _____ minutes. *(Your instructor will tell you what the percentage and time limits will be before you begin practicing.)*

KEY: 4 = Satisfactory   0 = Unsatisfactory   NA = This step is not counted

PROCEDURE STEPS	SELF	PARTNER	INSTRUCTOR
1. Wash your hands. Put on personal protective equipment.	☐	☐	☐
2. Assemble the equipment and supplies.	☐	☐	☐
3. Obtain a recently made dried blood smear.	☐	☐	☐
4. Place the slide on a stain rack blood side up.	☐	☐	☐
5. Place staining solution(s) onto slide according to manufacturer's instructions.	☐	☐	☐
6. Holding the slide with tweezers, gently rinse the slide with water. Wipe off the back of the slide with gauze. Stand the slide upright and allow it to dry.	☐	☐	☐
7. Properly care for or dispose of equipment and supplies. Clean the work area. Remove gloves and wash your hands. *Note:* Some manufacturers provide a simple one-step method that consists of dipping the smear in a staining solution, then rinsing. Directions provided by the manufacturer vary with the specific test.	☐	☐	☐

CALCULATION

Total Possible Points: _____

Total Points Earned: _____ Multiplied by 100 = _____ Divided by Total Possible Points = _____ %

PASS   **FAIL**   **COMMENTS:**

☐   ☐

Chart Documentation _____

Student's signature _____ Date _____

Partner's signature _____ Date _____

Instructor's signature _____ Date _____

PSY PROCEDURE 42-2 | Staining a Peripheral Blood Smear

Name: _____ Date: _____ Time: _____ Grade: _____

EQUIPMENT/SUPPLIES: Staining rack, Wright stain materials, prepared slide, tweezers, hand disinfectant, surface disinfectant, gloves

STANDARDS Given the needed equipment and a place to work, the student will perform this skill with _____% accuracy in a total of _____ minutes. *(Your instructor will tell you what the percentage and time limits will be before you begin practicing.)*

KEY: 4 = Satisfactory   0 = Unsatisfactory   NA = this step is not counted

PROCEDURE STEPS	SELF	PARTNER	INSTRUCTOR
1. Wash your hands. Put on personal protective equipment.	☐	☐	☐
2. Assemble the equipment and supplies.	☐	☐	☐
3. Obtain a recently made dried blood smear.	☐	☐	☐
4. Place the slide on a stain rack blood side up.	☐	☐	☐
5. Place staining solution(s) onto slide according to manufacturer's instructions.	☐	☐	☐
6. Holding the slide with tweezers, gently rinse the slide with water. Wipe off the back of the slide with gauze. Stand the slide upright and allow it to dry.	☐	☐	☐
7. Properly care for or dispose of equipment and supplies. Clean the work area. Remove gloves and wash your hands. *Note:* Some manufacturers provide a simple one-step method that consists of dipping the smear in a staining solution, then rinsing. Directions provided by the manufacturer vary with the specific test.	☐	☐	☐

CALCULATION

Total Possible Points: _____

Total Points Earned: _____ Multiplied by 100 = _____ Divided by Total Possible Points = _____ %

PASS   FAIL   COMMENTS:

☐   ☐

Chart Documentation _____

Student's signature _____ Date _____

Partner's signature _____ Date _____

Instructor's signature _____ Date _____

PSY PROCEDURE 42-3 Performing a Hemoglobin Determination

Name: _____ Date: _____ Time: _____ Grade: _____

EQUIPMENT/SUPPLIES: Hemoglobin meter, applicator sticks, whole blood, hand disinfectant, surface disinfectant, gloves, biohazard container

STANDARDS: Given the needed equipment and a place to work, the student will perform this skill with _____% accuracy in a total of _____ minutes. *(Your instructor will tell you what the percentage and time limits will be before you begin practicing.)*

KEY: 4 = Satisfactory   0 = Unsatisfactory   NA = This step is not counted

PROCEDURE STEPS	SELF	PARTNER	INSTRUCTOR
1. Wash your hands. Put on personal protective equipment.	☐	☐	☐
2. Assemble the equipment and supplies.	☐	☐	☐
3. Review instrument manual for your hemoglobin meter. Turn meter on and validate quality control before testing patient specimen.	☐	☐	☐
4. Obtain an EDTA (lavender-top tube) blood specimen from the patient, following procedures in Chapter 41.	☐	☐	☐
5. Place well-mixed whole blood into the hemoglobin meter chamber as described by the manufacturer.	☐	☐	☐
6. Slide the chamber into the hemoglobin meter.	☐	☐	☐
7. Record the hemoglobin level from the digital readout.	☐	☐	☐
8. Clean the work area with surface disinfectant. Dispose of equipment and supplies appropriately. Remove gloves and wash your hands. *Note:* This procedure may vary with the instrument.	☐	☐	☐

CALCULATION

Total Possible Points: _____

Total Points Earned: _____ Multiplied by 100 = _____ Divided by Total Possible Points = _____ %

PASS   **FAIL**   **COMMENTS:**

☐   ☐

Chart Documentation _____

Student's signature _____ Date _____

Partner's signature _____ Date _____

Instructor's signature _____ Date _____

PSY PROCEDURE 42-4 **Performing a Microhematocrit Determination**

Name: _____ Date: _____ Time: _____ Grade: _____

EQUIPMENT/SUPPLIES: Microcollection tubes, sealing clay, microhematocrit centrifuge, microhematocrit reading device, hand disinfectant, surface disinfectant, gloves, biohazard container, sharps container

STANDARDS: Given the needed equipment and a place to work, the student will perform this skill with_____% accuracy in a total of _____ minutes. *(Your instructor will tell you what the percentage and time limits will be before you begin practicing.)*

KEY: 4 = Satisfactory   0 = Unsatisfactory   NA = This step is not counted

PROCEDURE STEPS	SELF	PARTNER	INSTRUCTOR
1. Wash your hands. Put on personal protective equipment.	☐	☐	☐
2. Assemble the equipment and supplies.	☐	☐	☐

3. Draw blood into the capillary tube by one of two methods:
 	
  a. Directly from a capillary puncture (see Chapter 41) in which the tip of the capillary tube is touched to the blood at the wound and allowed to fill to three quarters or the indicated mark.
 	
  b. From a well-mixed EDTA tube of whole blood; again, the tip is touched to the blood and allowed to fill three-quarters of the tube.
	☐	☐	☐

4. Place the forefinger over the top of the tube, wipe excess blood off the sides, and push the bottom into the sealing clay.	☐	☐	☐
5. Draw a second specimen in the same manner.	☐	☐	☐
6. Place the tubes, clay-sealed end out, in the radial grooves of the microhematocrit centrifuge opposite each other. Put the lid on the grooved area and tighten by turning the knob clockwise. Close the centrifuge lid. Spin for 5 minutes or as directed by the centrifuge manufacturer.	☐	☐	☐
7. Remove the tubes from the centrifuge and read the results; instructions are printed on the device. Results should be within 5% of each other. Take the average and report as a percentage.	☐	☐	☐
8. Dispose of the microhematocrit tubes in a biohazard container. Properly care for or dispose of other equipment and supplies. Clean the work area. Remove gloves and wash your hands. *Note:* Some microhematocrit centrifuges have the scale printed in the machine at the radial grooves.	☐	☐	☐

CALCULATION

Total Possible Points: _____

Total Points Earned: _____ Multiplied by 100 = _____ Divided by Total Possible Points = _____ %

PASS   **FAIL**   **COMMENTS:**

☐   ☐

Chart Documentation _____

Student's signature _____ Date _____

Partner's signature _____ Date _____

Instructor's signature _____ Date _____

PSY PROCEDURE 42-5 Performing a Westergren Erythrocyte Sedimentation Rate

Name: _____ Date: _____ Time: _____ Grade: _____

EQUIPMENT/SUPPLIES: Hand disinfectant, gloves, EDTA blood sample less than 2 hours old, ESR kit, sedimentation rack, pipette, timer, surface disinfectant, biohazard disposal container, sharps container

STANDARDS: Given the needed equipment and a place to work, the student will perform this skill with _____% accuracy in a total of _____ minutes. *(Your instructor will tell you what the percentage and time limits will be before you begin practicing.)*

KEY: 4 = Satisfactory   0 = Unsatisfactory   NA = This step is not counted

PROCEDURE STEPS	SELF	PARTNER	INSTRUCTOR
1. Wash your hands. Put on personal protective equipment.	☐	☐	☐
2. Obtain an EDTA lavender-stoppered tube collected from your patient.	☐	☐	☐
3. Gently mix EDTA lavender-stoppered anticoagulation tube for 2 minutes.	☐	☐	☐
4. Using a vial from the ESR kit and a pipette, fill vial to the indicated mark. Replace stopper and invert vial several times to mix.	☐	☐	☐
5. Using an ESR calibrated pipette from the kit, insert the pipette through the tube's stopper with a twist and push down slowly but firmly until the pipette meets the bottom of the vial. The pipette will autozero with the excess flowing into the holding area. If the blood column does not reach the autozero point, discard used materials and start again at Step 4.	☐	☐	☐
6. Place the tube in a holder that will keep the tube vertical.	☐	☐	☐
7. Wait exactly 1 hour; use a timer for accuracy. Keep the tube straight upright and undisturbed during the hour.	☐	☐	☐
8. Record the level of the top of the RBCs after 1 hour. Normal results for men are 0–10 mL/hour; for women, 0–15 mL/hour.	☐	☐	☐
9. Properly care for or dispose of equipment and supplies. Clean the work area. Remove gloves, gown, and face shield. Wash your hands.	☐	☐	☐

CALCULATION

Total Possible Points: _____

Total Points Earned: _____ Multiplied by 100 = _____ Divided by Total Possible Points = _____ %

PASS   **FAIL**   **COMMENTS:**

☐   ☐

Chart Documentation _____

Student's signature _____ Date _____

Partner's signature _____ Date _____

Instructor's signature _____ Date _____

Cognitive Domain

1. Spell and define the key terms
2. Describe the methods of urine collection
3. List and explain the physical and chemical properties of urine
4. List confirmatory tests available and describe their uses
5. List and describe the components that can be found in urine sediment and describe their relationships to chemical findings
6. Analyze charts, graphs, and/or tables in the interpretation of health care results
7. Identify disease processes that are indications for CLIA-waived testing

Psychomotor Domain

1. Explain to a patient how and/or assist a patient to obtain a clean-catch mid-stream urine specimen (Procedure 43-1)
2. Explain the method of obtaining a 24-hour urine collection (Procedure 43-2)
3. Determine color and clarity of urine (Procedure 43-3)
4. Accurately interpret chemical reagent strip reactions (Procedure 43-4)
5. Prepare urine sediment for microscopic examination (Procedure 43-5)
6. Practice standard precautions
7. Perform handwashing
8. Use medical terminology, pronouncing medical terms correctly, to communicate information
9. Instruct patients according their needs to promote health maintenance and disease prevention

10. Prepare a patient for procedures
11. Document patient care
12. Respond to issues of confidentiality
13. Perform within scope of practice
14. Practice within the standard of care for a medical assistant
15. Document accurately in the patient record
16. Perform quality control measures
17. Perform urinalysis
18. Screen test results
19. Perform patient screening using established protocols
20. Report relevant information to others succinctly and accurately

Affective Domain

1. Distinguish between normal and abnormal test results
2. Display sensitivity to patient rights and feelings in collecting specimens
3. Explain the rationale for performance of a procedure to the patient
4. Show awareness of patients' concerns regarding their perceptions related to the procedure being performed
5. Demonstrate empathy in communicating with patients, family, and staff
6. Apply active listening skills
7. Use appropriate body language and other nonverbal skills in communicating with patients, family, and staff
8. Demonstrate awareness of the territorial boundaries of the person with whom you are communicating
9. Demonstrate sensitivity appropriate to the message being delivered

10. Demonstrate recognition of the patient's level of understanding in communications
11. Recognize and protect personal boundaries in communicating with others
12. Demonstrate respect for individual diversity, incorporating awareness of one's own biases in areas including gender, race, religion, age, and economic status
13. Demonstrate awareness of the consequences of not working within the legal scope of practice

ABHES Competencies

1. Use standard precautions
2. Screen and follow up patient test results
3. Perform selected CLIA-waived urinalysis testing that assist with diagnosis and treatment
4. Instruct patients in the collection of a clean-catch, midstream urine specimen

Name: _____   Date: _____   Grade: _____

COG MULTIPLE CHOICE

Circle the letter preceding the correct answer.

1. What color will be observed on the reagent pad if nitrites are present in urine?

    a. Blue

    b. Pink

    c. Red

    d. Yellow

    e. Green

2. How many tests are required to prove a positive drug result in a urine sample?

    a. One

    b. Two

    c. Three

    d. Four

    e. Five

3. Why is a 24-hour collection a better indicator of some values than a random specimen?

    a. Some substances are excreted with diurnal variation.

    b. Some bacteria do not develop fully for 24 hours.

    c. A 24-hour collection gives the physician a more accurate idea of the patient's diet.

    d. The higher the volume of urine tested, the more accurate the result.

    e. Some substances are excreted only at night.

4. The most common method of urine collection is:

    a. suprapubic aspiration.

    b. clean-catch midstream.

    c. random specimen.

    d. first morning void.

    e. postprandial specimen.

5. Which official body approves the drug test used to analyze urine samples?

    a. Clinical Laboratory Improvement Amendments

    b. Centers for Medicare and Medicaid Services

    c. Occupational Safety and Health Administration

    d. Food and Drug Administration

    e. Drug and Alcohol Testing Industry Association

6. Which of these conditions may cause a patient's urine to smell sweet?

    a. Urinary tract infection

    b. Kidney infection

    c. Diabetes

    d. Dehydration

    e. Yeast infection

7. What is the specific gravity of a normal urine specimen?

    a. 0.900–1.000

    b. 1.001–1.035

    c. 1.100–1.135

    d. 1.500–1.635

    e. 2.000–2.001

8. Why is a urinometer no longer used in a laboratory to test specific gravity?

    a. It requires a large volume of urine.

    b. It is not as accurate as other equipment.

    c. It is too expensive to use frequently.

    d. It takes longer to process a sample than other equipment.

    e. It takes up too much space in the laboratory.

9. What is the expected pH range for urine?

    a. 3.0–6.0

    b. 4.0–7.0

    c. 5.0–8.0

    d. 6.0–9.0

    e. 7.0–10.0

10. Increased numbers of epithelial cells in urine may indicate that:

    a. there is an irritation, such as inflammation, somewhere in the urinary system.

    b. the patient is overly hydrated.

    c. the patient is pregnant.

    d. the urine sample has sat for too long before examination.

    e. the testing was not performed correctly.

11. Which of the following statements is true about bilirubin?

    a. Bilirubin is formed in the kidneys.

    b. Bilirubin is a dark red pigment.

    c. Bilirubin is present in all urine crystals.

    d. Bilirubin will break down with exposure to light.

    e. Bilirubin in the urine usually results from a urinary tract infection.

12. Which group of people is most at risk of developing galactosuria?

    a. Teenagers

    b. Newborns

    c. Pregnant women

    d. Older adult men

    e. Older adult women

13. A patient with uric acid crystals in his or her urine possibly has:

    a. leukemia.

    b. a urinary tract infection.

    c. hepatitis.

    d. gout.

    e. gallbladder cancer.

14. A patient who has been asked to provide a 24-hour specimen should:

    a. void at exactly 24 hours and add it to the specimen.

    b. collect urine only after mealtimes.

    c. gently shake the container after each specimen is added.

    d. drink more water than usual during the collection period.

    e. avoid drinking soda or alcohol during the collection period.

15. Which of these should be included on a chain-of-custody document?

    a. The results of the urine test

    b. The reason for the chain of custody

    c. Instructions for providing a specimen

    d. The date the specimen was collected or transferred

    e. The volume of urine in the specimen

16. Which biological pigment gives urine its color?

    a. Melanin

    b. Hemoglobin

    c. Myoglobin

    d. Beta-carotene

    e. Urochrome

17. Why is a urine test preferable to a blood test for a routine drug test?

    a. It is less invasive and has national standards for testing.

    b. It is less expensive.

    c. There is less risk of contamination.

    d. It requires less equipment.

    e. A urine specimen will stay fresh longer than a blood sample.

18. Strenuous physical exercise may cause:

    a. increased protein in urine.

    b. decreased amounts of epithelial cells.

    c. increased quantities of ketones.

    d. increased glucose in urine.

    e. decreased concentration of phosphates.

19. Cast formation occurs in the:

   a. liver.

   b. small intestine.

   c. bladder.

   d. pathways of the digestive tract.

   e. tubules of the nephron.

20. Sulfosalicylic acid added to normal urine would cause the urine to:

   a. turn orange.

   b. remain clear.

   c. become cloudy.

   d. turn pink.

   e. form crystals.

cog MATCHING

Grade: _____

Match each key term with the correct definition.

Key Terms	Definitions
21. ____ acidic pH	**a.** variation during a 24-hour period
22. ____ acidosis	**b.** too much acid in the body
23. ____ albumbin	**c.** nonacidic pH
24. ____ bacteriuria	**d.** presence of glucose in the urine
25. ____ basic pH	**e.** abnormally high level of glucose
26. ____ Benedict reaction	**f.** most common test for reducing sugars
27. ____ bilirubin	**g.** group of chemicals produced during fat and protein metabolism
28. ____ bilirubinuria	**h.** blood in urine
29. ____ chain-of-custody procedure	**i.** large amount of blood in the urine
30. ____ Clinitest	**j.** formed during breakdown of hemoglobin
31. ____ conjugated bilirubin	**k.** one of the proteins that rarely passes through healthy kidneys
32. ____ diurnal variation	**l.** bilirubin in the urine
33. ____ glucose oxidase	**m.** the written policy for maintaining an accurate written record to track the possession, handling, and location of samples and data from collection through reporting
34. ____ glycosuria	**n.** copper reduction test
35. ____ gross hematuria	**o.** diazo tablet method to detect bilirubin
36. ____ hematuria	**p.** too much ketone in the blood and urine
	q. chemical reaction to detect the presence of glucose in the urine
	r. type of bilirubin that does dissolve into the bloodstream
	s. presence of bacteria in urine
	t. pH from 1–6

37. _____ hyperglycemia

38. _____ ictotest

39. _____ ketoacidosis

40. _____ ketones

COG **MATCHING**   Grade: _____

Match each key term with the correct definition.

Key Terms   **Definitions**

41. _____ leukocyte esterase   **a.** the external opening of the urethra

42. _____ lyse   **b.** a protein in heart and skeletal muscle

                                        c. cloudiness

43. _____ microalbumin   **d.** reflects the ability of the kidney to concentrate or dilute the urine

44. _____ microhematuria   **e.** neither an acid or a base

45. _____ myoglobin   **f.** the level that must be reached for an effect to be produced

                                        g. reagent test strip

46. _____ neutral pH   **h.** sugars including glucose

47. _____ nitrite   **i.** increased amounts of protein in the urine

48. _____ nitroprusside   **j.** white cells in urine

                                        k. the amount of blood in the urine is so small that the color of the specimen is not affected

49. _____ phagocytes

50. _____ proteinuria   **l.** rupture

                                        m. one of the parts of bilirubin when enzymes break it into parts

51. _____ pyuria   **n.** cells that fight the infection

52. _____ reducing sugars   **o.** enzyme reaction that detects pyuria

53. _____ sediment   **p.** tiny bits of albumin

                                        q. reaction is used to detect ketones

54. _____ specific gravity   **r.** common confirmation test for protein in urine

55. _____ sulfosalicylic acid   **s.** the button of cells and other particulate matter that collects in the bottom of the
            (SSA)   tube when centrifuging a urine specimen

56. _____ supernatant   **t.** urine above the sediment when the tube of urine is centrifuged

                                        u. mucoprotein that cements urinary casts together

57. _____ Tamm-Horsfall   **v.** positive test that indicates bacteriuria, which occurs with urinary tract infections
            mucoprotein

58. _____ threshold

59. _____ turbidity

60. _____ urethral meatus

61. _____ urine dipstick

62. _____ urobilinogen

COG **MATCHING**   Grade: _____

Match each type of specimen collection method with the correct description.

Collection Methods

63. _____ Random specimen

64. _____ First morning void

65. _____ Postprandial specimen

66. _____ Clean-catch urine specimen

67. _____ Suprapubic aspiration

68. _____ 24-hour collection

Descriptions

a. A specimen that is collected two hours after a patient consumes a meal

b. A specimen that is voided into a sterile container after the urinary meatus and surrounding skin have been cleansed

c. A specimen that is formed over a 6–8 hour period

d. A specimen voided into a clean, dry container

e. A specimen consisting of all urine voided over a 24-hour period

f. A specimen that is taken directly from the bladder using a needle

COG AFF **MATCHING**   Grade: _____

Read the descriptions of five of Dr. Philbin's patients. From your knowledge of chemical and physical properties of urine, match each patient with the correct diagnosis.

Patients

69. _____ Mr. Himmel is a 45-year-old father who is suffering from a stomach upset. His urine sample has a high specific gravity and is a deep yellow color.

70. _____ Mrs. Lincoln is a 33-year-old receptionist. Her urine sample is alkaline and contains leukocytes and a small amount of blood.

71. _____ Mr. Ackton is a 60-year-old gardener. His urine sample is dark yellow and contains bilirubin.

72. _____ Mrs. Franklin is a 75-year-old widow. Her urine sample has a high specific gravity, contains a high level of glucose, and is very acidic.

73. _____ Mrs. Taylor is a 29-year-old surgeon who has little time to exercise. She has a large quantity of protein in her urine.

74. _____ Ms. Sheffield is a 20 year-old college student. She has a large quantity of ketones in her urine.

75. _____ Mrs. Kotizky is a 43 year-old homemaker. Her urine is cloudy with a positive nitrite reaction.

76. _____ Mr. Kubik is a 67-year-old retiree. He has been a heavy drinker for 30 years and has increased his intake of alcohol significantly since retirement. His urine has an elevated urobilinogen level.

Diagnoses

a. Urinary tract infection

b. Diabetes mellitus

c. Dieting until protein breakdown

d. Pregnancy

e. Cirrhosis

f. Dehydration

g. Hepatitis

COG IDENTIFICATION

Grade: _____

List and explain the physical and chemical properties of urine.

PROPERTY	EXPLANATION
77.	
78.	
79.	
80.	
81.	
82.	
83.	
84.	
85.	
86.	
87.	

COG MATCHING

Grade: _____

Match each of the following types of confirmation tests with its correct description.

Tests

88. _____ Copper reduction method

89. _____ Nitroprusside test

90. _____ Precipitation test

91. _____ Diazo test

Descriptions

a. A test to confirm a protein on the reagent strip

b. A test that uses a tablet to detect bilirubin

c. A test used to detect any reducing sugar

d. A reaction test used to detect ketones

COG MATCHING   Grade: _____

Match the components that can be found in urine sediment to their related chemical findings (you may use items more than once or not at all).

Components

92. _____ Red blood cells

93. _____ White blood cells

94. _____ Bacteria

95. _____ Renal epithelial cells

96. _____ Calcium oxalate crystals

97. _____ Casts

Chemical Findings

a. Leukocyte esterase

b. Blood

c. pH >7.0

d. Protein

e. Nitrites

COG MATCHING   Grade: _____

As a medical assistant, you'll probably be asked to assist in the urinalysis procedure. Study the list of tasks below and decide which duties are within the scope of practice for a medical assistant. Place a check in the "Yes" box for tasks you would complete yourself and in the "No" box for tasks that would be completed by another member of the team.

Task	Yes	No
98. Prepare urine sediment for microscopic examination.		
99. Instruct patient on how to provide urine sample.		
100. Perform microscopic examination of urine sediment.		
101. Ensure that urine is tested or refrigerated within the correct time period.		
102. Use suprapubic aspiration to collect a urine sample.		
103. Perform confirmatory tests on urine samples.		
104. Label specimens for clear identification.		
105. Assemble equipment needed for urinalysis procedures.		

COG AFF SHORT ANSWER   Grade: _____

106. A patient provides a sample of urine for testing. You know that everyone in the medical office is extremely busy and that it will not get tested for at least three hours. What should you do with the sample?

_____

_____

_____

_____

107. A patient gives a urine sample at 11 AM, and the physician asks you to perform a urinalysis on the specimen. Before you can analyze the sample, there is an emergency situation in the office, and you become distracted. At 2 PM you remember that the specimen has still not been analyzed, and it is in a container that is not refrigerated. What should you do? Explain your answer.

_____

_____

_____

_____

108. A female patient visits the physician's office and tells you that she thinks she is pregnant. The physician tells her that it is possible to confirm this by from a urine sample. Which collection method would is easiest for you to determine the result? Explain your answer.

_____

_____

_____

_____

109. A severely underweight 15-year-old girl comes into the physician's office to give a urine sample. The test reveals that there are ketones in the patient's urine. Explain why this may be the case.

_____

_____

_____

_____

110. A urine sample has tested positive for protein. What procedure would be used to confirm the reagent strip reaction? Explain how the procedure works.

_____

_____

_____

_____

111. During an initial urine test, a specimen tests positive for ketones. The physician asks you to perform a confirmatory test on the specimen to make sure the diagnosis is correct. Explain what you would do to confirm the presence of ketones in urine and what you would expect to happen if the test is positive.

    _____

    _____

    _____

    _____

112. You are instructing your female patient how to collect a clean-catch specimen. She says she has diarrhea and is concerned about contaminating the specimen. How do you instruct her to collect the specimen? How do you use this information to coach her about her ongoing general health?

    _____

    _____

    _____

    _____

COG **IDENTIFICATION**

The chain-of-custody process is used to ensure that all urine specimens are identifiable and have not been tampered with. Read the scenarios in the table below and decide whether the correct chain-of-custody patient screening and procedure have taken place. Place a check mark in the appropriate box.

Scenario	Correct Procedure Used	Possibility of Contamination
113. A patient faxes you her identification in advance to save time at the reception desk.		
114. A patient enters the bathroom to give a urine sample wearing jeans and a T-shirt.		
115. A patient selects his own sealed collection container from the cupboard.		
116. A patient empties her pockets and enters the bathroom to give a urine sample while carrying a bottle of water.		
117. A patient enters the bathroom to give a urine sample wearing cargo pants, a sweater, and a baseball cap.		
118. A patient washes and dries his hands before entering the bathroom to give a urine sample.		
119. A patient has forgotten her ID, but an employer representative verifies that she is the correct person.		

COG PSY AFF **CASE STUDIES**

1. One of your patients needs to provide a 24-hour urine collection. She has never done it before and is unsure how to carry out the procedure. Write the patient a list of instructions, explaining what she should do in order to provide an accurate specimen. Why is it important that the patient thoroughly understands and complies with your instructions?

_____

_____

_____

_____

2. You instruct a patient how to perform a clean-catch midstream urine specimen. When you test the sample, you discover that the urine is cloudy, with a pH level of 7.5, and contains traces of red blood cells, nitrites, and leukocytes. How would you document this information on the patient's chart?

_____

_____

_____

_____

3. A patient asks you what types of drugs can be detected in urine. Two weeks later, the same patient comes into the office to provide a urine specimen. He appears to be acting suspiciously and you think you see him pick up a bottle before entering the bathroom. What should you do next?

_____

_____

_____

_____

4. Your patient, Sharon, has never collected a clean-catch midstream urine specimen before. As you describe the procedure, her facial expressions begin to change, and she becomes aloof. What are the possible reasons for her response? How do you adjust your behavior to support the patient's understanding of the procedure? How do you demonstrate empathy to this patient?

_____

_____

_____

_____

5. You are the patient at a medical office. The medical assistant greets you as you arrive in the laboratory to collect a specimen. The medical assistant is slumped and does not meet your gaze. The radio in the laboratory is blaring music. You ask questions about the collection process, and the medical assistant responds in a murmur. She looks over your head and grins at someone coming up behind you. She interrupts your questions and abruptly repeats the instructions. How does this make you feel? How would you suggest that the medical assistant change her body language? What expected skills is the medical assistant not using? What other coaching instructions would you provide the medical assistant?

_____

_____

_____

6. You call your next patient to give her instructions for collecting a 24-hour urine specimen. She enters the area and tosses her handbag into the phlebotomy chair. What is the patient conveying to you with her body language?

_____

_____

_____

_____

7. Performing a microscopic analysis of a urine specimen is not a CLIA-waived test. You complete a reagent stick analysis of the urine with a positive nitrite result. The physician tells you to perform a follow-up microscopic analysis of that urine. Why is he asking you to do this? What is the risk to the practice if you comply with that instruction?

_____

_____

_____

_____

8. In the laboratory, you perform a chemical reagent strip analysis. In the medical office, what should be completed prior to testing patients with this procedure? How do you analyze and respond to this action?

_____

_____

_____

_____

9. The results have come back from the testing laboratory on a drug screen test you collected. The medical assistant working the front office comes to you asking about this patient's test results. She says the woman babysits her children after school, and she wants to know if the patient is taking drugs. How do you respond?

_____

_____

_____

_____

PSY PROCEDURE 43-1 Obtaining a Clean-Catch Midstream Urine Specimen

Name: _____ Date: _____ Time: _____ Grade: _____

EQUIPMENT/SUPPLIES: Sterile urine container labeled with patient's name, cleansing towelettes (two for males, three for females), gloves if you are to assist patient, hand sanitizer

STANDARDS: Given the needed equipment and a place to work, the student will perform this skill with _____%
accuracy in a total of _____ minutes. *(Your instructor will tell you what the percentage and time limits will be before you begin practicing.)*

KEY: 4 = Satisfactory   0 = Unsatisfactory   NA = This step is not counted

PROCEDURE STEPS	SELF	PARTNER	INSTRUCTOR
1. Wash your hands. Put on personal protective equipment.	☐	☐	☐
2. Assemble the equipment and supplies.	☐	☐	☐
3. **AFF** Identify the patient and explain the procedure. Ask for and answer any questions.	☐	☐	☐
4. **AFF** Demonstrate recognition of the patient's level of understanding communications. Apply active listening skills. Modify communication to the patient's level of understanding, or obtain assistance with language differences. *Note:* Many offices prepare illustrated directions that may be helpful if the patient can see and read.	☐	☐	☐
5. If the patient is to perform the procedure, provide the necessary supplies.	☐	☐	☐
6. Have the patient perform the procedure. **a.** Instruct the male patient: **(1)** If uncircumcised, expose the glans penis by retracting the foreskin, then clean the meatus with an antiseptic wipe. The glans should be cleaned in a circular motion away from the meatus. A new wipe should be used for each cleaning sweep. **(2)** Keeping the foreskin retracted, initially void a few seconds into the toilet or urinal. **(3)** Bring the sterile container into the urine stream and collect a sufficient amount (about 30–60 mL). Instruct the patient to avoid touching the inside of the container with the penis. **(4)** Finish voiding into the toilet or urinal. **b.** Instruct the female patient: **(1)** Kneel or squat over a bedpan or toilet bowl. Spread the labia minora widely to expose the meatus. Using an antiseptic wipe, cleanse on either side of the meatus, then the meatus itself. Use a wipe only once in a sweep from the anterior to the posterior surfaces, then discard it.	☐	☐	☐

(2) Keeping the labia separated, initially void a few seconds into the toilet.			
(3) Bring the sterile container into the urine stream and collect a sufficient amount (about 30–60 mL).			
(4) Finish voiding into the toilet or bedpan.			
7. Cap the filled container and place it in a designated area.	☐	☐	☐
8. Transport the specimen in a biohazard container for testing.	☐	☐	☐
9. Properly care for or dispose of equipment and supplies. Clean the work area. Remove gloves and wash your hands.	☐	☐	☐

CALCULATION

Total Possible Points: _____

Total Points Earned: _____ Multiplied by 100 = _____ Divided by Total Possible Points = _____ %

PASS   **FAIL**   **COMMENTS:**

☐   ☐

Student's signature _____ Date _____

Partner's signature _____ Date _____

Instructor's signature _____ Date _____

PSY PROCEDURE 43-2 Obtaining a 24-Hour Urine Specimen

Name: _____ Date: _____ Time: _____ Grade: _____

EQUIPMENT/SUPPLIES: Patient's labeled 24-hour urine container (some patients require more than one container), preservatives required for the specific test, chemical hazard labels, graduated cylinder that holds at least 1 L, serological or volumetric pipettes, clean random urine container, fresh 10% bleach solution, gloves, hand disinfectant, surface disinfectant

STANDARDS: Given the needed equipment and a place to work, the student will perform this skill with _____% accuracy in a total of _____ minutes. *(Your instructor will tell you what the percentage and time limits will be before you begin practicing.)*

KEY: 4 = Satisfactory 0 = Unsatisfactory NA = This step is not counted

PROCEDURE STEPS	SELF	PARTNER	INSTRUCTOR
1. Wash your hands.	☐	☐	☐
2. Assemble the equipment.	☐	☐	☐
3. Identify the type of 24-hour urine collection requested and check for any special requirements, such as any acid or preservative that should be added. Label the container appropriately.	☐	☐	☐
4. Add to the 24-hour urine container the correct amount of acid or preservative using a serological or volumetric pipette.	☐	☐	☐
5. Use the provided label or make a label with spaces for the patient's name, beginning time and date, and ending time and date so that the patient can fill in the appropriate information.	☐	☐	☐
6. **AFF** Demonstrate recognition of the patient's level of understanding communications. Apply active listening skills. Modify communication to the patient's level of understanding, or obtain assistance with language differences. *Note:* Offices often prepare written instructions for the patient to take with them. This is helpful with some communication issues. Translations make this tool more versatile.	☐	☐	☐
7. Instruct the patient to collect a 24-hour urine sample as follows: **a.** Void into the toilet, and note this time and date as beginning. **b.** After the first voiding, collect each voiding and add it to the urine container for the next 24 hours. **c.** Precisely 24 hours after beginning collection, empty the bladder even if there is no urge to void and add this final volume of urine to the container. **d.** Note on the label the ending time and date.	☐	☐	☐
8. Explain to the patient that, depending on the test requested, the 24-hour urine may have to be refrigerated the entire time. Instruct the patient to return the specimen to you as soon as possible after collection is complete.	☐	☐	☐

9. Record in the patient's chart that supplies and instructions were given to collect a 24-hour urine specimen and the test that was requested.	☐	☐	☐
10. When you receive the specimen, verify beginning and ending times and dates before the patient leaves. Check for any acids or preservatives to be added before the specimen goes to the testing laboratory.	☐	☐	☐
11. Put on gloves.	☐	☐	☐
12. Pour the urine into a cylinder to record the volume. Pour an aliquot of the urine into a clean container to be sent to the laboratory. (Label the specimen with the patient's identification.) Record the volume of the urine collection and the amount of any acid or preservative added on the sample container and on the laboratory requisition. If permitted, you may dispose of the remainder of the urine.	☐	☐	☐
13. Record the volume on the patient's test requisition and chart.	☐	☐	☐
14. Clean the cylinder with fresh 10% bleach solution, then rinse with water. Let it air dry. If you are using a disposable container, be sure to dispose of it in the proper biohazard container.	☐	☐	☐
15. Clean the work area and dispose of waste properly. Remove protective equipment and wash your hands. *Note:* Some containers come with the preservative already added. In either case, be sure the patient is instructed not to discard preservative and not to allow it to be handled. *Warning!* Use caution when handling acids and other hazardous materials. Be familiar with the material safety data sheets for each chemical in your site.	☐	☐	☐

CALCULATION

Total Possible Points: _____

Total Points Earned: _____ Multiplied by 100 = _____ Divided by Total Possible Points = _____ %

PASS   **FAIL**   **COMMENTS:**

☐   ☐

Student's signature _____ Date _____

Partner's signature _____ Date _____

Instructor's signature _____ Date _____

Name: _____ Date: _____ Time: _____ Grade: _____

EQUIPMENT/SUPPLIES: Gloves, impervious gown, 10% bleach solution, patient's labeled urine specimen, clear tube, usually a centrifuge, white paper scored with black lines, hand disinfectant, surface disinfectant

STANDARDS: Given the needed equipment and a place to work, the student will perform this skill with _____% accuracy in a total of _____ minutes. *(Your instructor will tell you what the percentage and time limits will be before you begin practicing.)*

KEY: 4 = Satisfactory   0 = Unsatisfactory   NA = This step is not counted

PROCEDURE STEPS	SELF	PARTNER	INSTRUCTOR
1. Wash your hands.	☐	☐	☐
2. Assemble the equipment.	☐	☐	☐
3. Put on personal protective equipment.	☐	☐	☐
4. Verify that the names on the specimen container and the report form are the same.	☐	☐	☐
5. Pour about 10 mL of urine into the tube.	☐	☐	☐
6. In bright light against a white background, examine the color. The most common colors are straw (very pale yellow), yellow, dark yellow, and amber (brown-yellow).	☐	☐	☐
7. Determine clarity. Hold the tube in front of the white paper scored with black lines. If you see the lines clearly (not obscured), record as clear. If you see the lines but they are not well delineated, record as hazy. If you cannot see the lines at all, record as cloudy.	☐	☐	☐
8. Properly care for or dispose of equipment and supplies. Clean the work area using a surface disinfectant. Remove personal protective equipment. Wash your hands. *Notes:* Rapid determination of color and clarity is necessary because some urine turns cloudy if left standing. Bilirubin, which may be found in urine in certain conditions, breaks down when exposed to light. Protect the specimen from light if urinalysis is ordered but testing is delayed. If further testing is to be done but is delayed more than an hour, refrigerate the specimen to avoid alteration of chemistry.	☐	☐	☐

CALCULATION

Total Possible Points: _____

Total Points Earned: _____ Multiplied by 100 = _____ Divided by Total Possible Points = _____ %

PASS   **FAIL**   **COMMENTS:**

☐   ☐

Student's signature _____ Date _____

Partner's signature _____ Date _____

Instructor's signature _____ Date _____

PSY PROCEDURE 43-4 | Chemical Reagent Strip Analysis

Name: _____ Date: _____ Time: _____ Grade: _____

EQUIPMENT/SUPPLIES: Patient's labeled urine specimen, chemical strip (such as Multistix™ or Chemstrip™), manufacturer's color comparison chart, stopwatch or timer, personal protective equipment, hand disinfectant, surface disinfectant

STANDARDS: Given the needed equipment and a place to work, the student will perform this skill with _____% accuracy in a total of _____ minutes. *(Your instructor will tell you what the percentage and time limits will be before you begin practicing.)*

KEY: 4 = Satisfactory 0 = Unsatisfactory NA = This step is not counted

PROCEDURE STEPS	SELF	PARTNER	INSTRUCTOR
1. Wash your hands.	☐	☐	☐
2. Assemble the equipment.	☐	☐	☐
3. Put on personal protective equipment.	☐	☐	☐
4. Verify that the names on the specimen container and the report form are the same.	☐	☐	☐
5. Mix the patient's urine by gently swirling the covered container.	☐	☐	☐
6. Remove the reagent strip from its container and replace the lid to prevent deterioration of strips by humidity.	☐	☐	☐
7. Immerse the reagent strip in the urine completely, then immediately remove it, sliding the edge of the strip along the lip of the container to remove excess urine.	☐	☐	☐
8. Start your stopwatch or timer immediately.	☐	☐	☐
9. Compare the reagent pads to the color chart, determining results at the intervals stated by the manufacturer. Example: Glucose is read at 30 seconds. To determine results, examine that pad 30 seconds post dipping and compare with color chart for glucose.	☐	☐	☐
10. Read all reactions at the times indicated and record the results.	☐	☐	☐
11. Discard the reagent strips in the proper receptacle. Discard urine unless more testing is required.	☐	☐	☐
12. Clean the work area with surface disinfectant. Remove personal protective equipment. Wash your hands. *Warning:* Do not remove the desiccant packet in the strip container; it ensures that minimal moisture affects the strips. The desiccant is toxic and should be discarded appropriately after all of the strips have been used. *Notes:* The manufacturer's color comparison chart is assigned a lot number that must match the lot number of the strips used for testing. Record this in the quality assurance (QA/QC) log.	☐	☐	☐

False-positive and false-negative results are possible. Review the manufacturer's package insert accompanying the strips to learn about factors that may give false results and how to avoid them.			
Aspirin may cause false-positive ketones. Document any medications the patient is taking. If the patient is taking phenazopyridine (Pyridium™), do not use a reagent strip for testing, because the medication will interfere with the color. Outdated materials give inaccurate results. If the expiration date has passed, discard the materials.			

CALCULATION

Total Possible Points: _____

Total Points Earned: _____ Multiplied by 100 = _____ Divided by Total Possible Points = _____ %

PASS   **FAIL**   **COMMENTS:**

☐   ☐

Student's signature _____ Date _____

Partner's signature _____ Date _____

Instructor's signature _____ Date _____

PSY PROCEDURE 43-5 Preparing Urine Sediment

Name: _____ Date: _____ Time: _____ Grade: _____

EQUIPMENT/SUPPLIES: Patient's labeled urine specimen, urine centrifuge tubes, transfer pipette, centrifuge (1,500–2,000 rpm), personal protective equipment, hand disinfectant, surface disinfectant

STANDARDS: Given the needed equipment and a place to work, the student will perform this skill with _____% accuracy in a total of _____ minutes. *(Your instructor will tell you what the percentage and time limits will be before you begin practicing.)*

KEY: 4 = Satisfactory   0 = Unsatisfactory   NA = This step is not counted

PROCEDURE STEPS	SELF	PARTNER	INSTRUCTOR
1. Wash your hands.	☐	☐	☐
2. Assemble the equipment.	☐	☐	☐
3. Put on personal protective equipment.	☐	☐	☐
4. Verify that the names on the specimen container and the report form are the same.	☐	☐	☐
5. Swirl specimen to mix. Pour 10 mL of well-mixed urine into a labeled centrifuge tube or standard system tube. Cap the tube with a plastic cap or Parafilm.	☐	☐	☐
6. Centrifuge the sample at 1,500 rpm for 5 minutes.	☐	☐	☐
7. When the centrifuge has stopped, remove the tubes. Make sure no tests are to be performed first on the supernatant. Remove the caps and pour off the supernatant, leaving 0.5–1.0 mL of it. Suspend the sediment again by aspirating up and down with a transfer pipette, or follow manufacturer's directions for a standardized system.	☐	☐	☐
8. Properly care for and dispose of equipment and supplies. Clean the work area with surface disinfectant. Remove personal protective equipment. Wash your hands.	☐	☐	☐

Notes: If the urine is to be tested by chemical reagent strip, perform the dip test before spinning the urine. Preparing a urine specimen of less than 3 mL for sediment is not recommended because that is not enough urine to create a true sediment. However, some patients cannot provide a large amount of urine.

In such cases, document the volume on the chart under sediment to ensure proper interpretation of results. Centrifuge maintenance requires periodic checks to ensure that the speed and timing are correct.

Document this information on the maintenance log.

CALCULATION

Total Possible Points: _____

Total Points Earned: _____ Multiplied by 100 = _____ Divided by Total Possible Points = _____ %

PASS   **FAIL**   **COMMENTS:**

☐   ☐

Student's signature _____ Date _____

Partner's signature _____ Date _____

Instructor's signature _____ Date _____

Microbiology and Immunology

Cognitive Domain

1. Spell and define the key terms
2. List major types of infectious agents
3. Compare different methods of controlling the growth of microorganisms
4. Discuss quality control issues related to handling microbiological specimens
5. Describe the medical assistant's responsibilities in microbiological testing
6. Analyze charts, graphs, and/or tables in the interpretation of health care results

Psychomotor Domain

1. Collect throat specimens (Procedure 44-1)
2. Collect nasopharyngeal specimens (Procedure 44-2)
3. Collect wound specimens (Procedure 44-3)
4. Collect sputum specimens (Procedure 44-4)
5. Collect stool specimens (Procedure 44-5)
6. Collect blood specimens for culture (Procedure 44-6)
7. Collect genital specimens (Procedure 44-7)
8. Test stool specimen for occult blood (Procedure 44-8)
9. Prepare a smear for microscopic evaluation (Procedure 44-9)
10. Perform a Gram stain (Procedure 44-10)
11. Inoculate a culture (Procedure 44-11)
12. Perform mononucleosis testing (Procedure 44-12)
13. Perform HCG pregnancy testing (Procedure 44-13)

14. Perform rapid group A strep testing (Procedure 44-14)
15. Prepare patient for procedures
16. Document patient care
17. Respond to issues of confidentiality
18. Perform within scope of practice
19. Perform quality control measures
20. Screen test results
21. Practice standard precautions
22. Perform handwashing
23. Perform CLIA-waived microbiology testing
24. Practice within the standard of care for a medical assistant

Affective Domain

1. Distinguish between normal and abnormal test results
2. Display sensitivity to patient rights and feelings in collecting specimens
3. Explain the rationale for performance of a procedure to the patient
4. Show awareness of patient's concerns regarding their perceptions related to the procedure being performed
5. Analyze charts, graphs, and or tables in the interpretation of health care results
6. Demonstrate empathy in communicating with patients, family, and staff
7. Apply active listening skills
8. Use body language and other nonverbal skills in communicating with patients, family, and staff
9. Demonstrate awareness of territorial boundaries of the person with whom you are communicating
10. Demonstrate sensitivity appropriate to the message being delivered

11. Demonstrate recognition of the patient's level of understanding in communications
12. Recognize and protect personal boundaries in communicating with others
13. Demonstrate respect for individual diversity, incorporating awareness of one's own biases in areas including gender, race, religion, age, and economic status

ABHES Competencies

1. Document patient care
2. Perform quality control measures
3. Screen test results
4. Perform immunology testing
5. Practice standard precautions
6. Perform handwashing
7. Obtain specimens for microbiology testing
8. Perform CLIA-waived microbiology testing
9. Perform pregnancy test
10. Perform strep A test
11. Instruct patients in the collection of fecal specimens

COG MATCHING

Grade: _____

Match each key term with the correct definition.

| Key Terms | Definitions |

Key Terms

21. _____ aerobes

22. _____ agar

23. _____ anaerobes

24. _____ bacilli (singular, bacillus)

25. _____ biological agent

26. _____ biohazard symbol

27. _____ broth

28. _____ carbuncle

29. _____ cervix

30. _____ cocci

31. _____ cultures

32. _____ differential stain

33. _____ diplococci

34. _____ endometrium

35. _____ erector pili muscle

36. _____ erythrasma

37. _____ eyewashes

38. _____ folliculitis

39. _____ furuncle

40. _____ Gram negative

Definitions

a. bacteria that require oxygen to survive

b. bacteria that require a lack of oxygen to survive

c. the bacteria, viruses, and fungi that are submitted to microbiology as specimens

d. a universal warning of the presence of biological agents

e. used to irrigate and flush the eyes following a hazardous exposure

f. an environment that provides the bacteria a place to grow

g. liquid media in glass tubes or bottles

h. the most widely used solid media

i. stain used to identify differences in cells

j. bacteria that will lose the purple color in a Gram stain and stain red with safranin

k. bacteria that are spherical in shape

l. spherical cocci in pairs

m. bacteria that are rod shaped and are usually aerobic

n. an infection in the hair follicle

o. an infection of the pilosebaceous unit

p. the muscle which causes the hair to stand up when it contracts

q. a collection of multiple infected hair follicles

r. a bacterial skin infection occuring where skin touches skin, like between toes, in armpits, or groin

s. the part of the uterus that opens into the vagina

t. the inner layer of the uterine wall

COG MATCHING

Grade: _____

Match each key term with the correct definition.

Key Terms

41. _____ Gram positive

42. _____ Gram stain

43. _____ impetigo

44. _____ immunity

45. _____ inoculum

46. _____ isolate

47. _____ Kirby-Bauer method

48. _____ media

49. _____ mordant

50. _____ mycology

51. _____ mycoses

52. _____ normal flora

53. _____ nosocomial infection

54. _____ opthalmia neonatorum

55. _____ opportunistic

56. _____ pilosebaceous unit

57. _____ resistant

58. _____ sensitive

59. _____ sensitivity testing

60. _____ smear

61. _____ specificity

62. _____ spirochetes

63. _____ subcutaneous

64. _____ superficial

65. _____ systemic

Definitions

a. bacteria that normally live on the body and do not cause disease

b. infections acquired in a medical setting

c. a small sample placed into or onto the culture medium using a wire probe

d. a mixture of substances that nourish pathogens to support the growth of micro-organisms for identification

e. materials that have been dried on a glass slide

f. primary stain used in the microbiology lab

g. bacteria that keep the purple color even when exposed to the ethyl alcohol step of the Gram stain

h. Gram's iodine is one, used to fix the dye on the smear to make it more intense

i. long, spiral, flexible organisms

j. testing to determine if an antibiotic will be effective in stopping growth of an organism (also identifies antibiotics that will not stop the growth of an organism)

k. organisms that are inhibited by an antimicrobial agent

l. organisms that grow even in the presence of an antimicrobial agent

m. separate from any other microorganisms present

n. an eye infection acquired by infants passing through the birth canal of a mother infected with *N. gonorrhoeae*

o. manual technique for sensitivity testing

p. the study of fungi

q. diseases caused by fungi

r. skin, hair, nails

s. infection of the internal organs

t. infection only in the immunocompromised

u. bacterial infection of the top layer of the skin

v. the response to foreign bodies

w. an antibody combines with only one antigen

x. consists of the hair shaft, the hair follicle, the sebaceous gland, and the erector pili muscle

y. the dermis, subcutaneous tissue or adjacent structures

COG MATCHING

Grade: _____

Match each category of organisms to its description.

Organisms

66. _____ Rickettsia

67. _____ Chlamydia

68. _____ Mycoplasma

69. _____ Viruses

70. _____ Eukaryotic microorganisms

71. _____ Fungi

72. _____ Protozoa and helminths

73. _____ Nematodes

74. _____ Arthropods

75. _____ Prokaryotic cells

Descriptions

a. cause blindness, pneumonia, and lymphogranuloma venereum

b. cause atypical pneumonia and genitourinary infections

c. cells with no nuclei including bacteria

d. lice, fleas, and ticks

e. not susceptible to antibiotics and are extremely difficult to treat

f. pathogens include the groups fungi, algae, protozoans, and parasites

g. small organisms like bacteria with the potential to produce disease in susceptible hosts

h. parasites

i. round worm parasites

j. organisms carried on arthropods

COG IDENTIFICATION

Grade: _____

How does each method of control inhibit or prevent bacterial growth?

76. Temperature: _____

77. Desiccation: _____

78. Disinfectants and antiseptics: _____

79. Antimicrobial agents: _____

80. Filtration: _____

COG FILL IN THE BLANK

Grade: _____

81. The result of a laboratory test is only as good as the _____.

82. Positively _____ the patient before collecting a specimen.

83. _____ the specimen according to laboratory procedure.

84. If the specimen is not fully and correctly labeled, the laboratory may be required to _____ of the specimen.

85. Verify use of correct _____ _____, required _____ of specimen, and appropriate _____ of specimen collection.

86. Use the appropriate _____ media, if indicated.

87. _____ and _____ specimens appropriately and securely for travel.

88. Transport specimens at the _____ temperature.

89. Correct steps are important for keeping the pathogen _____ until it reaches the laboratory.

90. Most specimens for culture cannot be simply _____.

91. Handle all specimens as if _____. Follow standard precautions.

92. The laboratory needs to be aware of any _____ in transportation.

93. Confirm _____ and _____ of specimen receipt.

94. Document the _____ _____ before referral.

95. Follow laboratory disinfection and _____ policies.

COG IDENTIFICATION

Grade: _____

Identify the medical assistant's responsibilities in microbiological testing. Place MA in front of items that are CLIA approved for performance by the medical assistant. Place X in front of items that are outside the scope of practice for the medical assistant.

96. _____ Collection of most common microbiology specimens.

97. _____ Manage quality control in handling microbiological specimens.

98. _____ Use effective communication skills in educating the patient.

99. _____ Manage specimen transport that maintains the viability of the organism.

100. _____ Set up cultures for growth of pathogens.

101. _____ Maintain culture media.

102. _____ Read bacterial cultures.

103. _____ Report culture results.

104. _____ Prepare smears and slides.

105. _____ Read prepared slides under the microscope to identify organisms.

COG IDENTIFICATION   Grade: _____

Your office laboratory maintains a small supply of culture media. Using the media list provided, identify the media you would select for the cases below. Place the letter identifying the media in the blank provided in front of the case.

MEDIA LIST FOR ABC MEDICAL OFFICE		
A	TSA w/ 5% blood	General-purpose media for cultivation, isolation and determination of hemolytic activity of bacteria
B	SS agar (Salmonella and Shigella)	For the isolation and differentiation of Salmonella and Shigella species
C	MSA (manitol salt agar)	For the selective isolation and differentiation of Staphylococcus species
D	BE (bile esculin agar)	For the isolation and identification of Group D Streptococcus species
E	Chocolate agar	For the cultivation of pathogenic Neisseria and Haemophilus species
F	SAB (sabouraud dextrose agar)	Gold standard for cultivation of fungi on rich media; works well for isolation of fungi

106. _____ Your patient is a 10-year-old boy with a sore throat. You use two swabs to collect the throat speciment. The result of the rapid strep test on the first swab is negative. Your office confirms all negative Strep tests with a culture. What media do you choose?

107. _____ Your patient is a 3-year-old girl with severe diarrhea. The child's mother says that there is a Shigella outbreak at her daughter's daycare center. You instruct the mother to collect a stool specimen. What media do you choose?

108. _____ Your patient is an 18-year-old girl. The physician suspicions a gonorrhea infection and collects a vaginal culture. What media do you choose?

109. _____ Your patient is a 12-year-old boy. He just recovered from a severe case of poison ivy. Since those lesions healed, he has developed another skin outbreak. The doctor thinks it could be imeptigo. What media do you choose?

110. _____ Your patient is a 43-year-old woman. She is just recovering from a course of antibiotics to treat a urinary tract infection. She fears she may now have a vaginal infection. The physician collects a vaginal specimen for evaluation. He wants to confirm yeast he saw on the wet prep from the specimen. What media do you choose?

`COG` `AFF` **IDENTIFICATION**

111. List six autoimmune diseases.

_____

_____

_____

_____

112. How is an antigen–antibody reaction identified?

_____

_____

_____

_____

113. Using immunoassay test kits, how is a positive antigen indicated?

_____

_____

_____

_____

114. How does the medical assistant assure the accuracy of testing with an immunoassay test kit?

_____

_____

_____

_____

115. How does a medical assistant identify the expiration date on a test kit?

_____

_____

_____

_____

116. How are normal and abnormal test results identified using immunoassay test kits?

_____

_____

_____

_____

COG AFF **CASE STUDIES**

1. Your patient is concerned that others may learn of the results to her laboratory test. How do you reassure her this will not happen?

_____

_____

_____

_____

2. Your patient is a little girl being evaluated for sexual abuse by her father. How do you display sensitivity to the mother regarding her distress about collecting the specimens? How do you explain the rationale for performing the procedure? How do you demonstrate your awareness of the patient's concerns regarding perceptions related to the procedure being performed? How do you demonstrate empathy in communicating with the patient and her mother? How will you use active listening skills in this scenario? How will you demonstrate awareness of the territorial boundaries of the child and her mother? How will you demonstrate your sensitivity to the situation?

_____

_____

_____

3. Your patient is a 7-year-old boy. The doctor has ordered a throat culture, and the boy is obviously apprehensive. How do you use body language and other nonverbal skills to reassure the boy and also collect a good specimen?

_____

_____

_____

_____

PSY PROCEDURE 44-1 | Collect a Throat Specimen

Name: _____ Date: _____ Time: _____ Grade: _____

EQUIPMENT/SUPPLIES: Tongue blade, light source, sterile specimen container and swab, personal protective equipment, hand sanitizer, surface sanitizer and biohazard transport bag (if to be sent to the laboratory for analysis)

STANDARDS: Given the needed equipment and a place to work, the student will perform this skill with _____% accuracy in a total of _____ minutes. *(Your instructor will tell you what the percentage and time limits will be before you begin practicing.)*

KEY: 4 = Satisfactory   0 = Unsatisfactory   NA = This step is not counted

PROCEDURE STEPS	SELF	PARTNER	INSTRUCTOR
1. Wash your hands.	☐	☐	☐
2. Assemble the equipment and supplies.	☐	☐	☐
3. Put on personal protective equipment.	☐	☐	☐
4. **AFF** Greet and identify the patient. Explain the rationale of the performance of the collection to the patient.	☐	☐	☐
5. **AFF** If the patient is hearing impaired, you need to speak clearly and distinctly in front of the patient's face. Have an easy to read instruction guide for the patient to follow and point out where there are questions. If the patient can sign and you cannot, have someone proficient in sign language assist you in instructing the patient.	☐	☐	☐
6. **AFF** Use active listening to observe patients' body language and detect a lack of understanding of instructions. Obtain assistance when you realize that you are not able to communicate with the patient.	☐	☐	☐
7. **AFF** Leave time for the patient to ask questions.	☐	☐	☐
8. **AFF** Display empathy for the patient and family.	☐	☐	☐
9. Have the patient sit with a light source directed the throat.	☐	☐	☐
10. **AFF** Demonstrate awareness of the patient's territorial boundaries. Attempt to respect this comfort zone.	☐	☐	☐
11. Carefully remove the sterile swab from the container. If performing both the rapid strep and the culture to confirm negative results with a culture, swab with two swabs held together.	☐	☐	☐
12. Have the patient say "Ah" as you press down on the midpoint of the tongue with the tongue depressor. If the tongue depressor is placed too far forward, it will not be effective; if it is placed too far back, the patient will gag unnecessarily.	☐	☐	☐
13. Swab the mucous membranes, especially the tonsillar area, the crypts, and the posterior pharynx.	☐	☐	☐
14. Maintain the tongue depressor position while withdrawing the swab from the patient's mouth.	☐	☐	☐

15. Follow the instructions on the specimen container for transferring the swab or processing the specimen in the office using a commercial kit. Label the the specimen with the patient's name, the date and time of collection, and the origin of the material.	☐	☐	☐
16. Properly dispose of the equipment and supplies in a biohazard waste container. Remove personal protective equipment and wash your hands.	☐	☐	☐
17. Route the specimen or store it appropriately until routing can be completed.	☐	☐	☐
18. Document the procedure.	☐	☐	☐
19. Sanitize the work area.	☐	☐	☐

CALCULATION

Total Possible Points: _____

Total Points Earned: _____ Multiplied by 100 = _____ Divided by Total Possible Points = _____ %

PASS   **FAIL**   **COMMENTS:**

☐   ☐

Student's signature _____ Date _____

Partner's signature _____ Date _____

Instructor's signature _____ Date _____

PSY PROCEDURE 44-2 Collect a Nasopharyngeal Specimen

Name: _____ Date: _____ Time: _____ Grade: _____

EQUIPMENT/SUPPLIES: Penlight, tongue blade, sterile flexible wire swab, transport media, personal protective equipment, hand sanitizer, surface sanitizer and biohazard transport bag (if to be sent to the laboratory for analysis)

STANDARDS: Given the needed equipment and a place to work, the student will perform this skill with _____% accuracy in a total of _____ minutes. *(Your instructor will tell you what the percentage and time limits will be before you begin practicing.)*

KEY: 4 = Satisfactory   0 = Unsatisfactory   NA = This step is not counted

PROCEDURE STEPS	SELF	PARTNER	INSTRUCTOR
1. Wash your hands.	☐	☐	☐
2. Assemble the equipment and supplies.	☐	☐	☐
3. Put on personal protective equipment.	☐	☐	☐
4. **AFF** Greet and identify the patient. Explain the rationale of the performance of the collection to the patient.	☐	☐	☐
5. **AFF** If your patient is developmentally challenged, have the individual who transported the patient to the office assist you with communicating with the patient. The developmentally challenged patient may struggle if you have to proceed with something that he or she does not understand. Have another medical assistant available to help you should extra support be necessary to support the patient.	☐	☐	☐
6. **AFF** Leave time for the patient to ask questions.	☐	☐	☐
7. **AFF** Display empathy for the patient and family.	☐	☐	☐
8. Position the patient with his or her head tilted back.	☐	☐	☐
9. **AFF** Demonstrate awareness of the patient's territorial boundaries.	☐	☐	☐
10. Using a penlight, inspect the nasopharyngeal area.	☐	☐	☐
11. Gently pass the swab through the nostril and into the nasopharynx, keeping the swab near the septum and floor of the nose. Rotate the swab quickly, and then remove it and place it in the transport medium.	☐	☐	☐
12. Label the specimen with the patient's name, the date and time of collection, and the origin of the specimen.	☐	☐	☐
13. Properly dispose of the equipment and supplies in a biohazard waste container. Remove personal protective equipment, and wash your hands.	☐	☐	☐
14. Route the specimen or store it appropriately until testing can be completed.	☐	☐	☐
15. Document the procedure.	☐	☐	☐
16. Sanitize the work area.	☐	☐	☐

CALCULATION

Total Possible Points: _____

Total Points Earned: _____ Multiplied by 100 = _____ Divided by Total Possible Points = _____ %

PASS   **FAIL**   **COMMENTS:**

☐   ☐

Student's signature _____ Date _____

Partner's signature _____ Date _____

Instructor's signature _____ Date _____

PSY PROCEDURE 44-3 Collect a Wound Specimen

Name: _____ Date: _____ Time: _____ Grade: _____

EQUIPMENT/SUPPLIES: Sterile swab, transport media, personal protective equipment, hand sanitizer, surface sanitizer and biohazard transport bag (if to be sent to the laboratory for analysis)

STANDARDS: Given the needed equipment and a place to work, the student will perform this skill with _____% accuracy in a total of _____ minutes. *(Your instructor will tell you what the percentage and time limits will be before you begin practicing.)*

KEY: 4 = Satisfactory   0 = Unsatisfactory   NA = This step is not counted

PROCEDURE STEPS	SELF	PARTNER	INSTRUCTOR
1. Wash your hands.	☐	☐	☐
2. Assemble the equipment and supplies.	☐	☐	☐
3. Put on personal protective equipment.	☐	☐	☐
4. **AFF** Greet and identify the patient. Explain the procedure.	☐	☐	☐
5. **AFF** If your patient is struggling with dementia, he or she may have some trouble understanding your explanations and requests. Be prepared to gently repeat yourself as necessary until you have collected your specimen. You may have to physically adjust your patient as necessary to collect the specimen. Be gentle but remember to speak to the patient as an adult.	☐	☐	☐
6. If dressing is present, remove it and dispose of it in biohazard container. Assess the wound by observing color, odor, and amount of exudate. Remove contaminated gloves and put on clean gloves.	☐	☐	☐
7. Use the sterile swab to sample the exudate. Saturate swab with exudate.	☐	☐	☐
8. Avoid skin edge around wound.	☐	☐	☐
9. Place swab back into container and crush the medium ampule of transport medium.	☐	☐	☐
10. Label the specimen with the patient's name, the date and time of collection, and the origin of specimen.	☐	☐	☐
11. Route the specimen or store it appropriately until routing can be completed.	☐	☐	☐
12. Clean the wound and apply a sterile dressing using sterile technique.	☐	☐	☐
13. Properly dispose of the equipment and supplies in a biohazard waste container. Remove personal protective equipment, and wash your hands.	☐	☐	☐
14. Document the procedure.	☐	☐	☐
15. Sanitize the work area.	☐	☐	☐

CALCULATION

Total Possible Points: _____

Total Points Earned: _____ Multiplied by 100 = _____ Divided by Total Possible Points = _____ %

PASS **FAIL** **COMMENTS:**

☐ ☐

Student's signature _____ Date _____

Partner's signature _____ Date _____

Instructor's signature _____ Date _____

PSY PROCEDURE 44-4 · Collect a Sputum Specimen

Name: _____ Date: _____ Time: _____ Grade: _____

EQUIPMENT/SUPPLIES: Sterile swab, transport media, personal protective equipment, hand sanitizer, surface sanitizer and biohazard transport bag

STANDARDS: Given the needed equipment and a place to work, the student will perform this skill with _____% accuracy in a total of _____ minutes. *(Your instructor will tell you what the percentage and time limits will be before you begin practicing.)*

KEY: 4 = Satisfactory   0 = Unsatisfactory   NA = This step is not counted

PROCEDURE STEPS	SELF	PARTNER	INSTRUCTOR
1. Wash your hands.	☐	☐	☐
2. Assemble the equipment and supplies.	☐	☐	☐
3. Put on personal protective equipment.	☐	☐	☐
4. **AFF** Greet and identify the patient. Explain the procedure.	☐	☐	☐
5. **AFF** If English is not your patient's primary language, you will need to have someone available to translate. Often someone who speaks English will accompany the patient to the office. If this is not the case, use the assistance of someone else in the office who speaks the patient's language. Some offices subscribe to a telephone translation service.	☐	☐	☐
6. Provide the patient with a cup of water and instruct him or her to rinse his or her mouth with water.	☐	☐	☐
7. Ask the patient to cough deeply, using the abdominal muscles as well as lower muscles to bring secretions from the lungs and respiratory tract, not just the upper airways.	☐	☐	☐
8. Ask the patient to expectorate directly into the specimen container without touching the inside and without getting sputum on the outsides of the container. About 5–10 mL is sufficient for most sputum studies.	☐	☐	☐
9. Handle the specimen container according to the standard precautions. Cap the container immediately and put it into the biohazard bag for transport to the laboratory. Fill out a laboratory requisition slip to accompany the specimen.	☐	☐	☐
10. Label the specimen with the patient's name, date and time of collection, and the origin of the specimen.	☐	☐	☐
11. Route the specimen to the laboratory.	☐	☐	☐
12. Properly dispose of the equipment and supplies in a biohazard waste container. Remove personal protective equipment, and wash your hands.	☐	☐	☐
13. Document the procedure.	☐	☐	☐
14. Sanitize the work area.	☐	☐	☐

CALCULATION

Total Possible Points: _____

Total Points Earned: _____ Multiplied by 100 = _____ Divided by Total Possible Points = _____ %

PASS   **FAIL**   **COMMENTS:**

☐   ☐

Student's signature _____ Date _____

Partner's signature _____ Date _____

Instructor's signature _____ Date _____

PSY PROCEDURE 44-5 Collect a Stool Specimen

Name: _____ Date: _____ Time: _____ Grade: _____

EQUIPMENT/SUPPLIES: Specimen container dependent on test ordered (sterile container or Para-Pak collection system for C&S or ova and parasites, test kit or slide for occult blood testing: see laboratory procedure manual), tongue blade or wooden spatula, personal protective equipment, hand sanitizer, surface sanitizer and biohazard transport bag

STANDARDS: Given the needed equipment and a place to work, the student will perform this skill with _____% accuracy in a total of _____ minutes. *(Your instructor will tell you what the percentage and time limits will be before you begin practicing.)*

KEY: 4 = Satisfactory 0 = Unsatisfactory NA = This step is not counted

PROCEDURE STEPS	SELF	PARTNER	INSTRUCTOR
1. Wash your hands.	☐	☐	☐
2. Assemble the equipment and supplies.	☐	☐	☐
3. **AFF** Greet and identify the patient. Explain the procedure. Explain any dietary, medication, or other restrictions necessary for the collection. (These instructions for the patient are in the Patient Education box titled, "Patient Preparation for Fecal Occult Blood Testing.") Instruct patient to defecate.	☐	☐	☐
4. **AFF** If you are in a significantly different generation than the patient, you will need to take extra precautions with communication. First, remember that collecting a stool specimen is embarrassing for most patients. Watch the patient's facial expressions to note if he or she is understanding your instructions. This is one of the times you may find that your patient does not understand professional terminology.	☐	☐	☐
5. When obtaining a stool specimen for C&S or ova and parasites, the patient should collect a small amount of the first and last portion of the stool after the bowel movement with the wooden spatula or tongue blade and place it in the specimen container without contaminating the outside of the container. Fill Para-Pak until fluid reaches "fill" line, and recap the container.	☐	☐	☐
6. Upon receipt of the specimen, you should put on gloves and place the specimen into the biohazard bag for transport to the reference laboratory. Fill out a laboratory requisition slip to accompany the specimen.	☐	☐	☐
7. Label the specimen with the patient's name, the date and time of collection, and the origin of the specimen.	☐	☐	☐
8. Transport the specimen to the laboratory or store the specimen as directed. Refer to the laboratory procedure manual because some samples require refrigeration, others are kept at room temperature, and some must be placed in an incubator at a laboratory as soon as possible after collecting.	☐	☐	☐
9. Properly dispose of the equipment and supplies waste container. Remove personal protective equipment, and wash your hands.	☐	☐	☐
10. Document the procedure including patient instructions.	☐	☐	☐
11. Sanitize the work area.	☐	☐	☐

CALCULATION

Total Possible Points: _____

Total Points Earned: _____ Multiplied by 100 = _____ Divided by Total Possible Points = _____ %

PASS   **FAIL**   **COMMENTS:**

☐   ☐

Student's signature _____ Date _____

Partner's signature _____ Date _____

Instructor's signature _____ Date _____

PSY PROCEDURE 44-6 Collect Blood for Culture

Name: _____ Date: _____ Time: _____ Grade: _____

EQUIPMENT/SUPPLIES: Specimen container depends on testing site (yellow-top sodium polyanethol sulfonate Vacutainer tubes or aerobic and anaerobic blood culture bottles), blood culture skin prep packs (or 70% isopropyl alcohol wipes and povidone-iodine solution swabs or towelettes), venipuncture supplies (see Chapter 41), personal protective equipment, hand sanitizer, surface sanitizer

STANDARDS: Given the needed equipment and a place to work, the student will perform this skill with _____% accuracy in a total of _____ minutes. (Your instructor will tell you what the percentage and time limits will be before you begin practicing.)

KEY: 4 = Satisfactory   0 = Unsatisfactory   NA = This step is not counted

PROCEDURE STEPS	SELF	PARTNER	INSTRUCTOR
1. Wash your hands.	☐	☐	☐
2. Assemble the equipment and supplies, checking expiration dates.	☐	☐	☐
3. Put on personal protective equipment.	☐	☐	☐
4. **AFF** Greet and identify the patient. Explain the procedure. Verify that the patient has not started antibiotic therapy. If therapy has started, document antibiotic, strength, dose, duration, and time of last dose.	☐	☐	☐
5. **AFF** If the patient is hearing impaired, you need to speak clearly and distinctly in front of the patient's face. You should have an easy-to-read instruction guide for the patient to follow and point out where he or she has questions. If the patient can sign and you cannot, have someone proficient in sign language assist you in instructing the patient.	☐	☐	☐
6. Using skin preparation kits or supplies, apply alcohol to venipuncture site and allow to air dry. Apply povidone-iodine prep in progressively increasing concentric circles without wiping back over skin that is already prepped. Let stand for at least 1 minute and allow the site to air dry.	☐	☐	☐
7. Wipe bottle stoppers with povidone-iodine solution.	☐	☐	☐
8. Perform venipuncture as described in Procedure 41-1.	☐	☐	☐
9. Fill bottles or tubes according to the specific laboratory procedure. Invert each 8–10 times as soon as collected. If using culture bottles, fill the aerobic bottle first.	☐	☐	☐
10. Complete venipuncture. Use an isopropyl alcohol wipe to remove residual povidone-iodine from skin. Label the specimen with the patient's name, the date and time of collection, and the origin of the specimen.	☐	☐	☐
11. Remove gloves and wash hands. In preparation for the second collection 30 minutes after the first, put on new gloves between the two venipunctures. and repeat Steps 5–9 at a second venipuncture site.	☐	☐	☐
12. Label the specimens with the patient's name and the date and time of collection.	☐	☐	☐

13. Properly dispose of the equipment and supplies in a biohazard waste container. Remove personal protective equipment, and wash your hands.	☐	☐	☐
14. Document the procedure.	☐	☐	☐
15. Sanitize the work area.	☐	☐	☐

CALCULATION

Total Possible Points: _____

Total Points Earned: _____ Multiplied by 100 = _____ Divided by Total Possible Points = _____ %

PASS   **FAIL**   **COMMENTS:**

☐   ☐

Student's signature _____ Date _____

Partner's signature _____ Date _____

Instructor's signature _____ Date _____

PSY PROCEDURE 44-7 Collecting Genital Specimens for Culture

Name: _____ Date: _____ Time: _____ Grade: _____

EQUIPMENT/SUPPLIES: Specimen container depends on testing requested (bacterial, viral, and Chlamydia specimens require different media), personal protective equipment, hand sanitizer, surface sanitizer

STANDARDS: Given the needed equipment and a place to work, the student will perform this skill with _____% accuracy in a total of _____ minutes. *(Your instructor will tell you what the percentage and time limits will be before you begin practicing.)*

KEY: 4 = Satisfactory   0 = Unsatisfactory   NA = This step is not counted

PROCEDURE STEPS	SELF	PARTNER	INSTRUCTOR
1. Wash your hands.	☐	☐	☐
2. Assemble the equipment and supplies, checking expiration dates.	☐	☐	☐
3. Put on personal protective equipment.	☐	☐	☐
4. Your role will be to assist the physician in the collection and handling of these specimens. Be sure to verbally verify patient identification.	☐	☐	☐
5. **AFF** Be sensitive to indications that the patient is uncomfortable with your perception of him or her. Be reassuring with a gentle, professional demeanor. Be aware of your body language.	☐	☐	☐
6. **AFF** Assist the physician with patients having communication problems. Secure assistance as it is necessary.	☐	☐	☐
7. Accept specimens from the physician, securing in the appropriate medium follow the instructions for that particular medium.	☐	☐	☐
8. Label the specimen with the patient's name, the date and time of collection, and the origin of specimen.	☐	☐	☐
9. Repeat Steps 7 and 8 for each specimen.	☐	☐	☐
10. Store specimens per procedure instructions until transport. Transport to the testing facility as soon as possible.	☐	☐	☐
11. Properly dispose of the equipment and supplies in a biohazard waste container. Remove personal protective equipment and wash your hands.	☐	☐	☐
12. Document the procedure.	☐	☐	☐
13. Sanitize the work area.	☐	☐	☐

CALCULATION

Total Possible Points: _____

Total Points Earned: _____ Multiplied by 100 = _____ Divided by Total Possible Points = _____ %

PASS   **FAIL**   **COMMENTS:**

☐   ☐

Student's signature _____ Date _____

Partner's signature _____ Date _____

Instructor's signature _____ Date _____

PSY PROCEDURE 44-8 | **Testing Stool Specimen for Occult Blood – Guaiac Method**

Name: _____ Date: _____ Time: _____ Grade: _____

EQUIPMENT/SUPPLIES: Gloves, patient's labeled specimen pack, developer or reagent drops, personal protective equipment, hand sanitizer, surface sanitizer, contaminated waste container

STANDARDS: Given the needed equipment and a place to work, the student will perform this skill with _____% accuracy in a total of _____ minutes. *(Your instructor will tell you what the percentage and time limits will be before you begin practicing.)*

KEY: 4 = Satisfactory 0 = Unsatisfactory NA = This step is not counted

PROCEDURE STEPS	SELF	PARTNER	INSTRUCTOR
1. Wash your hands and put on clean examination gloves.	☐	☐	☐
2. Assemble the supplies and verify the patient identification on the patient's prepared test pack. Check the expiration date on the developing solution.	☐	☐	☐
3. Open the test window on the back of the pack and apply one drop of the developer or testing reagent to each window according to the manufacturer's directions. Read the color change within the specified time, usually 60 seconds.	☐	☐	☐
4. Apply one drop of developer as directed on the quality control monitor section or window of the pack. Note whether the quality control results are positive or negative as appropriate. If results are acceptable, patient results may be reported. If results are not acceptable, notify the physician.	☐	☐	☐
5. Properly dispose of the test pack and gloves. Wash your hands.	☐	☐	☐
6. Record the procedure.	☐	☐	☐
7. Sanitize the work area.	☐	☐	☐

CALCULATION

Total Possible Points: _____

Total Points Earned: _____ Multiplied by 100 = _____ Divided by Total Possible Points = _____ %

PASS **FAIL** **COMMENTS:**

☐ ☐

Student's signature _____ Date _____

Partner's signature _____ Date _____

Instructor's signature _____ Date _____

PSY PROCEDURE 44-9 Preparing a Smear for Microscopic Evaluation

Name: _____ Date: _____ Time: _____ Grade: _____

EQUIPMENT/SUPPLIES: Specimen, Bunsen burner, slide forceps, slide, sterile swab or inoculating loop, pencil or diamond-tipped pen, personal protective equipment, hand sanitizer, surface sanitizer, and contaminated waste container

STANDARDS: Given the needed equipment and a place to work, the student will perform this skill with _____% accuracy in a total of _____ minutes. *(Your instructor will tell you what the percentage and time limits will be before you begin practicing.)*

KEY: 4 = Satisfactory   0 = Unsatisfactory   NA = This step is not counted

PROCEDURE STEPS	SELF	PARTNER	INSTRUCTOR
1. Wash your hands. Put on personal protective equipment.	☐	☐	☐
2. Assemble the equipment and supplies, checking expiration dates.	☐	☐	☐
3. Label the slide with the patient's name and the date on the frosted edge with a pencil.	☐	☐	☐
4. Hold the edges of the slide between the thumb and index finger. Starting at the right side of the slide and using a rolling motion of the swab or a sweeping motion of the inoculating loop, gently and evenly spread the material from the specimen over the slide. The material should thinly fill the center of the slide within half an inch of each end.	☐	☐	☐
5. Do not rub the material vigorously over the slide.	☐	☐	☐
6. Dispose of the contaminated swab or inoculating loop in a biohazard container. If you are not using a disposable loop, sterilize it as follows: a. Hold the loop in the colorless part of the flame of the Bunsen burner for 10 seconds. b. Raise the loop slowly (to avoid splattering the bacteria) to the blue part of the flame until the loop and its connecting wire glow red. c. Cool it so the heat will not kill the bacteria that must be allowed to grow. Do not wave the loop in the air because doing so may expose it to contamination. Do not stab the medium with a hot loop to cool; this creates an aerosol.	☐	☐	☐
7. Allow the smear to air dry in a flat position for at least half an hour. Do not blow on the slide or wave it about in the air. Heat should not be applied until the specimen has been allowed to dry. Some specimens (e.g., Pap smear) require a fixative spray.	☐	☐	☐
8. Hold the dried smear slide with the slide forceps. Pass the slide quickly through the flame of a Bunsen burner three or four times. The slide has been fixed properly when the back of the slide feels slightly uncomfortably warm to the back of the gloved hand. It should not feel hot.	☐	☐	☐

9. Properly dispose of the equipment and supplies in a biohazard waste container. Remove personal protective equipment and wash your hands.	☐	☐	☐
10. Document the procedure.	☐	☐	☐
11. Sanitize the work area.	☐	☐	☐

CALCULATION

Total Possible Points: _____

Total Points Earned: _____ Multiplied by 100 = _____ Divided by Total Possible Points = _____ %

PASS   **FAIL**   **COMMENTS:**

☐   ☐

Student's signature _____ Date _____

Partner's signature _____ Date _____

Instructor's signature _____ Date _____

PSY PROCEDURE 44-10 | **Performing a Gram Stain**

Name: _____ Date: _____ Time: _____ Grade: _____

EQUIPMENT/SUPPLIES: Crystal violet stain, staining rack, Gram iodine solution, wash bottle with distilled water, alcohol-acetone solution, counterstain (e.g., Safranin), absorbent (bibulous) paper pad, specimen smear on glass slide labeled with a pencil or diamond-tipped pen (as prepared in Procedure 44-7), Bunsen burner, slide forceps, stopwatch or timer, personal protective equipment, hand sanitizer, surface sanitizer, and contaminated waste container

STANDARDS: Given the needed equipment and a place to work, the student will perform this skill with _____% accuracy in a total of _____ minutes. *(Your instructor will tell you what the percentage and time limits will be before you begin practicing.)*

KEY: 4 = Satisfactory   0 = Unsatisfactory   NA = This step is not counted

PROCEDURE STEPS	SELF	PARTNER	INSTRUCTOR
1. Wash your hands. Put on personal protective equipment.	☐	☐	☐
2. Assemble the equipment and supplies, checking expiration dates.	☐	☐	☐
3. Make sure the specimen is heat-fixed to the labeled slide and the slide is room temperature (see Procedure 44-7).	☐	☐	☐
4. Place the slide on the staining rack with the smear side up.	☐	☐	☐
5. Flood the smear with crystal violet. Time for 60 seconds.	☐	☐	☐

6. Hold the slide with slide forceps.
   a. Tilt the slide to an angle of about 45 degrees to drain the excess dye.
   b. Rinse the slide with distilled water for about 5 seconds and drain off excess water.
	☐	☐	☐

7. Replace the slide on the slide rack. Flood the slide with Gram iodine solution for 60 seconds.	☐	☐	☐
8. Using the forceps, tilt the slide at a 45-degree angle to drain the iodine solution. With the slide tilted, rinse the slide with distilled water from the wash bottle for about 5 to 10 seconds. Slowly and gently wash with the alcohol-acetone solution until no more stain runs off.	☐	☐	☐
9. Immediately rinse the slide with distilled water for 5 seconds and return the slide to the rack.	☐	☐	☐
10. Flood with Safranin or suitable counterstain for 60 seconds.	☐	☐	☐
11. Drain the excess counterstain from the slide by tilting it at a 45-degree angle. Rinse the slide with distilled water for 5 seconds to remove the counterstain. Gently blot the smear dry with bibulous paper. Take care not to disturb the smeared specimen. Wipe the back of the slide clear of any solution. It may be placed between the pages of a bibulous paper pad and gently pressed to remove excess moisture.	☐	☐	☐
12. Properly dispose of the equipment and supplies in a biohazard waste container. Remove personal protective equipment and wash your hands.	☐	☐	☐
13. Document the procedure.	☐	☐	☐
14. Sanitize the work area.	☐	☐	☐

CALCULATION

Total Possible Points: _____

Total Points Earned: _____ Multiplied by 100 = _____ Divided by Total Possible Points = _____ %

PASS   **FAIL**   **COMMENTS:**

☐   ☐

Student's signature _____ Date _____

Partner's signature _____ Date _____

Instructor's signature _____ Date _____

PSY PROCEDURE 44-11 | **Inoculating a Culture**

Name: _____ Date: _____ Time: _____ Grade: _____

EQUIPMENT/SUPPLIES: Specimen on a swab or loop, china marker or permanent laboratory marker, sterile or disposable loop, Bunsen burner, labeled Petri dish of culture medium (the patient's name should be on the side of the plate containing the medium, because it is always placed upward to prevent condensation from dripping onto the culture), personal protective equipment, hand sanitizer, surface sanitizer, and contaminated waste container

STANDARDS: Given the needed equipment and a place to work, the student will perform this skill with _____% accuracy in a total of _____ minutes. *(Your instructor will tell you what the percentage and time limits will be before you begin practicing.)*

KEY: 4 = Satisfactory   0 = Unsatisfactory   NA = This step is not counted

PROCEDURE STEPS	SELF	PARTNER	INSTRUCTOR
1. Wash your hands. Put on personal protective equipment.	☐	☐	☐
2. Assemble the equipment and supplies, checking expiration dates.	☐	☐	☐
3. Label the medium side of the plate with the patient's name, identification number, source of specimen, time collected, time inoculated, your initials, and date.	☐	☐	☐
4. Remove the Petri plate from the cover (the Petri plate is always stored with the cover down), and place the cover on the work surface with the opening up. Do not open the cover unnecessarily.	☐	☐	☐
5. Using a rolling and sliding motion, streak the specimen swab clear across half of the plate, starting at the top and working to the center. Dispose of the swab in a biohazard container.	☐	☐	☐
6. Use a disposable loop or sterilize the loop as described in Step 6 of Procedure 44-8.	☐	☐	☐
7. Turn the plate a quarter turn from its previous position. Pass the loop a few times in the original inoculum then across the medium approximately a quarter of the surface of the plate. Do not enter the originally streaked area after the first few sweeps.	☐	☐	☐
8. Turn the plate another quarter turn so that now it is 180 degrees to the original smear. Working in the previous manner, draw the loop at right angles through the most recently streaked area. Again, do not enter the originally streaked area after the first few sweeps. **FOR QUANTITATIVE CULTURES:** a. Streak the plate with the specimen from side to side across the middle. b. Streak the entire plate back and forth across the initial inoculate. This allows bacteria to grow in a way that colonies can be counted.	☐	☐	☐
9. Properly dispose of the equipment and supplies in a biohazard waste container. Remove personal protective equipment and wash your hands.	☐	☐	☐
10. Document the procedure.	☐	☐	☐
11. Sanitize the work area.	☐	☐	☐

CALCULATION

Total Possible Points: _____

Total Points Earned: _____ Multiplied by 100 = _____ Divided by Total Possible Points = _____ %

PASS   **FAIL**   **COMMENTS:**

☐   ☐

Student's signature _____ Date _____

Partner's signature _____ Date _____

Instructor's signature _____ Date _____

PSY PROCEDURE 44-12 | **Mononucleosis Testing**

Name: _____ Date: _____ Time: _____ Grade: _____

EQUIPMENT/SUPPLIES: Patient's labeled specimen (whole blood, plasma, or serum, depending on the kit), CLIA-waived mononucleosis kit (slide or test strip), stopwatch or timer, personal protective equipment, hand sanitizer, surface sanitizer, and contaminated waste container

STANDARDS: Given the needed equipment and a place to work, the student will perform this skill with _____% accuracy in a total of _____ minutes. *(Your instructor will tell you what the percentage and time limits will be before you begin practicing.)*

KEY: 4 = Satisfactory   0 = Unsatisfactory   NA = This step is not counted

PROCEDURE STEPS	SELF	PARTNER	INSTRUCTOR
1. Wash your hands. Put on personal protective equipment.	☐	☐	☐
2. Assemble the equipment and supplies, checking expiration dates.	☐	☐	☐
3. Verify that the names on the specimen container and the laboratory form are the same.	☐	☐	☐
4. Ensure that the materials in the kit and the patient specimen are at room temperature.	☐	☐	☐
5. Label the test pack or test strip (depending on type of kit) with the patient's name, positive control, and negative control. Use one test pack or strip per patient and control.	☐	☐	☐
6. Aspirate the patient's specimen using the transfer pipette and place volume indicated in kit package insert on the sample well of the test pack or dip test strip labeled with the patient's name.	☐	☐	☐
7. Sample the positive and negative controls as directed in Step 6.	☐	☐	☐
8. Set timer for incubation period indicated in package insert.	☐	☐	☐
9. Read reaction results at the end of incubation period.	☐	☐	☐
10. Verify the results of the controls before documenting the patient's results. Log controls and patient information on the worksheet.	☐	☐	☐
11. Properly dispose of the equipment and supplies in a biohazard waste container.	☐	☐	☐
12. Remove personal protective equipment and wash your hands.	☐	☐	☐
13. Document the procedure.	☐	☐	☐
14. Sanitize the work area.	☐	☐	☐

CALCULATION

Total Possible Points: _____

Total Points Earned: _____ Multiplied by 100 = _____ Divided by Total Possible Points = _____ %

PASS   **FAIL**   **COMMENTS:**

☐   ☐

Student's signature _____ Date _____

Partner's signature _____ Date _____

Instructor's signature _____ Date _____

PSY PROCEDURE 44-13 HCG Pregnancy Test

Name: _____ Date: _____ Time: _____ Grade: _____

EQUIPMENT/SUPPLIES: Patient's labeled specimen (plasma, serum, or urine depending on the kit), HCG pregnancy kit (test pack and transfer pipettes or test strip; kit contents will vary by manufacturer), HCG positive and negative control (different controls may be needed when testing urine), timer, personal protective equipment, hand sanitizer, surface sanitizer, and contaminated waste container

STANDARDS: Given the needed equipment and a place to work, the student will perform this skill with _____% accuracy in a total of _____ minutes. *(Your instructor will tell you what the percentage and time limits will be before you begin practicing.)*

KEY: 4 = Satisfactory   0 = Unsatisfactory   NA = This step is not counted

PROCEDURE STEPS	SELF	PARTNER	INSTRUCTOR
1. Wash your hands. Put on personal protective equipment.	☐	☐	☐
2. Assemble the equipment and supplies, checking expiration dates.	☐	☐	☐
3. Verify that the names on the specimen container and the laboratory form are the same.	☐	☐	☐
4. Ensure that the materials in the kit and the patient specimen are at room temperature. Note in the patient's information and in the control log whether you are using urine, plasma, or serum.	☐	☐	☐
5. Label the test pack or test strip (depending on type of kit) with the patient's name, positive control, and negative control. Use one test pack or strip per patient and control.	☐	☐	☐
6. Aspirate the patient's specimen using the transfer pipette and place volume indicated in kit package insert on the sample well of the test pack or dip test strip labeled with the patient's name.	☐	☐	☐
7. Sample the positive and negative controls as directed in Step 6.	☐	☐	☐
8. Set timer for incubation period indicated in package insert.	☐	☐	☐
9. Read reaction results at the end of incubation period.	☐	☐	☐
10. Verify the results of the controls before documenting the patient's results. Log controls and patient information on the worksheet.	☐	☐	☐
11. Properly dispose of the equipment and supplies in a biohazard waste container.	☐	☐	☐
12. Remove personal protective equipment and wash your hands.	☐	☐	☐
13. Document the procedure.	☐	☐	☐
14. Sanitize the work area.	☐	☐	☐

CALCULATION

Total Possible Points: _____

Total Points Earned: _____ Multiplied by 100 = _____ Divided by Total Possible Points = _____ %

PASS   **FAIL**   **COMMENTS:**

☐   ☐

Student's signature _____ Date _____

Partner's signature _____ Date _____

Instructor's signature _____ Date _____

PSY PROCEDURE 44-14 | Rapid Group A Strep Testing

Name: _____ Date: _____ Time: _____ Grade: _____

EQUIPMENT/SUPPLIES: Patient's labeled throat specimen, group A strep kit (controls may be included, depending on the kit), timer, personal protective equipment, hand sanitizer, surface sanitizer, and contaminated waste container

STANDARDS: Given the needed equipment and a place to work, the student will perform this skill with _____% accuracy in a total of _____ minutes. *(Your instructor will tell you what the percentage and time limits will be before you begin practicing.)*

KEY: 4 = Satisfactory   0 = Unsatisfactory   NA = This step is not counted

PROCEDURE STEPS	SELF	PARTNER	INSTRUCTOR
1. Wash your hands. Put on personal protective equipment.	☐	☐	☐
2. Assemble the equipment and supplies, checking expiration dates.	☐	☐	☐
3. Verify that the names on the specimen container and the laboratory form are the same.	☐	☐	☐
4. Label one extraction tube with the patient's name, one for the positive control, and one for the negative control.	☐	☐	☐
5. Follow the directions for the kit. Add the appropriate reagents and drops to each of the extraction tubes. Avoid splashing, and use the correct number of drops.	☐	☐	☐
6. Insert the patient's swab into the labeled extraction tube.	☐	☐	☐
7. Add the appropriate controls to each of the labeled extraction tubes.	☐	☐	☐
8. Set the timer for the appropriate time to ensure accuracy.	☐	☐	☐
9. Add the appropriate reagent and drops to each of the extraction tubes.	☐	☐	☐
10. Use the swab to mix the reagents. Then press out any excess fluid on the swab against the inside of the tube.	☐	☐	☐
11. Add three drops from the well-mixed extraction tube to the sample window of the strep A test unit or dip the test stick labeled with the patient's name. Do the same for each control.	☐	☐	☐
12. Set the timer for the time indicated in the kit package insert.	☐	☐	☐
13. A positive result appears as a line in the result window within 5 minutes. The strep A test unit or strip has an internal control; if a line appears in the control window, the test is valid.	☐	☐	☐
14. Read a negative result at exactly 5 minutes to avoid a false negative.	☐	☐	☐
15. Verify results of the controls before recording or reporting test results. Log the controls and the patient's information on the worksheet.	☐	☐	☐
16. Properly dispose of the equipment and supplies in a biohazard waste container.	☐	☐	☐
17. Remove personal protective equipment and wash your hands.	☐	☐	☐
18. Document the procedure.	☐	☐	☐
19. Sanitize the work area.	☐	☐	☐

CALCULATION

Total Possible Points: _____

Total Points Earned: _____ Multiplied by 100 = _____ Divided by Total Possible Points = _____ %

PASS **FAIL**   **COMMENTS:**

☐   ☐

Student's signature _____ Date _____

Partner's signature _____ Date _____

Instructor's signature _____ Date _____

Cognitive Domain

1. Spell and define the key terms
2. List the common electrolytes and explain the relationship of electrolytes to acid–base balance
3. Describe the nonprotein nitrogenous compounds and name conditions with abnormal values
4. List and describe the substances commonly tested in liver function assessment
5. Explain thyroid function and the hormone that regulates the thyroid gland
6. Describe how an assessment for a myocardial infarction is made with laboratory tests
7. Describe how pancreatitis is diagnosed with laboratory tests
8. Describe glucose use and regulation and the purpose of the various glucose tests
9. Describe the function of cholesterol and other lipids and their correlation to heart disease

Psychomotor Domain

1. Perform blood glucose testing (Procedure 45-1)
2. Perform blood cholesterol testing (Procedure 45-2)

3. Perform routine maintenance of a glucose meter (Procedure 45-3)
4. Use medical terminology, pronouncing medical terms correctly, to communicate information
5. Perform within scope of practice
6. Practice within the standard of care of a medical assistant
7. Screen test results
8. Analyze charts, graphs, and/or tables in the interpretation of health care results
9. Distinguish between normal and abnormal test results
10. Practice standard precautions
11. Perform handwashing

Affective Domain

1. Distinguish between normal and abnormal test results

ABHES Competencies

1. Perform CLIA-waived tests that assist with diagnosis and treatment
2. Perform chemistry testing
3. Perform routine maintenance of clinical equipment safely
4. Screen and follow up patient test results
5. Use standard precautions
6. Perform CLIA-waived tests

Name: _____   Date: _____   Grade: _____

COG **AFF** **MULTIPLE CHOICE**

Circle the letter preceding the correct answer.

1. Sodium is used to maintain:

    a. electrolytes.

    b. TSH stimulation.

    c. waste materials.

    d. fluid balance.

    e. blood oxygen.

2. An enzyme is a(n):

    a. cell that speeds up the production of proteins.

    b. protein that quickens chemical reactions.

    c. chemical reaction that ionizes electrolytes.

    d. ion that has an electrical charge.

    e. specialized cell that deals with blood levels.

3. Which of the following is formed in the liver?

    a. Urea

    b. TSH

    c. Creatinine

    d. Lipase

    e. Amylase

4. The kidneys are responsible for:

    a. releasing amylase and lipase into the bloodstream.

    b. ridding the body of waste products.

    c. producing bile and enzymes.

    d. removing worn-out red blood cells.

    e. regulating carbohydrate metabolism.

5. A patient's blood work shows her amylase level is found to be high. What other substance should you check to test for pancreatitis?

    a. Hemoglobin

    b. Triglycerides

    c. Potassium

    d. Lipase

    e. Lipoproteins

6. The function of LDLs is to:

    a. transport enzymes to the heart and lungs.

    b. assist in the production of lipoproteins.

    c. store energy in adipose tissue.

    d. move cholesterol from the liver to arteries.

    e. carry cholesterol from the cells to the liver.

7. Chloride, bicarbonate, and electrolytes are all a part of:

    a. maintaining thyroid function.

    b. bile formation.

    c. red blood cell maturation.

    d. glucose storage.

    e. acid-base balance.

8. The purpose of TSH is to:

    a. produce hormones in the thyroid gland.

    b. stimulate the thyroid gland.

    c. balance pH levels in the blood.

    d. provide warning of a system failure.

    e. carry cholesterol into the heart.

9. Women are screened for gestational diabetes:

    a. before they conceive.

    b. during the first month of pregnancy.

    c. during the second trimester.

    d. during the third trimester.

    e. after the baby is born.

10. When blood sugar levels go below 45 mg/dL, a person may experience:

    a. trembling.

    b. vomiting.

    c. diarrhea.

    d. chills.

    e. a high temperature.

11. A possible cause of waste-product buildup in the blood is:

   a. liver failure.

   b. renal failure.

   c. pancreatitis.

   d. hypokalemia.

   e. alkalosis.

12. If you are testing for a substance only found in serum, what should you do with a blood specimen?

   a. Use reagent strips to check for serum presence.

   b. Create a slide and analyze it under a microscope.

   c. Put the clotted specimen in the centrifuge to separate.

   d. Allow the specimen a few days to sit and separate.

   e. Run tests without doing anything to the specimen.

13. The pancreas functions in the:

   a. endocrine and exocrine systems.

   b. renal and endocrine systems.

   c. pulmonary and exocrine systems.

   d. digestive and renal systems.

   e. pulmonary and vascular systems.

14. The salivary glands produce:

   a. creatinine.

   b. phosphates.

   c. glucose.

   d. lipase.

   e. amylase.

15. What is the body's normal pH range?

   a. 6.0 to 6.5

   b. 6.9 to 7.35

   c. 7.0 to 7.5

   d. 7.35 to 7.45

   e. 7.45 to 8.25

16. People who exercise regularly, maintain normal weight, and eat mostly unsaturated fats will probably increase their level of:

   a. HDLs.

   b. LDLs.

   c. albumin.

   d. glucose.

   e. lipase.

17. Hemoglobin A1C is tested to measure the patient's:

   a. fasting glucose.

   b. level of anemia.

   c. glucose that is attached to hemoglobin molecules.

   d. hemoglobin attached to glucose molecules.

   e. glucose tolerance.

18. Why is fasting required to accurately measure lipid levels?

   a. To evaluate how the body handles fat intake

   b. To establish fasting glucose levels

   c. To measure how much water is in body fat

   d. To limit the action of digestion on increasing lipid levels

   e. To lower HDL levels

19. What is the number one environmental threat to children?

   a. Lead poisoning

   b. Carbon monoxide poisoning

   c. Glue sniffing

   d. Accidental fires

   e. High ozone levels

20. What effect does lead poisoning have on the body?

   a. Limits RBCs' ability to carry oxygen

   b. Increases production of blood cells

   c. Increases calcium absorption in bones

   d. Raises hemoglobin levels

   e. Causes uncontrollable bleeding

COG **MATCHING**

Match each key term with the correct definition.

Key Terms	**Definitions**

Key Terms

21. _____ acidosis

22. _____ alkalosis

23. _____ amylase

24. _____ atherosclerosis

25. _____ azotemia

26. _____ bicarbonate

27. _____ bile

28. _____ buffer systems

29. _____ catabolism

30. _____ creatinine

31. _____ electrolyte

32. _____ electrolyte balance

33. _____ endocrine

34. _____ enzyme

35. _____ exocrine

36. _____ ions

37. _____ lipase

38. _____ lipoproteins

39. _____ jaundiced

40. _____ metabolism

41. _____ urea

Definitions

a. electrically charged atoms

b. any substance containing ions

c. having electrolytes at the right levels

d. an electrolyte with a negative charge formed when carbon dioxide dissolves in the blood

e. set of chemical reactions that happen to sustain life

f. keeps the pH changes balanced

g. blood pH is below 7.4 caused by too much acid or too little base

h. blood pH is above 7.4 caused by too much base or too little acid

i. waste product from the body's metabolism of protein

j. abnormally high levels of nitrogen-containing compounds

k. breaks down fats in the stomach

l. a protein produced by living cells that speeds up chemical reactions

m. patient appears yellow

n. helps in the digestion of fats

o. breaks down starch into sugar

p. release hormones into the blood in order to cause a response from another organ in the body

q. release enzymes through ducts and include mammary glands, salivary glands, sweat glands, and glands that secrete digestive enzymes into the stomach and intestine

r. substances composed of lipids and proteins

s. buildup of plaques in the arteries

t. to break down molecules into smaller units

u. a waste product from making the energy muscles use to function

COG IDENTIFICATION

Grade: _____

Identify the electrolyte by the stated relationship to acid–base balance.

RELATIONSHIP	ELECTROLYTE
42. It causes the most problems when its level is not stable	
43. When the level is extremely low, it becomes difficult for the patient to breathe	
44. Can be made unstable if the patient is suffering diabetic ketoacidosis and metabolic acidosis	
45. Most important electrolyte used in acid–base balance	
46. Low levels are seen in patients experiencing a long-term severe illness	
47. Low levels result from inadequate absorption from the diet, GI losses, electrolyte shifts, and endocrine disorders	
48. A waste product of oxygen metabolism	

COG IDENTIFY

Grade: _____

The following table lists nonprotein nitrogenous compound descriptions and associated abnormal conditions. Identify the nonprotein nitrogenous compound that is described.

COMPOUND	DESCRIPTION	ABNORMAL CONDITION
49.	Waste product from the body's metabolism of protein	Dehydration, renal disease, inadequate dialysis, azotemia
50.	Waste product from making the energy muscles use to function	Kidney damage, kidney disease
51.	Waste product from breaking down protein	Gout, kidney stones

COG IDENTIFY

Grade: _____

Identify the substance by its use in liver function assessment.

RELATIONSHIP	SUBSTANCE
52. Two of the most useful measures of liver function	
53. Also seen in acute muscle injury	
54. Present in the bones, liver, intestines, kidneys, and placenta	
55. Elevated due to bile duct obstruction and primary biliary cirrhosis	
56. In addition to liver disease, drugs and alcohol cause increased levels	
57. Produced by the normal breakdown of hemoglobin	
58. If this is increased in the blood, it is due to liver disease	
59. Useful when all the liver test results are normal, except the total bilirubin	

COG **FILL IN THE BLANK**   Grade: _____

60. The _____ gland has two _____ that lie along the trachea and are joined together by a narrow band of thyroid tissue, known as the _____. The thyroid gland converts _____ into thyroid hormones: _____ and _____. The bloodstream carries T_3 and T_4 throughout the body where they control _____.

The thyroid gland is directed by the _____ gland at the base of the _____. When the levels of T_3 and T_4 _____, the pituitary gland is activated to produce _____. TSH activates the _____ gland to produce more _____. This production _____ the T_3 and T_4 blood levels. When the pituitary senses that the T_3 and T_4 are _____, it stops its _____ production. If the thyroid gland is malfunctioning, it cannot be _____ regardless of the amount of TSH secreted.

COG **FILL IN THE BLANK**   Grade: _____

61. No one test is completely sensitive and specific for _____.

62. Comparison of _____ with patient symptoms and electrocardiograms (EKGs) are important.

63. _____ is elevated in MI.

64. MI is not the only condition that causes _____ CK levels.

65. Most of the CK is located in _____ muscle.

66. CK has three parts: _____, _____, and _____.

67. The _____ _____ is present in both cardiac and skeletal muscle.

68. The _____ _____ is much more specific for cardiac muscle.

69. The CKMB fraction increases within _____ following MI.

70. CKMB results indicate heart involvement when they are _____ of the total CK result.

71. Troponin _____ are contained in cardiac muscle.

72. They are released into the bloodstream with _____.

73. Troponins will begin to rise following MI within _____.

74. _____ levels are the best indicator of MI.

75. _____ is used to evaluate the size of muscle injury.

76. Rise in myoglobin can help to determine the _____ of an infarction.

77. A negative myoglobin can help to rule out _____ _____.

78. _____ _____ is released from the myocardium in response to excessive stretching of heart muscle cells.

79. Since inflammation is part of MI, _____ _____ is tested to predict the diagnosis of MI.

COG SHORT ANSWER

Grade: _____

80. What is pancreatitis, and what two enzymes are elevated in this condition?

_____

_____

_____

_____

81. The pancreas makes two endocrine hormones that are important in diabetes. What are they and what do they do?

_____

_____

_____

_____

82. When you are testing for glucose, what is the puncture site, and why is it important to wash the surrounding area?

_____

_____

_____

_____

83. What are the two hormones that regulate the process of storing glucose as glycogen?

a. _____

b. _____

84. What glucose test is used for screening?

_____

_____

_____

_____

85. What glucose test is used to monitor insulin therapy?

_____

_____

_____

_____

86. Glucose tolerance testing is performed in obstetric patients to diagnose what condition?

_____

_____

_____

_____

87. How does hemoblogin A1C give the physician a picture of the patient's glucose levels over the past 3 months?

_____

_____

_____

_____

88. How are lipoproteins important to our bodies?

_____

_____

_____

_____

89. What are the four fats measured in a lipid panel?

_____

_____

_____

_____

90. What are four major responsibilities of the medical assistant in the chemistry laboratory?

_____

_____

_____

_____

COG SHORT ANSWER   Grade: _____

91. You are requested to use medical terminology to communicate information. Break these words down and use the definition of the parts to create a definition for the term.

a. Acidosis

_____

_____

_____

_____

b. Alkalosis

_____

_____

_____

_____

c. Atherosclerosis

_____

_____

_____

_____

d. Catabolism

_____

_____

_____

_____

e. Electrolyte

_____

_____

_____

_____

f. Endocrine

_____

_____

_____

_____

g. Exocrine

_____

_____

_____

_____

h. Lipoproteins

_____

_____

_____

_____

CASE STUDIES Grade: _____

1. Your patient is a 5-year-old girl. The physician has ordered a fingerstick glucose. Her mother brings her to the lab for the test. She has given the child a piece of candy because she thought her sugar might be low. You collect the specimen and run the test. The glucose is 60 mg/dl. You realize that you forgot to help the child wash her hands before the test. How could the result be affected if traces of the candy were on the child's finger? What do you do? What will make it difficult to do the right thing? How do you manage the parent and the child?

_____

_____

_____

_____

2. Your patient, Sarah Ingle, had an electrolyte panel ordered by Dr. Willis. The results are back from the reference lab. Your job is to screen the test results. What are the reference intervals (normal ranges) you expect to see for these tests: sodium, potassium, chloride, and CO_2? You find that the potassium level is 6.0 mmol/L, a panic value. What action do you take, and how do you document your action?

_____

_____

_____

_____

3. Melissa Woermann had a glucose tolerance test. The graph is below. Her fasting glucose was 90 mg/dL. Estimate Ms. Woermann's 1/2-hour, 1-hour, 2-hour, and 3-hour glucose levels. What are the criteria proposed by the National Diabetes Data Group and the World Health Organization and endorsed by the ADA for a diagnosis of diabetes? Does it appear from the graph that Ms. Woermann could be diagnosed with diabetes?

_____

_____

_____

_____

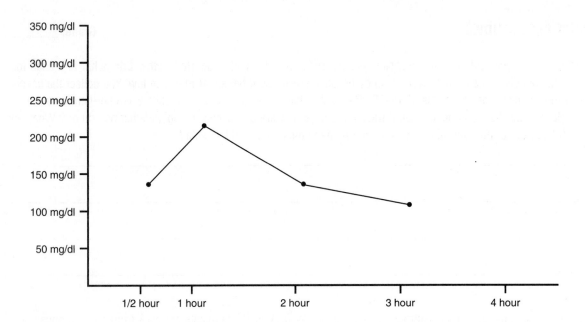

PSY PROCEDURE 45-1 | **Perform Blood Glucose Testing**

Name: _____ Date: _____ Time: _____ Grade: _____

EQUIPMENT/SUPPLIES: Glucose meter, glucose reagent strips, control solutions, capillary puncture device, personal protective equipment, gauze, paper towel, adhesive bandage, lancet, alcohol pad, hand sanitizer, surface sanitizer, contaminated waste container

NOTE: These are generic instructions for using a glucose meter. Refer to the manufacturer's instructions shipped with the meter for instructions specific to the instrument in use.

STANDARDS: Given the needed equipment and a place to work, the student will perform this skill with _____% accuracy in a total of _____ minutes. (Your instructor will tell you what the percentage and time limits will be before you begin practicing.)

KEY: 4 = Satisfactory   0 = Unsatisfactory   NA = this step is not counted

PROCEDURE STEPS	SELF	PARTNER	INSTRUCTOR
1. Wash your hands. Put on personal protective equipment.	☐	☐	☐
2. Assemble the equipment and supplies.	☐	☐	☐
3. Turn on the instrument, and ensure that it is calibrated.	☐	☐	☐
4. Perform the test on the quality control material. Record results. Determine whether QC is within control limits. If yes, proceed with patient testing. If no, take corrective action and recheck controls. Document corrective action. Proceed with patient testing when acceptable QC results are obtained.	☐	☐	☐
5. Remove one reagent strip, lay it on the paper towel, and recap the container.	☐	☐	☐
6. **AFF** Greet and identify the patient. Explain the procedure. Ask for and answer any questions.	☐	☐	☐
7. Have the patient wash his or her hands in warm water.	☐	☐	☐
8. Cleanse the selected puncture site (finger) with alcohol.	☐	☐	☐
9. Perform a capillary puncture, following the steps described in Chapter 41, Phlebotomy. Wipe away the first drop of blood.	☐	☐	☐
10. Turn the patient's hand palm down, and gently squeeze the finger to form a large drop of blood.	☐	☐	☐
11. Bring the reagent strip up to the finger and touch the pad to the blood. **a.** Do not touch the finger. **b.** Completely cover the pad or fill the testing chamber with blood.	☐	☐	☐
12. Insert the reagent strip into the analyzer. **a.** Meanwhile, apply pressure to the puncture wound with gauze. **b.** The meter will continue to incubate the strip and measure the reaction.	☐	☐	☐

13. The instrument reads the reaction strip and displays the result on the screen in mg/dL.	☐	☐	☐
14. Apply a small Band-Aid to the patient's fingertip.	☐	☐	☐
15. Properly care for or dispose of equipment and supplies.	☐	☐	☐
16. Clean the work area. Remove personal protective equipment and wash your hands.	☐	☐	☐

CALCULATION

Total Possible Points: _____

Total Points Earned: _____ Multiplied by 100 = _____ Divided by Total Possible Points = _____ %

PASS   **FAIL**   **COMMENTS:**

☐   ☐

Student's signature _____ Date _____

Partner's signature _____ Date _____

Instructor's signature _____ Date _____

PSY PROCEDURE 45-2 | **Perform Blood Cholesterol Testing**

Name: _____ Date: _____ Time: _____ Grade: _____

EQUIPMENT/SUPPLIES: Cholesterol meter and supplies or test kit, control solutions, capillary puncture equipment or blood specimen as indicated by manufacturer, personal protective equipment, hand sanitizer, surface sanitizer, contaminated waste container

NOTE: These are generic instructions for using a cholesterol meter or test kit. Refer to the manufacturer's instructions shipped with the testing tool for instructions specific for the instrument in use.

STANDARDS: Given the needed equipment and a place to work, the student will perform this skill with _____% accuracy in a total of _____ minutes. *(Your instructor will tell you what the percentage and time limits will be before you begin practicing.)*

KEY:　　　4 = Satisfactory　　　0 = Unsatisfactory　　　NA = this step is not counted

PROCEDURE STEPS	SELF	PARTNER	INSTRUCTOR
1. Wash your hands. Put on personal protective equipment.	☐	☐	☐
2. Assemble the equipment and supplies.	☐	☐	☐
3. Review instrument manual for your cholesterol meter or test kit.	☐	☐	☐
4. Perform the test on the quality control material. Record results. Determine whether QC is within control limits. If yes, proceed with patient testing. If no, take corrective action and recheck controls. Document corrective action. Proceed with patient testing when acceptable QC results are obtained.	☐	☐	☐
5. Obtain patient specimen per manufacturer's instructions.	☐	☐	☐
6. Perform the testing procedure following the manufacturer's instructions. Record results.	☐	☐	☐
7. Properly care for or dispose of equipment and supplies.	☐	☐	☐
8. Clean the work area. Remove personal protective equipment and wash your hands.	☐	☐	☐

CALCULATION

Total Possible Points: _____

Total Points Earned: _____ Multiplied by 100 = _____ Divided by Total Possible Points = _____ %

PASS **FAIL** **COMMENTS:**

☐ ☐

Student's signature _____ Date _____

Partner's signature _____ Date _____

Instructor's signature _____ Date _____

PSY PROCEDURE 45-3 **Perform Routine Maintenance of a Glucose Meter**

Name: _____ Date: _____ Time: _____ Grade: _____

EQUIPMENT: Glucose meter, maintenance and testing supplies, manufacturer's manual for glucose analyzer, control solutions, personal protective equipment, hand sanitizer, surface sanitizer, contaminated waste container

STANDARDS: Given the needed equipment and a place to work, the student will perform this skill with _____% accuracy in a total of _____ minutes. *(Your instructor will tell you what the percentage and time limits will be before you begin practicing.)*

KEY: 4 = Satisfactory   0 = Unsatisfactory   NA = this step is not counted

PROCEDURE STEPS	SELF	PARTNER	INSTRUCTOR
1. Wash your hands. Put on gloves.	☐	☐	☐
2. Assemble the equipment and supplies.	☐	☐	☐
3. Review the instrument manual for your glucose meter.	☐	☐	☐
4. Perform the maintenance procedures listed in the manufacturer's instructions. Document the performance of these procedures in the instrument maintenance log.	☐	☐	☐
5. Perform the test on the quality control material. Record results. Determine whether QC is within control limits. If yes, maintenance was successful and instrument is ready for patient testing. If no, take corrective action and recheck controls. Document corrective action. Instrument is available for patient testing when acceptable QC results are obtained.	☐	☐	☐
6. Properly care for or dispose of equipment and supplies.	☐	☐	☐
7. Clean the work area. Remove personal protective equipment, and wash your hands. *Note:* These are generic instructions for performing routine maintenance of a glucose analyzer. Refer to the manufacturer's manual for instructions specific to the particular instrument.	☐	☐	☐

CALCULATION

Total Possible Points: _____

Total Points Earned: _____ Multiplied by 100 = _____ Divided by Total Possible Points = _____ %

PASS   **FAIL**   **COMMENTS:**

☐   ☐

Student's signature _____ Date _____

Partner's signature _____ Date _____

Instructor's signature _____ Date _____

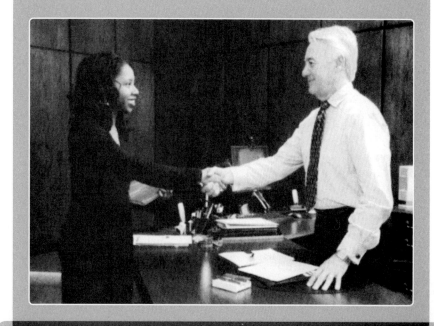

Career
Strategies

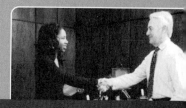
CHAPTER

46

Making the Transition: Student
to Employee

Learning
Outcomes

Cognitive Domain

1. Spell and define the key terms
2. Explain the purpose of the externship experience
3. Understand the importance of the evaluation process
4. List your professional responsibilities during externship
5. List personal and professional attributes necessary to ensure a successful externship
6. Determine your best career direction based on your skills and strengths
7. Identify the steps necessary to apply for the right position and be able to accomplish those steps
8. Draft an appropriate cover letter
9. List the steps and guidelines in completing an employment application
10. List guidelines for an effective interview that will lead to employment
11. Identify the steps that you need to take to ensure proper career advancement
12. Explain the process for recertification of medical assisting credentials
13. Describe the importance of membership in a professional organization
14. Recognize elements of fundamental writing skills
15. List and discuss legal and illegal interview questions
16. Discuss all levels of governmental legislation and regulation as they apply to medical assisting practice

Psychomotor Domain

1. Write a résumé to properly communicate skills and strengths (Procedure 46-1)
2. Compose professional/business letters

Affective Domain

1. Apply local, state, and federal health care legislation

ABHES Competencies

1. Comply with federal, state, and local health laws and regulations
2. Perform fundamental writing skills, including correct grammar, spelling, and formatting techniques when writing prescriptions, documenting medical records, etc.

Name: _____   Date: _____   Grade: _____

COG **MULTIPLE CHOICE**

1. Most externships range from:

    a. 160–240 hours a semester.

    b. 80–160 hours a semester.

    c. 200–240 hours a semester.

    d. 240–300 hours a semester.

    e. 260–300 hours a semester.

2. Preceptors are typically:

    a. physicians.

    b. nurses.

    c. graduate medical assistants.

    d. academic instructors.

    e. other students.

3. When responding to a newspaper advertisement, you should:

    a. mail your résumé and a portfolio.

    b. send your résumé by e-mail.

    c. phone right away to inquire about the job.

    d. follow the instructions in the advertisement.

    e. call to schedule an interview.

4. A CMA wishing to recertify must either retake the examination or complete:

    a. 60 hours of continuing education credits.

    b. 50 hours of continuing education credits.

    c. 100 hours of continuing education credits.

    d. 30 hours of continuing education credits.

    e. 75 hours of continuing education credits.

5. Two standard ways of listing experience on a résumé are:

    a. functional and chronological.

    b. functional and alphabetical.

    c. alphabetical and chronological.

    d. chronological and referential.

    e. referential and alphabetical.

6. During your externship, it is a good practice to arrive:

    a. a few minutes early.

    b. half an hour early.

    c. right on time.

    d. with enough time to beat traffic.

    e. as early as you can.

7. What is the appropriate length of a résumé?

    a. One page

    b. Two pages

    c. Three pages

    d. As long as it needs to be

    e. Check with the potential employer first

8. In addition to providing proof of general immunizations, what other vaccinations may be required before you begin your externship?

    a. Vaccination for strep throat

    b. Vaccination for cancer

    c. Vaccination for hepatitis B

    d. Vaccination for hepatitis C

    e. Vaccination for HIV

9. During your externship, you are expected to perform as:

    a. the student that you are; your preceptor will teach you the same skills as in the classroom.

    b. an experienced professional; your preceptor will expect you to perform every task perfectly.

    c. an entry-level employee; your preceptor will expect you to perform at the level of a new employee in the field.

    d. a patient; you have to see what it feels like to be on the receiving end of treatment.

    e. independently as possible; your preceptor will not have time to answer many questions.

10. Checking for telephone messages and arranging the day's appointments should be done:

    a. during your lunch break.

    b. at the close of the business day.

    c. after the office has opened.

    d. before the scheduled opening.

    e. between patients.

11. Fingernails should be kept short and clean to avoid:

    a. making your supervisor upset.

    b. accidentally scratching or harming a patient.

    c. transferring pathogens or ripping gloves.

    d. getting nail polish chips in lab samples.

    e. infecting sterile materials or surfaces.

12. Which document provides proof that tasks are performed and learning is taking place?

    a. Timesheet

    b. Journal

    c. Survey

    d. Evaluation

    e. Personal interview

13. Which document is used to improve performance and services offered to students?

    a. Timesheet

    b. Journal

    c. Survey

    d. Evaluation

    e. Personal interview

14. Membership in your professional allied health organization proves:

    a. that you are an allied health student.

    b. your level of professionalism and seriousness of purpose.

    c. that you will become a medical professional in 2 years.

    d. your willingness to network with other professionals.

    e. your interest in the medical field.

15. Which question should you avoid asking during an interview?

    a. Is there access to a 401(k) plan?

    b. Is tuition reimbursement available?

    c. How many weeks of vacation are available the first year?

    d. Are uniforms or lab coats worn?

    e. What are the responsibilities of this position?

16. If you decide to leave your job, it is a good idea to:

    a. tell your employer the day before you plan to leave.

    b. make sure your new job will pay more.

    c. get contact information for all of the new friends you made.

    d. finish all duties and tie up any loose ends.

    e. criticize employees during an exit interview.

17. If you are having a problem performing your assigned job duties, it is best to:

    a. volunteer for extra hours.

    b. inform your preceptor and instructor.

    c. ask for less challenging work.

    d. ask for a different externship site.

    e. switch your course of studies.

18. When anticipating calls from prospective employers, avoid:

    a. leaving silly or cute messages on your answering machine.

    b. telling family members or roommates that you are expecting important telephone calls.

    c. keeping a pen near the telephone at all times.

    d. checking messages on a regular basis.

    e. calling them every day after submitting your résumé.

19. If bilingual applicants are encouraged to apply for a position you want, you should:

   a. learn simple greetings and act as if you can speak several languages.

   b. learn simple greetings and admit that you know a few words but are not fluent.

   c. do nothing; being bilingual is not important.

   d. avoid applying since you do not fluently speak another language.

   e. learn how to answer possible interview questions in two different languages.

20. Being a lifelong learner is a must for all medical professionals because:

   a. medical professionals have to recertify every 5 years.

   b. medical professionals are widely respected.

   c. changes in procedures, medical technologies, and legal issues occur frequently.

   d. changes in medical technologies are decreasing the need for medical professionals.

   e. medical professionals are required to change legal statutes once a year.

COG MATCHING

Grade: _____

Match the following key terms to their definitions.

Key Terms	Definitions
21. _____ externship	**a.** a teacher; one who gives direction, as in a technical matter
22. _____ networking	**b.** an educational course that allows the student to obtain hands-on experience
23. _____ portfolio	**c.** a system of personal and professional relationships through which to share information
24. _____ preceptor	**d.** a document summarizing an individual's work experience or professional qualifications
25. _____ résumé	**e.** a portable case containing documents

COG SHORT ANSWER

Grade: _____

26. What is the purpose of an externship?

_____

_____

_____

_____

27. List three responsibilities you will have during an externship.

   a. _____

   b. _____

   c. _____

38. From the list of questions below, circle all that would be appropriate for a job applicant to ask a prospective employer.

　a. What are the responsibilities of the position offered?

　b. What is the benefit package? Is there access to a 401(k) plan or other retirement plan? Health insurance? Life insurance?

　c. Is it acceptable to take 3 weeks off during the holiday season?

　d. How does the facility feel about continuing education? Is time off offered to employees to upgrade their skills? Does the facility subsidize the expense?

　e. Do I have to work with physicians who have bad attitudes?

　f. How many potlucks and happy hours does this office usually have?

　g. Is there a job performance or evaluation process?

COG EXPLANATION　　　　　　　　　　　　　　　　　　　Grade: _____

39. Explain what it means to be a lifelong learner

_____

_____

_____

_____

40. How can you prepare for the process of recertification?

_____

_____

_____

_____

41. List two professional organizations you could join while you are a student.

　a. _____

　b. _____

Grade: _____

42. The office manager at your extern site does not allow CMAs to give injections. At an office meeting, the employees ask her why not. Her reply is, "it is illegal." The employees tell her that it is not illegal for medical assistants to give injections in the state where you are. She is surprised to hear this and asks the group to prove it to her. Because you are a student and have skills in researching topics, they ask you to find the legislation and bring it to the office manager. Choose all appropriate actions from the list below.

   a. Go to the state Web site and search "general assembly."

   b. Search for the information on the AAMA Web site by entering key words, "CMA scope of practice."

   c. Search for the information in general statutes by entering key words, "health care legislation in [name of your state]."

   d. Search for the information by entering key words, "unlicensed health personnel" under *general assembly* in your state.

   e. Search for the information by entering key words, "practice of medicine."

43. While working as an extern at a family care provider, you encounter an older adult patient who is uncomfortable with the fact that you as a student are participating in her care. What would you say to help her feel more comfortable?

   _____

   _____

   _____

   _____

44. There are multiple gaps in your work history, and your interviewer asks you to explain why. One of the gaps is from relocation, and other gaps are from taking time off to evaluate what you wanted to be doing. How would you explain this to your interviewer?

   _____

   _____

   _____

   _____

45. During an interview, you are asked to explain why your grades were low last semester. How would you answer this question honestly while still speaking about yourself fairly and objectively?

   _____

   _____

   _____

   _____

COG **TRUE OR FALSE?**   Grade: _____

Determine whether the following statements are true or false. If false, explain why.

46. When you see dangerous practices, it is usually best to confront the employee first.

_____

_____

47. Problems encountered at an externship site are best handled by site employees who have experience working with the office manager.

_____

_____

48. It is a good idea to include hobbies and personal interests on your résumé.

_____

_____

49. It is a good idea to write a long and detailed cover letter.

_____

_____

AFF **CASE STUDY FOR CRITICAL THINKING**   Grade: _____

It is the first day of your medical assisting externship.

50. Your externship preceptor has said that you cannot receive permission to draw blood and perform other phlebotomy procedures. However, you know this is an area that you are required to complete. Circle all of the appropriate actions from the list below.

   a. Tell your externship coordinator from your college at her next site visit.

   b. Tell the preceptor that you must perform these tasks and leave.

   c. Call your externship coordinator immediately.

   d. Call a classmate and ask her what to do.

51. Your school will likely request that you fill out an evaluation form to determine if your externship site was effective for training. This helps the school decide if it is a good site for future externships. Review the list of questions below and circle all you should consider when filling out your site evaluation form on your externship.

    a. Was the overall experience positive or negative?

    b. Was my preceptor fun to be around?

    c. Did the office have a good cafeteria or break room?

    d. Were opportunities for learning abundant and freely offered or hard to obtain?

    e. Was my preceptor flexible about taking personal time during the day for phone calls and breaks?

    f. Were staff personnel open and caring or unwelcoming?

    g. Was the preceptor available and easily approachable or preoccupied and distant?

52. Choose all appropriate ways to dress for your externship from the list below.

    a. Burgundy and navy scrubs along with a set of bangle bracelets, your favorite gemstone rings, and a pair of comfortable white clogs.

    b. The required scrubs with a pair of clean white sneakers. Dreadlocks placed in a neat ponytail above the shoulders.

    c. The required uniform and a pair of dark walking shoes. Hair with the tips of a spiked mohawk dyed burgundy to match.

    d. The required uniform with white sneakers and college nametag.

    e. Street clothes with lab coat and required nametag.

    f. Long sleeves to cover the tattoo on your arm.

PORTFOLIO

Grade: _____

Design and compile a portfolio to present at your upcoming job interviews. Refer to Chapter 46 for a list of possible contents of the portfolio. Remember, the purpose of a portfolio is to impress an interviewer. You have worked hard to earn your medical assisting certificate, diploma, or degree. This is your opportunity to show off your professional skills, abilities, and accomplishments.

PSY PROCEDURE 46-1 Writing a Résumé

Name: _____ Date: _____ Time: _____ Grade: _____

Equipment/Supplies: Word processor, paper, personal information

STANDARDS: Given the needed equipment and a place to work, the student will perform this skill with _____%
accuracy in a total of _____ minutes. *(Your instructor will tell you what the percentage and time limits will be
before you begin practicing.)*

KEY: 4 = Satisfactory 0 = Unsatisfactory NA = This step is not counted

PROCEDURE STEPS	SELF	PARTNER	INSTRUCTOR
1. At the top of the page, center your name, address, and phone numbers.	☐	☐	☐
2. List your education starting with the most current and working back. List graduation dates and areas of study. It is not necessary to go all the way back to elementary school.	☐	☐	☐
3. Using the chronological format, list your prior related work experience with dates, responsibilities, company, and supervisor's name.	☐	☐	☐
4. List any volunteer work with dates and places.	☐	☐	☐
5. List skills you possess, including those acquired in your program and on your externship.	☐	☐	☐
6. List any certifications or awards received.	☐	☐	☐
7. List any information relevant to a certain position (for example, competence in spreadsheet applications for a job in a patient billing department).	☐	☐	☐
8. After obtaining permission and/or notifying the people, prepare a list of references with their addresses and phone contact information.	☐	☐	☐
9. Carefully proofread the résumé for accuracy and typographical errors.	☐	☐	☐
10. Have someone else proofread the résumé for errors other than content.	☐	☐	☐
11. Print the résumé on high-quality paper.	☐	☐	☐
12. AFF You had only one job before finishing your medical assisting program. Should you try to "pad" your résumé by listing some anyway? Why or why not?	☐	☐	☐

_____

_____

_____

_____

CALCULATION

Total Possible Points: _____

Total Points Earned: _____ Multiplied by 100 = _____ Divided by Total Possible Points = _____ %

PASS   **FAIL**   **COMMENTS:**

☐   ☐

Student's signature _____ Date _____

Partner's signature _____ Date _____

Instructor's signature _____ Date _____

Capstone Activities: Applying What You Have Learned

Working in a medical office means dealing with situations as they arise in a professional, nonjudgmental manner. Your education and training has provided you with the information and tools to give you administrative competence as well as the clinical skills necessary to function in the medical office, but you must also use professional judgment and critical thinking when making decisions and interacting with patients, families, and staff. This chapter will provide opportunities for you to practice using professional judgment and critical thinking skills as would a practicing medical assistant in the physician office. Each section, containing documentation and active learning exercises, provides real-life scenarios followed by questions for you to think about and respond to according to directions from your instructor. Be sure to read carefully and, as usual, have fun!

COG PSY DOCUMENTATION

CHAPTER 1

Christopher Guest is waiting to see the physician, who has been called to the emergency room. You explain the situation to the patient, and he asks if you can perform his physical instead. You explain your scope of practice. Write a chart note to record the conversation.

_____

_____

_____

_____

CHAPTER 2

Your physician asks you to write a letter to Jean Mosley, a patient who has continued to be noncompliant. She wants to formally terminate the patient's care and refer her elsewhere. Write a note in the patient's chart documenting your actions.

_____

_____

_____

_____

CHAPTER 3

You are checking in a new patient who is obviously in acute pain. He is crying and pacing the floor. You take him to a private area to carry out the patient interview and help him complete his medical questionnaire. Write a note in the patient's chart documenting the fact that you assisted the patient with the questionnaire.

_____

_____

_____

_____

CHAPTER 4

Julia is an 8-year-old patient who has been diagnosed with juvenile diabetes. You supply the patient and her mother with educational materials about Julia's condition and how to manage her blood sugar. Write a chart note to document the conversation and actions.

_____

_____

_____

CHAPTER 5

Megan O'Conner is a patient who was discharged from the hospital a few hours ago. She calls the office to report that she is now feeling woozy and nauseous. She thinks it might be a side effect of the pain medication she was given. Per your office protocol, she is advised to stop taking the medication, and you will have the doctor e-prescribe a different medication. Ms. O'Conner is obviously very upset. She is crying and says she just wants to go back to the hospital. You reassure her. Write a note about the conversation to be included in the chart.

_____

_____

_____

_____

CHAPTER 6

Mr. Sheffield did not show up for his appointment. You call him, and he says he forgot. You reschedule his appointment for the next day at 10:00 a.m. Write a note to document this in the chart.

_____

_____

_____

_____

CHAPTER 7

The physician asks you to write a note to a patient, Nancy Chesnutt, informing her of her normal lab results. Construct the note that would be included as a copy in the patient's chart.

_____

_____

_____

_____

CHAPTER 8

A patient requests release of his records to another physician. What documentation is necessary for this release? Write a note to document the release in the patient's chart.

_____

_____

_____

_____

CHAPTER 9

You receive an e-mail from Mr. Hagler saying that his medication is working out well and is not causing any side effects. He will be in for this appointment next Tuesday. How do you document this information in Mr. Hagler's medical record?

_____

_____

_____

_____

CHAPTER 10

During a routine visit, Carlos Delgado, a 55-year-old male, complains of tightness in his chest and nausea. He is short of breath and appears hypoxic. You notify the physician, and, when you return, Mr. Delgado is in respiratory arrest. EMS is called. The physician orders bag-to-mouth respirations with 6 L supplemental oxygen, which you provide. An AED is not available. After 5 minutes of artificial respirations, the patient enters full cardiac arrest, and the physician begins chest compressions. Five minutes later, EMS arrives to take the patient. Use the space below to record the incident in the chart.

_____

_____

_____

_____

CHAPTER 11

Ms. Bailey has a large balance, and she is in today to see the doctor. You have a conversation with her about her unpaid bill. She promises to send $50.00 on the fifth of each month beginning next month. Write a note to record this agreement for her financial record.

_____

_____

_____

_____

CHAPTER 12

Tonya Sushkin's insurance company paid $25.00 for an office visit on 7/14/13. Your physician is a participating provider for this company. Your initial charge was $75.00. Post the payment and adjustment on a blank daysheet. Ms. Sushkin's previous balance is $75.00.

_____

_____

_____

CHAPTER 13

Laila Hildreath is a 4-year-old girl who needs to have tubes in her ears after failing conservative treatment for recurrent ear infections. Her father is a member of an HMO that requires preauthorization for surgery. You call the HMO and receive authorization for the in-patient procedure. You are given the following preauthorization number: 67034598 AB. Record your actions for the patient's financial record.

_____

_____

_____

_____

CHAPTER 14

The physician has asked you to write a letter to the insurance company requesting 1 more day for a patient to remain in the hospital due to the fact that she has an indwelling catheter.

_____

_____

_____

_____

CHAPTER 15

An 18-year-old woman is seen for a college physical. While being examined, she tells the physician's assistant that her boyfriend is abusive on occasion. The visit becomes predominantly counseling for the next 20 minutes of her 30-minute visit. How would you document this in the chart so that the visit can be coded accurately?

_____

_____

_____

_____

CHAPTER 16

A 40-year-old woman comes to talk to the physician because she would like to start a new exercise routine and change her diet to lose 15 pounds. She is currently 25 pounds overweight, so this is a great idea and a good move toward healthy living. The physician asks you to discuss exercise and diet changes with the patient. Write a narrative patient note describing your interaction with the patient to include in her chart.

_____

_____

_____

CHAPTER 17

Although you always take care to protect yourself from exposure to biohazardous materials, you spill a tube of a patient's blood while performing hematology testing. You have a fresh cut on your hand that came into contact with the blood. Following your office's Exposure Control Plan, you clean up and then document the incident. What information will you make sure to include in your report?

_____

_____

_____

_____

CHAPTER 18

You are interviewing a young patient during an assessment when you notice that he has three small burn marks on his arm. The burns are round and less than a centimeter in diameter. When you ask the patient about the burns, he suddenly turns solemn and avoids answering the question. You suspect that the patient has been abused. How should you document this interaction on the patient's chart?

_____

_____

_____

_____

CHAPTER 19

How should you record an axillary temperature, and why is it important to record it differently from other temperatures?

_____

_____

_____

_____

CHAPTER 20

A 45-year-old patient comes into the office for a routine physical examination. He has high blood pressure and is considerably overweight. The patient asks you for advice on healthy eating, and you provide him with several pamphlets and advise him to cut down on fatty foods. How would you document this interaction in the patient's chart?

_____

_____

_____

_____

CHAPTER 21

The autoclave in your office has not been working properly. It takes twice as long for the steam in the autoclave to reach an adequate temperature for sterilization. You realize that this may affect daily procedures within the office and could lead to bigger problems with the autoclave. You decide to have the autoclave serviced by a professional. What documentation will be needed in connection with this service request?

_____

_____

_____

_____

CHAPTER 22

A patient is recovering from a Caesarian section and returns to the office to have her staples removed. The physician asks you to remove the staples and apply adhesive skin closures over the incision site. The patient asks you when the strips should be removed, and you tell her that they should fall off on their own within 10 days. How would you document this interaction in the patient's chart?

_____

_____

_____

_____

CHAPTER 23

The physician has prescribed a patient 250 milligrams of amoxicillin for an ear infection.
The patient should take this medication three times a day by mouth for 9 days. Write a note to document this in the patient's chart.

_____

_____

_____

_____

CHAPTER 24

The physician has asked you to prepare an administration of gr iii Haldol IM for a patient. The dispenser is labeled in milligrams. How do you convert this dosage to the metric system, and how many milligrams of Haldol should you dispense? Write the preparation as a chart note.

_____

_____

_____

CHAPTER 25

You have just taken a chest x-ray to rule out pneumonia. Write a narrative note detailing this procedure to be included in the patient's chart.

_____

_____

_____

_____

CHAPTER 26

A patient received penicillin for a sexually transmitted infection, and this was the last event documented in the patient's chart. Fifteen minutes later, the patient began wheezing and gasping, and within 5 minutes was clearly suffering anaphylactic shock. A first injection of epinephrine administered SC at that time was ineffective, and the patient was in respiratory arrest when EMS arrived. Mask-to-mouth respirations were given with supplemental oxygen at 15 liters per minute for 2 minutes before EMS assumed care of the patient. How would you document this interaction in the patient's chart?

_____

_____

_____

_____

CHAPTER 27

Your patient is a 9-year-old girl who suffers from severe eczema. The physician has recommended that she wear bandages at night to protect against scratching. You demonstrate to the patient's mother how to apply the bandages. The patient's mother asks how often she should apply ointment to her daughter's skin, and you repeat the physician's instructions to use it twice a day. How would you document this interaction in the patient's chart?

_____

_____

_____

_____

CHAPTER 28

Your patient is an older adult man. The physician has determined that the patient requires an ambulatory assist device. You first attempt to teach the patient to use a cane. The patient is unsteady while using the cane, so you instead teach the patient to use a walker. The patient successfully learns how to use the walker and demonstrates stability and control. You explain to the patient how to use the aid safely, including how to maintain the aid and what changes the patient should make at home to operate the aid safely. The patient verbalizes that he is comfortable using the walker and that he understands his maintenance responsibilities. How would you document this interaction on the patient's chart?

_____

_____

_____

_____

CHAPTER 29

A patient has come in for ceruminosis treatment. Document the steps that were taken to complete this procedure as well as any complications that might have arisen during the procedure. Be sure to include any instructions that were given to the patient after the procedure.

_____

_____

_____

_____

CHAPTER 30

Write a patient care note for a patient recovering from bacterial pneumonia. Explain what her symptoms are as well as what remedies the physician recommends/prescribes. Also, indicate how these remedies are intended to combat specific elements of the disease. You do not need to explain the details of how a remedy works, only what it is intended to do (i.e., a glucocorticoid is prescribed to reduce inflammation).

_____

_____

_____

_____

CHAPTER 31

When interviewing a patient prior to a physical examination of the cardiovascular system, what should you ask the patient and document in his chart?

_____

_____

_____

_____

CHAPTER 32

A patient is being scheduled for a colonoscopy. You explain the preparation to him. Document your actions for inclusion in the patient's chart.

_____

_____

_____

_____

CHAPTER 33

A father brings in his 8-year-old daughter because she fell and hit her head while rollerblading. She was not wearing a helmet and seems to have lost consciousness for just a few seconds. The father is concerned about a possible traumatic brain injury. After a physical examination, the physician finds that the child has suffered a mild concussion. She is sent home, and you give her father instructions regarding her treatment. Write a narrative note documenting this visit for inclusion in the patient's chart.

_____

_____

_____

_____

CHAPTER 34

You have just spoken with a 20-year-old patient about cystitis and have given her tips on how to avoid cystitis in the future. Record what you would write on the woman's chart, and make a note of any handout materials you might give the patient.

_____

_____

_____

_____

CHAPTER 35

Ms. Molly Espinoza is a 43-year-old female patient. Dr. Cord ordered a routine screening mammogram for this patient. You confirm with her that she is not pregnant and explain the procedure. Then you prepare the patient, and two radiographs are taken of each breast, with repositioning the patient between each image. All four radiographs are developed and are readable and accurate. Record the incident in the chart.

_____

_____

_____

_____

CHAPTER 36

John Suiker is an athletic 38-year-old man scheduled for a routine visit. He arrives disoriented and appears to be drunk and unsteady on his feet. He presents with pale, moist skin; rapid, bounding pulse; and shallow breathing. You notify the physician, Dr. Burns, of the patient's condition, and she orders an immediate blood glucose test. The patient's blood glucose is 48 mg/dL. The patient is still conscious, so you provide him with fruit juice, which he accepts. Recovery is immediate. Record the incident in the chart.

_____

_____

_____

_____

CHAPTER 37

Rose Ryan is a 24-month-old girl visiting your office for a well-child visit. The physician directs you to obtain her length, weight, and head and chest circumference. You find the child measures 92 cm tall and weighs 15 kg. Her head circumference is 50 cm, and her chest circumference is 52 cm. Document these procedures. Use the space below to record the procedure in the chart. How would you document the above scenario on the child's chart? Be sure to document the interaction, as well as the education that was provided during her visit, and any scheduled follow-up appointments. How would you record the procedure in the chart?

_____

_____

_____

_____

CHAPTER 38

A 78-year-old patient visits the physician's office to ask about treatment for arthritis in his knees. While you are talking to the patient, you notice that his hearing has decreased considerably since the last time he was in the physician's office. How would you document this information in the patient's chart?

_____

_____

_____

_____

CHAPTER 39

How would you document the collection of a blood specimen and prepare it to be sent out for testing?

_____

_____

_____

_____

CHAPTER 40

You have just completed maintenance on the glucose meter. Document this maintenance as you would in the laboratory instrument maintenance log.

_____

_____

_____

_____

CHAPTER 41

Nicole Patton is a 35-year-old female inpatient receiving both a Lovenox injection and oral Coumadin. You are directed to obtain blood specimens by evacuated tube for platelet count, prothrombin time, and partial thromboplastin time tests. Document your collection as you would in the patient's chart. Include the type(s) of specimens you collected.

_____

_____

_____

_____

CHAPTER 42

You perform an ESR test on an older adult male patient with rheumatoid arthritis. You measure a rate of 16 mL/hour. How would you document the results of this test in the patient's chart?

_____

_____

_____

_____

CHAPTER 43

You instruct a patient how to perform a clean-catch midstream urine specimen. When you test the sample, you discover that the urine is cloudy, with a pH level of 7.5, and contains traces of red blood cells, nitrites, and leukocytes. Your office does not use laboratory report forms. How would you document this information in the patient's chart?

_____

_____

_____

_____

CHAPTER 44

The physician has ordered an influenza test on your patient. The influenza test requires a nasopharyngeal specimen. You collect the specimen. Document the collection as you would in a patient's chart.

_____

_____

_____

_____

CHAPTER 45

Dr. Ashanti asks you to perform a blood cholesterol test on a patient. The results are 282 mg/dL. Write a note to document this test and its results in the patient's chart as you would if your office does not use laboratory report forms.

_____

_____

_____

_____

CHAPTER 46

You just completed an interview with the office manager of a large family practice. Write a thank you note to the interviewer.

_____

_____

_____

_____

PSY ACTIVE LEARNING

CHAPTER 1

Talk with a grandparent or another older adult, and ask him or her to tell you about a medical discovery that he or she remembers well. Create a "before and after" chart, explaining what life was like before the discovery, and the changes and benefits that came about after the discovery.

CHAPTER 2

Go to the Health and Human Services Web site, http://www.hhs.gov/ocr/privacy. What is the mission statement of the Office for Civil Rights regarding the HIPAA Privacy Rule?

CHAPTER 3

Do a Web search for "anger management techniques." Are there suggestions that could help you communicate with an angry patient? Record your findings. Cite Web sites used.

CHAPTER 4

Go to the Council on Aging's Web site, http://www.ncoa.org. Describe the plan included in the *Falls Free Coalition* outlined in the Safety of Seniors Act of 2008.

CHAPTER 5

Go the Americans With Disabilities Web site, http://www.usdoj.gov/crt/ada. Go to the Primer for Small Businesses. Who is covered by the ADA?

CHAPTER 6

Memorize the days of the week in Spanish. Recite them for your classmates.

CHAPTER 7

When writing, it is important to know your audience. The way you write for a physician is different from the way you write for a patient. In the case of a physician, you can assume he or she understands medical terminology, but this is not so of a patient. Do some Internet research to better understand the possible digestive side effects of a common medication like simvastatin (Zocor) or esomeprazole (Nexium). Then, write two letters discussing the side effects, one to a physician and one to a patient. Think about what you must do differently when writing to a patient.

CHAPTER 8

If you were opening a new medical facility, consider whether you would want staff members using abbreviations in patient records. Then create a list of acceptable abbreviations that may be used in your new facility. Then create a "Do Not Use" list for abbreviations that may be confusing and should not be included in records. Visit the Web site for the Joint Commission (http://www.jointcommission.org) and include all of those abbreviations in addition to five other abbreviations of your own choice.

CHAPTER 9

Go to WebMD (http://www.webmd.com). Scroll down to the Symptom Checker. Think back to your last illness or pick an illness and answer the questions about the symptoms. What do you have?

CHAPTER 10

Prepare a list of emergency contacts in the area, including the contact information of local hospitals, poison control centers, and emergency medical services.

CHAPTER 11

Call two collection agencies in your local area. Compare services and fees. Record your findings.

CHAPTER 12

Research the banking services offered by your local bank. Gather brochures outlining the services. Share with classmates to compare services.

CHAPTER 13

When will/did ICD-10 CM codes go into effect? Search http://www.aapc.com/ICD-10 for the answer.

CHAPTER 14

Find the ICD-9-CM codes for the following diseases:

a. Acute gastric ulcer with hemorrhage and perforation without obstruction_____

b. Meningococcal pericardiitis_____

c. Impetigo_____

d. Benign essentiahypertension_____

CHAPTER 15

Research the subject of Current Procedural Coding. Write a paragraph describing the origin of the CPT codes. What was the original purpose of CPT coding?

CHAPTER 16

The Centers for Disease Control (CDC) offers a body mass calculator on its Web site. Visit http://www.cdc.gov and search for the BMI calculator. Determine whether your BMI is within normal limits for your gender, age, and height. Describe at least three things you can do to either maintain your current weight or lose/gain weight if necessary.

CHAPTER 17

You have been asked to select the best hand soap for use throughout the urgent care center where you work. Do Internet research to identify different types of antibacterial agents that are commonly used in hand soaps. Cite any evidence you can find as to the effectiveness of the agents. Determine which soap you believe is best. Write a letter to the office manager that gives your recommendation, clearly explaining why you chose that soap.

CHAPTER 18

Conduct a patient interview with a family member or friend. Use a sample patient history form such as the one found in this chapter from your textbook. Be sure to perform the interview in person so that you can observe the physical and mental status of your patient. When you are finished, ask your patient for feedback, such as demeanor and professionalism or comfort level of the patient. Use his or her comments to set one goal for yourself regarding your skills conducting patient interviews.

CHAPTER 19

With a partner, practice taking body temperature measurements with all the types of thermometers you have access to. For those you cannot access, mime the process so that you at least have the steps down the first time you are faced with the real thermometer. For all methods, go through all the steps from picking up the thermometer to returning it to the disinfectant or returning the unit to the charging base.

CHAPTER 20

Even though the physician is the person who is responsible for using most of the instruments discussed in this chapter, you should still be familiar with how all the instruments are used. Working with a partner, access at least three of the following instruments: tongue depressor, percussion hammer, tuning fork, nasal speculum, otoscope, and stethoscope. If you do not have access to these instruments, ask your teacher if he or she can assist you. Once you have the instruments, identify the main use of those instruments during a physical exam.

CHAPTER 21

Using the library and the Internet, research the instruments and equipment commonly used by the following medical specialties: endocrinology, rheumatology, palliative care, and radiology. Add to the list found in Chapter 21 of your text with the information you find. Include images of some of the instruments and equipment.

CHAPTER 22

One of the most common minor surgeries performed in your office is the excision of skin lesions and moles, often related to the possibility of skin cancer. Skin cancer is prevalent today, and you feel that it's important to educate young people on the importance of taking proper precautions to protect skin from harmful sunrays. You have been asked to prepare a one-page patient education handout highlighting the dangers of skin cancer and prevention techniques designed especially for young adults.

- Do Internet research to identify the leading causes of skin cancer and the dangers associated with harmful sun exposure. Gather any statistics that are available from reputable Web sites.
- Outline steps that can be taken to protect the skin when outside.
- Highlight issues that are especially important to teens (for example, summer jobs as lifeguards and outdoor sports practice during the day).
- Create a one-page handout to be given to teens in the office explaining how to protect their skin from the sun.

CHAPTER 23

You have just begun working in a medical office and are getting yourself acquainted with the types of medications that the physician frequently prescribes. You know that many medications interact with food; however, you don't know a lot about specific food–drug interactions. Choose 10 common drugs from different therapeutic classifications in Table 23-1 and then research any possible food interactions. Make a chart for patients showing how common drugs and foods interact with one another.

CHAPTER 24

Accidental needlesticks are one of the most frightening occupational hazards you will encounter as a medical assistant. The greatest fear is centered on human immunodeficiency virus (HIV) and hepatitis B (HBV). Research the incubation, signs and symptoms, treatment, and prognosis associated with these two diseases. Prepare a one-page handout on each.

CHAPTER 25

Research the current recommendations by the American Cancer Society for mammography. At what age does the ACS recommend that women get their first mammogram? What other important information do women need to know about breast cancer?

CHAPTER 26

Some medical professionals live on the front line of emergency medical care. Locate an EMT-Basic (EMT-B) textbook at a library, bookstore, or other source. Make a list of some basic emergency care that is expected of the EMT-B that may also be expected of the practicing medical assistant. Are there any skills that are similar? Different?

CHAPTER 27

Use the Internet to research the major causes of fungal infections and find out how they can be prevented. Produce a poster to display in the office, educating patients about the main types of fungal infection, how they are spread, and how patients can protect their families from outbreaks.

CHAPTER 28

School children, especially girls, are commonly screened for scoliosis. Research the methods used for this screening using the Internet or the library. Then, prepare a patient education pamphlet for school children who are about to undergo the screening. Explain the procedure in a way that will calm any anxieties. Include information about scoliosis as well as preventative measures the children can take and warning signs they should look for in the years following their school screening.

CHAPTER 29

The composer Beethoven was afflicted with hearing loss that left him completely deaf. Many music lovers today suffer from hearing loss as well, and they rely on the technology available to help them enjoy the subtle tones that are written into compositions. Research the new programs and software that are being installed in hearing aids that are specifically aimed toward listening to music. List differences between listening to music and listening to speech, and make a note of tips for listening to music that physicians can give to patients with hearing aids.

CHAPTER 30

Most people are aware of the dangers of smoking. However, it is still important to educate children about the long-term dangers of smoking. Create a pamphlet outlining the dangers of smoking to be presented to a group of middle school children.

CHAPTER 31

Pretend you are a patient who is keeping a Holter monitor diary. Create a diary based on experiences a patient is likely to have. What kinds of activities do you participate in during the day? How are these activities influencing your symptoms?

CHAPTER 32

One of the deadliest types of cancer is pancreatic cancer, which kills most patients within a year of diagnosis. Research the latest information about the suspected causes of pancreatic cancer on the Internet. Try to find out which treatments are proving the most effective and whether there have been any recent developments.

- Use the information you find to create an informational poster about pancreatic cancer, educating high-risk patients on how they can lower their chances of developing pancreatic cancer.
- Write a one-page leaflet for physicians, informing them of the latest treatments for pancreatic cancer.

CHAPTER 33

Safe use of car seats can reduce brain and spinal cord injuries in infants and young children. Research the guidelines for car seat use. Then research car seat ratings and find five car seats that receive high safety ratings in each category. Create a handout for parents of young children to promote car seat safety awareness.

CHAPTER 34

Prostate cancer is most common in men over age 50 years, and, like many other cancers, it is best treated in the early stages. Testicular cancer is another form of cancer, but it occurs most often in younger men, ages 15 to 34 years. Go online and research more information about these diseases. Design a presentation to be educational for both your classmates and patients alike. Be sure to include information about the causes, the symptoms, the ways to diagnose them, and the treatments available.

CHAPTER 35

With so many prenatal tests, procedures, and appointments at the physician's office, a pregnant patient can feel overwhelmed. Create a packet that can be distributed to a patient during the first prenatal visit. Include the schedule of prenatal visits and the procedures that will be done at each of these visits. Also include important information for the patient to consult throughout the duration of the pregnancy; especially include a list of signs and symptoms that may indicate a problematic condition.

CHAPTER 36

Make a list of common foods for a diabetes sufferer to avoid. Then create a poster to display in the office highlighting your findings. Be sure to stress the importance of proper nutrition.

CHAPTER 37

The physician has asked that you make a poster for the waiting room that shows important hygienic tips for children, such as washing hands, covering the mouth while sneezing, etc. Come up with a list of five hygienic tips that could be illustrated and design the poster. Use visuals so that children who are too young to read can understand the concepts being displayed.

CHAPTER 38

Research the latest information about Alzheimer disease on the Internet. Produce an informative poster to display in a physician's waiting room, educating people about the early warning signs of Alzheimer disease. Include information about the stages of Alzheimer disease and what friends and families can expect if a loved one develops it.

CHAPTER 39

Patient confidentiality is always an important part of your job, but so is safety. Research your state's rules and regulations in regard to the rights of a patient and the rights of the public. For instance, is someone with HIV/AIDS required by law to report his or her condition to his or her employer? What about other illnesses? After you have run a test and found a patient who tested positive for a specific disease, what are the obligations of your office in dealing with this?

CHAPTER 40

You perform an HCG pregnancy test for your patient. She has a weak positive result, which fails the QC, so you must administer the test again. The second time, the test shows a positive result, and the QC is acceptable. Document the QC results as you would in the office QC log.

CHAPTER 41

Familiarize yourself with phlebotomy equipment and draw a diagram of your blood-drawing station; detail on your diagram where supplies are kept. Think, in terms of safety, about where your blood station should be positioned in the office. Think about how the organization of your station will assist you in phlebotomy procedures and minimize the likelihood of accidents.

CHAPTER 42

White blood cells are the body's defense against foreign substances and objects that enter the bloodstream. However, there are cancers, diseases, and other ailments that attack white blood cells and their production. Research one of these diseases. How many people are reported to have this disease? Is there current treatment or therapy? What are some of the cures that are being developed to stop these diseases and to rebuild the immune system? After you have gathered the information, prepare a report on this disease to present to the class.

CHAPTER 43

Identify common features that patients can take note of in their own urine (e.g., dark color = possible dehydration). Make a brochure to raise patients' awareness of how their physical health can be reflected in the color and clarity of their urine.

CHAPTER 44

Many soaps and cleaning products today are antibacterial, meaning that they work to kill bacteria. People use these antibacterial products to wash and sanitize their hands as well as their homes, especially the kitchen and bathroom. Some studies have shown that the rise in popularity of antibacterial products may be creating strains of bacteria that are resistant to antibiotics. Perform research on this topic and present it to the class.

CHAPTER 45

A new patient says there is a history of heart attacks in his family, and he wants to know what he can do to prevent it. He is middle aged and slightly overweight; however, he has a healthy diet and exercises regularly. Search the Internet and list Web sites that could contain credible information for the patient. Compile a brochure for the prevention of heart disease.

CHAPTER 46

Do an Internet search of medical assisting job opportunities in your area. Now broaden your search to check jobs in any large metropolitan area. What are the differences and similarities in your local opportunities and those in the other city?